VOLUME NINETY TWO

ADVANCES IN PARASITOLOGY

Schistosomiasis in The People's Republic of China: from Control to Elimination

VOLUME NINETY TWO

ADVANCES IN PARASITOLOGY

Schistosomiasis in The People's Republic of China: from Control to Elimination

Edited by

XIAO-NONG ZHOU
Institute of Parasitic Diseases, Chinese Center for Disease Control and Prevention, Shanghai, The People's Republic of China

SHI-ZHU LI
National Institute of Parasitic Diseases, Chinese Center for Disease Control and Prevention, Shanghai, The People's Republic of China

JÜRG UTZINGER
Swiss Tropical and Public Health Institute, Basel, Switzerland

ROBERT BERGQUIST
Geospatial Health, University of Naples Federico II, Naples, Italy

ELSEVIER

AMSTERDAM • BOSTON • HEIDELBERG • LONDON
NEW YORK • OXFORD • PARIS • SAN DIEGO
SAN FRANCISCO • SINGAPORE • SYDNEY • TOKYO
Academic Press is an imprint of Elsevier

Academic Press is an imprint of Elsevier
125 London Wall, London EC2Y 5AS, UK
The Boulevard, Langford Lane, Kidlington, Oxford OX5 1GB, UK
50 Hampshire Street, 5th Floor, Cambridge, MA 02139, USA
525 B Street, Suite 1800, San Diego, CA 92101-4495, USA

First edition 2016

ISBN: 978-0-12-809466-2
ISSN: 0065-308X

For information on all Academic Press publications visit our website at https://www.elsevier.com

Publisher: Zoe Kruze
Acquisition Editor: Mary Ann Zimmerman
Editorial Project Manager: Helene Kabes
Production Project Manager: Magesh Kumar Mahalingam
Designer: Greg Harris

Typeset by TNQ Books and Journals

CONTENTS

CONTRIBUTORS

E.M. Abe
Key Laboratory of Parasite and Vector Biology of the Chinese Ministry of Health, Shanghai, The People's Republic of China; National Institute of Parasitic Diseases, Chinese Center for Disease Control and Prevention, Shanghai, The People's Republic of China; WHO Collaborating Center for Tropical Diseases, Shanghai, The People's Republic of China; Federal University Lafia, Lafia, Nasarawa, Nigeria

L. Ai
National Institute of Parasitic Diseases, Chinese Center for Disease Control and Prevention, Shanghai, The People's Republic of China; Key Laboratory of Parasite and Vector Biology of the Chinese Ministry of Health, Shanghai, The People's Republic of China; WHO Collaborating Center for Tropical Diseases, Shanghai, The People's Republic of China

R. Bergquist
Geospatial Health, University of Naples Federico II, Naples, Italy

S.-X. Cai
Hubei Provincial Center for Disease Control and Prevention, Wuhan, The People's Republic of China

C.-L. Cao
National Institute of Parasitic Diseases, Chinese Center for Disease Control and Prevention, Shanghai, The People's Republic of China; WHO Collaborating Center for Tropical Diseases, Shanghai, The People's Republic of China

Z.-G. Cao
Department of Pathogenic Biology and Immunology, Xi'an Jiaotong University Health Science Center, Xi'an, Shannxi Province, The People's Republic of China; Anhui Provincial Institute of Schistosomiasis Control, Hefei, Anhui Province, The People's Republic of China

J.-H. Chen
National Institute of Parasitic Diseases, Chinese Center for Disease Control and Prevention, Shanghai, The People's Republic of China; Key Laboratory of Parasite and Vector Biology of the Chinese Ministry of Health, Shanghai, The People's Republic of China; WHO Collaborating Center for Tropical Diseases, Shanghai, The People's Republic of China

L. Chen
Sichuan Provincial Center for Disease Control and Prevention, Chengdu, The People's Republic of China

S.-B. Chen
National Institute of Parasitic Diseases, Chinese Center for Disease Control and Prevention, Shanghai, The People's Republic of China; Key Laboratory of Parasite and Vector Biology of the Chinese Ministry of Health, Shanghai, The People's Republic of China; WHO Collaborating Center for Tropical Diseases, Shanghai, The People's Republic of China

S. Croft
London School of Hygiene and Tropical Medicine, London, United Kingdom

J.-R. Dai
Jiangsu Institute of Parasitic Diseases, Wuxi, Jiangsu, The People's Republic of China

Y. Du
Key Laboratory of Parasite and Vector Biology of the Chinese Ministry of Health, Shanghai, The People's Republic of China; WHO Collaborating Center for Tropical Diseases, Shanghai, The People's Republic of China; National Institute of Parasitic Diseases, Chinese Center for Disease Control and Prevention, Shanghai, The People's Republic of China

Y. Feng
Key Laboratory of National Health and Family Planning Commission on Parasitic Disease Control and Prevention, Jiangsu Provincial Key Laboratory on Parasite and Vector Control Technology, Wuxi, The People's Republic of China; Jiangsu Institute of Parasitic Diseases, Wuxi, Jiangsu Province, The People's Republic of China; Jiangsu Provincial Key Laboratory of Parasite Molecular Biology, Wuxi, The People's Republic of China; Public Health Research Center, Jiangnan University, Wuxi, Jiangsu Province, The People's Republic of China

J. Ge
Jiangxi Provincial Institute of Schistosomiasis Control, Nanchang, The People's Republic of China

J.-G. Guo
National Institute of Parasitic Diseases, Chinese Center for Disease Control and Prevention, Shanghai, The People's Republic of China; World Health Organization, Geneva, Switzerland

J. He
Jiangsu Institute of Parasitic Diseases, Key Laboratory of Parasitic Disease Control and Prevention (Ministry of Health), Jiangsu Provincial Key Laboratory of Parasite Molecular Biology, Wuxi, The People's Republic of China; Public Health Research Center, Jiangnan University, Wuxi, The People's Republic of China

W. Hu
Fudan University, Shanghai, The People's Republic of China; National Institute of Parasitic Diseases, Chinese Center for Disease Control and Prevention, Shanghai, The People's Republic of China; Key Laboratory of Parasite and Vector Biology of the Chinese Ministry of Health, Shanghai, The People's Republic of China; WHO Collaborating Center for Tropical Diseases, Shanghai, The People's Republic of China

X.-B. Huang
Hubei Provincial Center for Disease Control and Prevention, Wuhan, The People's Republic of China

T.-W. Jia
National Institute of Parasitic Diseases, Chinese Center for Disease Control and Prevention, Shanghai, The People's Republic of China; WHO Collaborating Centre for Tropical Diseases, Shanghai, The People's Republic of China

Q.-W. Jiang
Department of Epidemiology, School of Public Health, Fudan University, Shanghai, The People's Republic of China; Key Laboratory of Public Health Safety, Ministry of Education, Shanghai, The People's Republic of China; Center for Tropical Disease Research, Shanghai, The People's Republic of China

A. Lee Willingham
Ross University School of Veterinary Medicine, Basseterre, St Kitts, West Indies

R.-Z. Li
Sichuan Provincial Center for Disease Control and Prevention, Chengdu, The People's Republic of China

S.-Z. Li
National Institute of Parasitic Diseases, Chinese Center for Disease Control and Prevention, Shanghai, The People's Republic of China; WHO Collaborating Centre for Tropical Diseases, Shanghai, The People's Republic of China; Key Laboratory of Parasite and Vector Biology, MOH, Shanghai, The People's Republic of China; Key Laboratory of Public Health Safety, Ministry of Education, Shanghai, The People's Republic of China

W. Li
Jiangsu Institute of Parasitic Diseases, Key Laboratory of Parasitic Disease Control and Prevention (Ministry of Health), Jiangsu Provincial Key Laboratory of Parasite Molecular Biology, Wuxi, The People's Republic of China; Public Health Research Center, Jiangnan University, Wuxi, The People's Republic of China

Z.-J. Li
Jiangxi Provincial Institute of Parasitic Diseases, Nanchang, Jiangxi, The People's Republic of China

S. Liang
University of Florida, Gainesville, FL, United States

D.-D. Lin
Jiangxi Provincial Institute of Parasitic Diseases, Nanchang, Jiangxi, The People's Republic of China

L. Liu
Key Laboratory of National Health and Family Planning Commission on Parasitic Disease Control and Prevention, Jiangsu Provincial Key Laboratory on Parasite and Vector Control Technology, Wuxi, The People's Republic of China; Jiangsu Institute of Parasitic Diseases, Wuxi, Jiangsu Province, The People's Republic of China; Jiangsu Provincial Key Laboratory of Parasite Molecular Biology, Wuxi, The People's Republic of China; Public Health Research Center, Jiangnan University, Wuxi, Jiangsu Province, The People's Republic of China

Y. Liu
Sichuan Provincial Center for Disease Control and Prevention, Chengdu, The People's Republic of China

S. Lv
Key Laboratory of Parasite and Vector Biology of the Chinese Ministry of Health, Shanghai, The People's Republic of China; National Institute of Parasitic Diseases, Chinese Center for Disease Control and Prevention, Shanghai, The People's Republic of China; WHO Collaborating Center for Tropical Diseases, Shanghai, The People's Republic of China

H. Madsen
University of Copenhagen, Copenhagen, Denmark

D. Maybe
London School of Hygiene and Tropical Medicine, London, United Kingdom

R. Peeling
London School of Hygiene and Tropical Medicine, London, United Kingdom

Y.-J. Qian
National Institute of Parasitic Diseases, Chinese Center for Disease Control and Prevention, Shanghai, The People's Republic of China; WHO Collaborating Center for Tropical Diseases, Shanghai, The People's Republic of China; Key Laboratory of Parasite and Vector Biology, Ministry of Public Health, Shanghai, The People's Republic of China

Z.-Q. Qin
National Institute of Parasitic Diseases, Chinese Center for Disease Control and Prevention, Shanghai, The People's Republic of China; Key Laboratory of Parasite and Vector Biology of the Chinese Ministry of Health, Shanghai, The People's Republic of China; WHO Collaborating Center for Tropical Diseases, Shanghai, The People's Republic of China

D.-C. Qiu
Sichuan Provincial Center for Disease Control and Prevention, Chengdu, The People's Republic of China

D. Rollinson
Wolfson Wellcome Biomedical Laboratories, Life Sciences, The Natural History Museum, London, United Kingdom

L. Shi
Jiangsu Institute of Parasitic Diseases, Key Laboratory of Parasitic Disease Control and Prevention (Ministry of Health), Jiangsu Provincial Key Laboratory of Parasite Molecular Biology, Wuxi, The People's Republic of China; Public Health Research Center, Jiangnan University, Wuxi, The People's Republic of China

X.-X. Song
Department of Epidemiology, School of Public Health, Fudan University, Shanghai, The People's Republic of China; Key Laboratory of Public Health Safety, Ministry of Education, Shanghai, The People's Republic of China; Center for Tropical Disease Research, Shanghai, The People's Republic of China

P. Steinman
Swiss Tropical and Public Health Institute, Basel, Switzerland; Basel Universities, Basel, Switzerland

C.-S. Sun
Anhui Provincial Institute of Schistosomiasis Control, Hefei, Anhui Province, The People's Republic of China

J. Utzinger
Swiss Tropical and Public Health Institute, Basel, Switzerland; University of Basel, Basel, Switzerland

J.-J. Wan
Sichuan Provincial Center for Disease Control and Prevention, Chengdu, The People's Republic of China

M. Wang
Anhui Provincial Institute of Schistosomiasis Control, Hefei, Anhui Province, The People's Republic of China

Q. Wang
National Institute of Parasitic Diseases, Chinese Center for Disease Control and Prevention, Shanghai, The People's Republic of China; WHO Collaborating Center for Tropical Diseases, Shanghai, The People's Republic of China; Key Laboratory of Parasite and Vector Biology, Ministry of Public Health, Shanghai, The People's Republic of China

T.-P. Wang
Anhui Provincial Institute of Schistosomiasis Control, Hefei, Anhui Province, The People's Republic of China; Anhui Institute of Parasitic Disease, Hefei, The People's Republic of China

X.-Y. Wang
Jiangsu Institute of Parasitic Diseases, Key Laboratory of Parasitic Disease Control and Prevention (Ministry of Health), Jiangsu Provincial Key Laboratory of Parasite Molecular Biology, Wuxi, The People's Republic of China; Public Health Research Center, Jiangnan University, Wuxi, The People's Republic of China

B.L. Webster
Wolfson Wellcome Biomedical Laboratories, Life Sciences, The Natural History Museum, London, United Kingdom

L.-Y. Wen
Zhejiang Academy of Medical Sciences, Hangzhou, Zhejiang, The People's Republic of China; Institute of Parasitic Diseases, Zhejiang Academy of Medical Sciences, Hangzhou, The People's Republic of China

F. Wu
Jiangsu Institute of Parasitic Diseases, Key Laboratory of Parasitic Disease Control and Prevention (Ministry of Health), Jiangsu Provincial Key Laboratory of Parasite Molecular Biology, Wuxi, The People's Republic of China; Public Health Research Center, Jiangnan University, Wuxi, The People's Republic of China

S. Xia
National Institute of Parasitic Diseases, Chinese Center for Disease Control and Prevention, Shanghai, The People's Republic of China; WHO Collaborating Center for Tropical Diseases, Shanghai, The People's Republic of China; Key Laboratory of Parasite and Vector Biology, Ministry of Health, The People's Republic of China

J.-F. Xu
Hubei University for Nationalities, The People's Republic of China

J. Xu
National Institute of Parasitic Diseases, Chinese Center for Disease Control and Prevention, Shanghai, The People's Republic of China; Key Laboratory of Parasite and Vector Biology, Ministry of Public Health, Shanghai, The People's Republic of China; WHO Collaborating Center for Tropical Diseases, Shanghai, The People's Republic of China

X.-L. Yan
Zhejiang Academy of Medical Sciences, Hangzhou, Zhejiang, The People's Republic of China

G.-J. Yang
Key Laboratory of National Health and Family Planning Commission on Parasitic Disease Control and Prevention, Jiangsu Provincial Key Laboratory on Parasite and Vector Control Technology, Wuxi, The People's Republic of China; Jiangsu Institute of Parasitic Diseases,

Wuxi, Jiangsu Province, The People's Republic of China; Jiangsu Provincial Key Laboratory of Parasite Molecular Biology, Wuxi, The People's Republic of China; Swiss Tropical and Public Health Institute, Basel, Switzerland; University of Basel, Basel, Switzerland

K. Yang
Jiangsu Institute of Parasitic Diseases, Key Laboratory of Parasitic Disease Control and Prevention (Ministry of Health), Jiangsu Provincial Key Laboratory of Parasite Molecular Biology, Wuxi, The People's Republic of China; Public Health Research Center, Jiangnan University, Wuxi, The People's Republic of China

Y. Yang
Department of Epidemiology, School of Public Health, Fudan University, Shanghai, The People's Republic of China; Key Laboratory of Public Health Safety, Ministry of Education, Shanghai, The People's Republic of China; Center for Tropical Disease Research, Shanghai, The People's Republic of China

P. Yap
Swiss Tropical and Public Health Institute, Basel, Switzerland; University of Basel, Basel, Switzerland

L.-L. Yu
Zhejiang Academy of Medical Sciences, Hangzhou, Zhejiang, The People's Republic of China

Q. Yu
National Institute of Parasitic Diseases, Chinese Center for Disease Control and Prevention, Shanghai, The People's Republic of China; WHO Collaborating Center for Tropical Diseases, Shanghai, The People's Republic of China; Key Laboratory of Parasite and Vector Biology, Ministry of Public Health, Shanghai, The People's Republic of China

J.-F. Zhang
Zhejiang Academy of Medical Sciences, Hangzhou, Zhejiang, The People's Republic of China; Jiangsu Institute of Parasitic Diseases, Key Laboratory of Parasitic Disease Control and Prevention (Ministry of Health), Jiangsu Provincial Key Laboratory of Parasite Molecular Biology, Wuxi, The People's Republic of China; Public Health Research Center, Jiangnan University, Wuxi, The People's Republic of China

L.-J. Zhang
Key Laboratory of Parasite and Vector Biology of the Chinese Ministry of Health, Shanghai, The People's Republic of China; WHO Collaborating Center for Tropical Diseases, Shanghai, The People's Republic of China; National Institute of Parasitic Diseases, Chinese Center for Disease Control and Prevention, Shanghai, The People's Republic of China

S.-Q. Zhang
Anhui Provincial Institute of Schistosomiasis Control, Hefei, Anhui Province, The People's Republic of China

Y.-E. Zhao
Department of Pathogenic Biology and Immunology, Xi'an Jiaotong University Health Science Center, Xi'an, Shannxi Province, The People's Republic of China

B. Zhong
Sichuan Provincial Center for Disease Control and Prevention, Chengdu, The People's Republic of China

X.-N. Zhou
National Institute of Parasitic Diseases, Chinese Center for Disease Control and Prevention, Shanghai, The People's Republic of China; WHO Collaborating Center for Tropical Diseases, Shanghai, The People's Republic of China; Key Laboratory of Parasite and Vector Biology of the Chinese Ministry of Health, Shanghai, The People's Republic of China; Key Laboratory of Public Health Safety, Ministry of Education, Shanghai, The People's Republic of China

Y.-B. Zhou
Department of Epidemiology, School of Public Health, Fudan University, Shanghai, The People's Republic of China; Center for Tropical Disease Research, Shanghai, The People's Republic of China; Key Laboratory of Public Health Safety, Ministry of Education, Shanghai, The People's Republic of China

H.-Q. Zhu
National Institute of Parasitic Diseases, Chinese Centre for Disease Control and Prevention, Shanghai, The People's Republic of China; WHO Collaborating Center for Tropical Diseases, Shanghai, The People's Republic of China; Key Laboratory of Parasite and Vector Biology, Ministry of Health, Shanghai, The People's Republic of China

H. Zhu
Hubei Provincial Center for Disease Control and Prevention, Wuhan, The People's Republic of China

R. Zhu
Key Laboratory of Parasite and Vector Biology of the Chinese Ministry of Health, Shanghai, The People's Republic of China; National Institute of Parasitic Diseases, Chinese Center for Disease Control and Prevention, Shanghai, The People's Republic of China; WHO Collaborating Center for Tropical Diseases, Shanghai, The People's Republic of China

Preface

Elimination of Schistosomiasis Japonica in The People's Republic of China: The Last Leg

S.-Z. Li*,§,¶, J. Utzinger‖,#, R. Bergquist, X.-N. Zhou*,§,¶**

*National Institute of Parasitic Diseases, Chinese Center for Disease Control and Prevention, Shanghai, The People's Republic of China
§Key Laboratory of Parasite and Vector Biology, Ministry of Health, Shanghai, The People's Republic of China
¶WHO Collaborating Center for Tropical Diseases, Shanghai, The People's Republic of China
‖Swiss Tropical and Public Health Institute, Basel, Switzerland
#Basel Universities, Basel, Switzerland
**Geospatial Health, University of Naples Federico II, Naples, Italy

The corpse belonging to the wife of a local authority who lived in the Western Han Dynasty, found by Chinese archaeologists in Mawangdui, Changsha, Hunan Province in 1972, is the first evidence of schistosomiasis in this part of the world (Xu et al., 2016b). A number of eggs of *Schistosoma japonicum* in the lady remains from a well-to-do person indicate that the disease cannot have been uncommon at that time, while symptoms resembling those of schistosomiasis in 2500-year-old Chinese traditional medicine texts (Mao and Shao, 1982) underline that the disease has a much longer history. The first modern Chinese patient with schistosomiasis was diagnosed by Oliver Tracy Logan, an American physician working in a missionary hospital in Changde, Hunan Province (Logan, 1905). After his report, more and more field investigations or surveys were carried out in this region, which is resplendent with lakes and water courses providing habitats for the snail intermediate host. The first systemic study on the epidemiology of the disease covered only three provinces (Faust and Meleney, 1924) but when Hsu and Wu (1941) later reviewed the field surveys carried out in the 1930s, it became apparent that schistosomiasis was epidemic in 12 provinces south of the Yangtze River with the number of people infected estimated at around 10 million (Hsu and Wu, 1941). The highest published estimate (close to 12 million people) emanates from the 1950s (Chen and Feng, 1999; Mao and Shao, 1982). However, with 100 million people living in the endemic areas, the real figure must have been higher; perhaps as high as 20 million. Due to widespread morbidity of seriously infected people, such as advanced schistosomiasis cases, many places in southern China entered into a vicious cycle of disease and poverty, which has been vividly described by Chen (2014).

Through the never-interrupted control efforts, involving political levels down to the smallest communities and led by experts in schistosomiasis control, the disease has been efficiently controlled in the whole country and even eliminated in many places (Collins et al., 2012). The late Chairman Mao realized the threat posed by the disease early on, and when he in 1955 issued the slogan 'We must eliminate schistosomiasis' a vigorous national control programme was immediately established (Zhu et al., 2016) that has finally paid off spectacularly: schistosomiasis japonica has now been eliminated in 5 out of the 12 originally endemic provinces (or autonomous regions, cities), including Shanghai, Guangdong, Guangxi, Fujiang and Zhejiang; by the end of 2014, 98.9% of all endemic counties (448 out of 453) had interrupted or controlled the transmission of schistosomiasis (Lei and Zhou, 2015; Zhang et al., 2016). However, control of the disease in the remaining endemic areas has turned out to be the hardest to achieve and now represents the final obstacle for the national schistosomiasis elimination programme.

Supported by the Central Government of The People's Republic of China and the provincial governments in the endemic areas, the national schistosomiasis elimination programme has now been active for 60 years. During this time, the efforts to eliminate schistosomiasis both at the local and the country level by the control programme have taken place in collaboration with other sectors, including the Ministries of Agriculture, Water Conservation and Forest Administration with progress made in step with the strong social-economic development in The People's Republic of China (Cao et al., 2016; Li et al., 2016; Yang et al., 2016). The implementation of agreed approaches towards disease elimination, relying on the establishment of strong coordination mechanisms at all levels, has been increasingly successful. In the end of 2015, the schistosomiasis prevalence in The People's Republic of China reached the criteria for elimination as a public health problem set by the World Health Organization (WHO), and a new action plan for schistosomiasis eradication in The People's Republic of China by 2025 was proposed. There is no doubt that this final leg will require substantial, additional investments in the endemic areas over the next 10 years. However, in line with the words by the Chinese President Xi Jinping at the G20 summit of November 2015, 'The People's Republic of China, as the world's second largest economy, has the confidence and ability to sustain a medium-high growth rate and continue to create development opportunities for other countries', the way ahead is clear. Schistosomiasis is now on the top agenda of the Chinese

Government as one of six most important diseases targeted for control or elimination in next decade.

The total of 15 articles that make up this special issue of *Advances in Parasitology*, entitled 'Schistosomiasis in The People's Republic of China: from Control to Elimination', span the spectrum of activities from the national schistosomiasis control programme to the national schistosomiasis elimination programme, taking particular interest in the description of control and elimination strategies as well as more general epidemiological issues undertaken by Chinese schistosomiasis specialists together with international experts under the China–UK Global Health Support Programme (grant no. GHSP-CS-OP1-01) and the National Special Science and Technology Project for Major Infectious Diseases of The People's Republic of China (No. 2012ZX10004-220) since 2012 (Chen et al., 2016a,b; Feng et al., 2016; Liu et al., 2016; Shi et al., 2016; Wang et al., 2016; Zhang et al., 2016a,c). The lessons learnt and the experience gained with respect to schistosomiasis control and elimination are now sufficiently developed not only for national purposes, but also to be transferred to other endemic countries when needed (Xu et al., 2016a). Thus, this special issue not only distills national experiences, but also shares experience with other countries arriving at the stage when control has been reached and activities need to change into strategies for elimination (Xu et al., 2016c).

REFERENCES

Cao, Z.G., Zhao, Y.E., Willingham, A.L., Wang, T.P., 2016. Towards the elimination of schistosomiasis japonica through control of the disease in domestic animals in the People's Republic of China: a tale of over 60 years. Adv. Parasitol. 92, 269–306.

Chen, M.G., Feng, Z., 1999. Schistosomiasis control in China. Parasitol. Int. 48, 11–19.

Chen, L., Zhong, B., Xu, J., Li, R.Z., Cao, C.L., 2016a. Health education as an important component in the national schistosomiasis control programme in the People's Republic of China. Adv. Parasitol. 92, 307–339.

Chen, S.B., Ai, L., Hu, W., Xu, J., Bergquist, R., Qin, Z.Q., et al., 2016b. New anti-schistosome approaches in the People's Republic of China: development of diagnostics, vaccines and other new techniques belonging to the 'omics' group. Adv. Parasitol. 92, 385–408.

Chen, M.G., 2014. Assessment of morbidity due to *Schistosoma japonicum* infection in China. Infect. Dis. Poverty 3, 6.

Collins, C., Xu, J., Tang, S., 2012. Schistosomiasis control and the health system in P.R. China. Infect. Dis. Poverty 1, 8.

Faust, E.C., Meleney, H.E., 1924. Studies on schistosomasis japonica. Am. J. Hyg. 3, 219.

Feng, Y., Liu, L., Xia, S., Xu, J.F., Bergquist, R., Yang, G.J., 2016. Reaching the surveillance-response stage of schistosomiasis control in the People's Republic of China: a modelling approach. Adv. Parasitol. 92, 165–196.

Hsu, H.P.H., Wu, K., 1941. Schistosomiasis in China II: distribution. Natl. Med. J. China 27, 553–564.

Lei, Z.L., Zhou, X.N., 2015. Eradication of schistosomiasis:a new target and a new task for the national schistosomiasis control program in the People's Republic of China. Chin. J. Schisto Contr 27, 1–4.

Li, Z.J., Ge, J., Dai, J.R., Wen, L.Y., Lin, D.D., Madsen, H., et al., 2016. Biology and control of snail intermediate host of *Schistosoma japonicum* in the People's Republic of China. Adv. Parasitol. 92, 197–236.

Liu, Y., Zhou, Y.B., Li, R.Z., Wan, J.J., Yang, Y., Qiu, D.C., et al., 2016. Epidemiological features and control effectiveness of schistosomiasis in mountainous and hilly region of the People's Republic of China. Adv. Parasitol. 92, 73–95.

Logan, O.T., 1905. A case of dysentery in Hunan province ,caused by the trematoda, *Schistosoma japonicum*. Chin. Med. J. 19, 243–245.

Mao, S.P., Shao, B.R., 1982. Schistosomiasis control in the People's Republic of China. Am. J. Trop. Med. Hyg. 31, 92–99.

Shi, L., Li, W., Wu, F., Zhang, J.F., Yang, K., Zhou, X.N., 2016. Epidemiological features and control progress of schistosomiasis in waterway-network region in P.R. China. Adv. Parasitol. 92, 97–116.

Wang, X.Y., He, J., Yang, K., Liang, S., 2016. Applications of spatial technology in schistosomiasis control programme in the People's Republic of China. Adv. Parasitol. 92.

Xu, J., Bergquist, R., Qian, Y.J., Wang, Q., Yu, Q., Peeling, R., et al., 2016a. China-Africa and China-Asia collaboration on schistosomiasis control: a SWOT analysis. Adv. Parasitol. 92, 435–466.

Xu, J., Steinman, P., Maybe, D., Zhou, X.N., Lv, S., Li, S.Z., et al., 2016b. Evolution of the national schistosomiasis control programmes in the People's Republic of China. Adv. Parasitol. 92, 1–37.

Xu, J., Yu, Q., Tchuem-Tchuenté, L.A., Bergquist, R., Sacko, M., Utzinger, J., et al., 2016c. Enhancing collaboration between China and African countries for schistosomiasis control. Lancet Infect. Dis. http://dx.doi.org/10.1016/S1473-3099(1015)00360-00366. Published Online: February 03, 2016.

Yang, Y., Zhou, Y.B., Song, X.X., Li, S.Z., Zhong, B., Wang, T.P., et al., 2016. Integrated control strategy of schistosomiasis in the People's Republic of China: projects involving agriculture, water-conservancy, forestry, sanitation and environmental modification. Adv. Parasitol. 92, 237–268.

Zhang, J.F., Xu, J., Bergquist, R., Yu, L.L., Yan, X.L., Zhu, H.Q., et al., 2016a. Development and application of diagnostics in the national schistosomiasis control programme in the People's Republic of China. Adv. Parasitol. 92, 409–434.

Zhang, L.J., Li, S.Z., Wen, L.Y., Lin, D.D., Abe, E.M., Zhu, R., et al., 2016b. Establishment and function of schistosomiasis surveillance system towards elimination in the People's Republic of China. Adv. Parasitol. 92, 117–141.

Zhang, S.Q., Sun, C.S., Wang, M., Lin, D.D., Zhou, X.N., Wang, T.P., 2016c. Epidemiological features and control effectiveness of schistosomiasis in lake and marshland region in the People's Republic of China. Adv. Parasitol. 92, 39–71.

Zhu, H., Yap, P., Utzinger, J., Jia, T.W., Li, S.Z., Huang, X.B., et al., 2016. Policy support and resources mobilization for the national schistosomiasis control programme in the People's Republic of China. Adv. Parasitol. 92, 341–383.

CHAPTER ONE

Evolution of the National Schistosomiasis Control Programmes in The People's Republic of China

J. Xu*,§,¶, P. Steinman||,#, D. Maybe**, X.-N. Zhou*,§,¶,1, S. Lv*,§,¶, S.-Z. Li*,§,¶, R. Peeling**,1

*National Institute of Parasitic Diseases, Chinese Center for Disease Control and Prevention, Shanghai, The People's Republic of China
§Key Laboratory of Parasite and Vector Biology, Ministry of Health, Shanghai, The People's Republic of China
¶WHO Collaborating Center for Tropical Diseases, Shanghai, The People's Republic of China
||Swiss Tropical and Public Health Institute, Basel, Switzerland
#Basel Universities, Basel, Switzerland
**London School of Hygiene and Tropical Medicine, London, United Kingdom
[1]Corresponding authors: E-mail: zhouxn1@chinacdc.cn; Rosanna.Peeling@lshtm.ac.uk

Contents

Advances in Parasitology, Volume 92
ISSN 0065-308X
http://dx.doi.org/10.1016/bs.apar.2016.02.001

Abstract

Schistosomiasis japonica is caused by the parasitic trematode *Schistosoma japonicum*. It is endemic in The People's Republic of China and has significant impact on human health and socioeconomic development in certain regions. Over the last six decades, the national control programmes evolved in remarkable ways and brought schistosomiasis japonica largely under control. We describe the history and evolution of schistosomiasis control in The People's Republic of China, with an emphasis on shifts in control strategies that evolved with new insights into the biology of the parasite and its intermediate hosts, and the epidemiology of the disease in the country. We also highlight the achievements in controlling the disease in different socioecological settings, and identify persisting challenges to fully eliminate schistosomiasis japonica from the country. To reach the goal of schistosomiasis elimination, further integration of interventions, multisector collaboration, sensitive and effective surveillance are needed to strengthen.

1. INTRODUCTION

Intestinal schistosomiasis japonica is caused by *Schistosoma japonicum* infection and occurs in Indonesia, the Philippines and The People's Republic of China (Gryseels et al., 2006; Ross et al., 2002). The amphibious freshwater snail *Oncomelania hupensis* is the only intermediate host of *S. japonicum* but besides humans (Li et al., 2016), more than 40 mammals can serve as definitive hosts (Cao et al., 2016; McManus et al., 2009; Wang et al., 2008). People are infected during water contact due to economic, leisure and domestic activities. *Schistosoma japonicum* infections often cause more severe morbidity than infections with other schistosomes due to the high number of ova produced by the female worms. People from nonendemic areas and those infected with a large number of cercariae can have particularly acute manifestations such as cercarial dermatitis and Katayama fever (Chen, 2014; Ross et al., 2007). Bloody diarrhoea, abdominal pain, liver cirrhosis and portal hypertension are typical symptoms. Chronic schistosomiasis develops in inhabitants of endemic areas frequently exposed to cercariae. Chronic cases present without symptoms or with nonspecific intermittent abdominal pain, diarrhoea and rectal bleeding, with the frequency of symptoms related to the intensity of infection. If they are not treated promptly and adequately, cases may present as advanced schistosomiasis with symptoms such as splenomegaly, ascites, colonic tumouroid proliferations or growth retardation (Fig. 1) (Colley et al., 2014; Gryseels et al., 2006; Li, 2006).

Symptoms resembling early schistosomiasis or Katayama syndrome have been described in ancient Chinese medical publications where the disease was called water poison disease. Studies in the 1970s on two exhumed 2100-year-old corpses from the western Han dynasty identified schistosome

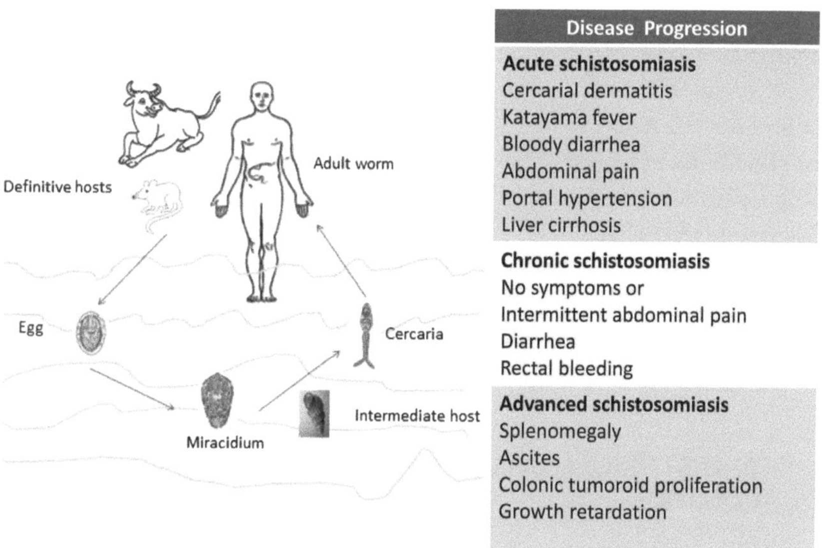

Figure 1 Life cycle of *Schistosoma japonicum* and disease progression.

eggs in their inner organs (Ross et al., 1997; Wei, 1973). The first modern medical description of schistosomiasis was published by Dr Logan in 1905 based on a case in Changde city of Hunan province (Logan, 1905). Over the subsequent 40 years, many missionary doctors and parasitologists conducted surveys and accumulated valuable information about the epidemiology of schistosomiasis japonica (Faust and Meleney, 1924; Kan and Yao, 1934; Kan and Kung, 1936; Tang, 1939). Mao (1948) reviewed these references and concluded that schistosomiasis japonica was prevalent in 138 counties in the mainland The People's Republic of China where an estimated 5 million people were infected, corresponding to an average infection rate of 21.1%. By 1949, the disease had been recognized in 12 provinces in mainland The People's Republic of China (Ling et al., 1949). The prevalence in some villages even exceeded 70% (Kuo, 1946; Lu et al., 1955; Mao, 1948; Totell, 1924) and many people died due to schistosomiasis as reflected in village names such as 'Big-belly village', 'Widows' village' and 'Village without villagers' (Chen, 1999; Mao and Shao, 1982). Efforts to control the disease were very limited at that time due to poverty, internal strife and a lack of effective tools (Chen et al., 2016).

Schistosomiasis control was a high priority for the leaders of The People's Republic of China soon after its foundation. Chairman Mao issued a slogan of 'Must eliminate schistosomiasis' in 1955 and a vigorous national control programme was established (Zhu et al., 2016). More than 60 years of continuous efforts resulted in the interruption of schistosomiasis japonica transmission in many areas in The People's Republic of China and its control in the remaining endemic areas (Xu et al., 2015; Zhou et al., 2005). By the end of 2014, 98.9% of all endemic counties (448/453) had interrupted or controlled the transmission of schistosomiasis (Lei and Zhou, 2015). In the present article, we review the evolution of the schistosomiasis control programmes in The People's Republic of China, with a focus on a description of the shift in strategies from controlling the intermediate host to preventing morbidity in humans and removing nonhuman end hosts, and finally integrated multisectoral approaches (Cao et al., 2016; Wan et al., 2016; Yang et al., 2016). Existing challenges to completely eliminate schistosomiasis are also explored to provide guidance for policy makers and research scientists.

2. HISTORICAL EVOLUTION OF SCHISTOSOMIASIS CONTROL

Over all of its 60-year history, schistosomiasis japonica control in The People's Republic of China was based on the basic policy of 'Prevention first, comprehensive management, mass control and prevention'. Based on the insight that blocking any step of the schistosome life cycle would interrupt the transmission, control strategies were developed and adapted over time to remain aligned with epidemiological insights, technological advances and the political environment (Fig. 2).

2.1 Preparation stage (1950–55)

In the early stages of the schistosomiasis control programme in The People's Republic of China, the treatment of patients with severe illness was the primary task. An instruction for schistosomiasis control was issued by the Ministry of Health in 1950, followed by the establishment of professional control system, treatment of patients and field surveys, thus providing the basis for future mass campaigns against schistosomiasis.

2.1.1 Set up of control infrastructure

To conduct treatment and control activities on a large scale, a national committee was established to organize the treatment of patients in known endemic regions, and a large number of control teams were formed in a short time (Wang et al., 1989). In 1950, the East Branch of the Central Institute of Health was established. This branch moved to Shanghai in 1957 and become the national agency for research and guiding schistosomiasis control. During 1950–55, schistosomiasis control stations at provincial, city and county levels were set up successively. 16 stations, 78 substations and 420 field units had been established by 1955 (Wang, 2011). The number of

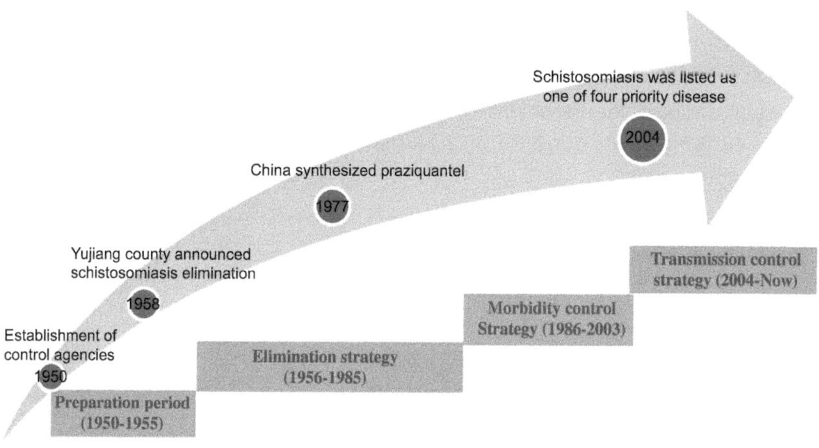

Figure 2 Strategies and key methods for schistosomiasis control in the national control program.

well-trained health workers focussing on schistosomiasis reached 3000 in East China alone (Lu, et al., 1955). Only in 1953, among 55,355 cases who received treatment, 60% of them were cured and health conditions improved in the remaining patients (Lu et al., 1955).

2.1.2 Understanding the epidemiology

During this period, field surveys on the distribution of intermediate host snails and human stool examinations were conducted to understand the endemic areas and epidemiology of schistosomiasis in The People's Republic of China (Chen, 1956; Sleigh et al., 1998; Tang, 1951; Wen and Tao, 2008; Zhuang, 1992). Knowledge about the schistosome life cycle, morbidity and prevention was disseminated through meetings, newspapers, leaflets, etc., providing peasants the basis for reporting the presence of snails or illnesses indicative of schistosomiasis to village leaders in their areas. Pilot studies in different endemic areas were implemented to explore effective approaches for controlling schistosomiasis. However, the achievements did not alter significantly the number of cases due to limited manpower and resources as well as lack of relevant tools and overall planning.

2.2 Mass campaign stage focussed on snail control (1956–85)

During this stage, the first national plan for schistosomiasis control was drafted and an elimination strategy based on snails control was implemented nationwide following the fully understanding of the endemic status of schistosomiasis across The People's Republic of China.

2.2.1 Understanding the endemic status and characteristics of schistosomiasis across The People's Republic of China

The first national schistosomiasis survey was initiated in 1956 and lasted 2 years. Its aim was to identify the true extent of schistosomiasis in The People's Republic of China. The results of the survey showed that schistosomiasis japonica was endemic in 373 counties in 12 provinces south of the Yangtze River. The endemic area was between 33°25′ N and 22°42′N and between 121°45′ E and 99°5′ E. Endemic areas were found from 0 to 3000 m above sea level (Chen and Feng, 1999). It was estimated that more than 10 million individuals were infected with *S. japonicum* and more than 100 million people were at risk of infection (Wang et al., 1989; Xia and Wang, 1989). The number of infected bovines was calculated at 1.2 million while the total area of *O. hupensis* habitat reached 14.5 billion m^2 (Chen, 1999). The most seriously affected areas were located in the delta of the Yangtze River including parts of Jiangsu, Shanghai and Zhejiang provinces, and in the marshland and lake regions along the Yangtze River including the Poyang and Dongting Lakes (Mao and Shao, 1982). The endemic areas were then classified according to eco-geographical characteristics into three categories: plain regions with waterway networks, mountainous and hilly regions, and marshland and lake regions (Fig. 3) (Mao and Shao, 1982).

2.2.2 Strengthening control agencies and guidance on control activities

In 1957, a bureau of schistosomiasis control was set up in the Ministry of Health, merging with the national leading group of schistosomiasis. By August 1957, there were 19 institutes, 236 stations and 1346 substations nationwide for schistosomiasis control, and the number of well-trained staff for schistosomiasis control reached over 17,000 (Daily, 1958). To strengthen the management of the national control programme, the national leading group was rebuilt up in 1970 and a national conference on schistosomiasis

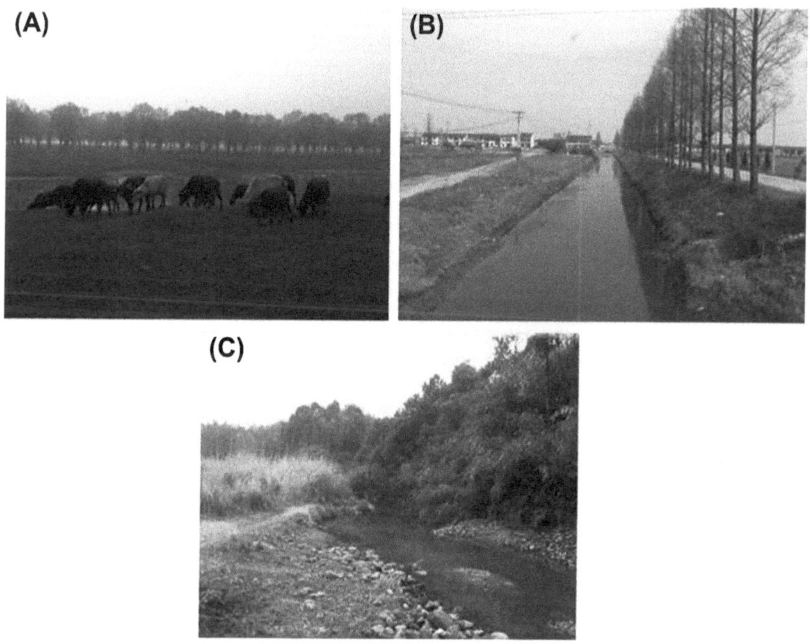

Figure 3 Categories of schistosomiasis japonica endemic areas in The People's Republic of China. (A) Marshland and lake region; (B) Plain region with waterway network; (C) Mountainous and hilly region.

control was organized each year. Furthermore, a national schistosomiasis research committee was established in 1956 to conduct studies on technologies and strategies for schistosomiasis control. The first version of the manual for schistosomiasis control was compiled and published in 1956 to guide the control of schistosomiasis. Criteria of schistosomiasis elimination were issued in 1958 and updated in 1980 by the Ministry of Health (Zhu et al., 2016).

2.2.3 Mass campaign focussed on snail control

In 1956, schistosomiasis was listed as one of five major parasitic diseases in the national programme for agricultural development (1956–67). The objective was set to eliminate schistosomiasis in any possible endemic areas within 12 years but the complexity of schistosomiasis transmission and its control had been neglected. The systematic control activities were affected 1966–69 by the culture revolution. Under the concerns of Chairman Mao and Prime Minister Zhou, several national conferences on schistosomiasis control were organized and control activities were implemented in subsequent years (Wang et al., 1989). The key tools to eliminate schistosomiasis were snail control through environmental modification and mollusciciding (Li et al., 2016). The basic principle of snail control was implementing activities from the upper to the lower reaches of a drainage system, with snail treatment strategies mainly determined by the environment, available resources and cost-effectiveness considerations (Yang et al., 2010, 2012; Yuan et al., 2005). A large number of people were mobilized to participate in the snail elimination campaign. As the most effective drugs at the time, potassium and sodium antimony tartrate was used to treat patients before the 1980s. The clinical use of praziquantel with its low toxicity and high cure rates started in 1978 and decreased the mortality and prevalence of late-stage schistosomiasis. By the end of 1984, a total of 11 million patients had received treatment (Zheng, 1986). Other control measures such as self-protection with chemical repellents or niclosamide impregnated clothes, safe water and sanitary toilets were also provided as complementary interventions (Wen and Tao, 2008).

2.2.4 Achievements and lessons learnt

Following three decades of intensive efforts, the schistosomiasis japonica prevalence and the number of patients with severe illness as well as the snail-infested area had decreased significantly. By 1981, 11 billion m^2 snail habitats were free of snails (Guo and Zheng, 1999). Guangdong Province and Shanghai Municipality had reached the criteria of schistosomiasis elimination in 1985 while Fujian Province and Guangxi Zhuang Autonomous Region eliminated schistosomiasis in 1987 and 1989, respectively (Pan et al., 2002; Sleigh et al., 1998; Wu et al., 2005). The experience showed that elimination of schistosomiasis with snail control could be achieved in areas where the water level was controlled and the economy was relatively developed. However, in 1986–88 the number of acute cases remained high (Xia and Wang, 1989) and the snail-infested area increased from 2.75 billion m^2 in 1980 to 3.47 billion m^2 in 1988 (Yuan, 1999) as an elimination strategy focused on snail control did not work well in places characterized by unstable water levels, a complicated environment or comparatively retarded economic development as it is found in the middle and lower reaches of the Yangtze River as well as in the mountainous areas of Sichuan and Yunnan provinces.

2.3 Morbidity control stage boosted by international cooperation (1986–2003)

2.3.1 Morbidity control strategy and pilot studies

Realizing elimination of schistosomiasis was difficult in poor countries, the WHO expert consultation committee adjusted its strategy and objective from transmission interruption or elimination to morbidity control in 1984 (WHO, 1985). This strategy focused on people and their behaviour rather than the snail and the environment, and had as its objective to reduce morbidity and mortality caused by schistosomiasis rather than focussing on halting transmission. Since 1980, The People's Republic of China carried out pilot studies on this new strategy in heavy endemic areas (Yuan et al., 1990; Zheng et al., 1996). In 1986, new policies were formulated that consisted of four items: to actively prevent and treat cases; to consider local and seasonal conditions; to integrate scientific techniques into mass campaign against schistosomiasis; to fight against schistosomiasis repeatedly (Mao, 1987). Since 1987, the morbidity control strategy intended to reduce the prevalence and intensities among local residents and livestock had been inaugurated in Hunan, Hubei, Jiangxi and Anhui provinces (Yuan et al., 2002).

2.3.2 World Bank loan project

The nationwide implementation of morbidity control was boosted by the World Bank Loan Project (WBLP) on schistosomiasis control which was initiated in 1992 in eight provinces, and ended in 1998 in five provinces and in 2001 in Hubei, Hunan and Yunnan provinces. The key aims of the project were to reduce morbidity caused by schistosomiasis and interrupt transmission in some regions were considered possible. Mass chemotherapy was used in endemic areas with a high prevalence (prevalence >15%) while selective chemotherapy was given to those with positive stool examinations or serological tests in areas with moderate (15% > prevalence > 3%) and low endemicity (prevalence < 3%). Praziquantel treatment of infected cattle along with chemotherapy for humans was also tested. In the frame of the project, almost 19 million treatments were given to humans while 1.7 million cattle and buffaloes were screened and those infected were treated (Chen et al., 2005).

Control through mollusciciding and/or environmental modification was reinforced as supplementary methods. Areas with infected snails were treated annually with niclosomide. Environmental modification was mainly conducted in low endemic areas with the goal to reach transmission interruption (Chen et al., 2005; Yuan et al., 2002). Health education aiming to change the behaviour of people at high risk was an important intervention measure in this strategy. By the end of 1995, there were more than 4000 full or part time staff conducting health education (Guo, 2006).

2.3.3 Achievements and lessons

Among the 219 counties covered by the WBLP, 47 had met the criteria of transmission control and 82 had met the criteria of transmission interruption by 2001. Zhejiang Province with 44 formerly endemic counties had reached the target of elimination in 1995 (Chen et al., 2005). Three national sampling surveys on schistosomiasis conducted before, during and after the WBLP in 1989, 1995 and 2004 demonstrated the impact of the WBLP but also showed the shortcomings of this morbidity control strategy (Fig. 4). The number of cases decreased from an estimated 1,638,103 in 1989 to 865,084 in 1995 while the average prevalence decreased from 9.7% to 4.9%. The prevalence

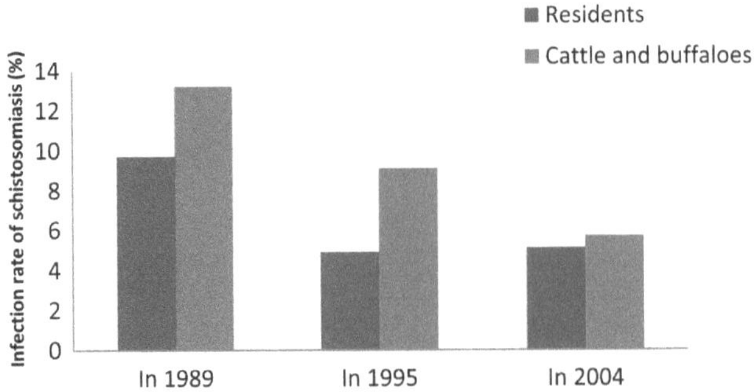

Figure 4 Prevalence of schistosomiasis in human beings and bovines in The People's Republic of China according to the three national sampling surveys.

in cattle and buffalos was reduced from 13.2% to 9.1% (Ministry of Health, 1993, 1998). However, the third national sampling survey conducted in 2004 after the termination of WBLP indicated that 726,112 individuals were estimated to be infected with schistosomes, and that the prevalence was 3.8% in the marshland and lake region (Zhou et al., 2007). Schistosomiasis had re-emerged in The People's Republic of China due to a shortage of financial support following the completion of the WBLP, devastating floods in 1998, important ecological changes caused by water conservancy projects, reforms in the economic and health systems, etc. (Bian et al., 2004; Liang et al., 2006; Xu et al., 2000; Yang et al., 2005; Zhou et al., 2002). The chemotherapy-based strategy could quickly decrease the prevalence of schistosomiasis but failed to interrupt transmission in the hyperendemic areas as it did not prevent reinfection.

2.4 Comprehensive strategy to block schistosomiasis transmission (2004–present)

2.4.1 Formulation of comprehensive strategy to block schistosomiasis transmission

Livestock, especially buffaloes, accounted for 70–90% of all new schistosomiasis cases in the marshland regions along the Yangtze River (Gray et al., 2007, 2008; Guo et al., 2001; Wang et al., 2005a,b). Pilot studies of a new strategy emphasizing health education, removing cattle from snail-infested grasslands, providing farmers with mechanized farm equipment, access to clean water and adequate sanitation and thus aiming to stop the contamination of the environment with schistosome eggs were conducted (Wang et al., 2009a,b; Zhou et al., 2009). While the human prevalence fluctuated in control villages, the infection rate decreased to less than 1% in two intervention villages after three transmission seasons. The prevalence of soil-transmitted helminthiases also gradually decreased (Wang et al., 2009a,b), supporting the public health relevance of this new strategy (Chen et al., 2014; Hong et al., 2013; Sun et al., 2011).

2.4.2 National control programme implementing comprehensive strategy

To curb the rebound of schistosomiasis in the new millennium and realize the final goal of eliminating schistosomiasis in The People's Republic of China, a national strategic plan for schistosomiasis control was issued in 2004. It aimed to reduce the prevalence in humans and livestock in all endemic counties to less than 5% by 2008 and then to below 1% by 2015 (Wang et al., 2009a,b). Two comprehensive multisectoral control projects adopting the comprehensive strategy to block the contamination of water bodies with schistosome eggs and thus prevent snail from being infected were conducted, covering 164 counties during 2004–08 and 189 counties during 2009–15, respectively.

The intervention approaches varied between counties according to the local conditions: (1) In endemic counties targeting infection control, interventions focused on infection resource control, including simultaneous chemotherapy of humans and livestock, snail control in high risk regions, agriculture mechanization to replace buffaloes with tractors, prohibiting pasturing animals in grasslands where infested snails exist, raising livestock in stables or on grasslands free of snails, etc. Environmental modification to destroy snail habitats was conducted in combination with farmland rehabilitation projects and forestry projects where possible (Yang et al., 2016). (2) In regions aiming to reach transmission control or transmission interruption, in addition to strengthening control interventions as described above and surveillance of remaining infection resources, snail control focussed on eliminating snail breeding areas through agriculture, water conservancy and forestry projects (Feng et al., 2016; Li et al., 2016).

2.4.3 Achievements and lessons learnt

After 10 years of implementing the comprehensive control strategy, the medium term goal of reaching infection control nationwide was achieved on schedule. Five provinces which had reached transmission interruption by 1995 consolidated their achievements and no new cases or infected snails had been found during this period. Hubei, Hunan, Anhui and Jiangxi provinces reached the criteria of infection control by 2008 simultaneously while Sichuan, Yunnan, Jiangsu and Hubei provinces reached the criteria of transmission control in 2008, 2009, 2010 and 2013, respectively (Fig. 5.). The estimated number of infected people decreased from 842,525 in 2004 to 184,943 in 2013, a reduction of 78.1%. The number of reported acute cases was nine in 2013 (Fig. 6) (Hao et al., 2005; Lei et al., 2014). These achievements suggested that the long-term target of the national programme drafted in 2004 could be achieved by the end of 2015.

3. DEVELOPMENT OF MAJOR CONTROL TOOLS AND TECHNIQUES

3.1 Drugs

3.1.1 Chemical drugs

In the 1950s, potassium and sodium antimony tartrate were considered the most effective drugs to treat schistosomiasis. However, they were toxic and

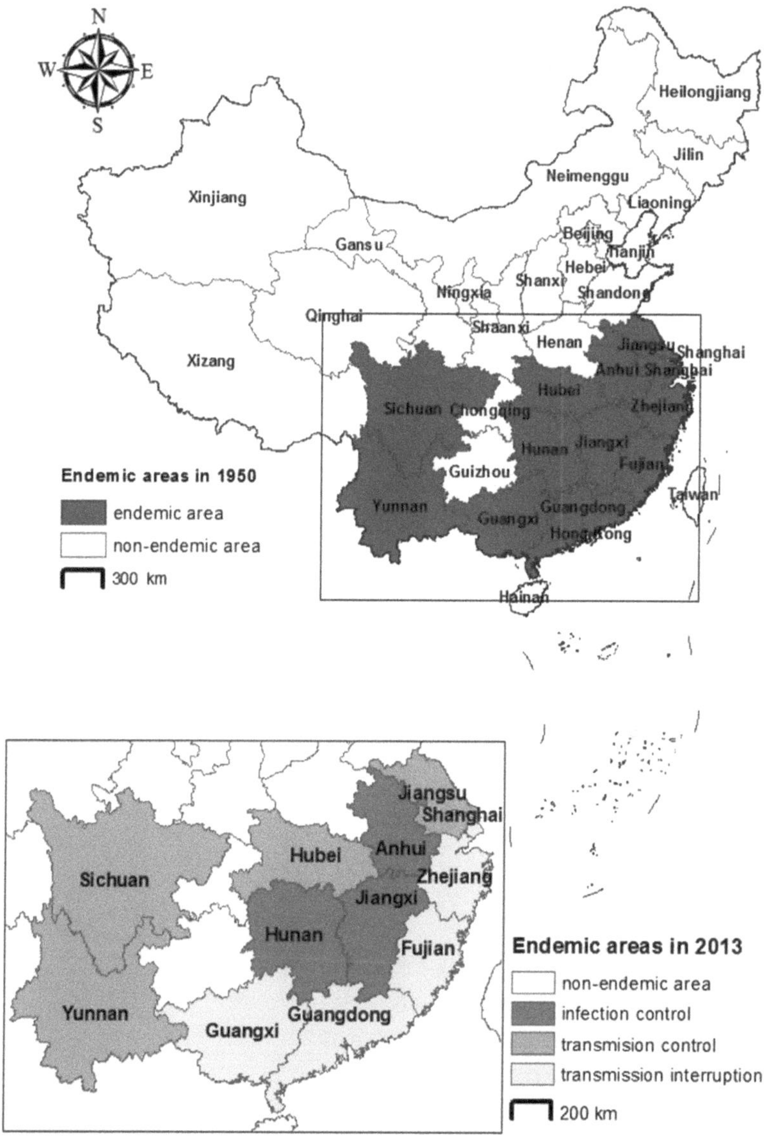

Figure 5 Distribution of schistosomiasis japonica in The People's Republic of China in the 1950s and in 2013.

could have serious side effects (Le et al., 1957; Lu et al., 1955). Furapromidum, the first nonantimonial oral drug against schistosomiasis japonica, was synthesized in The People's Republic of China in 1962 and used for acute cases (Hsiao et al., 1975; Lei et al., 1963). Treatment was only given to cases

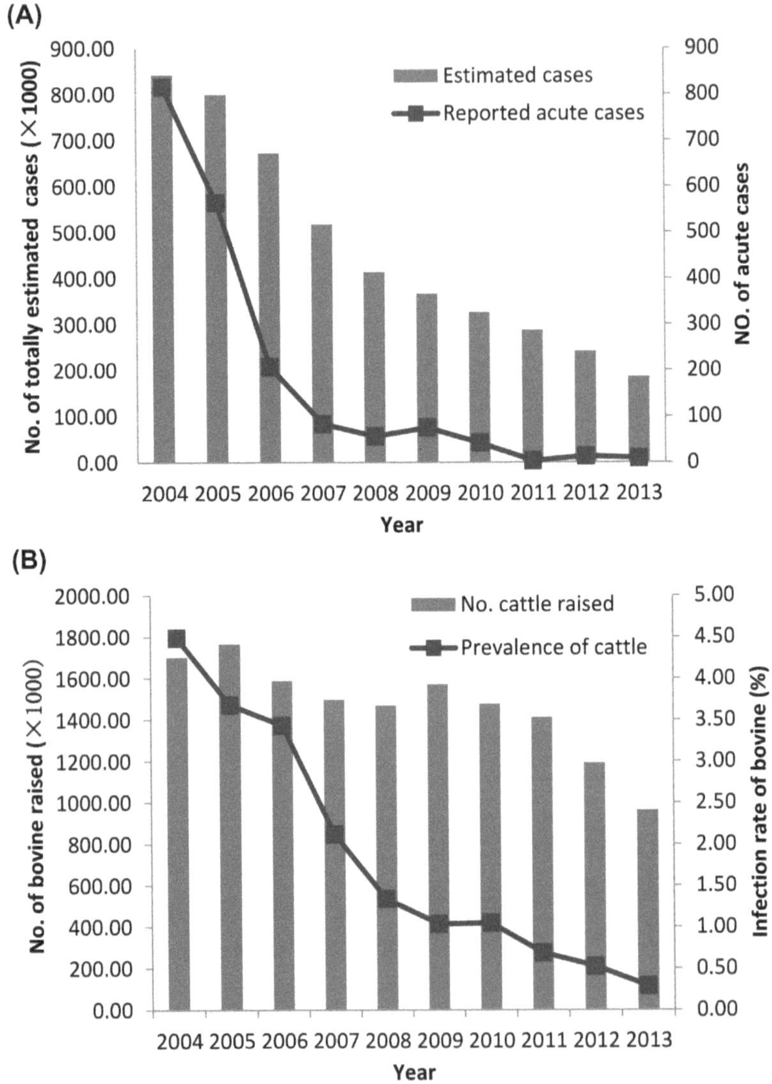

Figure 6 Changes in the prevalence of schistosomiasis japonica in humans and livestock during 2004–2013.

confirmed by direct stool parasitological tests (Maegraith, 1958). The first clinical trial with praziquantel conducted in the late 1970s in The People's Republic of China proved that the drug had a high efficacy against *S. japonicum* (Tambo et al., 2015; Yang et al., 1981). In 1977, praziquantel was synthesized in The People's Republic of China and later released for clinical use

(Fu et al., 1988). The significantly lower price compared to other drugs, high efficacy against acute and chronic schistosomiasis, and good safety profile of a single oral dose of usually 40–50 mg/kg body weight made praziquantel an ideal drug for large-scale use (Fu et al., 1988; Ojurongbe et al., 2014; Zhou et al., 2005). Chemotherapy with praziquantel became the backbone of the WBLP for schistosomiasis control in The People's Republic of China and also plays an important role in the current national control programme (Chen et al., 2005; Zhou et al., 2005).

3.1.2 Alternative treatments

Different antischistosomal drugs were developed based on traditional Chinese herbal medicine during the past six decades (Li et al., 2015). Pumpkin seeds exhibited antischistosomal activity especially against schistosomula (Chou et al.,1958; Shiao et al., 1959). Other herbs, although they showed activity against schistosomes, were finally abandoned due to toxic effects (Chen et al., 1962; Shiao et al., 1962; Wang et al., 1979; Shen et al., 1981; Yue et al., 1985). Herbs such as astragalus, angelica, paeoniflorin, salvia or their extracts were found to have high activity against liver fibrosis caused by chronic schistosomiasis when used alone or combined with other herbs (Li et al., 2009; Wang, 1984; Wu and Sun, 2014; Xie et al., 2002). In 1980, Chinese scientists first described the antischistosomal properties of artemisinin (Chen et al., 1980). Two years later, Le reported the antischistosomal activity of the derivatives of artemisinin, such as artemether and artesunate, which were found to be highly active against immature schistosomes (Le et al., 1982, 1983; Xiao et al., 2002; Xiao, 2005). The administration of these drugs effectively prevented the outbreak of schistosomiasis and was found to be especially useful during the unusual flood disaster in 1998 (Dai et al., 1999; Hu et al., 2000; Song et al., 1997). Considering that the derivatives of artemisinin and praziquantel exhibit high activity against schistosomula and adult worms, respectively, a combined treatment has been proposed to enhance the worm burden reduction and thus benefit the elimination of schistosomiasis but limited in use due to the high cost of the derivatives of artemisinin and afraid of the drug resistance against malaria (Hou et al., 2008; Liu et al., 2014; Villar et al., 2012; Xiao et al., 2000, 2010).

3.2 Diagnostic tools

3.2.1 Parasitological methods

The detection of eggs or miracidia in stool samples is the traditional way to confirm an infection with *S. japonicum*. Before the 1980s, direct smears, sedimentation, concentration and hatching tests and rectal biopsy were the main approaches to diagnose schistosome infection (Maegraith, 1958; Mao and Shao, 1982). Following its recommendation as a routine standard method for schistosomiasis diagnosis by WHO, the Kato–Katz thick smear method has been widely used in The People's Republic of China since the 1980s due to its favourable characteristics including a quantitative result, being cheap and technologically undemanding, and easy to use (Katz et al., 1972; WHO, 1985; Wu et al., 1995). The Kato–Katz test was most useful in high endemic areas as its sensitivity increased with the number of slides examined and the infection intensity (Lin et al., 2008; Yu et al., 2007). The miracidium hatching technique is another traditional method used in The People's Republic of China, arguably with a higher sensitivity than Kato–Katz due to the large volume of faeces examined (Ministry of Health, 2000). This technique is limited to use in low infection intensity areas due to its labour-intensive and time-consuming nature (Zhu et al., 2005). In the guidelines for schistosomiasis control and elimination in The People's Republic of China issued in 2006, the Kato–Katz method (three slides from one stool sample) or screening by serological tests followed by Kato–Katz method for antibody-positive individuals is recommended to evaluate whether a community has reached the infection control criteria while the miracidium hatching technique alone (3 hatching tests per stool sample) or in combination with serological tests was used to assess the endemic status where the aim was to achieve transmission control or transmission interruption (Collins et al., 2012; Ministry of Health, 2007).

3.2.2 Immunological assays

Immunological tests have a long history in the national schistosomiasis control programmes of The People's Republic of China due to advantages such as high sensitivity, easy use and rapidity (Chen et al., 2016; Zheng et al., 2013). Intradermal tests (ID) were the first successfully developed immunodiagnostic method. The strategy of screening a population by ID first followed by stool examination only for the ID positives made large-scale screening feasible and allowed understanding the distribution and approximate prevalence of schistosomiasis in a short time during the 1950s (Maegraith, 1958; Mao and Shao, 1982). Antibody-detection immunoassays such as the cercaria huellen reaction (CHR), circumoval precipitin test (COPT), indirect haemagglutination assay (IHA), enzyme-linked immunosorbent assay (ELISA) as well as rapid diagnostic assays such as the Dye Dipstick immunoassay (DDIA) and the Dot immunogold filtration assay (DIGFA) based on immunofiltration or immunochromatography principles were developed and some of them were widely used in The People's Republic of China (Wu, 2002; Zhu, 2005). Comprehensive assessments in the laboratory and in field settings conducted in recent years proved that most serological techniques to detect antibodies developed so far had a sensitivity of about 90% or more while showing only limited cross-reactions with other helminth infections (Xu et al., 2011a,b, Zhou et al., 2011). However, such tests cannot distinguish current from past infections. Still, they proved invaluable for the national control programmes when targeting chemotherapy, in epidemiological surveys, for surveillance and for the assessment of control strategies (Dang et al., 2014; Zhou et al., 2007, 2011). Research on antigen-based immunoassays for the detection of *S. japonicum* started in the late 1970s in The People's Republic of China (Wu, 2002). A number of monoclonal antibodies targeting circulating anodic antigen (CAA), circulating cathodic antigen (CCA) or membrane-associated antigen (MAA) were developed but such assays were not integrated into the national control programmes due to their unsatisfactory specificity and sensitivity in patients with light infections (Guan and Shi, 1996; Yi et al., 1995).

3.3 Snail control

3.3.1 Physical methods

Physical methods for snail control involve the environmental modification of snail habitats to make survival difficult for snails (Li et al., 2016).

3.3.1.1 Agricultural activities

Changing flood plains to farmland through construction of dykes and embankments, changing farmland to fish ponds, raising crawfish and rice alternately in paddy fields, planting rice in the mid-altitude lands and cotton in dry, high-altitude lands have played important roles in snail control by reducing snail habitats (Fan et al., 2009; Lei et al., 2000; Li, 2002; Wang et al., 2005a,b). These approaches have thus contributed to the gradual elimination of *S. japonicum* from vast formerly endemic areas of The People's Republic of China.

3.3.1.2 Water resources development projects

Water resources management projects lead to environmental changes and can have negative or positive impacts on the transmission of schistosomiasis depending on their nature and technical specifications (He et al., 2006; Steinmann et al., 2006; Su et al., 2004). Digging and dredging canals, water saving and irrigation schemes, provision of drinking water, river boundary modifications, concrete lining of riversides and canal banks, and construction of facilities to catch snails were all tried and tested to decrease the habitat and snail density of (Wang and Xia, 2006; Zhang et al., 2009; Zhu et al., 2009).

3.3.1.3 Forestry projects

Forestry projects for snail control include the planting of suitable trees such as poplar and Chinese tallow tree in marshlands or mountainous regions in combination with ploughing land and planting crops between forests. These methods change the ecology of snail habitats by decreasing the water level and thus soil moisture, changing the light intensity, etc. (Peng, 2006; Sun et al., 2007; Zhang et al., 2006). Snail densities and survival decrease over several years and significant impacts on human and livestock schistosomiasis prevalence have been documented (Li et al., 2014; Liu et al., 2011; Zhang et al., 2012a,b).

3.3.2 Chemical methods

Mollusciciding is an important tool for the control of snail populations as it is much cheaper, quicker and can save manpower compared with environmental modification. In the early stage of the Chinese schistosomiasis control programmes, chemicals including copper sulphate, DDT, 666, Paris green, calcium arsenate and calcium cyanamide as well as extracts from native herbs were tested to kill *O. hupensis* snails. However, none of them were widely used due to their high cost, serious environmental pollution, or low efficacy (Maegraith, 1958). Sodium pentachlorophenate was found to have high activity against snails and was produced in large quantity since 1959 as it was applied widely in The People's Republic of China before the WBLP. Niclosamide is also widely used in The People's Republic of China since the country started to produce it in 1967 (WHO, 1983). Different formulations have been developed over the past decades, adapted to different environments (Chen, 2003; Dai et al., 2008; He et al., 2007; Xia et al., 2014). Meanwhile, considerable efforts to explore and develop plant molluscicides were not successful (Yang et al., 2014).

3.4 Control of reservoir hosts

The role of livestock, especially buffaloes, in the transmission of schistosomes particularly in lake and mountain regions was realized early. Parasitological methods to diagnose infections in livestock, such as nylon sieve washing and concentrating techniques, and the miracidium hatching technique, were developed. Immunological tests such as IHA and Dot-ELISA kits were developed by Chinese scientists and approved by the Ministry of Agriculture. They are widely implemented for screening. The formulation, dosage, toxicity and pharmacology of different drugs such as antimonials, dipterex, amoscanate and praziqutantel were studied over the past 60 years. Treating infected livestock with oral praziquantel simultaneously when chemotherapy for humans was conducted is a standard procedure since the WBLP. Animal vaccination was regarded as an effective tool to accelerate efforts to reach the final goal of schistosomiasis elimination, and vaccines such as irradiation-attenuated vaccine, paramyosin, and DNA-based vaccines were assessed since the 1980s in The People's Republic of China (Chen et al., 2000; Hsu et al., 1984; Liu et al., 1995, 1998, 2004; Shi et al., 1990, 2001). In the current phase of the national control program initiated in 2004, other methods to decrease or interrupt the contamination of water bodies with eggs from the faeces of infected livestock were implemented: reforming agricultural structures through encouraging the poultry industry instead of raising susceptible livestock, prohibiting the grazing of bovines on snail-infected beaches, raising livestock in stables, replacing bovines by machines, construction of methane tanks to capture manure and improve the living conditions of humans (Chen et al., 2014; Wang et al., 2009a,b; Xu et al., 2015).

4. EXPERIENCE AND LESSONS LEARNT FROM SCHISTOSOMIASIS CONTROL PROGRAMME

The achievements of the schistosomiasis control programmes in The People's Republic of China can be attributed to the strong and stable political commitment of the government, the uninterrupted execution of the national control program, the progressive introduction of newly developed technologies and tools as well as continuous surveillance activities.

4.1 Strong political will and multisectoral collaboration

Since the founding of The People's Republic of China, schistosomiasis control has been given high priority in the public health agenda. A schistosomiasis leading group at national level and a full-time office were established by the end of 1955 to enhance schistosomiasis control since Chairman Mao Zedong issued the slogan to eliminate schistosomiasis (Wang et al., 1989). President Jiang Zemin ordered to take necessary steps to control schistosomiasis after an outbreak with more than 1000 acute schistosomiasis cases happened in Wuchang district of Hubei province in 1989 (Chen, 1990). A schedule of conducting field investigations in spring and organizing a conference in autumn with participants from different sectors was established. With the resurgence of schistosomiasis at the beginning of the new millennium, schistosomiasis was listed as one of four major communicable diseases given high priority (the others being HIV/AIDS, tuberculosis and hepatitis B) in 2004 (Wang et al., 2008). The leading group on schistosomiasis at the State council level was re-established and a notice to further strengthening the schistosomiasis control was issued by the State council in 2004 to strengthen the collaboration between sectors. The promulgation of the Schistosomiasis Prevention and Control Regulations in 2006 accelerated the implementation of the integrated control strategy in endemic areas, making resource mobilization easier.

4.2 Scientific control strategies and effective intervention measures

Big difference exists between different endemic areas in terms of local epidemiology, environment and socioeconomic conditions. Strategies for schistosomiasis control had shifted from the initial elimination strategy before the mid-1980s, to morbidity control during the WBLP and to the current comprehensive strategy of blocking transmission. Research pertaining to schistosomiasis was listed as a key research program in the ministries of health, agriculture and water resources. The introduction of praziquantel, artemether and artesunate to kill schistosomula, transfer from bench to the field of sensitive and easy-to-use diagnostic tool, new chemicals for mollusciciding and livestock treatment were developed in the frame of research projects and promoted the progress of schistosomiasis control in The People's Republic of China (Xin and Dai, 2010; Yang et al., 2012; Zhang et al., 2013; Zhou et al., 2013a,b). Along with the shift of control strategies, criteria for schistosomiasis control and elimination were formulated and modified six times, providing guidance for control activities and to assess the effect of the interventions (Zhou et al., 2013a,b). Technical support to different endemic areas improved their capacity to implement and combine the appropriate interventions.

4.3 Vertical control program and sufficient workforce

The reliance on a professional workforce contributed to the success of schistosomiasis control in The People's Republic of China. The Ministry of Health played an important role in managing and monitoring the national control program. Antischistosomiasis institutions or stations were established at all levels (national, provincial, municipal, county and township) in the

1950s. They are well funded to take the main responsibility for disease control, treatment and prevention (Collins et al., 2012). By the end of 2011, except one national institute, 365 agencies for schistosomiasis control existed in seven provinces including Jiangsu, Anhui, Jiangxi, Hubei, Hunan, Sichuan and Yunnan. Among them 282 are responsible for schistosomiasis prevention and control and the others are in charge of prevention and clinical case management. Although many antischistosomiasis stations were integrated into general centre for disease control (CDC) institutions or other disease-specific facilities due to the decreased prevalence and scale down of programs, the workforce dedicated to schistosomiasis control full time has been maintained (Ross et al., 2013).

4.4 Epidemiological surveys and surveillance

National surveys conducted since the 1950s and three national sampling surveys conducted in the frame of the WBLP provided basic information on the epidemiological features and updated the endemic status of schistosomiasis in The People's Republic of China (Wu et al., 2007; Zhou et al., 2005). To monitor changes in the epidemiological status and assess the effectiveness of control strategies, systematic cohort monitoring and surveillance of schistosomiasis have been conducted since the 1990s (Zhou, 2009, Zhu et al., 2011). Other surveillance projects focussing on the impact of climate changes and large water conservancy projects on schistosomiasis transmission at the border of nonendemic and endemic areas, and sentinel mice-based surveillance in high risk water bodies are regularly conducted in The People's Republic of China (Dang et al., 2014; Zhang et al., 2012a,b; Zhu et al., 2011). New technologies such as remote sensing, geographical information system and predictive statistical modelling, and xeno-monitoring based on loop-mediated isothermal amplification technique are also implemented (Tong et al., 2015; Yang et al., 2006; Zhang et al., 2005). These activities provide basic information for decision-makers when they draft control programmes or design control activities and allow the assessment of the achievements obtained through decades of efforts (Tambo et al., 2014).

5. CHALLENGES

5.1 Extensive and complicated snail habitats

Over the past decade, the snail-infested areas nationwide remained at 3.6–3.8 billion m^2. In 2013, 96.5% of all snail habitats were located in the marshland and lake regions. Among these areas, 94.3% were distributed outside embankments where they are easily influenced by water level fluctuations (Lei et al., 2014). Big challenge exists to eliminate snails from such extensive areas with complicated ecological characteristics such as unstable water level or flourish vegetation. Furthermore, agricultural activities, flooding and water conservancy projects may spread snails to urban regions or previously uncolonized areas. Between 2002 and 2010, snails were found in areas previously free of snails measuring 125 million m^2 (Wang et al., 2015).

5.2 Management of different sources of infection

The schistosomiasis prevalence in bovines has been reduced to a very low level, but the number of livestock including bovines and goats in endemic areas is significant. Other species, especially rodents, which also play important roles in some lake and mountainous regions, make it difficult to completely eliminate schistosomiasis (Guo et al., 2013; Lu et al., 2010). Fishermen and boat people are currently at highest risk of schistosome infection, but control programs among such migrating populations are difficult to implement. They may also spread schistosomes to other places where intermediate host snails exist. Medical services also need to become aware of other forms of schistosomiasis, eg, in travellers and workers returning from African countries (Zhou et al., 2013a,b, Zhu and Xu, 2014).

5.3 Unbalanced implementation of integrated strategy

Despite the significant economic growth occurred in The People's Republic of China since the reform of the economic system in 1978, big differences exist between urban and rural areas, western and eastern regions, and lake and mountainous regions (Bian et al., 2004; Tang et al., 2008). Many of the proposed integrated measures such as improving safe water supply and sanitation, mechanization of agriculture, building methane tanks, environmental modification, etc. need large funds which are not available in poor areas. Particularly problematic is the Chinese system that programs and interventions are centrally planned but implementation and financing are largely up to local governments. Prohibiting grazing in snail habitats has also encountered resistance in some regions as it impacts farmers' benefits since such pastures are communal land requiring no or very limited investments for use (He, 2011).

5.4 Unavailability of sensitive diagnostic tools

As the prevalence in intermediate and end hosts decreases to a very low level, moving forward towards elimination requires sensitive diagnostic tools. The current strategy of conducting stool examination only for antibody-positive individual increases feasibility and compliance but risks missing infected individuals also increase due to the relative insensitivity of the Kato–Katz method and/or miracidium hatching technique in identifying light infections. Consequently, the current prevalence of schistosomiasis is probably underestimated and the undetected cases continue to serve as infection sources (Zhou et al., 2011). Snail surveys and dissection are labour intensive approaches and require trained technicians. Diagnostic tools and snails examination based on molecular techniques have a higher sensitivity and specificity than traditional approaches but they are expensive and their performance and applicability need further field assessment (Tong et al., 2015; Xia et al., 2009, 2014; Xu et al., 2010).

5.5 Weak surveillance and active response system

The biological and social factors promoting the transmission of schistosomiasis still exist in many areas where active transmission has ceased. Thus, a rebound or re-emergence of schistosomiasis can easily happen once infection sources or intermediate hosts are imported. Although systematic surveillance has been conducted since the 1990s and the current surveillance system covers all endemic counties, the tools did not change fundamentally and shortcomings such as simple monitored contents, insensitive indicators, obsolete technologies and insufficient use of collected data become ever more pressing with the decrease of the prevalence. In counties which had reached transmission control or interruption for many years, the diagnostic and epidemiological survey capacity and the ability to respond to outbreaks decreases due to staff turnover, weak infrastructure, sliding consciousness and low training levels. During 2011–13, most acute cases that were ultimately reported were initially misdiagnosed and new cases are regularly seen from areas where transmission was thought to have ceased (Lei et al., 2014; Li et al., 2013; Zheng et al., 2012). The surveillance and particularly the ability to actively respond need to be strengthened to ensure early detection and correct handling of schistosomiasis outbreaks and thus accelerate progress towards schistosomiasis elimination nationwide (Zhang et al., 2016).

6. PROSPECT

The raise in awareness for the importance of schistosomiasis control and in view of the achievements gained in several countries, resolution WHA65.21 on the elimination of schistosomiasis was adopted by World Health Assembly (WHA) in 2012. It calls for increased investment in schistosomiasis control using multiple approaches, support for countries to initiate elimination programs where appropriate and the creation of a process to verify interruption of transmission (WHO, 2013). The action plan drafted by the WHO Western Pacific Region (WPRO) in 2012 expects The People's Republic of China to eliminate schistosomiasis as a public health problem (prevalence in human beings and livestock <1%) by 2016 (WPR/RC63/6, 2012). According to the current trends, the target could be reached in 2015 (the Chinese criteria for transmission control are equal to the criteria for eliminating schistosomiasis as a public health problem set by WHO).

As the current phase of the national schistosomiasis control program will be successfully completed by the end of 2015, elimination of schistosomiasis must be the next target. In November 2014, the national schistosomiasis control conference at state council level was organized in Hunan Province. Based on the current achievements, a new goal was put forward to eliminate schistosomiasis nationwide following the approaches laid out in another two consecutive five year plans (Lei and Zhou, 2015). Systematic assessments will be conducted to understand the endemic status of schistosomiasis in the country and evaluate the efficacy of the current integrated strategy in The People's Republic of China. As changes existed to achieve elimination in current situation, full integration of interventions including chemotherapy, snail control, safe water supply, improving sanitation, environmental modification through water conservancy, agriculture, and forestry projects is required. Intersectoral cooperation needs to be strengthened. More sensitive and effective diagnostic and surveillance tools and techniques need to be explored to monitor the declination or cessation of transmission and verify elimination of schistosomiasis transmission. Risk assessments should be conducted to identify hotspots of transmission and guide policy makers. Capacity building in surveillance should be strengthened to consolidate achievements and prevent re-emergence of schistosomiasis.

APPENDIX

Milestones of schistosomiasis japonica control process in The People's Republic of China

Year	Political will	National program or plan	Instructive materials	Endemicity	Drugs development
1950	Instruction of schistosomiasis control issued by Ministry of Health		First version of manual for schistosomiasis control	1335 people died in an outbreak of schistosomiasis in Gaoyou county	
1955	Set up national leading group for schistosomiasis control				
1956	Chairman Mao issued a slogan of eliminating schistosomiasis	National plan for agricultural development (1956–65)	Second version of manual for schistosomiasis control	Estimated 11.6 million people infected with schistosomes and 1.2 million bovines infected	
1958	Chairman Mao wrote the poem of 'Farewell to the god of plague'		First version of criteria for schistosomiasis elimination	Yujiang county first announced schistosomiasis elimination	
1959					Production of sodium pentachlorophenate
1962					First nonantimonial oral drug synthesized by The People's Republic of China
1967					Production of niclosamide

(Continued)

Milestones of schistosomiasis japonica control process in The People's Republic of China—cont'd

Year	Political will	National program or plan	Instructive materials	Endemicity	Drugs development
1970	Reset up of national leading group for schistosomiasis control				
1977			Second version of criteria for schistosomiasis elimination		Praziquantel synthesized by The People's Republic of China
1978		National plan of eliminating schistosomiasis in 13 provinces	Third version of criteria for schistosomiasis elimination		
1980					Found the antischistosomal properties of artemisinin
1984	Chairman Deng Xiaopeng issued the instruction of schistosomiasis prevention and control				
1986	Dismissed the national leading group and set up Bureau of Eendemic Diseases in Ministry of Health		Fourth version of criteria for schistosomiasis elimination		

1987		Seventh five year plan for schistosomiasis control		
1989	Chairman Jiang Zemin put forward that control and elimination of schistosomiasis is the responsibility of government			1604 cases attacked by acute schistosomiasis in Wuhan city in Hubei Province
1990	State council issued the notice of strengthening schistosomiasis control and prevention			
1991		Eighth five year plan for schistosomiasis control		
1992		Started WBLP		Acute cases and snails found in Guangdong Province again
1995			Fifth version of criteria for schistosomiasis elimination	Five provinces eliminated schistosomiasis
1997		Ninth five year plan for schistosomiasis control		

(Continued)

Milestones of schistosomiasis japonica control process in The People's Republic of China—cont'd

Year	Political will	National program or plan	Instructive materials	Endemicity	Drugs development
2001		Termination of WBLP tenth five year plan for schistosomiasis control	Third version of manual for schistosomiasis control		
2004	Schistosomiasis was listed as one of four priority disease and a strategic plan was issued Reset up of national leading group for schistosomiasis control	National key project for schistosomiasis comprehensive control (2004–08)			
2006	Promulgation of the schistosomiasis prevention and control regulations		Sixth version of criteria for schistosomiasis elimination		
2008				The whole country reached the criteria of infection control	
2009		National key project for schistosomiasis comprehensive control (2009–15)			

ACKNOWLEDGEMENTS

This manuscript was supported by the China UK Global Health Support Programme (Grant no. GHSP-CS-OP1-01) and the National Special Science and Technology Project for Major Infectious Diseases of China (No. 2012ZX10004-220). We acknowledge partial financial support by the National Natural Science Foundation of China (Grant no. 81301454).

REFERENCES

Bian, Y., Sun, Q., Zhao, Z., Blas, E., 2004. Market reform: a challenge to public health—the case of schistosomiasis control in China. Int. J. Health Plan. Manag. 19, S79—S94.

Cao, Z.G., Zhao, Y.E., Willingham, A.L., Wang, T.P., 2016. Towards the elimination of Schistosomiasis japonica through control of the disease in domestic animals in the People's Republic of China: a tale of over 60 years. Adv. Parasitol. 92.

Chen, C., Zheng, X.Y., Quian, Y.F., Xiao, S.H., Shao, B.R., Huang, L.S., 1962. Studies on *Hemerocallis thunbergii Baker* III. isolation and characterization of active principle against schistosomiasis japonica. Acta Pharm. Sin. 40, 579—586.

Chen, M.G., Feng, Z., 1999. Schistosomiasis control in China. Parasitol. Int. 48, 11—19.

Chen, D.J., Fu, L.F., Shao, P.P., Wu, F.Z., Shu, H., Ren, C.S., et al., 1980. Experimental studies on antischistosomal activity of qinghaosu. Zhong Hua Yi Xue Zha Zhi 60, 422—425.

Chen, H.G., Nara, T., Zeng, X.J., Satoh, M.S., Wu, G.C., Jiang, W.S., et al., 2000. Vaccination of domestic pig with recombinant paramyosin: against *Schistosoma japonicum* in China. Vaccine 18, 2142—2146.

Chen, X.Y., Wang, L.Y., Jiming, C., Zhou, X.N., Zheng, J., Guo, J.G., et al., 2005. Schistosomiasis control in China: the impact of a 10-year World Bank Loan Project (1992—2001). Bull. World Health Organ. 83, 43—48.

Chen, Y.Y., Liu, J.B., Huang, X.B., Cai, S.X., Su, Z.M., Zhong, R., et al., 2014. New integrated strategy emphasizing infection source control to curb Schistosomiasis japonica in a marshland area of Hubei Province, China: findings from an eight-year longitudinal survey. PLoS One 9, e89779.

Chen, S.B., Ai, L., Hu, W., Xu, J., Bergquist, R., Qin, Z.Q., et al., 2016. New anti-schistosome approaches in the People's Republic of China: development of diagnostics, vaccines and other new techniques belonging to the 'omics' group. Adv. Parasitol. 92.

Chen, G.X., 1956. Endemic status of schistosomiasis in Hunan Province. In: data compilation on schistosomiasis research. Shanghai Health Publ. House 36—44.

Chen, M.Z., 1990. Control schisotosomiasis by strengthening leadershiping and conducting effective measures. Chin. J. Schistosomiasis Control 2, 8.

Chen, M.G., 1999. Progress in schistosomiasis control in China. Chin. Med. J. Engl. 112, 930—933.

Chen, C., 2003. Molluscicides and their application in China. Chin. J. Schistosomiasis Control 321—322.

Chen, M.G., 2014. Assessment of morbidity due to *Schistosoma japonicum* infection in China. Infect. Dis. Poverty 3, 6.

Chou, H.J., Hu, S.G., Jue, T.E., 1958. China congress on parasitic diseases. In: Abstract of Papers Presented in November 1958. China Scientific Publishing House, Beijing, p. 16.

Colley, D.G., Bustinduy, A.L., Secor, W.E., King, C.H., 2014. Human schistosomiasis. Lancet 383, 2253—2264.

Collins, C., Xu, J., Tang, S., 2012. Schistosomiasis control and the health system in P.R. China. Infect. Dis. Poverty 1, 8.

Department of Disease Control, Ministry of Health, 2000. Textbook for Schistosomiasis Control. Shanghai Publishing House for Science and Technology, Shanghai.

Dai, Y.H., Lv, G.Y., Liu, Z.Y., Zhang, D.P., 1999. Analysis of efficacy of artesunate against schistosomiasis during flood. Chin. J. Schistosomiasis Control 143–145.
Dai, J.R., Wang, W., Liang, Y.S., Li, H.J., Guan, X.H., Zhu, Y.C., 2008. A novel molluscicidal formulation of niclosamide. Parasitol. Res. 103, 405–412.
Daily, P.S., 1958. Strengthening the leadership of Ministry of Health and more than 300 counties conduct schistosomiasis prevention and control. In: People's Daily. People's Daily Publishing House, Beijing.
Dang, H., Xu, J., Li, S.Z., Cao, Z.G., Huang, Y.X., Wu, C.G., et al., 2014. Monitoring the transmission of *Schistosoma japonicum* in potential risk regions of China, 2008-2012. Int. J. Environ. Res. Public Health 11, 2278–2287.
Fan, C.B., Li, Y.B., Xiong, Y.Q., Dai, Z.W., 2009. Effect of comprehensive measures with an emphasis on raising crawfish and rice alternatively in paddy field for schistosomiasis control. Chin. J. Schistosomiasis Control 21, 422–423.
Faust, E.C., Meleney, H.E., 1924. Studies on Schistosomiasis japonica. Am. J. Hyg. 3, 219.
Feng, Y., Liu, L., Xia, S., Xu, J.F., Bergquist, R., Yang, G.J., 2016. Reaching the surveillance-response stage of schistosomiasis control in the People's Republic of China: a modelling approach. Adv. Parasitol. 92.
Fu, S., Xiao, S.H., Catto, B.A., 1988. Clinical use of praziquantel in China. Parasitol. Today 4, 312–315.
Gray, D.J., Williams, G.M., Li, Y., Chen, H., Li, R.S., Forsyth, S.J., et al., 2007. A cluster-randomized bovine intervention trial against *Schistosoma japonicum* in the People's Republic of China: design and baseline results. Am. J. Trop. Med. Hyg. 77, 866–874.
Gray, D.J., Williams, G.M., Li, Y., McManus, D.P., 2008. Transmission dynamics of *Schistosoma japonicum* in the lakes and marshlands of China. PLoS One 3, e4058.
Gryseels, B., Polman, K., Clerinx, J., Kestens, L., 2006. Human schistosomiasis. Lancet 368, 1106–1118.
Guan, X.H., Shi, Y.E., 1996. Collaborative study on evaluation of immunodiagnostic assays in schistosomiasis japonica by treatment efficacy assessment. Chin. Med. J. 109, 659–664 (in Chinese).
Guo, J.G., Zheng, J., 1999. Epidemiology of schistosomiasis and progress of control and research. Chin. J. Parasitol. Parsit. Dis. 17, 260–263.
Guo, J.G., Ross, A.G., Lin, D.D., Williams, G.M., Chen, H.G., Li, Y., et al., 2001. A baseline study on the importance of bovines for human *Schistosoma japonicum* infection around Poyang Lake, China. Am. J. Trop. Med. Hyg. 65, 272–278.
Guo, Y., Jiang, M., Gu, L., Qiao, Y., Li, W.G., 2013. Prevalence of *Schistosoma japonicum* in wild rodents in five islands of the west Dongting Lake, China. J. Parasitol. 99, 706–707.
Guo, J.G., 2006. Historical and current comprehensive control of schistosomiasis in P.R. China. Chin. J. Prev. Med. 40, 225–228.
Hao, Y., Wu, X.H., Xia, G., Zheng, H., Guo, J.G., Wang, L.Y., et al., 2005. Endemic status of schistosomiasis in P.R. China in 2004. Chin. J. Schistosomiasis Control 17, 401–404.
He, J.F., Yan, T., Lin, D.D., 2006. Studies on impact of "National 32 zi Policy" on schistosomiasis transmission along Yangtz River region. Int. J. Med. Parasit. Dis. 33, 191–194.
He, J.X., Wang, H., Wu, M.Y., Chen, X.F., Shu, Q.M., Tao, W., et al., 2007. Observation on the molluscicidal effect of niclosamide ethanolamine salt dustable powder by dusting in fields. J. Trop. Dis. Parasitol. 5, 153–154.
He, H.B., 2011. Thought of schistosomiasis control strategy with emphasis on controlling sources of infection in lake and marshland endemic regions. Chin. J. Schistosomiasis Control 23, 710–713.
Hong, X.C., Xu, X.J., Chen, X., Li, Y.S., Yu, C.H., Yuan, Y., et al., 2013. Assessing the effect of an integrated control strategy for schistosomiasis japonica emphasizing bovines

in a marshland area of Hubei Province, China: a cluster randomized trial. PLoS Negl. Trop. Dis. 7, e2122.

Hou, X.Y., McManus, D.P., Gray, D.J., Balen, J., Luo, X.S., He, Y.K., et al., 2008. A randomized, double-blind, placebo-controlled trial of safety and efficacy of combined praziquantel and artemether treatment for acute schistosomiasis japonica in China. Bull. World Health Organ. 86, 788–795.

Hsiao, S.H., Liu, J.C., Chan, C.C., 1975. Combined oral F-30066 and rectal dipterex in treatment of experimental schistosomiasis japonica. Chin. Med. J. 88, 51–59.

Hsu, S.Y., Xu, S.T., He, Y.X., Shi, F.H., Shen, W., Hsu, H.F., et al., 1984. Vaccination of bovines against schistosomiasis japonica with highly irradiated schistosomula in China. Am. J. Trop. Med. Hyg. 33, 891–898.

Hu, S.Y., Liu, J., Wang, B., Hu, Z.D., Xiao, C.J., 2000. The effect of artesunate in preventing the population from *Schistsoma japonicum* infection during flood-control. Chin. J. Parasitol. Parasit. Dis. 18, 113–114.

Kan, H.C., Kung, J.C., 1936. Incidence of *Schistosomiasis japanica* in an endemic area in Chekiang. Chin. Med. J. (Suppl.), 449–456.

Kan, H.C., Yao, Y.T., 1934. Some notes on the anti-schistosomiasis japonica campaign in Chih-huai-pan, Kaihua, Chekiang. Chin. Med. J. Engl. 23, 323–336.

Katz, N., Chaves, A., Pellegrino, J., 1972. A simple device for quantitative stool thick-smear technique in *Schistosomiasis mansoni*. Rev. Inst. Med. Trop. Sao Paulo 14, 397–400.

Kuo, S.C., 1946. Further studies on distribution of schistosomiasis japonica in Szechwan Province, China. J. Parasitol. 32, 367.

Le, W.J., Xiao, S.H., Mao, S.B., 1957. Comparison of efficacy against schistosomiasis in mice treated by potassium and sodium antimony tartrate. Chin. Med. J. 43, 523–524.

Le, W.J., You, J.Q., Yang, Y.Q., Mei, J.Y., Guo, H.F., Yang, H.Z., et al., 1982. Studies on the efficacy of artemether in experimental schistosomiasis. Acta Pharm. Sin. 17, 187–193.

Le, W.J., You, J.Q., Mei, J.Y., 1983. Chemotherapeutic effect of artesunate in experimental schistosomiasis. Acta Pharm. Sin. 18, 619–621.

Lei, Z.L., Zhou, X.N., 2015. Eradication of schistosomiasis: a new target and a new task for the national schistosomiasis control program in the People's Republic of China. Chin. J. Schistosomiasis Control 27, 1–4.

Lei, X.H., Chang, L.C., Hsu, M.L., Chang, S.P., Cheng, K.C., Lu, M.C., et al., 1963. A new class of chemotherapeutic agents orally effective against Schistosomiasis japonica. Chin. Med. J. 82, 90–91.

Lei, J.Q., Shen, H.Z., Shao, S.Y., 2000. Trial of digging fish pond to control snail at lakes area. Chin. J. Vet. Parasitol. 8, 61–62.

Lei, Z.L., Zheng, H., Zhang, L.J., Zhu, R., Xu, Z.M., Xu, J., et al., 2014. Endemic status of schistosomiasis in People's Republic of China in 2013. Chin. J. Schistosomiasis Control 26, 591–597.

Li, X.Y., Shen, J.L., Zhong, Z.R., Wen, H.Q., Luo, Q.L., Wei, W., 2009. Paeoniflorin: a monomer from traditional Chinese medical herb ameliorates *Schistosoma japonicum* egg-induced hepatic fibrosis in mice. J. Parasitol. 95, 1520–1524.

Li, S.Z., Zheng, H., Gao, J., Zhang, L.J., Zhu, R., Xu, J., et al., 2013. Endemic status of schistosomiasis in People's Republic of China in 2012. Chin. J. Schistosomiasis Control 25, 557–563.

Li, Q.Y., Huang, Y., Cao, Z.G., Zhang, S.Q., 2014. Impact of the afforestation project for schistosomiasis control on the inhibition of *Oncomelania* snails: a longitudinal study. J. Trop. Dis. Parasitol. 12, 129–132.

Li, X.X., Chen, J.X., Wang, L.X., Sun, J., Chen, S.H., Chen, J.H., et al., 2015. Profiling B and T cell immune responses to co-infection of Mycobacterium tuberculosis and hookworm in humans. Infect. Dis. Poverty 4, 20.

Li, Z.J., Ge, J., Dai, J.R., Wen, L.Y., Lin, D.D., Madsen, H., et al., 2016. Biology and control of snail intermediate host of *Schistosoma japonicum* in the People's Republic of China. Adv. Parasitol. 92.

Li, Q., 2002. Observation of schistosomiasis control in areas by changing rice field to dry land. Chin. J. Vet. Parasitol. 10, 40–41.

Li, Y.S., 2006. Diagnosis and Treatment of Schistosomiasis. People's Health Publishing House, Beijing.

Liang, S., Yang, C., Zhong, B., Qiu, D., 2006. Re-emerging schistosomiasis in hilly and mountainous areas of Sichuan, China. Bull. World Health Organ 84, 139–144.

Lin, D.D., Liu, J.X., Liu, Y.M., Hu, F., Zhang, Y.Y., Xu, J.M., et al., 2008. Routine Kato-Katz technique underestimates the prevalence of *Schistosoma japonicum*: a case study in an endemic area of the People's Republic of China. Parasitol. Int. 57, 281–286.

Ling, C.C., Cheng, W.J., Chung, H.L., 1949. Clinical and diagnostic features of schistosomiasis japonica. Chin. Med. J. 67, 347–360.

Liu, S.X., Song, G.C., Xu, Y.X., Yang, W., McManus, D.P., 1995. Anti-fecundity immunity induced in pigs vaccinated with recombinant *Schistosoma japonicum* 26 kDa glutathione-S-transferase. Parasite Immunol. 17, 355–400.

Liu, S.X., Song, G.C., Xu, Y.X., McManus, D.P., Hotez, P.J., 1998. Progress in the development of a vaccine against schistosomiasis in China. Int. J. Infect. Dis. 2, 176.

Liu, J.M., Cai, X.Z., Lin, J.J., Fu, Z.Q., Yang, G.Z., Shi, F.H., et al., 2004. Gene cloning, expression and vaccine testing of *Schistosoma japonicum* SjFABP. Parasite Immunol. 26, 351–358.

Liu, G.F., Li, K., Zhang, C.H., 2011. Snail control effect and economical benefit of forest for snail control and schistosomiasis prevention in mountainous regions. Chin. J. Schistosomiasis Control 23, 386–389.

Liu, Y.X., Wu, W., Liang, Y.J., Jie, Z.L., Wang, H., Wang, W., et al., 2014. New uses for old drugs: the tale of artemisinin derivatives in the elimination of schistosomiasis japonica in China. Molecules 19, 15058–15074.

Logan, O.T., 1905. A case of dysentery in Hunan province, caused by the trematoda, *Schistosoma japonicum*. Chin. Med. J. 19, 243–245.

Lu, Z.H., Zhong, H.L., Ling, Z.S., Wu, Z.J., 1955. Some aspects of research in the prevention and treatment of schistosomiasis japonica in new China. Chin. Med. J. 73, 100–106.

Lu, D.B., Wang, T.P., Rudge, J.W., Donnelly, C.A., Fang, G.R., Webster, J.P., 2010. Contrasting reservoirs for *Schistosoma japonicum* between marshland and hilly regions in Anhui, China – a two-year longitudinal parasitological survey. Parasitology 137, 99–110.

Maegraith, B., 1958. Schistosomiasis in China. Lancet 1, 208–214.

Mao, S.P., Shao, B.R., 1982. Schistosomiasis control in the people's Republic of China. Am. J. Trop. Med. Hyg. 31, 92–99.

Mao, C.P., 1948. A review of the epidemiology of schistosomiasis japonica in China. Am. J. Trop. Med. Hyg. 28, 659–672.

Mao, S.P., 1987. Epidemiology and control of schistosomiasis in the People's Republic of China. Mem. Inst. Oswaldo Cruz 82 (Suppl. 4), 77–82.

McManus, D.P., Li, Y., Gray, D.J., Ross, A.G., 2009. Conquering 'snail fever': schistosomiasis and its control in China. Expert Rev. Anti Infect. Ther. 7, 473–485.

Ministry of Health, 1993. Epidemiological Situation of Schistosomiasis in China: Results from a Nationwide Sampling Survey in 1989. Press of Chengdu Science and Technology University, Chengdu.

Ministry of Health, 1998. Epidemic Status of Schistosomiasis in China-a Naitonwide Sampling Survey in 1995. Nanjing University Press, Nanjing.

Ministry of Health, 2007. Criteria for Schistosomiasis Control and Elimination in P.R. China. China Standards Press, Beijing.

Ojurongbe, O., Sina-Agbaje, O.R., Busari, A., Okorie, P.N., Ojurongbe, T.A., Akindele, A.A., 2014. Efficacy of praziquantel in the treatment of *Schistosoma*

haematobium infection among school-age children in rural communities of Abeokuta, Nigeria. Infect. Dis. Poverty 3, 30.
Pan, H.D., Huang, D.S., Wang, K.T., 2002. Approach to surveillance and consolidation during past 15 years after elimination of schistosomiasis in Shanghai. Acta Trop. 82, 301–303.
Peng, Z.H., 2006. Techniques of afforestation in the beaches of Yangtze River for Snail (*Oncomelania hupensis*) Control and Schistosomiasis Prevention. Wetl. Sci. Manag. 1.
Ross, A.G., Li, Y.S., Sleigh, A.C., McManus, D.P., 1997. Schistosomiasis control in the People's Republic of China. Parasitol. Today 13, 152–155.
Ross, A.G., Bartley, P., Sleigh, A., Olds, G.R., Li, Y.S., Williams, G., et al., 2002. Schistosomiasis. N. Engl. J. Med. 346, 1212–1220.
Ross, A.G., Vickers, D., Olds, G.R., Shah, S.M., McManus, D.P., 2007. Katayama syndrome. Lancet Infect. Dis. 7, 218–224.
Ross, A.G., Olveda, R.M., Acosta, L., Harn, D.A., Chy, D., Li, Y., et al., 2013. Road to the elimination of schistosomiasis from Asia: the journey is far from over. Microbe. Infect./Institut Pasteur 15, 858–865.
Shen, J.F., Liu, B.Q., Huang, L.S., 1981. Isolation and identification of the active principle against schistosome from Dryopteris crassirhizoma. Chin. Pharm. Bull. 16, 79–80.
Shi, Y.E., Jiang, C.F., Han, J.J., Li, Y.L., Ruppel, A., 1990. *Schistosoma japonicum*: an ultraviolet-attenuated cercarial vaccine applicable in the field for water buffaloes. Exp. Parasitol. 71, 100–106.
Shi, F.H., Zhang, Y.B., Ye, P., Lin, J.J., Cai, Y.M., Shen, W., et al., 2001. Laboratory and field evaluation of *Schistosoma japonicum* DNA vaccines in sheep and water buffalo in China. Vaccine 20, 462–467.
Shiao, S.H., Yang, Y.Q., Loh, W.C., Chow, H.Y., Mao, S.P., 1959. Studies on the effect of pumpkin seed on experimental schistosomiasis japonica. Acta Pharm. Sin. 7, 300–308.
Shiao, S.H., Shao, B.R., He, Y.X., Yang, Y.Q., Yang, H.Z., Chang, Y.C., 1962. Studies on *Hemerocallis thunbergii Baker* II. Effectiveness of *Hemerocallis thumbergii* in oral treatment of experimental schistosomiasis in mice. Acta Pharm. Sin. 19, 218–224.
Sleigh, A., Li, X., Jackson, S., Huang, K., 1998. Eradication of schistosomiasis in Guangxi, China. Part 1: Setting, strategies, operations, and outcomes, 1953-92. Bull. World Health Organ. 76, 361–372.
Song, Y., Xiao, S.H., Wu, W., Zhang, S.J., Xie, H.Q., Xu, X.P., et al., 1997. The preventive effect of artemether in protection of people from schistosome infection during fighting against flood. Chin. J. Parasitol. Parasit. Dis. 15, 133–137.
Steinmann, P., Keiser, J., Bos, R., Tanner, M., Utzinger, J., 2006. Schistosomiasis and water resources development: systematic review, meta-analysis, and estimates of people at risk. Lancet Infect. Dis. 6, 411–425.
Su, Z.M., Wei, F.H., He, H., Fan, H.P., Tu, Z.W., Xu, X.J., 2004. Dynamic observations on snail situation and wild faeces pollution in marshlands in pilot areas of Hubei Province. Chin. J. Schistosomiasis Control 16, 47–50.
Sun, Q.X., Peng, Z.H., Zhou, J.X., 2007. Strategies and mechanisms on shistosomiasis eco-control with forest of snail control and shistosomiasis prevention. J. Anhui Agric. Univ. 34, 338–341.
Sun, L.P., Wang, W., Liang, Y.S., Tian, Z.X., Hong, Q.B., Yang, K., et al., 2011. Effect of an integrated control strategy for schistosomiasis japonica in the lower reaches of the Yangtze River, China: an evaluation from 2005 to 2008. Parasites Vectors 4, 243.
Tambo, E., Ai, L., Zhou, X., Chen, J.H., Hu, W., Bergquist, R., et al., 2014. Surveillance-response systems: the key to elimination of tropical diseases. Infect. Dis. Poverty 3, 17.
Tambo, E., Khater, E.I., Chen, J.H., Bergquist, R., Zhou, X.N., 2015. Nobel prize for the artemisinin and ivermectin discoveries: a great boost towards elimination of the global infectious diseases of poverty. Infect. Dis. Poverty 4, 58.

Tang, S., Meng, Q., Chen, L., Bekedam, H., Evans, T., Whitehead, M., 2008. Tackling the challenges to health equity in China. Lancet 372, 1493–1501.
Tang, C.C., 1939. Further investigation on schistosomiasis japonica in Futsing, Fukien Province. Chin. Med. J. Engl. 56, 452–473.
Tang, C.C., 1951. Epidemiology of schistosomiasis japonica in Futsing, Fukien province. Peking. Nat. Bull. 19, 225–247.
Tong, Q., Chen, R., Zhang, Y., Yang, G., Kumagaid, T., Shimogawarad, R., et al., 2015. A new surveillance and response tool: risk map of infected *Oncomelania hupensis* detected by Loop-mediated isothermal amplification (LAMP) from pooled samples. Acta Trop. 141, 170–177.
Totell, G.T., 1924. A preliminary survey of schistosomiasis infection in the region of Changteh. Chin. Med. J. Engl. 38, 270–274.
Villar, L.P.R., Burguillo, F.J., LÃ3pez-AbÃ¡n, J., Muro, A., 2012. Systematic review and meta-analysis of artemisinin based therapies for the treatment and prevention of schistosomiasis. PLoS One 7.
Wan, L., Song, X.X., Sun, Q.X., Jiang, J.M., Zhang, X.D., Tang, Y.X., et al., 2016. Control of schistosomiasis japonica through afforestation in the People' Republic of China. Adv. Parasitol. 92.
Wang, G., Yang, Y., Le, W., Yang, H., You, J., Xie, R., 1979. The effect of agrimophol and its combination with niridazole in experimental schistosmiasis. Acta Pharm. Sin. 14, 379–384.
Wang, P., Xia, Z.P., 2006. Major techniques in the water conservancy projects for schistosomiasis prevention. Yangtz River 37, 84–85.
Wang, H.Z., Jia, Y.D., Guo, J.P., Xia, C., 1989. A historic review or 40 years' control on schistosomiasis in P.R. China. Chin. J. Schistosomiasis Control 1, 1–4.
Wang, T.P., Vang Johansen, M., Zhang, S.Q., Wang, F.F., Wu, W.D., Zhang, G.H., et al., 2005a. Transmission of *Schistosoma japonicum* by humans and domestic animals in the Yangtze River valley, Anhui province. China. Acta Trop. 96, 198–204.
Wang, W.L., Zhang, H.Z., Xu, Q.C., Zhang, Y.Q., Qin, Q., Liu, F.C., et al., 2005b. Relationship between agriculture adjustment and schistosomiasis transmission in lake regions. Chin. J. Schistosomiasis Control 17, 454–456.
Wang, L.D., Utzinger, J., Zhou, X.N., 2008. Schistosomiasis control: experiences and lessons from China. Lancet 372, 1793–1795.
Wang, L.D., Chen, H.G., Guo, J.G., Zeng, X.J., Hong, X.L., Xiong, J.J., et al., 2009a. A strategy to control transmission of *Schistosoma japonicum* in China. N. Engl. J. Med. 360, 121–128.
Wang, L.D., Guo, J.G., Wu, X.H., Chen, H.G., Wang, T.P., Zhu, S.P., et al., 2009b. China's new strategy to block *Schistosoma japonicum* transmission: experiences and impact beyond schistosomiasis. Trop. Med. Int. Health 14, 1475–1483.
Wang, Q., Xu, J., Zhang, L.J., Zheng, H., Ruan, Y., Hao, Y.W., et al., 2015. Analysis of endemic changes of schistosomiasis in China from 2002 to 2010. Chin. J. Schistosomiasis Control 27.
Wang, R.Y., 1984. Treatment of late-stage schistosomiasis with injection of astragalus and salvia: clinical observation and preliminary investigation. Acta Acad. Med. Nanjing 2, 14.
Wang, G.Z., 2011. The practice and enlightment of schistosomiasis control by Chinese Communist Party through integrating human power in 1950s. Study Teach. Hist. Communist Party 221, 89–96.
Wei, O., 1973. Internal organs of a 2100-year-old female corpse. Lancet 2, 1198.
Wen, L.Y., Tao, H.Q., 2008. Progress and prospect on schistosomiasis control in Zhejiang Province. Int. J. Epidemil. Infect. Dis. 6, 361–364.
WHO, 1983. The role of mollusciciding in schistosomiasis control. In: WHO (Ed.), Geneva, pp. 72–73.

WHO, 1985. The control of schistosomiasis. In: Report of a WHO Expert Committee. Geneva.
WHO, 2013. Schistosomiasis: Progress Report 2001–2011 Strategic Plan 2012–2020.
WPR/RC63/6, 2012. In: Draft Regional Action Plan for Neglected Tropical Diseases in the Western Pacific (2012–2016). Hanoi, Viet Nam.
Wu, Z., Sun, X., 2014. Treatment methods of traditional Chinese medicine for schistosomiasis and other trematode infections. In: Treatment of Human Parasitosis in Traditional Chinese Medicine. Springer, pp. 141–154.
Wu, X.H., Li, Y.S., Zeng, J., 1995. The application Kato–Katz smear technique in the research and control of schistosomiasis. Chin. J. Schistosomiasis Control 7, 382–384.
Wu, X.H., Chen, M.G., Zheng, J., 2005. Surveillance of schistosomiasis in five provinces of China which have reached the national criteria for elimination of the disease. Acta Trop. 96, 276–281.
Wu, X.H., Wang, X.H., Utzinger, J., Yang, K., Kristensen, T.K., Berquist, R., et al., 2007. Spatio-temporal correlation between human and bovine schistosomiasis in China: insight from three national sampling surveys. Geospatial Health 2, 75–84.
Wu, G.L., 2002. A historical perspective on the immunodiagnosis of schistosomiasis in China. Acta Trop. 82, 193–198.
Xia, C., Wang, H.Z., 1989. The endemic status and control of schistosomiasis. Bull. Biol. 9, 26–27.
Xia, C.M., Rong, R., Lu, Z.X., Shi, C.J., Xu, J., Zhang, H.Q., et al., 2009. *Schistosoma japonicum*: a PCR assay for the early detection and evaluation of treatment in a rabbit model. Exp. Parasitol. 121, 175–179.
Xia, J., Yuan, Y., Xu, X., Wei, F., Li, G., Liu, M., et al., 2014. Evaluating the effect of a novel molluscicide in the endemic schistosomiasis japonica area of China. Int. J. Environ. Res. Public Health 11, 10406–10418.
Xiao, S.H., You, J.Q., Mei, J.Y., Guo, H.F., Jiao, P.Y., Tanner, M., 2000. Effect of praziquantel together with artemether on *Schistosoma japonicum* parasites of different ages in rabbits. Parasitol. Int. 49, 25–30.
Xiao, S.H., Tanner, M., N'Goran, E.K., Utzinger, J., Chollet, J., Bergquist, R., et al., 2002. Recent investigations of artemether, a novel agent for the prevention of schistosomiasis japonica, mansoni and haematobia. Acta Trop. 82, 175–181.
Xiao, S.H., Keiser, J., Chen, M.G., Tanner, M., Utzinger, J., 2010. Research and development of antischistosomal drugs in the People's Republic of China a 60-year review. Adv. Parasitol. 73, 231–295.
Xiao, S.H., 2005. Development of antischistosomal drugs in China, with particular consideration to praziquantel and the artemisinins. Acta Trop. 96, 153–167.
Xie, K.M., Ju, S.G., Gu, Y.P., Hu, Y.M., 2002. Inhibition of in vitro and in vivo granulomatous responses surrounding schistosome eggs by administration of Angelicae Sinensis. Chin. J. Pathophysiol. 9, 30.
Xin, Y.T., Dai, J.R., 2010. Progress of research on molluscicide niclosomide. Chin. J. Schistosomiasis Control 22, 504–508.
Xu, X.J., Wei, F.H., Yang, X.X., Dai, Y.H., Yu, G.Y., Chen, L.Y., et al., 2000. Possible effects of the Three Gorges dam on the transmission of *Schistosoma japonicum* on the Jiang Han plain, China. Am. J. Trop. Med. Hyg. 94, 333–341.
Xu, J., Rong, R., Zhang, H.Q., Shi, C.J., Zhu, X.Q., Xia, C.M., 2010. Sensitive and rapid detection of *Schistosoma japonicum* DNA by loop-mediated isothermal amplification (LAMP). Int. J. Parasitol. 40, 327–331.
Xu, J., Feng, T., Lin, D.D., Wang, Q.Z., Tang, L., Wu, X.H., et al., 2011a. Performance of a dipstick dye immunoassay for rapid screening of *Schistosoma japonicum* infection in areas of low endemicity. Parasites Vectors 4, 87.

Xu, J., Peeling, R.W., Chen, J.X., Wu, X.H., Wu, Z.D., Wang, S.P., et al., 2011b. Evaluation of immunoassays for the diagnosis of *Schistosoma japonicum* infection using archived sera. PLoS Negl. Trop. Dis. 5, e949.

Xu, J., Xu, J.F., Li, S.Z., Zhang, L.J., Wang, Q., Zhu, H.H., et al., 2015. Integrated control programmes for schistosomiasis and other helminth infections in P.R. China. Acta Trop. 141, 332–341.

Yang, Y., Shen, G.R., Mei, Y.S., Zhang, C.H., Ying, L.Z., You, B.Y., et al., 1981. Study on the new drug praziquantel for schistosomiasis. New Med. 12, 5–9.

Yang, G.J., Vounatsou, P., Zhou, X.N., Tanner, M., Utzinger, J., 2005. A potential impact of climate change and water resource development on the transmission of *Schistosoma japonicum* in China. Parassitologia 47, 127–134.

Yang, G.J., Vounatsou, P., Tanner, M., Zhou, X.N., Utzinger, J., 2006. Remote sensing for predicting potential habitats of *Oncomelania hupensis* in Hongze, Baima and Gaoyou lakes in Jiangsu province, China. Geospatial Health 1, 85–92.

Yang, G.J., Li, W., Sun, L.P., Wu, F., Yang, K., Huang, Y.X., et al., 2010. Molluscicidal efficacies of different formulations of niclosamide: result of meta-analysis of Chinese literature. Parasites Vectors 3, 84.

Yang, G.J., Sun, L.P., Hong, Q.B., Zhu, H.R., Yang, K., Gao, Q., et al., 2012. Optimizing molluscicide treatment strategies in different control stages of schistosomiasis in the People's Republic of China. Parasites Vectors 5, 260.

Yang, F., Long, E., Wen, J., Cao, L., Zhu, C., Hu, H., et al., 2014. Linalool, derived from *Cinnamomum camphora* (L.) Presl leaf extracts, possesses molluscicidal activity against *Oncomelania hupensis* and inhibits infection of *Schistosoma japonicum*. Parasites Vectors 7, 407.

Yang, Y., Zhou, Y.B., Song, X.X., Li, S.Z., Zhong, B., Wang, T.P., et al., 2016. Integrated control strategy of schistosomiasis in the People's Republic of China: projects involving agriculture, water-conservancy, forestry, sanitation and environmental modification. Adv. Parasitol. 92.

Yi, X.Y., He, Y.K., Li, Y.S., 1995. Collaborative studies on circulating antigen detection against *Schistosoma japonicum*. Chin. J. Parasitol. Parasit. Dis. 13, 277–283.

Yu, J.M., De Vlas, S.J., Jiang, Q.W., Gryseels, B., 2007. Comparison of the Kato-Katz technique, hatching test and indirect hemagglutination assay (IHA) for the diagnosis of *Schistosoma japonicum* infection in China. Parasitol. Int. 56, 45–49.

Yue, W.J., You, J.Q., Mei, J.Y., 1985. The activity of *Dryoteris crassirhizoma Nakai* against *Schistosoma japonicum*. Information Chin. Pharmacol. Soc. 2, 31–33.

Yuan, H.C., Zhuo, S.J., Zhang, S.J., Al, E., 1990. Studies on the epidemic factors and principles in beaches of rivers and lakes. Chin. J. Schistosomiasis Control 2, 14–21.

Yuan, H.C., Jiang, Q.W., Zhao, G.M., He, N., 2002. Achievements of schistosomiasis control in China. Mem. Inst. Oswaldo Cruz 97 (Suppl. 1), 187–189.

Yuan, Y., Xu, X.J., Dong, H.F., Jiang, M.S., Zhu, H.G., 2005. Transmission control of schistosomiasis japonica: implementation and evaluation of different snail control interventions. Acta Trop. 96, 191–197.

Yuan, H.C., 1999. Achievements and experience on schistosomiasis control in P.R. China. Chin. J. Epidemiol. 20, 3–6.

Zhang, Z.Y., Xu, D.Z., Zhou, X.N., Zhou, Y., Liu, S.J., 2005. Remote sensing and spatial statistical analysis to predict the distribution of *Oncomelania hupensis* in the marshlands of China. Acta Trop. 96, 205–212.

Zhang, X.D., Peng, Z.H., Zhou, J.X., 2006. A review on the research advances of snail controlling mechanism of the snail control and schistosomiasis prevention forest ecosystem. World For. Res. 19, 38–43.

Zhang, S.Q., Zhang, G.H., Bao, J.G., Qiang, G.X., 2009. Cohort study on snail controlling effect of water conservancy projects for schistosomiasis prevention. Yangtz River 40, 100–102.

Zhang, C.H., Tang, G.Y., Liu, F.Y., Kun, L., 2012a. Effect of agroforestry model on inhibition of *Oncomelania* snails in plateau mountainous area of Yunnan Province. Chin. J. Schistosomiasis Control 24, 514–517.
Zhang, L.J., Zhu, R., Dang, H., Xu, J., Li, S.Z., Guo, J.G., 2012b. Analysis of surveillance of schistosomiasis in China in 2011. Chin. J. Schistosomiasis Control 24, 627–631.
Zhang, Z., Fang, R., Yu, B., Liu, Z., Zhao, Z., Xu, X., et al., 2013. Field evaluation of a novel plant molluscicide"Luo-wei"against *Oncomelania hupensis* snails II Molluscicidal effect in the field of lake areas in Hanchuan City, Hubei Province. Chin. J. Schistosomiasis Control 25, 481–484.
Zhang, L.J., Li, S.Z., Wen, L.Y., Lin, D.D., Abe, E.M., Zhu, R., et al., 2016. Establishment and function of schistosomiasis surveillance system towards elimination in the People's Republic of China. Adv. Parasitol. 92.
Zheng, J., Gu, X.G., Qiu, Z.L., et al., 1996. Study on the strategy for schistosomiasis control for mountainous regions. Chin. J. Schistosomiasis Control 8, 65–71.
Zheng, H., Zhang, L.J., Zhu, R., Xu, J., Li, S.Z., Guo, J.G., et al., 2012. Schistosomiasis situation in People's Republic of China in 2011. Chin. J. Schistosomiasis Control 24, 621–626.
Zheng, Q., Vanderslott, S., Jiang, B., Xu, L.L., Liu, C.S., Huo, L.L., et al., 2013. Research gaps for three main tropical diseases in the People's Republic of China. Infect. Dis. Poverty 2, 15.
Zheng, G., 1986. Progress of Schistosomiasis Epidemiology in P.R. China (1980–1985). Jiangsu Medical Publishing House, Nanjing.
Zhou, X.N., Lin, D.D., Yang, H.M., Chen, H.G., Sun, L.P., Yang, G.J., et al., 2002. Use of landsat TM satellite surveillance data to measure the impact of the 1998 flood on snail intermediate host dispersal in the lower Yangtze River Basin. Acta Trop. 82, 199–205.
Zhou, X.N., Wang, L.Y., Chen, M.G., Wu, X.H., Jiang, Q.W., Chen, X.Y., et al., 2005. The public health significance and control of schistosomiasis in China—then and now. Acta Trop. 96, 97–105.
Zhou, X.N., Guo, J.G., Wu, X.H., Jiang, Q.W., Zheng, J., Dang, H., et al., 2007. Epidemiology of schistosomiasis in the People's Republic of China, 2004. Emerg. Infect. Dis. 13, 1470–1476.
Zhou, X.N., Wang, T.P., Lin, D.D., Wu, X.H., 2009. Current strategy and its effect on control of schistosomiasis transmission in P.R. China. Int. J. Med. Parasit. Dis. 36, 266–272.
Zhou, X.N., Xu, J., Chen, H.G., Wang, T.P., Huang, X.B., Lin, D.D., et al., 2011. Tools to support policy decisions related to treatment strategies and surveillance of schistosomiasis japonica towards elimination. PLoS Negl. Trop. Dis. 5, e1408.
Zhou, X.N., Xu, J., Lin, D.D., Wang, T.P., Liang, Y.S., Zhong, B., et al., 2013a. Role of the new version of the control and elimination criteria for Schistosomiasis in acceleration of the schistosomiasis elimination program in China. Zhongguo Xue Xi Chong Bing Fang. Zhi Za Zhi (Chin. J. Schistosomiasis Control) 25, 1–4 (in Chinese).
Zhou, Y., Wang, Z., Zhang, B., Xie, D., Mei, Z., Jia, T., et al., 2013b. Field evaluation of a novel plant molluscicide "Luo-wei" against the snail *Oncomelania hupensis* III Molluscicidal effect by spraying method in hilly regions. Chin. J. Schistosomiasis Control 25, 495–497.
Zhou, X.N., 2009. Surveillance and forecast of schistosomiasis in China. Chin. J. Schistosomiasis Control 21, 341–344.
Zhu, R., Xu, J., 2014. Epidemic situation of oversea imported schistosomiasis in China and thinking about its prevention and control. Chin. J. Schistosomiasis Control 26, 111–114.
Zhu, H.Q., Cao, C.L., Gao, F.H., Guo, J.G., Bao, Z.P., Wang, X.H., et al., 2005. Evaluation of effectiveness of modified Kato-Katz technique for diagnosis of schistosomiasis japonica. Chin. J. Schistosomiasis Control 17, 273–277.
Zhu, Y., Peng, X., Liang, X.Y., Yuan, X.B., Xiong, X.H., Dong, Y., et al., 2009. Effect of hydraulic schistosomiasis control projects on disease prevention. Chin. J. Schistosomiasis Control 21, 227–229.

Zhu, R., Zhao, G.M., Li, H.Z., Guo, J.G., 2011. Development and prospect of surveillance network of schistosomiasis in China. Chin. J. Schistosomiasis Control 23, 14–17.
Zhu, H., Yap, P., Utzinger, J., Jia, T.W., Li, S.Z., Huang, X.B., et al., 2016. Policy support and resources mobilization for the national schistosomiasis control programme in the People's Republic of China. Adv. Parasitol. 92.
Zhu, Y.C., 2005. Immunodiagnosis and its role in schistosomiasis control in China: a review. Acta Trop. 96, 130–136.
Zhuang, B.J., 1992. History of Schistosomiasis Control in Zhejiang Province. Shanghai Health Publishing House, Shanghai.

CHAPTER TWO

Epidemiological Features and Effectiveness of Schistosomiasis Control Programme in Lake and Marshland Region in The People's Republic of China

S.-Q. Zhang*,[1], C.-S. Sun*, M. Wang*, D.-D. Lin[§], X.-N. Zhou[¶,||,#], T.-P. Wang*,**

*Anhui Provincial Institute of Schistosomiasis Control, Hefei, Anhui Province, The People's Republic of China
[§]Jiangxi Provincial Institute of Schistosomiasis Control, Nanchang, The People's Republic of China
[¶]National Institute of Parasitic Diseases, Chinese Center for Disease Control and Prevention, Shanghai, The People's Republic of China
[||]WHO Collaborating Center for Tropical Diseases, Shanghai, The People's Republic of China
[#]Key Laboratory of Parasite and Vector Biology of the Chinese Ministry of Health, Shanghai, The People's Republic of China
**Anhui Institute of Parasitic Disease, Hefei, The People's Republic of China
[1]Corresponding author: E-mail: zhangsq2820@163.com

Contents

Advances in Parasitology, Volume 92
ISSN 0065-308X
http://dx.doi.org/10.1016/bs.apar.2016.02.018

Abstract

Schistosomiasis is one of neglected tropical diseases in the world. The People's Republic of China has made great achievements in schistosomiasis control through integrated interventions. Although the morbidity and mortality have been reduced to the lowest level in all three endemic regions, namely lake and marshland regions, hilly and mountainous regions and plains with waterway networks regions, the endemic status in lake and marshland region is still that of implementing the interventions in the higher endemicity areas towards elimination of schistosomiasis transmission. This review explores and analyses the endemic characteristics, control measures and its effectiveness in the course of schistosomiasis control programme, in order to provide more theoretical information and experiences for development of appropriate strategies leading to schistosomiasis elimination in the next stage in the country.

1. INTRODUCTION

Schistosomiasis is one of neglected tropical diseases in the world, which has been targeted as one of diseases to be eliminated by World Health Organization (WHO). There are four major types of human schistosomiasis: schistosomiasis mansoni, schistosomiasis haemetobia, schistosomiasis japonica and schistosomiasis mekongi (Chitsulo et al., 2000; Collins et al., 2012). Schistosomiasis japonica is prevalent in the south of the Yangtze River basin and 12 provinces (municipalities and autonomous regions) in The People's Republic of China (Xu et al., 2016). According to the environmental characteristics of snail habitats, the endemic areas are divided into three types, namely lake and marshland regions, plain regions with waterway networks, and hilly and mountainous regions (Collins et al., 2012; Chen, 2014). Due to differences in the endemic factors and geographical characteristics, the control process was faster in the provinces dominated by waterway networks, while in the provinces with lake and marshland regions, the control process is relatively slow and tortuous. The five endemic areas dominated by waterway networks, namely Guangdong, Guangxi, Shanghai, Zhejiang and Fujian provinces achieved the standard of transmission interruption in 1985, 1988, 1985, 1995 and 1987, respectively (Shi et al., 2016). Hilly and mountainous areas such as Sichuan and Yunnan provinces, as well as mainly lake and marshland areas such as Hunan, Hubei, Jiangxi, Anhui and Jiangsu provinces have not yet reached the standard of transmission interruption (Liu et al., 2014, 2016). After more than 60 years of active and effective prevention and control measures, 124 counties achieved the standard of transmission control and 34 counties were not able to achieve the standard of transmission control in The People's Republic of China by the end of 2013; and all the 34 counties were distributed in lake and marshland regions (Lei et al., 2014). Therefore, lake and marshland region is the focus on schistosomiasis control, and it also is the key to realize the target of transmission interruption and elimination of schistosomiasis in The People's Republic of China. By analysing the epidemic characteristics in lake and marshland region, the achievements or experiences from the national schistosomiasis programme has been summarized for more than six decades, highlighting the problems and challenges of the current schistosomiasis control programme. This chapter aims to provide an important reference for the development of The People's Republic of China's 'Thirteen Five-Year' plans on schistosomiasis control and provide reference for schistosomiasis control in the world.

2. BACKGROUND

Lake and marshland regions are mainly distributed in Hunan, Hubei, Jiangxi, Anhui and Jiangsu provinces located in the middle and lower reaches of Yangtze River. At the beginning of the national schistosomiasis control programme, the infection rate of people and bovine was very high in those areas. The infection rate of people was as high as about 70% and a large number of acute schistosomiasis cases occurred every year. The infection rate of cattle and pig had reached up to 80–90% in some places (Chen, 2014). Snails are widely distributed in marshland regions, and the habitat of snails is so complex that the effect of mollusciciding is difficult to consolidate (Li et al., 2016). The process on schistosomiasis control is relatively slow and tortuous due to the special features of geographical environment and characteristic of prevalent situation in lake and marshland regions. At the beginning of prevention and control programme, the area of snail habitat accounted for 82.1% and the number of cases accounted for 43.9% of the total schistosomiasis patients in The People's Republic of China (Mao and Shao, 1982). In the 1960s and 1970s, the strategy on schistosomiasis control was emphasized on snails elimination. These measures including reclamation planting, changing paddy fields into dry land, environmental modification and mollusciciding were implemented in Hunan, Hubei, Jiangxi, Anhui and Jiangsu provinces, that is, 'five provinces in the lake regions'. Meanwhile, mass examination and treatment of people and bovine were carried out widely in the five provinces. Snail areas decreased substantially and the prevalent situation of schistosomiasis was controlled effectively. Snail areas were reduced 1.873 billion m^2 in Hubei by 1983, nearly 60% in Hunan, 920 million m^2 in Jiangxi combined with large-scale agricultural development in Poyang Lake, up to 78% in Anhui by the end of 1981, more than 97% of snail areas were eliminated in Jiangsu and reached the standard of transmission control by 1976 (Wang, 2006). Since the 1980s, with the advent of praziquantel that has safe and efficient therapeutic effect, the comprehensive measures with emphasis on chemotherapy on human and livestock were taken in The People's Republic of China. The infection rate of people and livestock decreased rapidly with the implementation of chemotherapy measures. However, acute schistosomiasis infection and reinfection were very serious due to the complexity of snail habitats, flood disasters and frequent contact with contaminated water for the production and living in lake and marshland regains. In the 1980s and 1990s, the prevalence of schistosomiasis presented up and down in The People's Republic of China, and even seriously rose in some areas. The snail areas increased from 2.75 billion m^2 in 1980 to 3.47 billion m^2 in 1988. The first national sample survey of schistosomiasis was conducted in 1989, which indicated that snail areas in lake and marshland regions accounted for 95.5% of the total snail areas in The People's Republic of China, the number of schistosomiasis patients accounted for 85.6% of the total patients, the average infection rate of people was 12.94% in the lake and marshland regions and a large number of acute schistosomiasis occurred every year along the Yangtze River (MOH, 1993). World Bank Loan Project on schistosomiasis control in The People's Republic of China was carried out in eight provinces from 1992 to 2001, in order to curb the upward trend of schistosomiasis. Chemotherapy for humans and livestock by praziquantel was adopted as the main measure. Mollusciciding, health education and limited environmental modification were taken as the supplemental measures. For chemotherapy on a large scale with high intensity, the prevalence of schistosomiasis was controlled effectively, the number of patients dropped by 50% and the number of infected cattle declined by 70% in the eight provinces. However, the change in snail situation was not significant, and the density of infected snails still remained at a certain level (MOH, PR China, 2002). To accelerate the process of schistosomiasis control further in The People's Republic of China, and protect the health of people to promote economic and social development in endemic regions, Ministry of Health, Development and Reform Commission, Ministry of Finance and six other central ministries jointly issued the 'Outline on national long-term plan for prevention and control of schistosomiasis (2004–15)', which aimed at achieving the target of transmission control by 2015 (Zhu et al., 2016). For this purpose, according to the prevalence situation of schistosomiasis in lake and marshland regions, comprehensive control measures that emphasized on infection source control (replacing cattle with machine for cultivation, forbidding depasturage of livestock on marshland and so on) were adopted in combination with the adjustment of farming and aquaculture in rural areas, water conservancy project, afforestation for schistosomiasis prevention, wetland protection projects to change the habitat of snail in the highlighted areas and reduce the endemic range. With the implementation of the Outline, the process of schistosomiasis control in The People's Republic of China received great impetus. The infection rate of people and livestock, the inventory of infected livestock, the number of acute schistosomiaisis and the area of infected snails dropped significantly. By the end of 2013, only nine acute cases occurred nationwide, the calculated number of patients dropped to 184,900, infected cattle were found to be 633, snail areas fell to 3.655 billion m^2 with infected snails scattered in the local environment, and the prevalence of schistosomiasis was reduced to the lowest level historically. However, 96.49% of snail areas were distributed in lake and marshland regions; 96.34% of the estimated patients were in Jiangxi, Hubei, Hunan and Anhui provinces which are mainly the lake and marshland endemic regions (Lei et al., 2014). Presently, the lake and marshland endemic regions are still the key districts for schistosomiasis control. To summarize, the experience of prevention and control, the epidemiological characteristics and the systematic achievements in lake and marshland endemic regions have implication for interrupting transmission or eliminating of schistosomiasis as soon as possible.

3. ENDEMIC CHARACTERISTICS

3.1 Natural environmental factors

Lake and marshland endemic regions are located on both sides of the Yangtze River and the adjacent areas of lakes interlinked with Yangtze River, for example Dongting Lake in Hunan Province, Poyang Lake in Jiangxi Province, lakes in Jianghan Plain in Hubei Province and lakes in the lower reaches of outlet of river in Jiangxi Province. The remarkable natural environmental feature of lake and marshland endemic area is the significant seasonal variation. The regions of 'water in summer and land in winter' are the potential snail habitats, which are covered with water when annual floods occur and snails are likely to breed on the water coverage regions. The marshland become exposed with large scale of lush vegetation after the flood subsides in the autumn. Thus, the annual floods play an important role in marshland deposition, formation of new marshlands and spread of snails in the lake and marshland endemic areas.

Snails immigrate and multiply quickly as the vegetation (weed and bulrush, etc.) grows with the accumulation of silty sand to a certain height, and the snail would be found in this region about 4 or 5 years later, resulting in the steady increase of snail area in lake and marshland regions. In the 150 km stretch between Jiangning and Jingjiang in Jiangsu Province, about 233.4 hm^2 of beach land was formed every year since 1985. The area of beach increased from 99.9 hm^2 in 1990 to 233.1 hm^2 in 1995 in Jiangan district of Wuhan city. The area of snail habitat increased 34.7 hm^2 every year in Dongting Lake due to the accumulation of silty sand. A total of 40.43 hm^2 of snail area was increased in 1988 in Hunan Province, and 929.2 hm^2 in Anhui Province (Zhang et al., 2002). The fluctuation of the flood provided appropriate environment for the growth and reproduction of snails, and the coverage of flood promoted the development and hatching of snail eggs. The surface of marshland would retain long-term moisture after being covered by water for 3–8 months, especially in the regions overgrown with weeds and bulrush, which was conducive to the growth and reproduction of snails. Lake and marshland endemic area was divided into four subtypes, namely fork-beach, marshland, inner embankment and embankment according to the variability of water level, the type of snail habitat, geographical position of the residential districts and endemic characteristics (Chen, 1980).

3.2 Infectious sources

It has been proved that livestock was the main source of schistosomiasis infection in lake and marshland endemic regions (Fig. 1). At the beginning of schistosomiasis control, more than 50% of cattle were detected positive for schistosomiasis (Shen, 1992). Epidemiologically, cattle played an important role in the transmission of schistosomiasis due to a large number of cattle pasturing frequently in the beach, which discharge a large quantity of excreta containing schistosome eggs. Because there is a wide range of lake and marshland endemic areas in The People's Republic of China, the type of infectious sources and their implication for schistosomiasis transmission varied in different regions. The marshland outer embankment of Dongting Lake is a natural ranch that is full of lush vegetation, where the mean infection rate was 20.63% for the cattle (Li et al., 2002). The cattle rowed faeces and

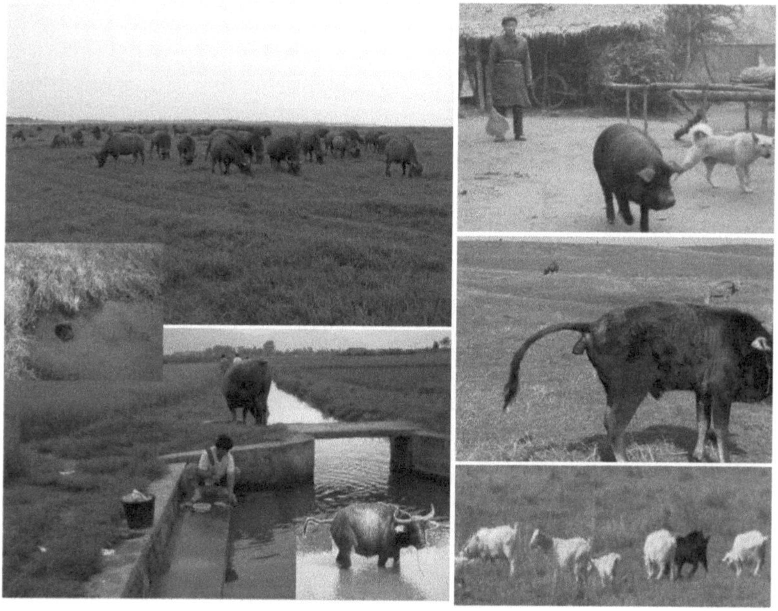

Figure 1 The main infectious sources in lake and marshland endemic regions (including more than 40 species of mammals).

contaminated the marshland. Cattle was the main infection source and accounted for 83.64% of annual actual contamination index (AACI); followed by swine (9.37%) (Wu et al., 1990). Xu et al. (1985) conducted five surveys on field stool in Muping Lake from 1979 to 1982; of the 5017 samples collected in the field, livestock's stools accounted for 99.58% and those of humans accounted for 0.42%. AACI is an objective indicator for determining the epidemic intensity of schistosomiasis, which can perceivably reflect the infectivity of the infectious sources.

Of the infectious sources in the south Dongting Lake, domestic pigs had the highest infection rate. The infection rate of domestic pigs was 45.94% in local areas. After the domestic pigs were checked and treated monthly for a year, the new infection rate of domestic pigs was 12.75% monthly, and the reinfection rate was 50% yearly. The highest positive rate (23.29%) and the highest density (22.46/10,000 m^2) of wild stool were found to be domestic pigs. Domestic pigs accounted for 89.83% of annual actual contamination index, which were 9 times higher than that of cattle and 200 times higher than that of humans (Hu et al., 1996). The activity of domestic pigs was in a relative narrow range and concentrated in place within 300 m distance of dike. The shorter to the dike, the higher the density of wild stool and the density of infected snails, and there was positive correlation between the density of wild stool and the density of infected snails (Chen et al., 1999). Therefore, domestic pigs might play much more important role in schistosomiasis transmission and bringing more serious harm to people in some places.

There were plenty of cattle and domestic pigs near the dike in Poyang Lake area, where the infection rate of schistosomiasis was 20–50% in domestic pigs, 20–30% in cattle and more than 30% in people (Xie, 1990). Some studies on contamination index of wild stool in marshland revealed that bovine faeces accounted for more than 90%, domestic pigs accounted for 6–8% and other livestock accounted for a smaller proportion. The infected cattle, domestic pigs and people (eg, fishing, mowing and swimming) in the marshland of Poyang Lake were all sources of schistosomiasis infection, while the infected cattle was the main infectious sources (Lin et al., 2003). More than 90% of endemic areas were located in Jianghan plain in Hubei Province; a survey conducted in Hanbei river revealed that the bovine faeces were severely infected by schistosomiasis, which accounted for 97.5% of wild stool and 89.5% of eggs per day (EPD) (Huang, 1998).

With the development of livestock husbandry, the amount of sheep is on the rise. Sheep is a susceptible host for schistosomiasis with higher infection rate and likely to defecate in the wild. Furthermore, sheep always dispersively defecate granulated faeces, which results in easy contact with snail. Therefore, the role of the faeces of infected sheep in contaminating environment and diffusion of pathogens should not be neglected. The infection rate of sheep was 7.5–17.5% in Jingzhou district and Honghu Lake; the positive rate of sheep faeces was significantly higher than that of cattle faeces, and sheep might become the new main infectious source (Yuan et al., 2003). Dog is also one of the definitive hosts, but it plays only a small role in the course of schistosomiasis transmission. However, the infection rate of dog was found to be 75.0% and EPD result was 80.4 in three pilot studies in the lower reaches of Dongjing lake; in some areas, the infection rate of dog was found to be more than 90% and relative contamination index was 46.6%. Dog might be one of the most important infectious sources due to its wide range of activities and freely spreading of eggs (Su et al., 1994).

There is large-scale marshland along Yangtze River in Anhui and Jiangsu provinces, where the cattle grazed freely on the beach. The infection rate of cattle generally was very high, reaching to as high a level as 77.3% in some places. The mean infection rate of cattle was 45.42% and the proportion of contamination index was 99.8% in beach areas in Anhui Province (He et al., 1995). Despite many years of active control, the infection rate of cattle was still very high due to the reinfection of schistosomes.

Sun et al. (1997) conducted a 5-year prospective study and reported a mean infection rate of 8.23% in cattle, and bovine faeces accounted for 85.15% of wild stool in river beach areas. The characteristics of water level in the lake and marshland endemic area, including water-rising stage and drought period, has direct effect on the activity of domestic animals and people on the beach. In general, livestock are the main infectious source in the drought period for it they are freely active in a large range, especially the cattle and pigs infected with schistosomiasis. While during the water-rising period, the fishermen may act as an important infectious source, who, living on the fishing boat, contaminate the water easily, and the infection rate of snail is generally higher in the moorings. In different seasons, there are some differences in the types and implication of the main infectious sources in the lake and marshland endemic area; the free-ranging cattle and pig are the main source of infection during drought period in Dongting Lake, while infected fishermen are the main infectious source during water-rising period (Wu, Xie, 1991).

3.3 Distribution of snails

The distribution of snails is associated with the annual flooding duration and vegetation in marshland. Snail often presents a planar distribution with wide range and large scale in the marshland. The 'water in summer and land in winter' appears in the snail habitats due to the uncontrollable water level, which results in the specific characteristics of the distribution of snails, namely 'two lines and three belts'. The 'two lines' represent the lowest and highest snail hypsometric curve, and the 'three belts' represent the upper rare snail areas, the middle dense snail areas and lower rare snail areas. Snails are generally distributed at a certain elevation in lake and marshland area, while dense snail areas are scattered in the beach covered by flood for 3–5 months. The height of attitude for 'two lines and three belts' varied in different beaches. Snails are widely distributed in Poyang Lake areas. While no snails were found in the marshland at an altitude of less than 13 m and over than 18 m above sea level, 5.4% of snail areas were found in the marshland at an altitude between 13 and 14 m and between 17 and 18 m, and 94.6% of snail areas were located in marshland at an altitude between 14 and 17 m above sea level. The dense snail areas were majorly distributed in the range from 27 to 29 m above sea in Dongting Lake, and from 24 to 27 m in Hubei Province. The snails were distributed along the new channel similar to the typical waterway networks regions in the dam-circled marsh region.

The infected snail plays an important role in the course of schistosomiasis transmission, which has remarkable aggregation in lake and marshland area

(Collins et al., 2012). The infection rate of snails was higher in the areas closer to village or the place with frequent activity of people and livestock. The infected snail can be easily found in the areas close to village or the places seriously contaminated by wild stool (Wang and Wang, 2000a). Generally, there was slight variation of the distribution of infected snails yearly, but infection rate of snails might increase with the rise of snail density. Because livestock was the main infectious source in the lake and marshland areas, the distribution of infected snail was closely related to the distribution of cattle in these areas. In Dongting Lake area, the width of distribution zones for the infected snails was closely related to the width of distribution zones of living snails, vegetation type, topography level, flow velocity and the type of infectious sources. In the high transmission areas with cattle faeces as the main contaminating source, the distribution range of infected snail could be as far as 1000 m to the dike due to a wider range of activity. While in the berth which can easily be contaminated by fisherman, the distribution zones of infected snail was narrow and concentrated in the range of 300 m away from bridge of dam and hill, and residential houses (Zhuo et al., 1991). To understand the distribution characters of infected snails it is necessary to focus on transmission as well as provide important information for molluscicciding. Generally, the areas with the density of infected snail more than 0.005/0.11 m^2 are deemed as highly susceptible or dangerous zone for the infection with schistosomes. It was proposed that the classification of high transmission zones be based on the density of infected snails as the criteria. The areas with the density of infected snails more than 0.005/0.1 m^2 with easily occurring acute schistosomiasis are classified as high focus areas of transmission, which account for about 25% in lake and marshland regions, the areas with the density of infected snails less than 0.005/0.1 m^2 are classified as the next focus areas of transmission zones, which also account for 25% of marshland, and infected snails were not found in more than half of the marshland (Zhang et al., 1996). Practically, carrying out mollusciciding in high-transmission areas and the strategy guided by the classification as above have led to remarkable achievements in lake and marshland regions (Zhou et al., 2013).

3.4 Water contact

Contacting cercariae-infested water is the essential step for the transmission of schistosomiasis. To understand the residents' habit of contacting affected water can provide the basis for making out specific control measures. There were significant variations in the mode and frequency of contacting affected water in the lake and marshland areas based on the differences of geographical environment, socioeconomic and cultural and living habits. The frequency (times/person-day) of contacting affected water in marshland areas was 10 times higher than that in fork-beach areas and embankment areas. The frequency in marshland was stable except for the month of February. While there was remarkable seasonal variation on the frequency of contacting affected water in fork-beach and embankment areas, April, May, October and November usually with the higher frequency of contact, presented a bimodal pattern. People who frequently contacted affected water were 15–29 year-olds in marshland, and 30–35 year-olds in fork-beach and embankment areas. The mode of contacting affected water included fishing, laundry and dabbling in marshland, and wading, grazing and fishing in fork-beach and embankment areas (He et al., 1997). The adult males contacted affected water mainly through working in paddy field in the inner embankment areas. Except for working in paddy field, the adult females might contact affected water through other manner, for example washing clothes and washing dishes. The main manner of contacting affected water among teenagers included washing clothes and dishes, fishing and playing in the water (Guan et al., 1999). The distance from their houses to dam impacted on contacting affected water; for example, the frequency of contacting infected water was significantly higher for people living within 200 m than the residents living more than 200 m away from the dike in Dongting Lake area. Generally, the seasons with highest frequency of contacting infected water were spring and summer, followed by autumn and winter in lake and marshland area. The manner of contacting affected water mainly included mowing grass in spring, washing clothes, swimming and catching fish/shrimp in summer and autumn. Contacting affected water is closely related to economic status. Poverty is a promoting factor in contacting affected water as the poor families tend to more frequently contact the affected water.

3.5 Infection with schistosomes

People living in lake and marshland areas can be infected by schistosome in a variety of manners. Infection can occur throughout the year except winter, and the outbreak of acute schistosomiasis might take place when a large number of people contact affected water due to floods, harvest and swimming. The infection was variable among different types of epidemic areas; the people living on island and inner embankment have the highest infection rate. At the beginning of schistosomiasis control, the infection rate was 57.9% in Nanji village, an island endemic area in Jiangxi Province, and 49.7% in Mingshan village in Hubei Province; the infection rate was more than 35% in inner embankment in Hubei Province. The mean infection rate was 20% in marshland and embankment endemic areas. In lake and marshland endemic areas, the infection rate was positively correlated with the distance from residential houses to the marshland. The infection rate of people in marshland regions was 15–30% when the distance was less than 500 m, 5% when the distance was from 500 to 1000 m and less than 3% when the distance was more than 1000 m (Lin and Zhang, 2002). The infection rate in embankment endemic areas was similar to that in marshland endemic areas. The infection rate of people in island endemic areas was significantly higher than that in other types of endemic areas and the infection rate could be as higher as 50–80% for the people living with the distance less than 500 m away from marshland, while the infection rate was about 30% when the distance was from 500 to 1000 m. The infection rate was similar between female and male in island-type and inner embankment endemic area. There were two age peaks for the infection of schistosome, namely teenager and adult, which present typical 'bimodal curve'. The infection rate of male was commonly higher than that of female in embankment and marshland endemic areas, and there was only one age peak in marshland endemic regions, namely 15–20 years of age, which presents typical 'unimodal type', with the infection rate in a higher level maintained constant for the older people. The fishermen were very easily infected by schistosome for their frequent and long duration contact with affected water.

Reinfection is very common in lake and marshland endemic areas. The prevalence situation rebounds once the intervention measures are reduced or stopped. Wu, Po, et al. (1995) conducted a survey along the Dongting Lake and revealed that the reinfection rate was 12.9% after treatment with PQT; the male reinfection rate was higher than that of female; and the people aged from 10 to 40 years had the highest reinfection rate. Wu et al. (1994) conducted a survey in island-type endemic area and revealed that the reinfection rate increased to 47.1% in September after a periodic flood, and increased to 54.5% in January in the second year, very nearly to the infection rate before chemotherapy (64.3%). The heavier the prevalence situation before chemotherapy was, the higher was the reinfection rate. The reinfection rate in the lower age group (<20 years) was significantly higher than that in the higher age group. Ceng et al. (1996) conducted a 3-year prospective study in an island-type endemic area and reported that the reinfection rate was 22.6% in 1990, 47.8% in 1991 and 40% in 1992. Qin et al. conducted a survey in a marshland epidemic area and reported reinfection rate of 13.49% after an epidemic season, which was similar to the infection rate before therapy (13.37%). The reinfection rate was 9.52% from June to September, and 3.97% from October to December. The reinfection rate in the lower age group (<20) was significantly higher than that in the older age group (≥20) (Qin et al., 2000). Carrying out effective intervention measures in heavy endemic areas could reduce reinfection. The reinfection rate has slight change if only single chemotherapy measure is taken in serious endemic areas, and the reinfection rate decreased year by year when environmental modification measures were taken. The reinfection rate was closely related with the intensity of transmission in endemic areas. The more serious the previous prevalence, the higher the reinfection rate of people and the shorter the period of rebound, and so is the contrary.

Acute infection was hard to avoid in lake and marsh epidemic areas due to the frequent exposure to contaminated water. Studiers have revealed that acute infection was positively correlated with water level, and the outbreak of acute schistosomiasis might take place in flood year. Acute schistosomiasis outbreak in Yangtze River valley in 1989 had the number of acute cases 2.97 times more than that in 1988, and 99.38% of the patients were in 'five provinces in lake regions'. As for Anhui Province, 96.5% of the acute patients in 1989 occurred in 18 counties mainly lake and marshland endemic areas, teenagers accounting for the majority of patients; the number of male patients was higher than that of female, and the main infection modes were fishing and paddling. Analysis on acute schistosomiasis occurred from 1987 to 1989 in Dongting Lake and Poyang Lake showed that the male cases accounted for 86.1% and the female cases for 13.9% in Dongting Lake areas, and 76.4% of cases in male and 23.6% of cases in female were found in Poyang Lake areas. The adolescent (<20 year-olds) accounted for 58.3% in Dongting Lake and 57.0% in Poyang Lake. The main infection modes were swimming (51.8%) and fishing (20.8%) in Dongting Lake, and fishing (44.9%), swimming (14.1%) and grazing (11.2%) in Poyang Lake regions.

4. PREVENTION AND CONTROL MEASURES

4.1 Snail control

Snail control is always one of the important measures in The People's Republic of China in the course of 60 years of schistosomiasis control. Shanghai, Zhejiang, Guangdong, Guangxi and Fujian provinces have achieved the goal of transmission interruption mainly by snail control measures. Due to wide distribution of sail areas and complex environment of snail habitats in lake and marshland regions, appropriate methods of snail control according to the local conditions can achieve better results. At present, 70% of snail habitats have been changed by means of reclamation and cultivation in low dyke or reclamation and cultivation without dam, aquaculture in low dyke, reclaiming farmland from lakes and other measures in lake and marshland regains in The People's Republic of China (Fig. 2), which are not only conducive to production, but also achieved significant snail control and elimination of snails. Environmental modification measures is an important experience for the elimination of snails in the long history of schistosomiasis control in lake and marshland regions in The People's Republic of China.

4.1.1 Reclamation and cultivation for eliminating snail

The best method for eliminating *Oncomelania* snail is to change the habitat and make it unsuitable for snails to survive. According to the environmental features of snail habitats in lake and marshland epidemic areas, we can control and eliminate *Oncomelania hupensis* by means of changing the environment of snail habitats, for example reclamation with low embankment, reclamation without embankment, reclamation with high embankment, filling lakes

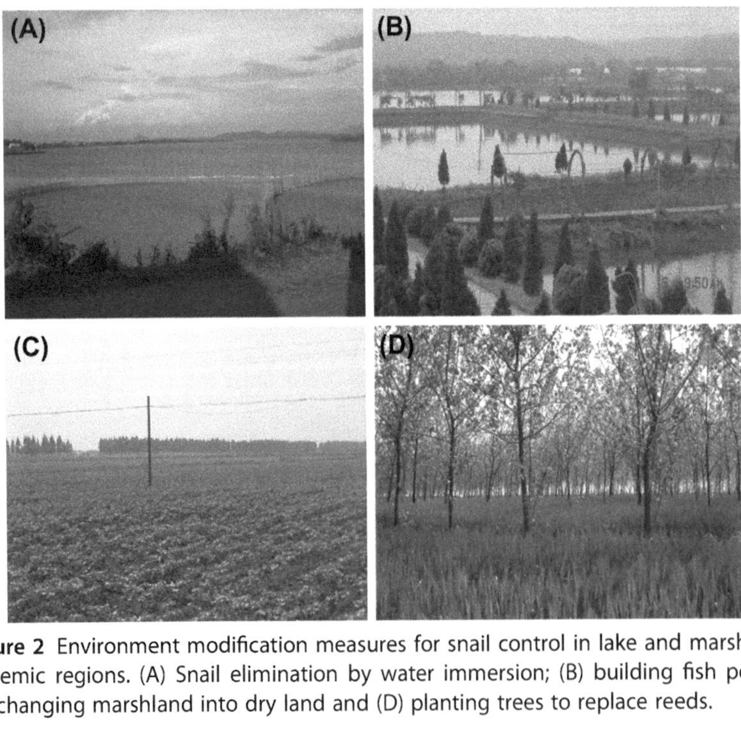

Figure 2 Environment modification measures for snail control in lake and marshland endemic regions. (A) Snail elimination by water immersion; (B) building fish ponds; (C) changing marshland into dry land and (D) planting trees to replace reeds.

and reclaiming land from lakes, and so on. In the 20 years, two-thirds of lake had been reclaimed in Hubei Province, including two-fifths in Dongting Lake, one-thirds in Poyang Lake and large area in the middle and lower section along Yangtze River in Anhui and Jiangsu provinces. Reclaiming and planting in marshland has a good effect on eliminating oncomelania snail, which reduced two-thirds of the total snail areas in lake and marshland regions in The People's Republic of China (Wang and Wang 2000a,b). The snails were in patchy distribution in Poyang Lake and Dongting Lake. Reclaiming and planting by using large machinery directly to change the environment of snail habitats could get better effect on snail control and elimination of snails in the places with relatively higher elevation. A survey conducted in 21 places on land reclaimed and planted by machinery revealed that the occurrence rate of frames with living snails and the density of living snails decreased over 80% in 15 places, between 30% and 80% in 2 places and less than 10% in 4 places (Tu et al., 1992). For the environment with higher density of living snails, mollusciciding should be carried out prior to reclaiming by machinery or reclaiming combined with planting crops to further enhance the effect of snail control. More than 3 years of continuous ploughing and planting can ensure the quality and effect of eliminating snails. If reclaiming by machinery is not implemented successively, the density of living snails would rise again. The effect of snail control by different methods in Dongting Lake regions showed that the mean density of living snails reduced by 86.6% and the occurrence rate of farms with living snails decreased by 92.95% after reclaiming for 3 years; the mean density of living snails reduced by 93% and the occurrence rate of frames with living snails decreased by 83.4% after building lower embankment and mollusciciding by immersion for 3 years. However, the effect was not remarkable by single mollusciciding only; the density of living snails only decreased by 17.78% and the occurrence rate of farms with living snails was similar to that 3 years ago. In recent years, with the development of the city along Yangtze River, the environment of snail habitat changed greatly since the areas were filled with sand, especially some low-lying areas that were not suitable for ploughing and inter-planting (Huang et al., 2013).

4.1.2 Storing water to raise aquatic products for eliminating oncomelania snail

As protection against floods, storing water to raise aquatic products by constructing low embankment in low-lying marsh areas and then mollusciciding in the inner and outer of the embankment, not only brought economic benefits, but also played the role of elimination of snails. Hu et al. (2003) conducted a prospective study in 41 projects of building dike and revealed that 50% of projects reached the standard of elimination of snails in 7 years, all projects reached the standard of elimination of snails in 15 to 17 years, the number of schistosome patients and snails declined simultaneously and no rebound was reported showing that ultimately we can achieve the aim of controlling or eliminating of schistosomiasis. Hubei Province is one of the larger lake and marsh epidemic areas in The People's Republic of China, it had significant changes on the environment by hydrographic engineering projects since 1956, including reclamation of 81 lakes, that provides favourable conditions for snail control. Xinmin beach which is located between Gaoyou lake and Shaobo lake in Jiangsu Province, the infection rate of residents was more than 80%; 4019 peoples were infected with acute schistosomiasis of which 1335 peoples died and 45 households had been extinct due to acute schistosomiasis in 1950. Building low embankment and mollusciciding with sodium pentachlorophenate since 1971, the density of living snails decreased to 0 in 1979 and the infection rate of people reduced from 36.59% in 1971 to 0.17% in 1980.

4.1.3 Forestry engineering for schistosomiasis control

Peng (2001) put forward the concept of construction of forestry ecological engineering after extensive investigation and evaluation in the 1980s. The mechanism is to construct forestry-based complex ecological systems comprising forestry, agriculture, animal husbandry, fishery and so on according to eco-environment speciality, improve the natural environment and enhance biodiversity so as to achieve ecological improvement and economic benefits. By strengthening management of the forestry project, it could prevent livestock and nonprofessional people from entering forestry, reduce faeces containing schistosome eggs that contaminate environment with snails and decrease probability for the infection of people and livestock to realize the objective of snail control and schistosomiasis prevention. The forestry engineering for schistosomiasis control provides a new way for snail control in lake and marshland regions. It was considered in 1044 spots with snails in lake and marshland areas in Anhui Province and 43.8% of the spots implemented forestry ecological project for snail control and schistosomiasis prevention. The main afforestation model was pure forestry and accounted for 57.8% of the total spots. The occurrence rate of frames with living snails in the environment with afforestation (14.9%) was lower than that in the environment without afforestation (19.7%) ($\chi^2 = 2219.42$, $P < 0.01$). Of the different engineering modes, agroforestry pattern had the lowest occurrence rate of frames with living snails. The mean density of living snails was 0.552/0.1 m^2 in marshland with afforestation and 0.989/0.1 m^2 without afforestation (Huang et al., 2010) in the survey. At present, forestry ecological projects for snail control and schistosomiasis prevention have been promoted widely in Hunan, Hubei, Jiangxi, Anhui and Jiangsu provinces. For it to be a systematic engineering, the project should be designed specifically, implemented strictly and managed carefully to play a better role in schistosomiasis control.

4.2 Chemotherapy measure

Praziquantel is one of anti-schistosoma drugs with low toxicity, high efficiency and low price (Tambo et al., 2015). Since the late 1980s, chemotherapy measure for schistosomiasis control had been taken extensively in The People's Republic of China and it was very important for schistosomiasis control especially in the early phase. The measure of mass chemotherapy with praziquantel was carried out once a year for three consecutive years in marshland area of Guifan, Anhui Province, and the infection rate of people decreased from 19.2% to 8.9%, 6.8% and 7.2% yearly after 3 years of chemotherapy, but it rose to 13.6% after 2 years' interruption (Jiang et al., 1991). Wu, Yuan, et al. (1991) carried out the selective population chemotherapy trials with praziquantel once a year for two consecutive years in island area of Jishan, Jiangxi Province, and the infection rate of people changed a little, from 39.3% to 32.6%. It was thus clear that the annual mass chemotherapy was difficult to reduce the reinfection in severely affected marshland areas. Extending mass chemotherapy in the severe endemic areas of Dongting Lake, the infection rate of local residents reduced from 17.2% to 6.5% in 3 years and decreased by 62.2% after which it was stable under 5%, but the positive rate of wild faeces, the density of infected snails and the infection rate of sentinel mice remained at a high level and it was difficult to achieve the effect of blocking transmission of schistosomiasis (Wu et al., 1995). Due to the high missing rate of faecal examination, single strategy of individual chemotherapy could not control the infectious sources fully. In the middle of 1980s, expanding chemotherapy strategy was carried out to treat people with positive of serum immunological screening, obvious symptoms or signs and clear history of contacting infected water by praziquantel, except for positive of stool examination. This extended chemotherapy for three consecutive years was carried out in serious endemic villages where the infection rate of residents was 57.5% and the infection rate of residents and children decreased by 74.9% and 87.7%, respectively. This chemotherapy strategy had low inputs and could control the disease soon (Wang et al., 1989). A strategy that including treating patients and infected cattle in combination of killing of snails for 3 years was implemented. The prevalence of infection in residents did not decrease but slightly increased from 33.1% to 34.7%; however, it reduced by 80.2% after extending chemotherapy strategy for one more year (Tian et al., 1996). Therefore, the coverage of chemotherapy and selecting appropriate chemotherapy targets were very important in serious endemic areas. Since 1992, World Bank Loan Project for schistosomiasis control was implemented in eight provinces of The People's Republic of China. The mass chemotherapy strategy for three consecutive years was carried out widely in the endemic villages where the infection rate of residents was above 15%. Until 1998, the number of serious endemic villages in The People's Republic of China where the infection rate of residents was above 15% reduced by 47.40% compared to that in 1992. But the consecutive mass chemotherapy measure not only wasted drugs but also involved in ethical issues; moreover, the compliance of chemotherapy drive reduced year by year. Therefore, the intermittent mass chemotherapy strategy research was launched in Hubei, Sichuan, Jiangxi and Anhui provinces from 1996 to 2000. The effect on schistosomiasis control was also better and the positive testing rate of faecal examination for residents decreased by 39.3% with 1 year interval mass chemotherapy and 54.7% with every year mass chemotherapy, respectively, in serious endemic areas in Hubei Province. This strategy considered to alleviate the complicated process of pathogenic and serological test was implemented in the endemic villages where the infection rate of residents was below 20% to control schistosomiasis gradually, but the coverage of chemotherapy should not be less than 70% each time in order to get better effect (Wang et al., 1998).

Mass chemotherapy for cattle was very important to maintain the prevalence at a low level in marshland endemic areas, but the single measure for livestock was insufficient to block the reinfection of schistosomiasis (Chen et al., 1996). The infection rate of cattle still remained at around 10% after six consecutive years of mass chemotherapy by longitudinal observation at Dongliu township, Dongzhi County, Anhui Province. The infection rate of cattle still remained as high as 42% after four consecutive years of treatment by longitudinal observation at Wucheng township, Yongxiu County, Jiangxi Province. The pigs that grazed in south Dongting Lake areas were tested and treated 12 times a year, but the infection rate was still above 10% (Wang and Wang, 2000b). Since 1987, in order to investigate the effect of chemotherapy on decreasing the infection rate of livestock and the role in transmitting schistosoma, 30 villages in Dongting Lake area were selected for trial pilots and the potential contamination indexes of all kinds of infectious sources were calculated by longitudinal observation for 8 years. The results showed that the actual contamination indexes of all kinds of infectious sources reduced but the proportion remained unchanged. The infection rate of cattle and pig declined definitely in the early phase of chemotherapy, but could only be controlled at a certain level after consecutive chemotherapy and it was hard to continue decreasing the infection rate of livestock. The effect of cleansing the marshland of snails was difficult to achieve by livestock chemotherapy alone (Guo and Zheng, 2000). Chemotherapy effect on controlling cattle infected by schistosoma was positively correlated with the coverage of chemotherapy. Expanding the coverage of chemotherapy on cattle from 35% to 50% resulted in reduction of the positive rate of cattle by 77.52% with the coverage of 50%, and 48.25% with the coverage of 35% (Xu et al., 1999). The effect of chemotherapy was associated with the environmental characteristics of marshland regions. The closed type of endemic areas was the best, semi-open type was the second and open type endemic area was the worst.

Synchronization chemotherapy for people and livestock was adopted in the closed type of marshland areas for six consecutive years and the prevalence of infection among residents reduced from 15.6% in 1980 to 0.9% in 1985, a decrease by 94.2%. But once the measures paused, the infected snails reappeared and the infection rate of people also began to rebound 4 years later. Synchronization chemotherapy measures for people and livestock were carried out in Dongting Lake regions and in the second year the infection rate of residents, fishermen, cattle and pigs decreased by 65.17%, 30.18%, 62.62% and 26.85%, respectively. However, the infection rate of people and livestock remained at a certain level in the subsequent years. The infection rate of snails and the density of infected snails in susceptible zones declined significantly 1 year after chemotherapy and fluctuated in the subsequent years (Liu et al., 2003). The coverage of chemotherapy was related to the positive rate of stool examination directly. The positive rate of stool examination reduced significantly while the coverage was above 80%. Continuous mass chemotherapy could reduce the incidence of patients, delay onset time, reduce the number of advanced schistosomiasis cases and protect the labour force.

4.3 Synchronization chemotherapy for people and livestock plus other control measures

Chemotherapy was an effective method for schistosomiasis control in marshland areas. This measure could decrease the infection rate and the degree of infection for residents and control the prevalence situation at a certain level, but it was still difficult to block the transmission of schistosomiasis (Chen et al., 2000). To improve the effect of chemotherapy, National Research Committee of Schistosomiasis selected 22 pilots in marshland areas to launch the study on comprehensive control strategy based on chemotherapy for 5 years since 1980. These pilots were divided into three types and the corresponding control measures were implemented respectively. The measures for eliminating infectious sources and killing snails in susceptible zones were carried out in the first type regions, eliminating infectious sources and killing snails in large areas in the second type regions and eliminating infectious sources thoroughly (that is, expanding to chemotherapy) in the third type regions. The results showed all the measures had remarkable effects after 5 years of observation. In marshland areas, the measures implemented in first type of pilots were good and feasible for schistosomiasis control and had the most remarkable effect. The second type of measures controlled the disease well with relatively stable effect, but there was low feasibility and high cost for killing snails in large areas. Moreover, the third type of measure was easy to carry out but susceptible to external factors; the prevalence situation rebounded fast and the control effect was influenced by the coverage of chemotherapy and mobility of infectious sources. On this basis, the study on optimization control strategy was carried out in serious marshland areas, including chemotherapy for people and livestock, health education and killing snails in susceptible zones combined with environment improvement. The comparative field study was launched to eliminate infectious sources and block transmission of schistosomiasis by different control measures from 1989 to 1990 in Bailang Lake areas, Anhui Province. Simply extending chemotherapy could reduce the prevalence at a certain degree but it was hard to block the transmission. General control measures could only retain the prevalence at a certain level. The effect of extending chemotherapy supplemented with killing the snails one time in the susceptible zones was remarkable and the prevalence of infection among residents decreased from 15.39% to 0.30%, reduced by 98.05% after 4 years (Xu et al., 1990). The control measures were carried out in marshland areas including expanding chemotherapy for people and livestock, health education and environment improvement. The infection rate of people and livestock decreased by 93.1% and 72.6%, while the density of infected snails and infection rate of snails reduced by 66.7% and 77.3% respectively. The comparative study on three categories of measures was implemented in serious endemic areas of Dongting Lake, including selective mass chemotherapy, selective mass chemotherapy combined with killing snails in susceptible zones and simple treatment for positive cases of stool examination. After 3-year investigation, the actual contamination indexes reduced by 74.7%, 84.6% and 36.2% respectively, but the density of infected snails and infection rate of sentinel mice all remained at higher levels and the threshold of blocking transmission was not reached (Wu et al., 1993). Comparative experiments of three strategies were once launched in Guichi, Anhui Province. The first type strategy was simple mass chemotherapy, the second was killing snails in susceptible zones combined with mass chemotherapy and the third was comprehensive measures including those based on killing of snails. In Guifan pilot with the first strategy, the infection rate of residents reduced from 19.2% in 1981 to 7.2% in 1984, decreased by 62.5% in 3 years. There were acute schistosomiasis cases occurring every year and the infectious sources could not be controlled effectively by this measure. The density of infected snails was 0.0465/0.11 m^2 in 1981 and 0.0989/0.11 m^2 in 1984. The infection rate of sentinel mice was 100% in 1984 and the transmission of schistosomiasis still existed. The infection rate of residents rebounded to 13.6% in 1987 after the termination of intervention measures. In Sanlian pilot with the second strategy, the population prevalence reduced from 21.0% to 1.7%, decreased by 91.9% in 3 years. The density of snails decreased from 1.51/0.11 m^2 to 0.22/0.11 m^2, the density of infected snails reduced under 0.002/0.11 m^2 in the 3-year period of experiment and no case of acute schistosomiasis occurred. After 2 years' pause of intervention measures, the density of snails rebounded from 0.22/0.11 m^2 in 1984 to 4.01/0.11 m^2 in 1986. It was obvious that snails could not be eliminated only by chemicals and snails would reproduce fast once the intervention ceased. The prevalence of infection among people would rebound 1~2 years later than snails, the infection rate of residents was 10.2% and cases of acute schistosomiasis occurred in 1988. Integrated control strategy could maintain the prevalence at a trough for 2~3 years. In Jijiaba pilot with the third strategy, the mollusciciding effect was consolidated by constructing low embankment and storing water for fish-farming in marshland areas with snails. The infection rate of residents in 1981, 1984 and 1988 were 17.4%, 1.36% and 0.4%, respectively. No acute case occurred after intervention measures and the disease was controlled effectively in this region (Jiang et al., 1991). The study on control strategies and effect was carried out in five serious endemic villages of lake regions from 1995 to 1999. In the villages implemented with chemotherapy and killing snails, the infection rates of people and livestock reduced by 68.62% and 84.01% in 5 years, and the area of snails, the average density of live snails and infected snails decreased remarkably. In the villages implemented with health education and expanding chemotherapy, the prevalence decreased by 66.31% which was significantly higher than the villages implemented with single expanding chemotherapy, but the indexes of snails reduced unremarkably. In the villages implemented with single expanding chemotherapy, the indexes of the disease and snails both decreased unremarkably. Comprehensive control effect indexes showed that the effect on villages implemented with chemotherapy and killing snails was evident and stable, long-term effect of health education and chemotherapy was better than single chemotherapy and the comprehensive control effect of villages implemented with single chemotherapy was the worst. The results showed that chemotherapy was the major measure for schistosomiasis control in marshland areas, but in order to achieve the best control effect, chemotherapy must combine with snails control and health education. Therefore, the strategy of chemotherapy combined with killing of snails should be the preferred measure for schistosomiasis control (Huang et al., 2002).

Conventional chemotherapy measure was difficult to control schistosomiasis in marshland areas and simple chemotherapy could only control the disease to a certain extent. The effect of chemotherapy combined with killing of snails was maintained only for 2~3 years once the measures were terminated and this strategy was also hard to block the transmission. The control effect of improving the ecological environment on snails was permanent and the prevalence situation did not rebound after the termination of intervention measures. Through the comprehensive comparison of the effects of different measures for schistosomiasis control and cost-effectiveness analysis, chemotherapy for people and livestock combined with health education should be chosen when schistosomiasis control is the major target at hand, and meanwhile the measure of environment improvement could be added in the regions with appropriate economic conditions. In the areas with prevalence situation almost under control, the achievement of schistosomiasis control should be consolidated by the measures as follow: repeated examination and chemotherapy for people and livestock combined with eliminating infected snails, chemotherapy for susceptible people and cattle, health education, killing the snails in susceptible zones and individual protection (Xu et al., 1996).

4.4 Infectious sources control

To control the faeces of infected people and livestock is the key for schistosomiasis control in The People's Republic of China (Wang et al., 2009). It was difficult to eliminate snails in marshland areas and protect cattle from being infected and reinfected with schistosoma by praziquantel. Contamination to environment with snails, from livestock especially cattle, as one of infectious sources of schistosoma, persistently existed and it was difficult to block the transmission of schistosomiasis. So, an integrated control strategy for schistosomiasis with emphasis on infectious sources control was proposed in 2004 in The People's Republic of China. Under this strategy, the measures including replacing cattle with machine for cultivation and forbidding livestock pasturing on marshland were implemented for eliminating contamination of marshland from faeces of cattle and other livestock effectively and to cut off the transmission chain. Moreover, to achieve the purpose of blocking transmission, these measures were supplemented by conventional measures, for example, chemotherapy, killing of snails, health education and so on (Fig. 3).

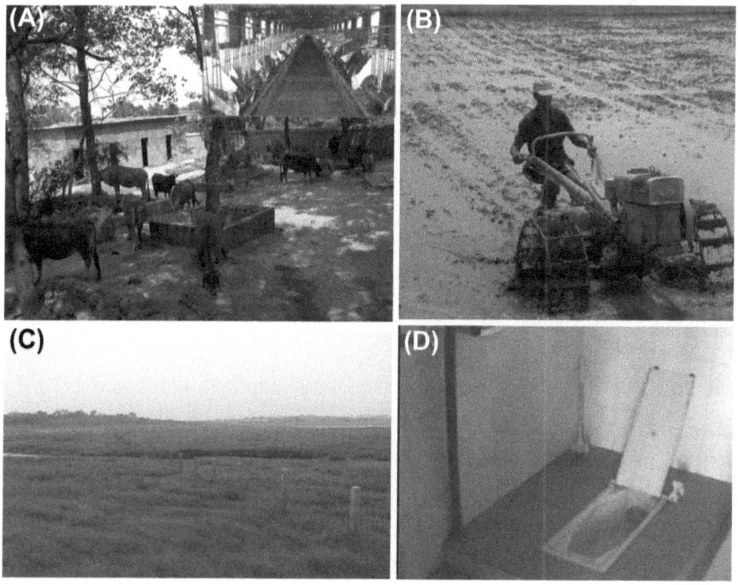

Figure 3 Infectious sources control measures in lake and marshland regions. (A) Raising animals in fen; (B) replacing bovine with machine; (C) building barrier to hind herding and (D) safe treatment of night-soil.

Forbidding livestock pasturing on marshland by setting up fences in the marshland with snails, deterring cattle and other livestock from grazing there, cutting off pathogen and cleansing the marshland aimed at achieving the goal of schistosomiasis control without killing snails. In the 1990s, X.Y. Wang, X.H. Wang and K.D. Zhang carried out the studies on the measure of forbidding livestock pasturing on marshland in Poyang Lake. Their results showed, respectively, that after 2 years the infection rate of residents reduced by 75.67%, 79.25% and 56.72%, the infection rate of cattle decreased by 88.53%, 97.14% and 87.7%, and the density of infected snails declined by 100%, 99.26% and 75.0%. The results of the three pilots proved it was an immediate and effective measure (Wang et al., 1999, 2003; Zhang et al., 2003). With the measures of constructing fences and forbidding livestock pasturing implemented on marshland, the number of livestock reduced by 73.6%, activities of residents in marshland decreased by 83.21%, the wild faeces reduced obviously and the infection rate of people, livestock and snails decreased remarkably, and the transmission of schistosomiasis was controlled effectively (Liu et al., 2010).

With the development of social economy and changes in production methods in rural areas, cattle were no longer the major way for cultivation and replacing cattle with machine became a trend gradually. The measure of replacing cattle with machine was promoted in marshland areas and the number of cattle decreased greatly, the role of cattle as major infectious source in the transmission of schistosomiasis was eliminated gradually. Meanwhile, the labour productivity was improved and the process of mechanization of agriculture was accelerated. The field experiments in marshland areas of Hunan, Hubei, Jiangxi, Anhui and Jiangsu provinces showed that schistosomiasis could be controlled effectively by comprehensive strategies with emphasis on eliminating cattle and replacing cattle with machine. The measure of replacing cattle with machine was implemented in six villages of Hubei Province and forbidding livestock pasturing on marshland was enforced in seven villages of Hunan Province. The results showed that the infection rate of people in the two groups decreased by 83.08% and 81.62%, respectively, there being no significant difference between them. But the infected cattle were still detected in the pilot with the measure of forbidding livestock pasturing on marshland and the prevalence of infection in cattle was 0.65%. The density and positive rate of wild faeces in seven villages with the measure of forbidding livestock pasturing on marshland were all higher than the six villages with the measure of replacing cattle with machine. The density of wild faeces in two groups of villages was

$25.73/hm^2$ and $0.1/hm^2$ and the positive rates were 1.15% and 0, respectively (Cao et al., 2014). To maximize the effectiveness of replacing cattle with machine and forbidding livestock pasturing on marshland on blocking the transmission of schistosomiasis, the measures of infectious sources control should be promoted in whole village, town and county, otherwise the effectiveness of infectious sources control would be influenced by the existence of cattle in adjacent domains and their activities in environment with snails. Moreover, the later management of infectious sources control should be strengthened for preventing the return of livestock. The fences should be protected by specially assigned persons for preventing the facilities from being destroyed. Control and elimination of infectious sources is one of the important measures for schistosomiasis control. It is hard to eliminate snails in lake regions of The People's Republic of China at present and the integrated strategy with emphasis on forbidding livestock pasturing on marshland should be adopted based on epidemiology of schistosomiasis, biology of schistosoma, ecology of *Oncomelania* snails, hydrology and the activities characteristics of people and livestock. This measure not only protects the people and livestock from being infected by schistosoma, but also cuts off pathogen and cleanses the marshland.

5. CONTROL EFFECTIVENESS

The People's Republic of China has seen remarkable achievements in schistosomiasis control after 60 years of active and effective control. The snail area in marshland regions reduced from 11.3 billion m^2 in the early stage to 3.627 billion m^2 in 2013, a decrease by 67.9%, while, the snail area of Poyang Lake regions reduced from 1.4 to 0.63 billion m^2 by the measures of reclamation, storing water for fish-farming and killing snails in susceptible zones (Lin and Zhang, 2002). The snail area of Dongting Lake regions reduced from 3.333 to 1.77 billion m^2 by the snails control measures of large-scale construction of conservancy and farmland, reclamation and killing snails by drugs, a decrease by 46.89% (Li et al., 2014a). In early stage, the prevalence of infection among residents along the Yangtze River and lakes was very high, generally above 20%, and in some villages as high as 70%. There were large number of acute schistosomiasis and more cases of new and reinfection occurred every year. For example, the positive rate of stool examination of villagers near Poyang Lake was mostly more than 30%, even up to 80%; the infection rate of residents was more than 10%

in 79.3% of the villages and 5~10% in 14.5% of the villages in Dongting Lake areas. The prevalence of infection among livestock including cattle and pigs was also very high. Schistosomiasis was one of the important public health problems in endemic areas and restricted the development of rural economy seriously. Schistosomiasis was controlled effectively as the snail distribution area decreased greatly in marshland areas. The results of epidemiological sampling survey on national schistosomiasis in 1989, 1995 and 2004 showed that the prevalence of the infection among people in 1989 in marshland areas was still as high as 12.94%, the infection rate of livestock including cattle, buffalo and sheep was overall higher than people and the prevalence in sheep was as high as 43.59%. But in the present century, the prevalence of infection among people in 2004 decreased below 5%, reduced by 70.32%, compared to that in 1989. Moreover, the infection rate of cattle, buffaloes, pigs and sheep decreased by 72.14%, 61.53%, 93.72% and 93.85%, respectively (Table 1). Jiangsu and Hubei provinces reached the standard of schistosomiasis transmission control in 2011 and 2013 respectively; Anhui and Jiangxi provinces passed the assessment and achieved the goal of transmission control during the end of 2014 and April of 2015; Hunan Province was expected to achieve the target of transmission control for schistosomiasis by the end of 2015.

6. CHALLENGES

6.1 Influence of the Three Gorges Dam on schistosomiasis transmission

After the construction of the Three Gorges Dam, the temporal and spatial distribution of water and sand and the ecological environment of related areas in the middle and lower reaches of the Yangtze River underwent changes which influenced the distribution of snails and the prevalence of schistosomiasis in marshland areas. The highest and lowest water lever of flooding outer embankment with snails in Dongting Lake regions changed and the flooding time of altitude above 27 m reduced. In drought period, the phenomenon of shortage of water continuously occurred in upper and middle reaches of the Xiangjiang River, but the reproduction ability of snails in Dongting Lake regions was not influenced by the Three Gorge Project. The highest and lowest altitude of snails' distribution fell down. The altitude of high-density snails' zone and the density of living snails decreased, and the snail area increased when the water level rose (Guo et al., 2012).

Table 1 Results of stool examination for residents and domestic animals in different subtypes of lake and marshland endemic regions (nationwide sampling survey on schistosomiasis in 1989, 1995 and 2004 in The People's Republic of China)

Year	Subtype	Infection rate of residents (%)	Infection rate of cattle (%)	Infection rate of buffaloes (%)	Infection rate of pigs (%)	Infection rate of sheep (%)
1989	Fork-beach	10.33	19.51	10.28	5.25	—
	Islet without embankment	10.41	20.0	15.8	1.79	53.33
	Islet with embankment	13.29	17.89	15.85	6.38	88.24
	Inner embankment	15.44	3.57	20.05	3.66	9.68
	Total	12.94	17.03	16.56	3.98	43.59
1995	Fork-beach	7.72	1.08	8.82	1.92	—
	Islet without embankment	5.95	15.73	19.07	5.0	5.91
	Islet with embankment	7.13	7.18	6.66	0.88	—
	Inner embankment	6.67	21.28	8.65	1.89	4.48
	Total	6.63	7.74	11.84	2.73	5.73
2004	Fork-beach	3.36	8.57	8.65	0.56	1.95
	Islet without embankment	2.71	10.26	2.87	0	0
	Islet with embankment	4.28	0.36	13.07	0	6.87
	Inner embankment	4.25	3.83	5.54	0	0
	Total	3.84	4.55	6.37	0.25	2.68

After the Three Gorges Project became operational, the spatial distribution pattern of vegetation in marshland of Poyang Lake regions changed, the dominant population and distribution of vegetation occurred succession, and the natural meadow vegetation and snails presented a trend of slowly migrating to the lower altitude areas of the marshland (Li et al., 2014b). Earlier, the flood submerged partial marshland of Jiangsu and Anhui provinces along the middle and lower reaches of the Yangtze River in spring and receded in autumn, leading to the downtrend of the density of snails and the prevalence of schistosomiasis (Li et al., 2013). But the changes of water level led to the reduction of flooding time in partial marshland which was appropriate for snails reproduction and had became the potential, expanding areas of snails. Some embankments became the regions with snails distribution and the snail area appeared on an increasing trend as the measures of returning farmland to lake and detruding embankments for flood discharge were implemented.

6.2 Complexity of snails' habitats

Since the mid-1990s, the snail area in The People's Republic of China was maintained at around 3.5 billion m^2, of which 95% was distributed in marshland regions. Because of the large area of marshland, wide distribution and complicated habitats of snails and influence factors from water conservancy, environment and ecological aspects, the past experience of large-scale reclamation was no longer suitable for eliminating snails in order to maintain the ecological balance and water level (Zheng et al., 2013). The water level in marshland areas of the middle and lower reaches along the Yangtze River was difficult to control and molluscicidng effect was not ideal. Furthermore, snails drifted with streams and attachment for long distance, resulting in the expanding trend of snails and increasing the difficulty and complexity of snail control (Li et al., 2016).

6.3 Remaining infectious sources

In recent years, through the integrated control strategy including forbidding livestock pasturing on marshland, replacing cattle with machine and eliminating cattle, the number of cattle and the prevalence of livestock in marshland areas decreased year by year. There were abundant grass resources in marshland areas that were the ideal place for grazing. In spite of replacing cattle with machine for cultivation, the number of cattle for beef and sheep were present for utilizing the grass resources fully and promoting economy in epidemic areas. However, the effect of the measure of forbidding livestock pasturing on the marshland was not ideal because the later management of fences was not enough, resulting in damage. Besides human, there are more than 40 kinds of mammal as the reservoir hosts of *Schistosoma japonicum* and the wild animals living in marshland areas are often infected with schistosoma (Tambo et al., 2014). In addition, a large number of fishermen can play an important role in the transmission of schistosomiasis during the flood season. The persistent existence of many infectious sources and contamination of the environment by their faeces and by snails are important potential risks for further consolidating the achievement of schistosomiasis control.

7. PROSPECTS

The Chinese government has always attached great importance to the control and elimination of infectious diseases, including schistosomiasis (Collins et al., 2012; Tambo et al., 2015). In order to further consolidate the success of schistosomiasis control, the Chinese government held the National Conference of Schistosomiasis Control in November 2014, proposed the goals of blocking transmission of schistosomiasis by 2020 and eliminating schistosomiasis by 2025 in whole country, and confirmed the targets of the national schistosomiasis elimination programme in the next 10 years (Zhu et al., 2016). Based on the comprehensive analysis of epidemic characteristics in marshland areas and distilling experiences on schistosomiasis control, in the next decade of the national schistosomiasis elimination programme will be developed around the goal of eliminating schistosomiasis. The integrated control strategy with emphasis on infectious sources control will be continuously implemented along with the strengthening of the epidemic situation surveillance, constantly improving the ability of scientific control in order to block the route of transmission effectively through a decade-long battle against schistosomiasis, and finally achieve the goal of eliminating schistosomiasis.

REFERENCES

Cao, C.L., Bao, Z.P., Yang, P.C., et al., 2014. Schistosomiasis control effect of measures of replacing cattle with machine for cultivation and forbidding depasturage of livestock on marshlands in marshland and lake regions. Chin. J. Schistosomiasis Control 26 (6), 602–607 (in Chinese).

Ceng, X.J., Wu, F.D., Zhang, S.J., et al., 1996. Observation on reinfection of *Schistosoma japonicum* by selective chemotherapy on inhabitants in heavy islet endemic region. Chin. J. Schistosomiasis Control 8, 83–86 (in Chinese).

Chen, W., Fu, Y., Liu, L.M., et al., 1996. Observation on the role of control the transmission of schistosomiasis by mass chemotherapy on cattle. Hubei J. Prev. Med. 7 (3), 23–25 (in Chinese).

Chen, K.X., 1980. Sub-type of habitats of *Oncomelania hupensis* in marshland endemic regions. Acta Hunan Med. Coll. 5, 129–130 (in Chinese).

Chen, M.G., 2014. Assessment of morbidity due to *Schistosoma japonicum* infection in China. Infect. Dis. Poverty 3, 6.

Chen, X.Y., Jiang, Q.W., Guo, J.P., et al., 2000. Analysis of effectiveness of chemotherapy on schistosomiasis control in marshland regions. Chin. J. Schistosomiasis Control 12 (1), 8–11 (in Chinese).

Chen, Y., Xie, M.S., Yang, R.Q., et al., 1999. Study on the relationship between the field stool and density of infected snails in endemic foci of schistosomiasis outside Dongting Lake. Prac. Prev. Med. 6, 11–13 (in Chinese).

Chitsulo, L., Engels, D., Montresor, A., Savioli, L., 2000. The global status of schistosomiasis and its control. Acta Trop. 77, 41–51.

Collins, C., Xu, J., Tang, S., 2012. Schistosomiasis control and the health system in P.R. China. Infect. Dis. Poverty 1, 8.

Guan, W.H., Yuan, H.C., Zhao, G.M., et al., 1999. A quantitative study on human water contact in dam circled marsh region of *Schistosoma japonicum*. Chin. J. Schistosomiasis Control 11, 211–214 (in Chinese).

Guo, F.Y., Zhao, Z.Y., Ren, M.Y., et al., 2012. Impact of marshland changes on snail distribution in Dongting Lake after the construction of the Three Gorge Dam. Trop. Dis. Parasitol. 14 (3), 125–127 (in Chinese).

Guo, J.G., Zheng, J., 2000. Prevalence and prevention of schistosomiasis in China. J. Dis. Control 4 (4), 289–293 (in Chinese).

He, J.C., Wang, E.M., Wang, T.P., et al., 1995. The prevalence situation of schistosomiasis of cattle and transmission role in river beach region in Anhui Province. Chin. J. Schistosomiasis Control 7, 288–289 (in Chinese).

He, N., Yuan, H.C., Zhang, S.J., et al., 1997. Quantitative research on human water contact after reclamation in an islet region of *Schistosoma japonicum*. Chin. J. Parasitol. Parasit. Dis. 5, 410–414.

Hu, F., Lin, D.D., Zhang, B.L., et al., 2003. Study on the influence of the project of building dike for storing water to schistosomiasis trasmission in Duchang County. Chin. J. Schistosomiasis Control 15, 177–181 (in Chinese).

Hu, S.G., Qin, S.T., Shi, Z.G., et al., 1996. Investigation on prevalence situation and harmless of schistosomiasis of pig in Dongting Lake. Hunan J. Anim. Sci. Vet. Med. 4, 25–26 (in Chinese).

Huang, X.B., Fang, T.Q., Li, S.H., et al., 2002. Evaluation on control strategies and effectiveness in schistosomiasis hyper endemic marshland areas. Chin. J. Parasit. Control 15 (3), 166–168 (in Chinese).

Huang, Y., Zhang, S.Q., He, J.C., et al., 2010. Investigation on the status of afforestation for schistosomiasis prevention in marshland regions in Anhui Province. Trop. Med. Parasitol. 8, 198–200 (in Chinese).

Huang, Y.J., 1998. Characteristic of wild feces contamination in the river beach. Parasitol. Parasit. Dis. 6, 86 (in Chinese).

Huang, Y.J., Tang, H.P., Hang, D.R., et al., 2013. Effect of sand buried on elimination of *Oncomelania hupensis* snails in marshland along the Yangtze River in Jiangdu District, Jiangsu Province. Chin. J. Schistosomiasis Control 25, 672–673 (in Chinese).

Jiang, Q.W., Yuan, H.C., Zhong, D.M., et al., 1991. A longitudinal evaluation of efficacy on control of schistosomiasis by comparative study of different control measures. Chin. J. Schistosomiasis Control 3 (5), 260–263.

Lei, Z.L., Zheng, H., Zhang, L.J., et al., 2014. Endemic status of schistosomiasis in People's Republic of China in 2013. Chin. J. Schistosomiasis Control 26, 591–594 (in Chinese).

Li, S.M., Ren, G.H., Huo, H.B., et al., 2014a. The impact of development in the ecological economic zone of Dongting Lake on transmission of schistosomiasis. Trop. Dis. Parasitol. 12 (1), 10–14 (in Chinese).

Li, W., Hang, D.R., You, B.R., et al., 2013. Effect of environmental change in marshland after implementation of Three Gorges Reservoir Project on schistosomiasis in Jiangsu Province. Chin. J. Schistosomiasis Control 25 (6), 576–580 (in Chinese).

Li, Y.Y., Liu, Z.C., Huo, H.B., et al., 2002. Study on the characteristics of grazing and chemotherapy strategies on bovine in endemic area of Dongting Lake. Chin. J. Schistosomiasis Control 14, 270–272 (in Chinese).

Li, Z.J., Chen, H.G., Ceng, X.J., et al., 2014b. Studies on changes of vegetation and *Oncomelania hupensis* snails in Poyang Lake after impoundment of Three Gorges Project. Chin. J. Schistosomiasis Control 26 (2), 115–120 (in Chinese).

Li, Z.J., Ge, J., Dai, J.R., Wen, L.Y., Lin, D.D., Madsen, H., et al., 2016. Biology and control of snail intermediate host of *Schistosoma japonicum* in the People's Republic of China. Adv. Parasitol. 92.

Lin, D.D., Liu, Y.M., Hu, F., et al., 2003. Animal host of *Schistosoma japonicum* and transmission of schistosomiasis in Poyang Lake regions. J. Trop. Med. 3, 383–387 (in Chinese).

Lin, D.D., Zhang, S.J., 2002. Geographical environment and schistosomiasis transmission in Poyang Lake regions. Chin. J. Epidemiol. 23, 90–93 (in Chinese).

Liu, L., Yang, G.J., Zhu, H.R., Yang, K., Ai, L., 2014. Knowledge of attitudes towards, and practice relating to schistosomiasis in two subtypes of a mountainous region of the People's Republic of China. Infect. Dis. Poverty 3, 16.

Liu, Q.L., Zhao, Z.Y., Yang, G.F., et al., 2003. Schistosomiasis control effect by chemotherapy in Dongting Lake area. Parasit. Infect. Dis. 1 (3), 119–120 (in Chinese).

Liu, Y., Zhou, Y.B., Li, R.Z., Wan, J.J., Yang, Y., Qiu, D.C., et al., 2016. Epidemiological features and control effectiveness of schistosomiasis in mountainous and hilly region of the People's Republic of China. Adv. Parasitol. 92.

Liu, Z.C., Huo, H.B., Wang, Z.X., et al., 2010. Effect of marshland isolation and grazing prohibition on schistosomiasis control in Dongting Lake region. Chin. J. Schistosomiasis Control 22 (5), 459–463 (in Chinese).

Mao, S.B., Shao, B.R., 1982. Schistosomiasis control in People's Republic of China. Am. J. Trop. Med. Hyg. 31, 92–99.

MOH, PR China, 1993. Epidemiological Situation of Schistosomiasis in China-Results from a National-Wide Sampling Survey in 1989. Chengdu University of Science and Technology Publishing House, Chengdu, pp. 16–30 (in Chinese).

MOH, PR China, 2002. World Bank Loan Project Completion Report on Infectious and Endemic Disease Control Project Schistosomiasis Control Component (1992–2001), pp. 1–15 (in Chinese).

Peng, Z.H., 2001. Study on the beaches snails outwipping forest ecological engineering. Eng. Sci. 3 (7), 12–16 (in Chinese).

Qin, X.Y., Xiao, X., Wang, T.P., et al., 2000. A prospective cohort study on human infection and reinfection with *Schistosoma japonicum* in river beach area. J. Pract. Parasit. Dis. 8, 1–5 (in Chinese).

Shen, W., 1992. Review and suggestion on animal schistosomiasis control. Chin. J. Schistosomiasis Control 4, 82–85 (in Chinese).

Shi, L., Li, W., Wu, F., Zhang, J.F., Yang, K., Zhou, X.N., 2016. Epidemiological features and control progress of schistosomiasis in waterway-network region in P.R. China. Adv. Parasitol. 92.

Su, Z.W., Hu, C.Q., Fu, Y., 1994. Role of several hosts in transmission of schistosomiasis japonica in lake region. Chin. J. Parasitol. Parasit. Dis. 12, 248–251 (in Chinese).
Sun, L.P., Zhang, Y.P., Cao, Q., et al., 1997. Schistosomiasis transmission role of farm cattle in marshland region in Jiangsu Province. Prac. J. Parasit. Dis. 5, 66–68 (in Chinese).
Tambo, E., Ai, L., Zhou, X., Chen, J.H., Hu, W., Bergquist, R., et al., 2014. Surveillance-response systems: the key to elimination of tropical diseases. Infect. Dis. Poverty 3, 17.
Tambo, E., Khater, E.I., Chen, J.H., Bergquist, R., Zhou, X.N., 2015. Nobel prize for the artemisinin and ivermectin discoveries: a great boost towards elimination of the global infectious diseases of poverty. Infect. Dis. Poverty 4, 58.
Tian, Z.Y., Xiao, J.W., Liu, D.S., et al., 1996. The effect of three different strategies on schistosomiasis control at Wuyi village. Chin. J. Schistosomiasis Control 8, 96–98 (in Chinese).
Tu, Z.X., Liu, Z.D., Sun, Y.S., et al., 1992. Observation on the Effect of Reclaiming and Planting by Machinery for Snail Control on a Large Scale in Lake Region. Data Compilation on Schistosomiasis Research (1986–1990). Shanghai Science and Technology Publishing House, p. 262 (in Chinese).
Wang, L.D., 2006. The Progress and Prospect of Schistosomiasis Control in People's Republic of China. The People's Medical Publishing House, Beijing, pp. 133–176 (in Chinese).
Wang, L.D., Chen, H.G., Guo, J.G., et al., 2009. A strategy to control transmission of *Schistosoma japonicum* in China. New Eng. J. Med. 360 (2), 121–128.
Wang, X.H., Liu, W., Zhou, H., et al., 2003. Study on schistosomiasis control with "marshland isolation and farming prohibition" but no snail control in Lake marshland. Chin. J. Schistosomiasis Control 15 (4), 259–261 (in Chinese).
Wang, X.Y., Wang, X.H., 2000a. Consideration and suggestion on the control strategies of schistosomiasis in marshland endemic regions in China. Jiangxi Sci. 18, 45–50 (in Chinese).
Wang, X.Y., Wang, X.H., 2000b. Strategies on schistosomiasis control in Lake regions in China. Chin. J. Vet. Parasit. Dis. 8 (4), 40–45 (in Chinese).
Wang, X.Y., Wang, X.H., Wu, G.C., 1999. Studies on the purification of meadow and control of schistosomiasis in Lake area by means of isolating the meadow and prohibiting pasture farming. Jiangxi Sci. 17 (3), 163–167 (in Chinese).
Wang, Z.H., Yi, Z.H., Zhang, Y.H., et al., 1998. Studies on the effectiveness of varied chemotherapy strategies with praziquantel for schistosomiasis control. Chin. J. Schistosomiasis Control 10 (4), 203–206 (in Chinese).
Wang, Z.H., Zhang, J.W., Yi, Z.H., et al., 1989. Studies on expanding chemotherapy measures with praziquantel for schistosomiasis control. Chin. J. Schistosomiasis Control 1 (2), 19–22, 37 (in Chinese).
Wu, G.L., Yuan, J.H., He, Q., et al., 1991. Clinical epidemiological investigation on liver and spleen swelling of schistosomiasis japonica. Chin. J. Parasitol. Parasit. Dis. 9, 274–277 (in Chinese).
Wu, Z.W., Peng, X.S., Li, W.C., et al., 1995. A longitudinal pilot study of chemotherapy effect for schistosomiasis control in Dongting Lake region. Pract. Prev. Med. 2 (1), 5–7 (in Chinese).
Wu, Z.W., Po, K.M., Liu, Q.L., et al., 1993. The effect of chemotherapy with praziquantel on morbidity and transmission of schistosomiasis japonica in Dongting lake region. Chin. J. Schistosomiasis Control 5 (6), 325–328 (in Chinese).
Wu, Z.W., Po, K.M., Yuan, L.P., et al., 1995. Analysis on reinfection factors of *Schistosoma japonicum* in lake region. Pract. Prev. Med. 2 (2), 87–88 (in Chinese).
Wu, Z.W., Xie, M.S., Zhuo, S.J., et al., 1991. The relevance of human behavior to the endemicity and control of schistosomiasis japonica in Dongting Lake region. Chin. J. Schistosomiasis Control 3, 7–11 (in Chinese).

Wu, Z.D., Zhang, S.J., Hu, L.S., et al., 1994. Observation on reinfection of schistosomiasis after chemotherapy at Gaojia village. Chin. J. Schistosomiasis Control 6, 252–253 (in Chinese).

Wu, Z.W., Zhuo, S.J., Po, K.M., et al., 1990. Application and calculation on the index of actual contamination for the infectious resources in Dongting Lake. Chin. J. Schistosomiasis Control 2, 31–34 (in Chinese).

Xie, Z.M., 1990. Discussion on schistosomiasis control measures in Poyang Lake. Chin. J. Schistosomiasis Control 2, 69–71 (in Chinese).

Xu, F.N., Wang, T.P., Qin, X.Y., et al., 1990. Study on the interruption of transmission of schistosomiasis by the elimination of infection source. Chin. J. Schistosomiasis Control 2 (3), 11–16 (in Chinese).

Xu, F.N., Wu, Z.X., Wu, W.D., et al., 1996. Study on epidemiological factors and control strategies of schistosomiasis in beach regions Yangtze River. Chin. J. Schistosomiasis Control 8 (6), 325–330 (in Chinese).

Xu, J., Steinman, P., Maybe, D., Zhou, X.N., Lv, S., Li, S.Z., et al., 2016. Evolution of the national schistosomiasis control programmes in the People's Republic of China. Adv. Parasitol. 92.

Xu, S.T., Dai, Y.H., Wu, W.M., et al., 1985. Study on Epidemiology of Animal Schistosomiasis and Control Strategies in Area of Pingmuhu. Single Copy, Hunan Province (in Chinese).

Xu, X.J., Yang, X.X., Chen, L.Y., et al., 1999. Evaluation on the effect of expanded chemotherapy on farm cattle in middle endemic region of *Schistosoma japonicum*. Chin. J. Zoonoses 5 (3), 106–107 (in Chinese).

Yuan, Y.S., He, H.S., Chen, W.X., et al., 2003. The survey of epidemilogy of sheep's schistosomiasis in Jingzhou city along the Changjiang River-line. Chin. J. Vet. Parasit. 11, 48–50 (in Chinese).

Zhang, K.D., Wang, S.Z., Li, F., et al., 2003. Observation on the effect of control and prevention for schistosomiasis by marshland isolation and farming prohibition in lake region. Chin. Vet. Parasit. Dis. 11 (3), 38–39 (in Chinese).

Zhang, S.J., Wu, Z.D., Lin, D.D., 1996. Progress on epidemiology and control strategy of schistosomiasis in Poyang Lake region. Acta Nanchang Univ. (Nat. Sci.) 20 (Suppl.), 98–102 (in Chinese).

Zhang, S.Q., Jiang, Q.W., Ge, J.H., 2002. Influence of flood on schistosomiasis transmission. Chin. J. Schistosomiasis Control 14, 315–317 (in Chinese).

Zheng, Q., Vanderslott, S., Jiang, B., Xu, L.L., Liu, C.S., Huo, L.L., et al., 2013. Research gaps for three main tropical diseases in the People's Republic of China. Infect. Dis. Poverty 2, 15.

Zhou, X.N., Bergquist, R., Tanner, M., 2013. Elimination of tropical disease through surveillance and response. Infect. Dis. Poverty 2, 1.

Zhu, H., Yap, P., Utzinger, J., Jia, T.W., Li, S.Z., Huang, X.B., et al., 2016. Policy support and resources mobilization for the national schistosomiasis control programme in the People's Republic of China. Adv. Parasitol. 92.

Zhuo, S.J., Wu, Z.W., He, Y.K., 1991. Study on factors affecting the prevalence and epidemiological patterns of schistosomiasis in Dongting Lake region. Chin. J. Schistosomiasis Control 3, 133–137 (in Chinese).

CHAPTER THREE

Epidemiological Features and Effectiveness of Schistosomiasis Control Programme in Mountainous and Hilly Region of The People's Republic of China

Y. Liu*, Y.-B. Zhou[§,¶,||], R.-Z. Li*, J.-J. Wan*, Y. Yang[§], D.-C. Qiu*, B. Zhong*[,1]

*Sichuan Provincial Center for Disease Control and Prevention, Chengdu, The People's Republic of China
[§]Department of Epidemiology, School of Public Health, Fudan University, Shanghai, The People's Republic of China
[¶]Key Laboratory of Public Health Safety, Ministry of Education, Shanghai, The People's Republic of China
[||]Center for Tropical Disease Research, Shanghai, The People's Republic of China
[1]Corresponding author: E-mail: zhongbo1968@163.com

Contents

Abstract

Schistosomiasis is a parasitic disease that affects over 200 million people worldwide in at least 76 countries, ranking second only after malaria in terms of its socio-economic

Advances in Parasitology, Volume 92
ISSN 0065-308X
http://dx.doi.org/10.1016/bs.apar.2016.02.019

and public health importance in tropical and subtropical areas of the world. Chinese surveillance data since the mid-1950s have shown that endemic areas are divided into three types based on geographical, ecological and epidemiological factors, such as marshland and lake region, plain region with waterway networks and hilly and mountainous region. As confirmed by numerous epidemiological investigations, schistosomiasis endemic areas of the mountainous type are distributed in 178 counties in 11 provinces of The People's Republic of China. Over the past several decades great success in transmission control has been achieved by implementation of control strategies that were suitable for the mountainous and hilly endemic region.

1. INTRODUCTION

Schistosomiasis, caused by human infection with *Schistosoma* spp., such as *S. mansoni*, *S. hematobia*, *S. japonicum*, *S. menkongi*, is a parasitic disease that affects over 200 million people worldwide in at least 76 countries, ranking second only after malaria in terms of its socio-economic and public health importance in tropical and subtropical areas, mostly in Asia and Africa (Chitsulo et al., 2000; Salam et al., 2014; Dabo et al., 2015). In addition to humans, over 40 species of mammals are definitive hosts of *S. japonicum* which is distributed in The People's Republic of China, Philippines and Indonesia. Surveillance data in the mid-1950s in The People's Republic of China have shown that there have been 12 provinces (autonomous regions and municipalities directly under the central government) and 427 counties located in the basin south of the Yangtze River that have experienced widespread transmission (Collins et al., 2012). Evidence of human infection extends back for over 2000 years, but the first mention in any type of literature dates only back to the 1920s. The first domestic efforts to estimate the extent and severity of the disease and to address control began in the mid-1950s (Chen, 2014). Over the past five decades, almost all endemic areas of the country have had notable success in schistosomiasis control efforts.

There are four control stages in the national schistosomiasis control programme based on the *National Criteria for Schistosomiasis Control and Elimination*, ie, morbidity control, transmission control, transmission interruption and elimination. All stages clearly indicated the effort determinants on human, animal and snail prevalence of infection and very substantial reductions in snail habitat as well as special attention to infections in children and over increasing time periods (Zhu et al., 2016). The specific criteria issued in 1995 were as follows:

- Morbidity control: Prevalence in both human and cattle less than 3%; acute cases of human infection occur with low frequency.

- Transmission control: Prevalence in human and cattle less than 1% by parasitological examination; no new infections in children less than 12 years old and in cattle less than 3 years old; no acute cases of human infection; snail habitat reduced by 98% of precontrol level.
- Transmission interruption: Prevalence in human and/or cattle less than 0.2% by parasitological examination; no new infection of human and/or cattle found continuously for 5 years; no snails found for more than 1 year.
- Elimination: No new infection of human and/or cattle found continuously for 5 years after attaining transmission interruption.
- Re-emerging schistosomiasis: Infection reported since the declaration of disease elimination.

At the end of 2013, schistosomiasis transmission had been interrupted in 296 counties and controlled in 124 counties. The schistosomiasis transmission has been interrupted in three provinces (ie, Fujian, Guangdong and Zhejiang), the municipality of Shanghai and the autonomous region of Guangxi province (Zheng, 2003). The number of endemic provinces has been reduced to seven, including five in the lake region of the lower Yangtze River (ie, Jiangsu, Hubei, Hunan, Anhui and Jiangxi provinces) and two (ie, Sichuan and Yunnan provinces) achieved transmission control criterion. In addition, symptomatic and advanced cases were significantly reduced, falling to the lowest level in history (Collins et al., 2012).

Schistosomiasis endemic areas in The People's Republic of China are divided into three types based on geographical, ecological and epidemiological factors, such as marshland and lake region, plain region with waterway networks and hilly and mountainous region (Zhou, 2007). Mountainous habitats account for 12.6% of all snail habitat regions in The People's Republic of China. This type is distributed in 10 provinces and one autonomous region. Snail habitat areas of Zhejiang and Jiangxi provinces account for more than 20%; Anhui, Sichuan and Yunnan, between 10% and 20%; the total numbers in Hubei, Jiangsu, Fujian, Guangxi, Hunan and Guangdong provinces account for less than 10%, respectively (Mao, 1991; Zhong et al., 2011) (Fig. 1).

In 2013, it was reported that the total snail habitat in The People's Republic of China covered a land area of 365,468 hm^2 with marshlands totalling 352,627 hm^2, lakes 216 hm^2 and mountains 12,624 hm^2. The mountainous endemic area that is the focus of this report accounted for 3.45% of the total habitat land area (Lei et al., 2014) but 23.6% of all human infections. These areas are now mainly distributed in Sichuan and Yunnan provinces subsequent to Guangdong, Guangxi, Fujian and Zhejiang provinces meeting transmission interruption criterion (Zheng et al., 2012, 2013).

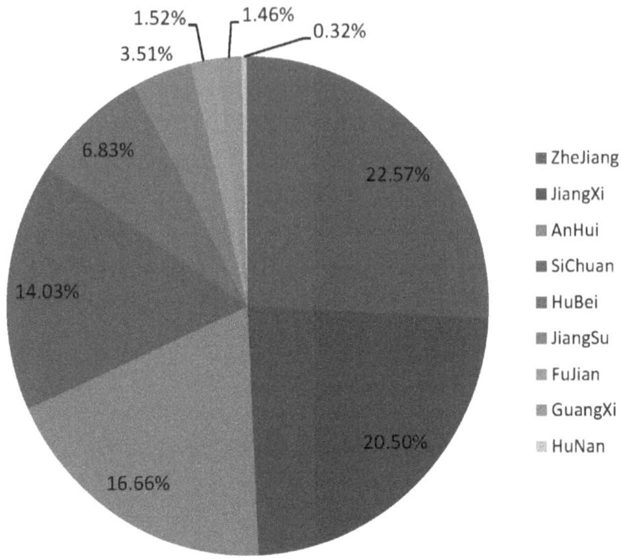

Figure 1 Distribution of snail habitat areas for mountainous and hilly region in The People's Republic of China.

2. EPIDEMIOLOGICAL FEATURES OF SCHISTOSOMIASIS IN MOUNTAINOUS AND HILLY REGION

2.1 Epidemiological distribution

As confirmed by numerous epidemiological investigations, schistosomiasis endemic areas of the mountainous type are distributed in 178 counties in 11 provinces of The People's Republic of China (Table 1). The mountainous-type environment is complex, including lofty mountain ranges, intermountain basins and rolling hills. The differing epidemiological characteristics of schistosomiasis transmission, snail habitat features and prevention and control strategies have led to the division of the mountainous endemic areas into three subtypes: flatlands, hills and high mountains (Mao, 1991; Liu et al., 1991).

2.2 Classification of endemic areas and epidemiological features

2.2.1 The flatland subtype

The flatland subtype (Fig. 2) is mainly located in the basin areas of Sichuan and Yunnan provinces (Mao, 1991). Flatlands in Sichuan account only for 41% of snail-infested areas, but contribute to 68% of all schistosomiasis cases.

Table 1 Distribution of snail habitat areas in The People's Republic of China, 2014

Province	Area (hm^2)	Marshland and lake region (hm^2)		Plain region with waterway networks (hm^2)	Hilly and mountainous region (hm^2)
Shanghai	1.74	0	0	1.74	0
Jiangsu	2253.75	0	2094.53	145.14	14.08
Zhejiang	69.47	0	0	0.4	69.07
Anhui	27,279.93	0	24,341.19	0	2938.79
Fujian	3.17	0	0	0	3.17
Jiangxi	78,720.95	0	76,907.04	0	1813.90
Hubei	76,165.12	21,516.28	52,219.69	0.00	2429.15
Hunan	175,910.47	829.02	174,096.01	0.00	985.44
Guangdong	0	0	0	0	0
Guangxi	5.430	0	0	0	5.430
Sichuan	2525.29	0	0	0	2525.29
Yunnan	1389.06	0	0	0	1389.06
Total	364,324.38	22,345.30	329,658.46	147.28	12,173.38

However, in Yunnan province, the flatland subtype is characterized by arable land, abundant water resources in lowlands, sparse population density, isolated communities and lack of water in highland. It causes 90% of cases and *Oncomelania* spp. snail habitat in flatland areas (Sun, 1981). In Sichuan province, habitat is primarily distributed in the counties of the Chengdu Plain and some townships in the drainage basin of the Anning River which lies in the Panzhihua-Xichang region (Jin and Yao, 1989). In Yunnan province, the flatland subtype is in Dali, Midu, Gejiu, Xiangyun, Xiaguan, Weishan, Eryuan, Jianchuan, Heqing and Lijiang counties (Sun, 1981). These environments are characterized by subtropical climate and developed water systems in which the preferred breeding sites of *Oncomelania* snails are in irrigation ditches (Dong et al., 2008). As a result of the nature of the

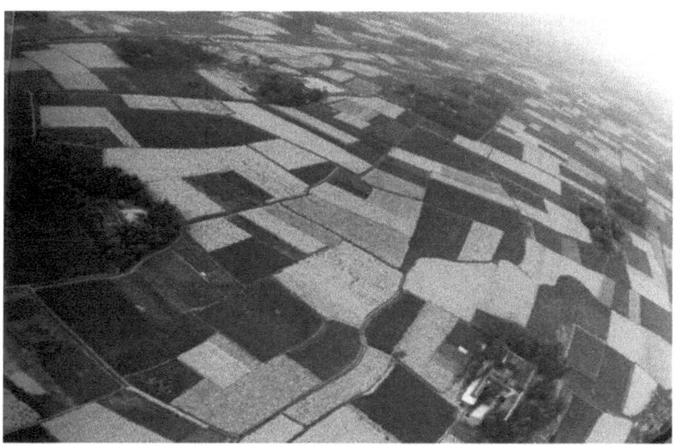

Figure 2 Geographical pattern of the flatland subtype for snail habitat in mountainous and hilly region.

agriculture, residents have frequent water contact, contributing to a high burden of disease. About 50% of the endemic villages in Sichuan province belong to the flatland subtype (Wu et al., 2008; Yin et al., 2002). In flatland areas, infected *Oncomelania* spp. are also distributed in the vicinity of residential areas, adjacent to sidewalks and near septic tanks, but the infection rate is generally not more than 1%.

The flatland areas are characterized by rich fertile soil crisscrossed by canals and gullies, which results in snail habitat in clustered distributions. The irrigation water flows through main canals to branch and lateral canals, and then to ditches and sublateral canals. The canal width gradually narrows and water velocity also decreases. The weeds in the waterways also increase as the water velocity decreases and it has also been found that ditches and sublateral canals are the most suitable living environment for snails (Gu, 1987). The flatland areas are mainly employed for rice cultivation and 95% of the paddy fields that contain snails are connected with ditches that also contain snails. The snails in the paddy fields are generally located along the edge within 5 m of the inlet or along the edge close to the ditches that contain snails. In wetlands, the highest density of snails is distributed around these paddy fields. As for other environments such as graveyard, water pools, springs, ponds, dry land, bamboo forests, etc., snails can also be found but in smaller numbers. Owing to the simple topography and improvements in economic, irrigation and agricultural conditions, lining ditches with concrete has achieved good effects in reducing snail habitat with the number of snails in the flatland areas having been greatly reduced. At present, the flatland area is no longer of high priority for snail prevention and control (Yin et al., 2002).

In the flatland areas at higher elevations, highly developed agriculture has led to a decrease of farm cattle. Hence, humans are responsible for up to 88% of the schistosome egg excretion to the environment, with cattle being responsible for most of the remainder. Dogs and voles have been found to be infected, but contribute little to the transmission cycle due to their low infection rate and small amount of faeces (Gu,1993; Xu et al., 1995, 2001).

2.2.2 The hill subtype

In the hill subtype areas (Fig. 3), because of increasing altitude and corresponding lower temperatures, the characteristics of the schistosomiasis epidemic change (Yang and Chen, 2011). Research carried out in Sichuan and Yunnan provinces showed that the *Oncomelania* spp. natural infection rate and the schistosomiasis infection rate of people and animals both

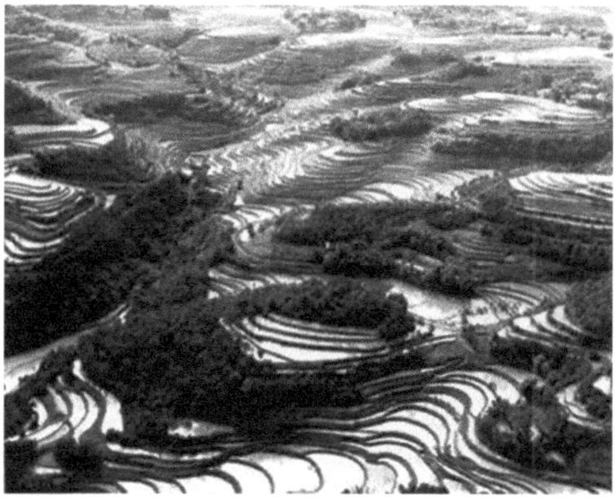

Figure 3 Geographical pattern of the hill subtype for snail habitat in mountainous and hilly region.

gradually declined with increasing altitude. However, infection rates remain difficult to predict between regions, even at the same altitude. For instance, there are 97 endemic villages and towns in Sichuan distributed below 1800 m (Dong et al., 2008) while in Weishan county of Yunnan province, 95% of *Oncomelania* spp. habitat and 97% of infected *Oncomelania* spp. are distributed between 1800 and 2150 m above sea level. In areas where the annual average temperature is below 16°C and the monthly average temperature does not exceed 20°C for more than 3 months, uninfected *Oncomelania* spp. populations can be observed.

In the hill subtype, due to these large differences in altitude and rugged and scattered terrain, most cultivated areas support terrace-style farming of rice and upland crops (Wu et al., 2008). This subtype is mainly distributed on the border of flatlands and central basins of the 11 schistosomiasis endemic provinces except Shanghai (Lu et al., 2013). Snail distribution is scattered among bamboo gardens, rice paddies and untilled land, where more serious epidemic conditions have occurred (Jin and Yao, 1989; Guo, 2008). In Sichuan province, hilly endemic villages are mainly found surrounding the Chengdu plain. The hill subtype accounts for 43% of endemic villages, 23% of snail habitat areas and 29% of schistosomiasis cases in 1980s (Jin and Yao, 1989; Yin et al., 2002). No endemic areas are classified as hilly in Yunnan province.

Hill subtype areas have the most widely distributed snail populations primarily located at the edge of the flatland areas or of the central basins. Isolated snails are scattered in various environments such as terraced fields, ditches, dry land, ponds, wooded land, etc. (Institute of Parasitic Diseases

Control, 1961, 1978a; Gu et al., 1986). Fields and dry land are the major living environment for most snails with more than 50% of the snails in such places, while there are only about 10% living in irrigation furrows, wild grassland or ditches near houses. Due to uneven topography, most of the lowland fields are irrigated by the surplus water from the upland fields and the snails in the lowland fields are affected by those in the upland fields. Furthermore, the snails in the fields and ditches also affect each other since the snails in the ditches can flow into the fields during high water flow events and vice versa. Due to the relatively complicated topography in the hill areas, snail control continues to be difficult.

In hilly regions with uneven terrain, infected *Oncomelania* spp. are distributed in an isolated and scattered fashion, not discriminating between water ditches close or far from residential habitation (Gu et al., 1993; Yin et al., 2003; Guo et al., 1999). However, this distribution is related to local human activities and animal grazing habits and it tends to be stable over time. *Oncomelania* spp. infection rates and human infection rates are positively related (Liu et al., 1992). But due to the different densities in paddy fields and on dry land, opportunities for residents to contact contaminated water in agriculture and in daily life are also different, and even in neighbouring villages, infection rates of residents can differ. An important factor is that the local people use farmyard manure, a mixture of human and animal waste, which is washed into the ditches where both snails and humans are exposed to the free swimming forms of the parasite; the villagers are exposed, for example, while washing clothes and the like (Liu et al., 1992; Mao et al., 2004, 2006; Guo et al., 1999; Wu et al., 2004).

In the hill areas, large numbers of cattle and horses are needed for agricultural cultivation. As a result, cattle and humans are the major mammalian hosts of the parasite followed by pigs and dogs, while sheep, cats and voles are minor targets of infection (Liu et al., 1992). Due to frequent trading of domestic animals in these areas, infected animals can easily spread schistosome eggs. The local residents are exposed by water contact in daily life and in agricultural activities while the children and teenagers are exposed by water contact while playing in or near water. The infection sites are mainly terraced fields and ditches. In the early 2000s, a case of acute schistosomal infection was detected in the hill areas in Sichuan province (Wu et al., 2006) and the result showed that the infection source was domestic animals and the rate of schistosome infection was relatively high both among local residents and animals (Yin et al., 2002; Wu et al., 2005a,b; Gu et al., 1993).

2.2.3 The high mountain subtype

The high mountain subtype (Fig. 4) is mainly distributed in lofty mountains and steep hills of Sichuan and Yunnan provinces (Mao, 1991). In Sichuan, it is mainly in the mountains on the western margin of the Sichuan basin and the Panzhihua-Xichang area (Jin and Yao, 1989) which accounts for 36% of the total snail habitat areas. In Yunnan province, this subtype is mainly distributed in Nanjian, Ningbo, Binchuan, Lufeng, Yangmo, Yunlong, Chuxiong, Yongsheng and other counties which only account for 5% of snail habitat areas in Yunnan (Sun, 1981). These areas are characterized by complex geographical environments, water independence, open hillside terraces and grassy slopes overgrown with weeds. Terrace agriculture uses water from natural precipitation or mountain streams or springs (Yin et al., 2002). Awareness of schistosomiasis is low among minority populations in these areas due to economic difficulties and cultural differences (Jin and Yao, 1989). Furthermore, low resident living standards and poor working conditions, as well as poor transportation, make schistosomiasis control extremely difficult. The State Council's pilot implementation of integrated schistosomiasis control in this region is targeted at the difficulties in high mountain valley endemic areas, which include poor living and sanitary conditions, and scattered populations living in marginal lands mixed with livestock. Under such conditions, infection rates can be as high as 30% (Wu et al., 2009). Owing to socio-economic development and water conservancy, agriculture and land improvement projects, snail habitats in the Pingba area have been greatly reduced, and have ceased to be the

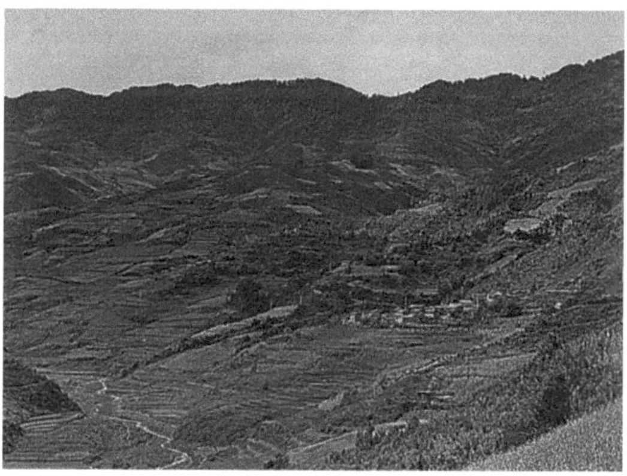

Figure 4 Geographical pattern of the high mountain subtype for snail habitat in mountainous and hilly region.

primary focus of prevention efforts (Yin et al., 2002), which now focus on the high mountain and hillside areas with entrenched poor economic situations and unfavourable environmental conditions.

In high mountain areas, snail habitats occur in highly complex topological environments, but with limited scope of activity and dispersal ability. The snails occur in a clustered or dotted distribution (Yang et al., 2001). Their major living environment includes terrace edges, small transverse furrows, waste lands, mud fields, permeable rocks, slopes with water seepage, valleys and graveyards (Jin and Yao, 1989; Dong et al., 2008). The snail habitat on the slopes is in an isolated and dispersed state with the area ranging from dozens to hundreds of square metres. Those habitats spread downwards and, again, form clusters. The snails on the top of the mountain can also spread downwards under the force of rainstorms. In the mountain areas with a high degree of reclamation and rice cultivation, terraced fields are the major living environment for snails which, while distributed around the whole field, are mainly concentrated in the higher end of the edge. In the mountain areas where dry land crops are mainly cultivated, the wild lands and drainage ditches are the major living environment for the snails. In the vast and sparsely populated areas with a low degree of reclamation, major living environments of snails include vast areas of virgin slopes, grassland, river basin and swamp-shaped regions which are soaked in water all the year round (Institute of Parasitic Diseases Control, 1978b).

Due to limited arable land in high mountain areas, pastoral agriculture is the major economic activity. Thus, the number of domestic animals such as cattle, sheep, horses and goats is enormous and in some regions, the number of domestic animals exceeds that of the local residents. A study was conducted in Sichuan province to explore the major infection sources of schistosomiasis in the hill regions and it was found that the index of potential contamination (IPC) reached 87.70% (Yin et al., 2003). Another study undertaken from 2001 to 2005 and carried out in six key counties of Yunnan province found that the infection rate among farm cattle was about 2.7%, but in some villages it was more than 10%, which was significantly higher than the human infection rate (Li et al., 2007). From this study, it was concluded that domestic animals were the major infection source in this environment followed by humans (Dong et al., 2008; Xu et al., 1995). Trade of livestock and other domestic animals spreads infected animals throughout entire regions, which further promotes the enlargement of epidemic regions (Zheng et al., 2000; Wang and Zheng, 1995). In the hills, the major infection sites are terraced fields and the prevention and control work in these areas is relatively more difficult. A historical review shows that local residents and domestic animals had a higher infection rate of schistosome than those living in the flatland areas (Yin et al., 2002; Wu et al., 2005a,b, 2007).

In summary, mountain areas are characterized by low population density, large land areas, complex topology and high infection rates of *Oncomelania*. Infected *Oncomelania* are mainly distributed in barren pastures, water pools and rice paddies, and there is no obvious relationship to distance from the residential areas. The infection rate of *Oncomelania* is comparatively high in regions of cattle grazing. The exposure of residents is influenced by the terrain and the extent of rural development which varies by region.

In summary, because of the scarcity of arable lands in the high mountain areas, semi-farming and semi-husbandry is the main economic base, livestock populations often exceed human populations, the source of infection is mainly domestic animals and *Oncomelania* spp. are mainly distributed in noncultivated and reclaimed lands (Tables 2 and 3). In mountain bench terraces and flatlands, traditional agriculture is predominant. Infection source are given priority to farmers which are infected by using human waste as an agricultural fertilizer. (Meng et al., 2001). In the suburbs of rural industrialization, the suitable *Oncomelania* spp. is reduced, farm cattle almost disappear and infection of residents is also sharply reduced (Huang et al., 1957). Here, schistosomiasis presents strong seasonal trends in infection. Surveys show that in hilly-type endemic areas, schistosomiasis infection presents two peaks, namely in June and in September. In the regions with different social and economic structures, the epidemic characteristics of schistosomiasis are also different to some degree. Studies have shown that schistosome infection is closely linked with the degree of educational attainment, family income and degree of water contact, and that these features vary by ethnic region (Liu et al., 2014). The infection rate of residents who are engaged in economic crop cultivation is significantly higher than that of the other workers (Meng et al., 2001). Schistosomiasis clustering characteristics can reduce spatial clustering due to changes in the environment, the changed economic conditions can reduce family clustering and the implementation of the prevention and control works seasonal can reduce temporal clustering so as to achieve the purpose of reducing schistosomiasis epidemic (Wang, 2006).

Table 2 Result of human infection survey in different endemic regions[a]

Region	Serological test		Etiological test		Average infection rate	Epg of patient		Epg of people	
	No. examined	No. positive	No. examined	No. positive		Mean	Geometric mean	Mean	Geometric mean
Flatland subtype	52,126	4672	4246	107	0.27	76.71	27.54	1.93	0.09
Mountain subtype	13,400	4516	4131	549	7.1	71.81	24.59	9.54	0.54
Hill subtype	59,909	5985	5816	402	1.01	82.57	35.85	5.71	0.28
Total	125,435	15,173	14,193	1058	1.06	76.39	28.71	5.69	0.29

[a]The third National Epidemiological Survey in 2004. Epg = The number of eggs per gram faeces.

Table 3 Result of bovine infection survey in different endemic regions[a]

	Cattle			Water buffalo		
Region	**No. examined**	**No. positive**	**(%)**	**No. examined**	**No. positive**	**(%)**
Flatland subtype	789	17	2.15	822	6	0.73
Mountain subtype	627	23	3.67	412	13	3.16
Hill subtype	544	14	2.57	1,693	48	2.84
Total	2,136	72	3.37	2,999	82	2.73

[a]The third National Epidemiological Survey in 2004.

3. PREVENTION AND CONTROL STRATEGY

Schistosomiasis control strategy changed with time, shifted from single measure to comprehensive control efforts (Xu et al., 2016a,b,c). Control in the 1950s focused on humans and livestock (Huang et al., 1957), shifting to snail elimination in the 1960s to the early 1980s. With the advent of the drug praziquantel, chemotherapy was the primary strategy. However, single measures could not consolidate the effect of control. With the re-emergence of schistosomiasis at the beginning of 21st century in some regions of The People's Republic of China, a government-directed and multi-department strategy was implemented, which showed the important place of the government in schistosomiasis control (Zheng et al., 2006). The comprehensive strategy now emphasizes infection source control.

3.1 First phase (1950s–1980s)

From the 1950s to the 1960s, after broad investigations of the schistosomiasis epidemic, preliminary data of key areas of distribution and prevalence features came to light. Sources of infection were controlled, patient treatment was carried out and decontamination of waste was implemented. Because of the significant cardiovascular and hepatic toxic side effects of antimonial agents, this chemotherapeutic was eliminated until the early 1980s (Zhang et al., 2005). Owing to the limited national financial ability during those years, funding for the harmless decontamination of human excrement was lacking; therefore, the government mobilized rural people to eradicate the *Oncomelania* spp., the intermediate snail host of *S. japonicum*, to block the transmission route. Thus, in the 1970s, extensive *Oncomelania* spp. eradication was executed in reclamation areas in concert with developing basic agricultural exploitation (Li et al., 2016). Meanwhile the professional team in disease control departments in charge of this issue in hilly endemic areas of The People's Republic of China found and concluded many effective methods for the eradication of *Oncomelania* snail, for example, the irrigation aqueduct system was redeveloped and improved, affected farmlands were sterilized and the land surfaces containing *Oncomelania* were deeply buried in Dujiangyan (dam area in northwest Chengdu plain). Mianzhu Center for Disease Control (CDC) in Sichuan province was more experienced in the management of human excrement and optimal antiparasitic therapy for local patients; in mountainous and hill areas they developed agriculture in terraced fields which was not the most suitable breeding area for *Oncomelania* snail. In high mountain regions as Tianquan, Lushan and Xichang, the local CDC investigated many special methods for the eradication of *Oncomelania* snails and antiparasitic therapy for local patients to be applied in the special environment of high mountain regions in western Sichuan (Wu et al., 2008). Despite early success, inevitable mistakes and setbacks were encountered; during the Cultural Revolution period (1970s), the local government implemented unscientific agricultural development, leading to introduction of *Oncomelania* snails to non-endemic hill areas through forest reclamation, inadvertently spreading schistosomiasis in wider regions (Wang et al., 2009; Yang et al., 2016).

3.2 Second phase (1980s–2000)

After the 1980s, morbidity control became the focal point of schistosomiasis control strategy, owing to the success of praziquantel for the clinical treatment (Wang et al., 2009). The strategy concluded to implement chemotherapy for both humans and livestock. The investigation for treatment and snail elimination in Sichuan and Yunnan provinces showed that new infection rate fell down from 17.3% to 0 (Guo, 2006), and the stool positive rate in Zongguan residents was reduced from 62.2% in 1980 to 0 in 1985 in Yongsheng county of Yunnan province. The stool positive rate of Guishan residents was reduced from 17.4% in 1981 to 3.0% in 1984 in Qionglai county of Sichuan province. The stool positive rate of cattle was reduced from 18.3% to 0. These results demonstrated the strategy was very effective with regards to schistosomiasis control (Xiao et al., 2004; Chen et al., 2005).

In the 1990s, support from the World Bank Loan Project (WBLP) for schistosomiasis control made massive chemotherapy possible in hilly areas. After implementation of strategies with an emphasis on human and livestock control, the epidemic came under effective control. The number of chronic schistosomiasis patients was reduced to 12,000 in Sichuan and Yunnan provinces, 14.92% of the national burden. In this period, Guangdong, Fujian Guangxi and Zhejiang provinces reached transmission interruption.

With the WBLP finished, the number of infected individuals remained steady at 800,000 between 2002 and 2004 (Xiao et al., 2004; Hao et al.,2005, 2006). After much study, scholars found that reinfection was the primary cause of the high rate of schistosomiasis infection (Utzinger et al., 2005; Guo et al., 2006; Balen et al., 2007). Chemotherapy focused on clinical treatment failed to interrupt transmission, which was facilitated by untreated stool, allowing for reinfection of people and livestock. Stool management is a key point for schistosomiasis control (Wang, 2005).

3.3 Third phase (2004 to now)

Benefitting from prevention and control work, epidemic situations in hilly regions is in decline. An epidemiological survey has shown (Department of Disease Control, 2006) that human and cattle infection rates fell by 55.21% and 56.61% in 1995 to 60.6% and 72.56% in 2004, in Sichuan and Yunnan provinces, respectively. Nonetheless, the human infection rate of the mountain subtype endemic area increased by 20% (Department of Disease Control, 2006). The study by Wang Rubo et al. on the re-emerging situation of schistosomiasis epidemics in 2004 showed that re-emergence was seen in 52.94% (9/17) and 71.43% (15/21) of hilly region in the counties which previously achieved transmission control or interruption status (Wang et al., 2004). This indicated difficulties in epidemic control and suggests efforts be focused on hilly endemic areas which are economically underdeveloped and with more serious epidemic situations.

National Health and Family Planning Commission (NHFPC, formerly the Ministry of Health) put forward a new strategy since 2004 to control infection sources: using tractor instead of cattle farming, the prohibition on grazing livestock in snail habitat areas and creation and use of livestock pens, conversion of sanitary latrines, construction of biogas digesters and other measures, strengthen the management and decontamination of human and animal waste (Qi and Lian, 2002). In flatland regions, where agriculture is the primary source of livelihood, better economic situation results in tractors taking precedence over cattle for farming, construction of sanitary latrines and digesters, land modulation, transformation of snail habitats in some areas and monitoring of the imported source to consolidate schistosomiasis control (Liu et al., 1992). In hill and mountain subtype areas, owing to complex topology, agricultural production is less developed than in the flatland subtype area. Since livestock is a major transportation and agricultural tool, livestock is a significant reservoir of infection (Yang and Chen, 2011; Liu et al., 1992). Under such conditions, replacement of livestock with tractors is difficult and schistosomiasis control is best accomplished by implementation of comprehensive control measures, including combination of programs lead by water affairs, forestry, agriculture sectors and so on (Liu et al., 1992; Wang et al., 2004; Cao et al., 2016).

4. EFFECTIVENESS OF SCHISTOSOMIASIS CONTROL

4.1 Changes of epidemic status

Owing to a combination of scientific research and control and prevention efforts, and adjustment of control strategies, the schistosomiasis epidemics in hilly type areas in western The People's Republic of China has gradually been decreased, infection rate declined year by year. National schistosomiasis epidemiology survey data showed (Department of Disease Control, 2006) that human and cattle infection rates have fallen from 55.21% and 56.61% in 1995 to 60.6% and 72.56% in 2004 in Sichuan and Yunnan provinces, respectively. However, there is still 8.48% human infection rate in mountain subtype areas, with higher cattle infection rates (Department of Disease Control, 2006). These statistics indicate the difficulties of the control efforts; given rapid economic development in flatland endemic areas, further control and prevention work should focus on serious epidemic regions with less economic development.

By the end of 2013, the actual snail area was 365,468.00 hm^2 in the hilly and mountainous region, with the hilly type epidemic region of 12,624.23 hm^2 which accounted for 3.45% of the national snail habitat areas (Lei et al., 2014). The proportion of patients with schistosomiasis in Sichuan and Yunnan provinces fell from 29.34% to 0.2% in 1981 (Mao, 1991; Lei et al., 2014), revealing effective control of the epidemic situation.

4.2 Achievements toward control goal

Since 2004, with The People's Republic of China's overall strategy adjustment, great strides have been achieved in Sichuan and Yunnan provinces by means of implementation of comprehensive control measures with emphasis on infection source control (Wang et al., 2009), resulting in achievement of transmission control in 2008 and 2010, respectively (Lei et al., 2014). Zhejiang, Fujian, Guangdong and Guangxi provinces, where priority is given to hilly type epidemic areas, have achieved transmission interruption. As of 2014, among the 178 counties belonging to hilly subtype epidemic regions, 110 have reached transmission control status and another 64 have reached transmission interruption. Resulting from efforts based on guidelines set by The People's Republic of China CDC, Sichuan province will likely be able to achieve complete transmission interruption by 2015.

4.3 Case studies

Schistosomiasis control strategies have proven success in Sichuan and Yunnan provinces through application of comprehensive methods closely integrated with social and economic development, which are summarized in the following case studies:

1. Pujiang mode – Small watershed harness
   The main characteristic of this model is to conduct small and mini water source projects combined with human and animal drinking water projects in hilly regions, such as mountain plateau pond regulation, water pipe hardening, etc. and cooperation with the reform of the middle-and-low-yielding fields, construction of ecological agriculture to significantly compress *Oncomelania* snail habitat environment and control schistosomiasis transmission (Gu, 1987; Yang et al., 2001; Gong, 2003).
2. Xichang mode – The overall development of agriculture
   Combined with the comprehensive agricultural development, including hardening of canal systems, development of hillside terraces, wet field transformation and structural adjustment of farming, transformation of rice fields into dry land, etc., have effectively controlled the snail habitat area and achieved the goal of schistosomiasis elimination (Spear et al., 2006; Xu, 1996).
3. Eryuan mode – Control of infectious sources
   Based on the conventional measures of infection control, source control such as prohibiting grazing in snail area, fixed-point livestock grazing, stable cattle, toilets amelioration, building biogas digesters, etc., should be carried out (Li et al., 2001; Yang et al., 2009; Zheng, 1990; Zheng, 1999; Qiu et al., 2001). Promotion of these measures has changed local ecosystems, traditional living and production habits, aided in the compression of snail habitats, effectively controlled sources of infection and transmission, reduced contamination and lowered probability of infection. The development in local economies, as a result of the control programme, suggested this is a sustainable method for combating schistosomiasis in local settings.

5. LOOKING FORWARD

Through the efforts of multiple generations of professionals over decades in the mountainous and hilly endemic areas of The People's Republic of China, great progress has been made towards elimination of the disease. Such efforts protect the welfare and health of people and livestock, enhance their productivity and quality of life in endemic areas and lead to great social and economic benefits. However, challenges remain in areas with complex environmental features and less developed socioeconomic settings, especially in the context of ethnic minority populations, where emergence may occur sometimes (Zhang et al., 2016a,b). Implementation of comprehensive control measures with emphasis on infection source control is a significant strategic adjustment in The People's Republic of China at the present stage (Qi and Lian, 2002). It is also an effective way to control and eliminate schistosomiasis in mountainous and hilly endemic regions. In this context, it is meaningful to monitor infection sources in both human and animals. Since the disease has re-emerged in areas previously considered controlled, we should pay close attention to the surveillance, strengthening cooperation among multiple related departments, identifying and controlling epidemics on time and promoting schistosomiasis awareness among the public (Tambo et al., 2014). At the same time, we should actively explore diagnosis technologies with high sensitivity and specificity, suitable for mass screening of people which is more targeted to treat and eliminate the source of infection. In addition, we should also actively implement snail control work in high-risk areas to prevent expansion of *Oncomelania* snail areas to reduce the risk of infection.

New strategy which can adapt to the current social and economic development need to be further explored in the region, in order to promote control work effectively, and strive to achieve the goal of elimination in 2025. It is the time to continuously improve strategies, or create new and more effective ones, to form sustainable methods for interruption of schistosomiasis transmission in the region.

At the same time, in the face of the contradiction between the generally low level of prevalence and technology which have not meet the goal of the national schistosomiasis elimination programme, we need to actively explore new methods such as sensitive diagnostic techniques, early warning monitoring systems and digital database construction (Zheng et al., 2013; Tambo et al., 2015; Wiwanitkit et al., 2015; Feng et al., 2016; Wang et al., 2016; Zhang et al., 2016a,b). Such advancements would be of great significance for interrupting transmission and ensuring improvement of health and welfare, and could further promote economic and social development in the regions. Finally, those experiences may also able to transfer into other low- and middle-income countries of the world (Xu et al., 2016a,b,c).

ACKNOWLEDGEMENTS

This work was supported by China UK Global Health Support Programme (GHSP-OP101)-China's Experiences in Control of Malaria and Schistosomiasis: Relevant to LMICs through Distillation, Synthesis and Dissemination Approaches.

REFERENCES

Balen, J., Zhao, Z.Y., Williams, G.M., et al., 2007. Prevalence, intensity and associated morbidity of *Schistosoma japonicum* infection in the Dongting Lake region, China. Bull. World Health Organ. 85 (7), 519–526.

Cao, Z.G., Zhao, Y.E., Willingham, A.L., Wang, T.P., 2016. Towards the elimination of schistosomiasis japonica through control of the disease in domestic animals in the People's Republic of China: a tale of over 60 years. Adv. Parasitol. 92.

Chen, M.G., 2014. Assessment of morbidity due to *Schistosoma japonicum* infection in China. Infect. Dis. Poverty 3, 6.

Chen, X.Y., Wang, L.Y., Cai, J.M., et al., 2005. Schistosomiasis control in China: the impact of a 10 year World Bank Loan Project (1992–2001). Bull. World Health Organ. 83 (1), 43–48 (in Chinese).

Chitsulo, L., Engels, D., Montresor, A., Savioli, L., 2000. The global status of schistosomiasis and its control. Acta Trop. 77, 41–51.

Collins, C., Xu, J., Tang, S., 2012. Schistosomiasis control and the health system in P.R. China. Infect. Dis. Poverty 1, 8.

Dabo, A., Diarra, A.Z., Machault, V., Toure, O., Niambele, D.S., Kante, A., et al., 2015. Urban schistosomiasis and associated determinant factors among school children in Bamako, Mali, West Africa. Infect. Dis. Poverty 4, 4.

Department of Disease Control, 2006. Prevalence of Schistosomiasis in China–Report on Randon Survey in 2004. Shanghai Scientific and Technological Literature Press, 2006, Shanghai (in Chinese).

Dong, X.Q., Feng, X.G., Dong, Y., 2008. Epidemiological characteristics and control strategies of schistosomiasis in mountainous areas of Yunnan Province. Chin. J. Schistosomiasis Control 20 (2), 135–137 (in Chinese).

Feng, Y., Liu, L., Xia, S., Xu, J.F., Bergquist, R., Yang, G.J., 2016. Reaching the surveillance-response stage of schistosomiasis control in the People's Republic of China: a modelling approach. Adv. Parasitol. 92.

Gong, Q., 2003. Snail control effect by small-size irrigation works in Pujiang County. Parasit. Infect. Dis. 1 (3), 126–127 (in Chinese).

Gu, X.G., 1993. Study on prevalence regulations and control strategies of schistosomiasis in Sichuan Province. J. Prev. Med. Inf. S1, 21–22 (in Chinese).

Gu, X.G., Zhao, W.X., Xu, F.S., et al., 1986. Cause from snail-existent non-endemic areas in Sichuan Province. Progress on the epidemiology of schistosomiasis. Jiangsu Med. J. 249–253 (in Chinese).

Gu, X.G., Zhao, W.X., Xu, F.S., et al., 1993. Typical epidemiological survey of schistosomiasis in mountainous areas of Sichuan Province. Chin. J. Schistosomiasis Control 5 (2), 82–85 (in Chinese).
Gu, X.G., 1987. Compilation of Schistosomiasis Reasearch Data (1980–1985), 404(Unpublished).
Guo, J., Li, Y., Gray, D., et al., 2006. A drug-based intervention study on the importance of buffaloes for human *Schistosoma japonicum* infection around Poyang Lake, People's Republic of China. Am. J. Trop. Med. Hyg. 74 (2), 335–341.
Guo, J.G., 2006. Status and role of strategy for control of sources of infection of schistosomiasis in China. Chin. J. Schistosomiasis Control 18 (3), 3 (in Chinese).
Guo, J.G., 2008. Prevalence and control of schistosomiasis in hilly regions in China. Chin. J. Prev. Med. 42 (8), 2 (in Chinese).
Guo, W.Y., Lai, J., Wu, Z.S., et al., 1999. Characteristics of infected snail distribution in Xichang schistosomiasis epidemiological demonstration area. J. Pract. Parasit. Dis. 7 (1), 40 (in Chinese).
Hao, Y., Wu, X.H., Xia, G., et al., 2005. Schistosomiasis situation in People's Republic of China in 2004. Chin. J. Schistosomiasis Control 7 (6), 401–404.
Hao, Y., Wu, X.H., Xia, G., et al., 2006. Schistosomiasis situation in People's Republic of China in 2005. Chin. J. Schistosomiasis Control 8 (5), 321–324.
Huang, M.X., Pan, R.S., Hong, S.J., 1957. Schistosoma and Schistosomiasis. People's Medical Publishing House, Beijing, pp. 130–140 (in Chinese).
Institute of Parasitic Diseases Control, 1961. Parasitic Research Materials (1956–1960), pp. 133–137.
Institute of Parasitic Diseases Control, 1978a. Parasitic Research Materials (1965–1960), pp. 161–167.
Institute of Parasitic Diseases Control, 1978b. The Relationship Between Characteristics of Snail Distribution and Schistosomiasis Endemic (1965–1977), pp. 183–185 (in Chinese).
Jin, J.M., Yao, M.J., 1989. Endemic features of schistosomiasis in Sichuan Province. Chin. J. Schistosomiasis Control 01, 13–15 (in Chinese).
Lei, Z.L., Zhen, H., Zhang, L.J., Zhu, R., Xu, Z.M., Xu, J., Fu, Q., Wang, Q., Li, S.Z., Zhou, X.N., 2014. Endemic status of schistosomiasis in People's Republic of China in 2013. Chin. J. Schistosomiasis Control 06, 591–597 (in Chinese).
Li, Z.J., Ge, J., Dai, J.R., Wen, L.Y., Lin, D.D., Madsen, H., et al., 2016. Biology and control of snail intermediate host of *Schistosoma japonicum* in the People's Republic of China. Adv. Parasitol. 92.
Li, J., Duan, G., Dong, G., 2007. Investigation on domestic animal schistosomiasis in Yunnan Province, 2001–2005. China Anim. Husb. Vet. Med. 34 (8), 107–109 (in Chinese).
Li, X.B., Yang, L.G., Yang, C.S., Lan, E.X., 2001. Four years' schistosomiasis control effect in a village in hyper-endemic plain area of Yunnan Province. J. Pract. Parasit. Dis. 01, 33 (in Chinese).
Liu, L., Yang, G.J., Zhu, H.R., Yang, K., Ai, L., 2014. Knowledge of, attitudes towards, and practice relating to schistosomiasis in two subtypes of a mountainous region of the People's Republic of China. Infect. Dis. Poverty 3, 16.
Liu, B.Z., Liu, C.Y., Zhang, G.S., et al., 1992. Epidemiological characteristics of schistosomiasis in mountainous areas. Chin. J. Schistosomiasis Control 4 (4), 305–307 (in Chinese).
Liu, B.Z., Wei, J.B., Wang, F.H., et al., 1991. Analysis of two kinds of control strategies for schistosomiasis. Chin. J. Schistosomiasis Control 3 (5), 292–294 (in Chinese).
Lu, L.T., Zhu, R., Zhang, L.J., 2013. Evolution of schistosomiasis control and prevention strategies in hilly regions with schistosomiasis endemic in China. Chin. J. Schistosomiasis Control 05, 528–532 (in Chinese).

Mao, S.B., 1991. Schistosoma Biology and Schistosomiasis Control. People's medical publishing house, Beijing, p. 636 (in Chinese).
Mao, Y., Liang, L., Shan, J.Z., et al., 2006. Snail screen in ditches of Changqiu Mountain area, Sichuan from 2003 to 2004. Parasit. Infect. Dis. 4 (4), 180–181 (in Chinese).
Mao, Y., Meng, X.H., Yang, C.H., et al., 2004. To fit infected snail in Xichang City, Sichuan mountainous terrace area with negative binomial distribution. Parasit. Infect. Dis. 2 (1), 44 (in Chinese).
Meng, X.H., Yang, Y., Wu, Z.S., et al., 2001. Research on family clustering of schistosomiasis in Meishan City of Sichuan province. J. Pract. Parasit. Dis. 9 (2), 70 (in Chinese).
Qi, Y.L., Lian, Z.Q., 2002. Study on the strategy of maintain schistosomiasis control results in Yunnan plateaus. Chin. J. Schistosomiasis Control 04, 279–280 (in Chinese).
Qiu, Y.f., Li, J.R., Xu, L., 2001. Surveillance on schistosomiasis for 8 years in hilly regions. Chin. J. Schistosomiasis Control 13 (5), 315 (in Chinese).
Salam, R.A., Maredia, H., Das, J.K., Lassi, Z.S., Bhutta, Z.A., 2014. Community-based interventions for the prevention and control of helmintic neglected tropical diseases. Infect. Dis. Poverty 3, 23.
Spear, R.C., Seto, E., Remais, J., Carlton, E.J., Davis, G., Qiu, D., et al., 2006. Fighting waterborne infectious diseases. Science 314, 1081–1082 (in Chinese).
Sun, D.L., 1981. A brief history of discovery and prevalence of schistosomiasis in Yunnan Province. Med. Pharm. Yunnan 03, 51–54 (in Chinese).
Tambo, E., Ai, L., Zhou, X., Chen, J.H., Hu, W., Bergquist, R., et al., 2014. Surveillance-response systems: the key to elimination of tropical diseases. Infect. Dis. Poverty 3, 17.
Tambo, E., Khater, E.I., Chen, J.H., Bergquist, R., Zhou, X.N., 2015. Nobel Prize for the artemisinin and ivermectin discoveries: a great boost towards elimination of the global infectious diseases of poverty. Infect. Dis. Poverty 4, 58.
Utzinger, J., Zhou, X.N., Chen, M.G., et al., 2005. Conquering schistosomiasis in China: the long march. Acta Trop. 96 (2–3), 69–96.
Wang, X.Y., He, J., Yang, K., Liang, S., 2016. Applications of spatial technology in schistosomiasis control programme in the People's Republic of China. Adv. Parasitol. 92.
Wang, L.D., 2005. Management of human and animal feces is a key element for effective control of endemic schistosomiasis in China. Chin. J. Epidemiol. 26 (12), 929–930 (in Chinese).
Wang, L.D., 2006. Promotion of strategy transition for national schistosomiasis control programme by implementation of the regulation of schistosomiasis control in China. Chin. J. Prev. Med. 40 (4), 219–220 (in Chinese).
Wang, R.B., Wang, T.P., Wang, L.Y., et al., 2004. Study on the re-emerging situation of schistosomiasis epidemics in areas already under control and interruption. Chin. J. Epidemiol. 25 (7), 564–567 (in Chinese).
Wang, T.P., Chao, Z.G., Chen, H.G., et al., 2009. Changes of control strategy and improvement of schistosomiasis control in China. Chin. J. Schistosomiasis Control 21 (4), 241–242 (in Chinese).
Wang, X.F., Zhen, J., 1995. Relationship of the development of the livestock to schistosomiasis transmission in Yunnan Province. Chin. J. Schistosomiasis Control 7 (5), 262–266 (in Chinese).
Wiwanitkit, V., Tambo, E., Ugwu, E.C., Ngogang, J.Y., Zhou, X.N., 2015. Are surveillance response systems enough to effectively combat and contain the Ebola outbreak? Infect. Dis. Poverty 4, 7.
Wu, Z.S., Qian, X.H., Xu, L., et al., 2005a. Analysis on surveillance of schistosomiasis in Sichuan Province in 2005. J. Trop. Dis. Parasitol. 4 (4), 212–214 (in Chinese).
Wu, Z.S., Zhang, X.S., Zhong, B., et al., 2006. Analysis of acute schistosomiasis in Sichuan Province, 2003–2005. Chin. J. Schistosomiasis Control 17 (3), 386–387 (in Chinese).

Wu, Z.S., Xu, F.S., Qiu, D.C., 2008. Epidemiological characteristics and control strategies of schistosomiasis in Sichuan Province. Parasit. Infect. Dis. 01, 1–4 (in Chinese).
Wu, Z.S., Yihuo, W.L., Qiu, D.C., 2009. Schistosomiasis epidemic characteristic and effectiveness for comprehensive measure with emphasis on infectious resource control in high mountainous area in Sichuan Province. Parasit. Infect. Dis. 03, 126–130 (in Chinese).
Wu, Z.S., Yihuo, W.L., Wang, S.A., et al., 2007. Comprehensive measures for schistosomiasis control: analysis of epidemic situation in Tezi, Puge county, 2005–2006. Parasit. Infect. Dis. 5 (1), 43–44.
Wu, Z.S., Yin, H.Z., Zhao, L.G., et al., 2005b. Field study on ecology of *Oncomelania hupensis* using mark-recapture method. Chin. J. Schistosomiasis Control 17, 2089–2092 (in Chinese).
Wu, Z.S., Zhao, L.G., Mao, Y., 2004. Report on *Oncomelania* snail survey in ditches in basin around Qionghai Lake, Xichang, Sichuan Province. China 2002–2003. Chin. J. Schistosomiasis Control 16 (5), 359–361 (in Chinese).
Xiao, D.L., Yu, Q., Dang, H., et al., 2004. Schistosomiasis situation in People's Republic of China in 2003. Chin. J. Schistosomiasis Control 16 (6), 401–404 (in Chinese).
Xu, J., Bergquist, R., Qian, Y.J., Wang, Q., Yu, Q., Peeling, R., et al., 2016a. China-Africa and China-Asia collaboration on schistosomiasis control: a SWOT analysis. Adv. Parasitol. 92.
Xu, J., Steinman, P., Maybe, D., Zhou, X.N., Lv, S., Li, S.Z., et al., 2016b. Evolution of the national schistosomiasis control programmes in the People's Republic of China. Adv. Parasitol. 92.
Xu, J., Yu, Q., Tchuem-Tchuenté, L.A., Bergquist, R., Sacko, M., Utzinger, J., et al., 2016c. Enhancing collaboration between China and African countries for schistosomiasis control. Lancet Infect. Dis. http://dx.doi.org/10.1016/S1473-3099(1015)00360-00366. Published Online: 03 February 2016.
Xu, F.S., 1996. Effect of schistosomiasis control and prevention in Chuanxing County, Xichang, 1987–1995. J. Pract. Parasit. Dis. 129–130 (in Chinese).
Xu, F.S., Gu, X.G., Qiu, D.C., 2001. A quantitative study of schistosomiasis infection status in Chuanxing township of Xichang City. J. Pract. Parasit. Dis. 9 (4), 159–160 (in Chinese).
Xu, F.S., Gu, X.G., Zhao, W.X., 1995. The function of different sources of infection in schistosomiasis transmission in moutainous area. J. Pract. Parasit. Dis. 3 (3), 129 (in Chinese).
Yang, Y., Zhou, Y.B., Song, X.X., Li, S.Z., Zhong, B., Wang, T.P., et al., 2016. Integrated control strategy of schistosomiasis in the People's Republic of China: projects involving agriculture, water-conservancy, forestry, sanitation and environmental modification. Adv. Parasitol. 92.
Yang, A.G., Mao, G.Q., Xie, Z.M., 2001. Application and dissemination of detecting three parasites of a blood-paper by Dot-ELISA technology. Chin. J. Vet. Parasitol. 9 (1), 28–30 (in Chinese).
Yang, K.L., Li, H.J., Yang, W.C., Shi, X.W., Qi, Y.L., 2009. Effect of comprehensive schistosomiasis control measures with emphasis on infectious source control in dam areas of mountainous region, Yunnan province. Chin. J. Schistosomiasis Control 04, 272–275 (in Chinese).
Yang, Y.L., Chen, Q.S., 2011. Epidemiological characteristics and control strategies of schistosomiasis in mountainous areas. Livest. Poult. Ind. 04, 76–77 (in Chinese).
Yin, Z.C., Gu, X.G., Qiu, D.C., 2002. Prevalence of schistosomiasis in Sichuan Province—report on Randon Survey in 2001. J. Pract. Parasit. Dis. 10 (3), 97–103 (in Chinese).
Yin, Z.C., Qian, X.H., Wu, Z.S., 2003. Analysis of schistosomia infection in bovine in Sichuan Province in 2001. Parasit. Infect. Dis. 1 (3), 104–107.

Zhang, J.F., Xu, J., Bergquist, R., Yu, L.L., Yan, X.L., Zhu, H.Q., et al., 2016a. Development and application of diagnostics in the national schistosomiasis control programme in the People's Republic of China. Adv. Parasitol. 92.

Zhang, L.J., Li, S.Z., Wen, L.Y., Lin, D.D., Abe, E.M., Zhu, R., et al., 2016b. Establishment and function of schistosomiasis surveillance system towards elimination in the People's Republic of China. Adv. Parasitol. 92.

Zhang, F., Fang, D., Peng, C.Y., et al., 2005. Study overview of drugs for resisting Bilharziasis. Guid. J. TCM 20 (12), 79–81 (in Chinese).

Zheng, H., Zhang, L.J., Zhu, R., Xu, J., Li, S.Z., Guo, J.G., Xiao, N., Zhou, X.N., 2012. Endemic status of schistosomiasis in People's Republic of China in 2011. Chin. J. Schist. Control 01, 10–13 (in Chinese).

Zheng, J., 2003. Schistosomiasis control and its prospect in China. Chin. J. Schistosomiasis Control 15, 1–2 (in Chinese).

Zheng, J., Guo, J.G., Wang, X.F., et al., 2000. Relationship of the livestock trade to schistosomiasis transmission in moutainous area. Chin.J.Parasitol. Parasit.Dis. 18 (3), 146–148 (in Chinese).

Zheng, J., Wu, X.H., Wang, R.B., et al., 2006. Challenges and control strategies of schistosomiasis in China. Process and prospect of combat against schistosomiasis in China. People's Medical Publishing House, Beijing, pp. 245–249 (in Chinese).

Zheng, J., Gu, X.G., Qiu, Z.L., et al., 1996. Study on control strategies of schistosomiasis in plateau mountainous areas. Chin. J. Schistosomiasis Control 8 (2), 65–71 (in Chinese).

Zheng, Q., Vanderslott, S., Jiang, B., Xu, L.L., Liu, C.S., Huo, L.L., et al., 2013. Research gaps for three main tropical diseases in the People's Republic of China. Infect. Dis. Poverty 2, 15.

Zheng, J., 1990. Investigation and Prevention Strategy of Schistosomiasis in Mountainous Area (in Chinese).

Zheng, J., 1999. Mobile population and transmission of schistosomiasis. Chin. J. Schistosomiasis Control 11 (2), 25–127 (in Chinese).

Zhong, B., Wu, Z.S., Chen, L., Liang, S., Dong, X.Q., Qiu, D.C., 2011. Strengthening the achievements of schistosomiasis control in hilly regions of China. Chin. J. Schistosomiasis Control 01, 10–13 (in Chinese).

Zhou, X.Z., 2007. Distribution of schistosomiasis and prevention in China. J. Anhui Agric. Sci. 3766–3768 (in Chinese).

Zhu, H., Yap, P., Utzinger, J., Jia, T.W., Li, S.Z., Huang, X.B., et al., 2016. Policy support and resources mobilization for the national schistosomiasis control programme in the People's Republic of China. Adv. Parasitol. 92.

CHAPTER FOUR

Epidemiological Features and Control Progress of Schistosomiasis in Waterway-Network Region in The People's Republic of China

L. Shi*,§, W. Li*,§, F. Wu*,§, J.-F. Zhang*,§,**, K. Yang*,§,1, X.-N. Zhou¶,||,#,1

*Jiangsu Institute of Parasitic Diseases, Key Laboratory of Parasitic Disease Control and Prevention (Ministry of Health), Jiangsu Provincial Key Laboratory of Parasite Molecular Biology, Wuxi, The People's Republic of China
§Public Health Research Center, Jiangnan University, Wuxi, The People's Republic of China
¶National Institute of Parasitic Diseases, Chinese Center for Disease Control and Prevention, Shanghai, The People's Republic of China
||Key Laboratory of Parasite and Vector Biology of the Chinese Ministry of Health, Shanghai, The People's Republic of China
#WHO Collaborating Center for Tropical Diseases, Shanghai, The People's Republic of China
**Zhejiang Academy of Medical Sciences, Hangzhou, Zhejiang, The People's Republic of China
[1]Corresponding authors: E-mail: jipdyk76@hotmail.com; zhouxn1@chinacdc.cn

Contents

Advances in Parasitology, Volume 92
ISSN 0065-308X
http://dx.doi.org/10.1016/bs.apar.2016.02.002

Abstract

Schistosomiasis was one of the most serious parasitic diseases in The People's Republic of China, and the endemic region was classified into three types according to the epidemiological characteristics and living conditions of the intermediate host. After more than 60 years of efforts, schistosomiasis control programme has made great strides in waterway-network regions. We analyse the epidemic changes of schistosomiasis and its control progress through the schistosomiasis regions' documents and investigation data to evaluate the efficacy of the schistosomiasis control strategies in the waterway-network–type endemic region, which provides the basis for refinement of efforts, as well as summary of the Chinese schistosomiasis control experience in the waterway-network areas.

1. INTRODUCTION

Schistosomiasis was one of the most serious parasitic diseases in The People's Republic of China with a documented history of over 2100 years. During the mid-1950s, at the beginning of the national control programme, schistosomiasis was endemic in 12 provinces, with estimated 11.6 million people (Zhou et al., 1994) and 1.2 million cattle infected, and an area of 14,300 km^2 infested by the intermediate host snail, *Oncomelania hupensis* (Xianyi et al., 2005). According to the epidemiological characteristics and living conditions of the intermediate host, the endemic regions were classified into three types, namely (1) waterway-network regions, (2) marshlands and lakes regions and (3) the mountainous and hilly regions (Chen and Zheng, 1999).

Compared with the marshland and lake regions, waterway-network regions constitute 7.9% of the total area and had 33% of the total accumulative number of patients in the whole country in 1950s (Table 1, Fig. 2). There are two main reasons for this: the high density of the district population and the high infection rate of residents. Shanghai, Jiangsu and Zhejiang provinces are few of the major growing regions along the Yangtze River delta in The People's Republic of China; therefore, schistosomiasis has affected the development and production of the country. For instance, in Qingpu County, located in Shanghai, during 1950s, nearly 92% (23/25) townships were infected with schistosomiasis. Residents' faecal positive test rate was 45.90% and accumulated snail area was 74,297,000 m^2, whereby snails infection rate was 8.88% (Cheng and Song, 1997). In a break out of acute infection in Gaoyou, a waterway-network–type city located in the middle of Jiangsu Province, 4019 residents were infected and 1335 residents died of schistosomiasis (Xu, 1994).

Waterway-network–type endemic areas in The People's Republic of China were mainly distributed in Shanghai, Jiangsu, Zhejiang, Anhui and

Table 1 Constituent ratio of different types of the distribution in The People's Republic of China in 1950s

	Waterway-network region	Marshlands and lakes region	Mountainous regions
Province	Constituent ratio (%)	Constituent ratio (%)	Constituent ratio (%)
Shanghai	14.84		
Jiangsu	59.06	5.91	3.51
Zhejiang	20.32	0.09	22.57
Anhui	5.44	7.9	16.66
Fujian		17.7	1.52
Jiangxi		36.46	20.5
Hubei		31.16	6.83
Hunan		0.77	0.73
Guangdong	0.35		0.32
Guangxi			1.46
Sichuan			14.03
Yunnan			11.88
Total	7.89	79.52	12.59

Guangdong provinces. All the schistosomiasis endemic areas in Shanghai were in the waterway-network region; 47.55%, 35.91% and 4.01% of the Jiangsu, Zhejiang and Guangdong provinces, respectively, were the waterway-network regions (Fig. 3). Shanghai, Jiangsu and Zhejiang had the most serious outbreaks of the epidemic in the waterway-network–type regions (Fig. 1). The results of a study by Shanghai Research Institute showed that in 1953, 9 of 10 country regions had the epidemic and 51.1% population was infected with schistosomiasis. The average prevalence was 24.7%, and about a third of the total villages and towns had high levels of prevalence with the infection rate over 30% (Jinli et al., 1982).

After the liberation of The People's Republic of China, the Communist Party of The People's Republic of China (CPC) Central Committee attached great importance to control schistosomiasis (Xu et al., 2016a,b). Professional management institutions were established in the epidemic area on the principle of 'integrated scientific control adjusting measures to local conditions, classification and guidance'. After more than 60 years of efforts, schistosomiasis control program has made great strides in the waterway-network regions. Shanghai, Jiangsu, Zhejiang and other waterway-network regions of the county (city) have achieved schistosomiasis transmission interruption standard and have entered the stage of surveillance and consolidation. In this chapter, we analyse the epidemic changes of schistosomiasis and its control progress through the schistosomiasis regions' documents and investigation data to evaluate the efficacy of the schistosomiasis control strategies in the

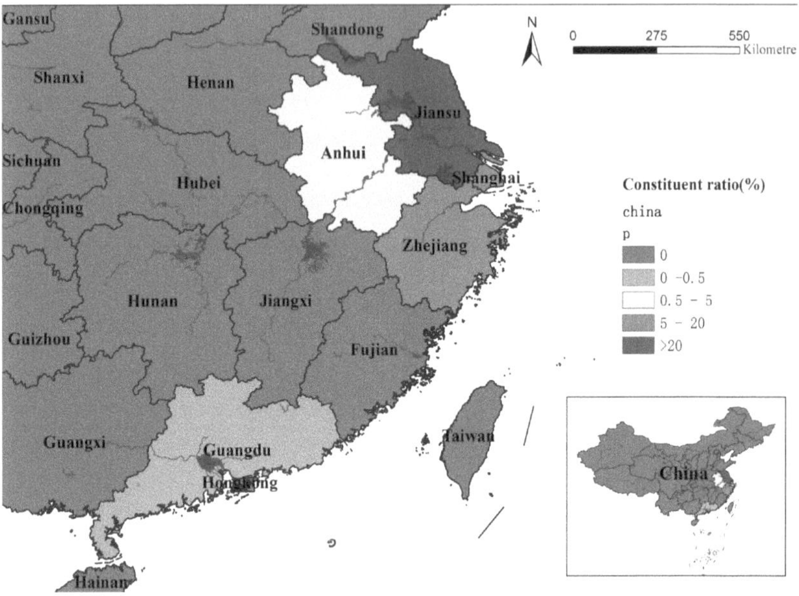

Figure 1 Constituent ratio of waterway-network regions of different provinces in The People's Republic of China during 1950s.

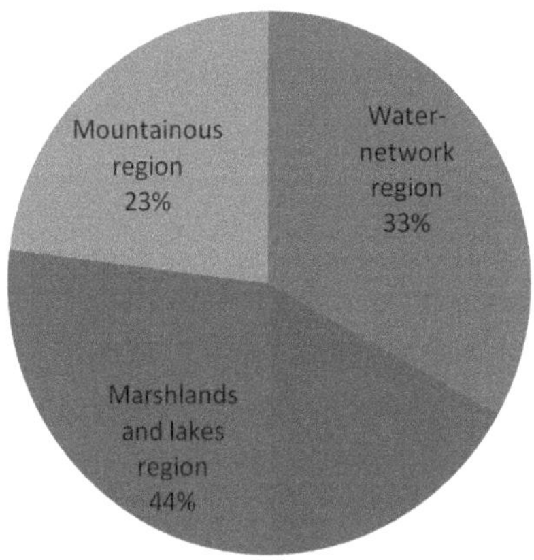

Figure 2 Constituent ratio of people infections in different types of regions in 1963.

waterway-network type endemic region, which provides the basis for refinement of efforts, as well as summary of the Chinese schistosomiasis control experience in the waterway-network areas.

2. WATERWAY-NETWORK AREAS: GEOGRAPHICAL FEATURE

Water-network areas, also called plain regions with waterway networks, mainly refer to the broad plains between the Yangtze River and

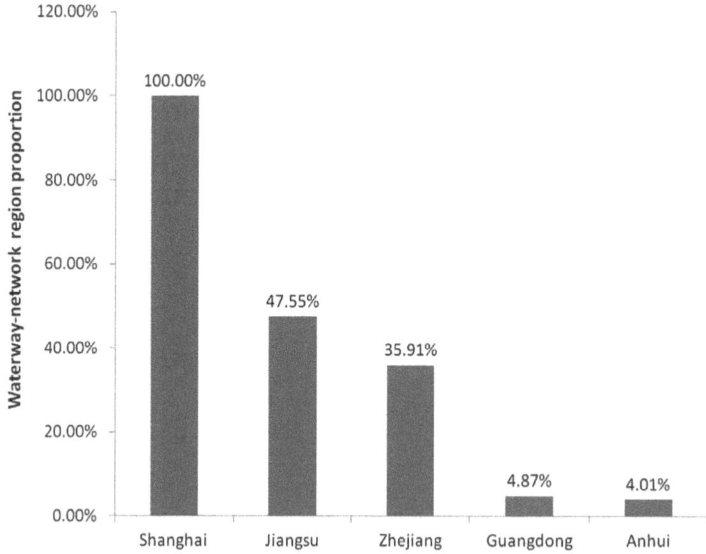

Figure 3 Proportion of waterway-network region areas in different provinces in 1950s.

the Qiantang River or belong to the Yangtze River delta region. This area belongs to subtropical climate zone, spring and winter rainy areas, where the annual rainfall is about 1200 mm. These areas are characterized by dense population, rivers and lakes, low altitude and many rice fields. Furthermore, the water levels have not changed significantly, there is slow or sluggish flow of water and the shore weeds along the river provide a conducive breeding environment for the snails responsible for schistosomiasis.

3. EPIDEMIOLOGICAL FEATURES OF SCHISTOSOMIASIS IN WATERWAY-NETWORK REGION

The waterway-network regions are different from the other two types of regions due to snail ecology, infected ways of population, reservoir type and geography.

3.1 Ecology and distribution of characteristics of snail

Structurally, the snail in waterway-network epidemic area is medium sized, 5.5–7.5 mm height and with shallow ribs. Each spiral has 15 ribs, but this is not always the case, as snails in north Jiangsu coastal plain have no ribs (Li et al., 2016; MOH, 2000) (Fig. 4).

Snail distribution is linear along the irrigation water system, but the snail density in the linear region sometimes is uniform. Usually the snails are

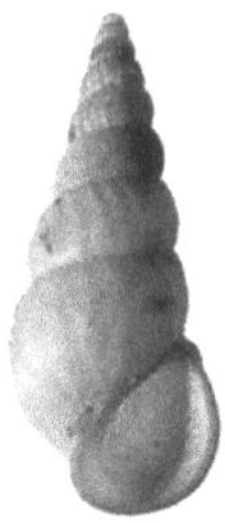

Figure 4 Waterway-network region snail.

found within the irrigation ditch where water flows slowly and it is full of grass. Sometimes the snails are also found in the ponds that interlink the river and the ditch, but the population density is scanty. In the fields, the snails are mainly distributed at the inlets and outlets of the ridge waterways.

3.2 Ways of infected and characteristic of patient distribution

Residents of waterway-network region live alongside the river, for the convenience to get water for domestic use and transportation to another area. They, also defaecate into cylinders from where faeces containing eggs of *Schistosoma* escape and contaminate the water. Daily life of the villagers brings them into frequent contact with the contamination: children swim in the contaminated water and local cattle drink at these water bodies.

In 1963 (Fig. 2), 34.3% of the total patients came from the water-network area. The prevalence was typically higher in men than in women and the prevalence also increased with age peaking at 15–19 or 20–24 years (Chen, 2014). Fishermen, boatmen and farmers had the highest infection rate, followed by rural children who bathed in the river.

3.3 The Reservoir Host

Sources of infection in the water-network regions were mainly infected persons and infected animals (cattle, dogs and rats) with schistosomiasis. Schistosomes infect animals mainly through skin and oral mucosa. Epidemiological investigations proved that infection of the human is related to animal's infection such as murine or bovine. There were examples found in two neighbouring villages in the suburbs of Shanghai; infection of cattle and rats in North-Ma village were higher than South-Ma village (Xu, 1985) (Table 2). In the waterway-network area, the number of infected animals is an indicator that affects the significance of the animals as a source of

Table 2 Comparison of people and animal infection in Shanghai in 1959

	North-Ma village			South-Ma village		
Statistical indicators	**People**	**Cattle**	**Ditch mouse**	**People**	**Cattle**	**Ditch mouse**
The number of survey	617	28	68	951	23	61
Number of infections	428	14	63	369	5	6
Infection rate (%)	69.4	50	92.6	41.6	21.7	9.8

infection due to the amount of the feces of the animals frequenting and polluting the water bodies. In general, the number of schistosomiasis eggs in cow dung (per unit weight) is far lower than that in the faeces of the patients, but the quantity of cow dung is nearly a 100 times that of the human feces. Livestock is often housed in the homes of local residents, so the impact of livestock infection on the residents is relatively straightforward. Wild animals being far away from the residential area had a less direct impact. Considering the nearness to the residential area the, ditch rat, although not a livestock, was also an important source of infection (Cao et al., 2016).

3.4 Snail control strategies and measures in the waterway-network region

In accordance with the human living conditions and occurrences of infection (contacting water frequently, high repeated infection rate), the integrated schistosomiasis control strategy with emphasis on snail control was taken up in the waterway-network region.

Rivers, ditches, paddy fields and beach were the main breeding grounds for snails in waterway-network regions. According to the snail ecology, the spring and autumn were the right seasons to survey and control the snails, especially in late March and early April. The experience gained proved that most snail habitats can be eliminated by snail control through environmental management as the main measure and drug as the auxiliary measure. Normally, the snail control method through environmental management in these areas was combined with farmland capital construction, water conservancy and aquatic production. There are various kinds of environmental management methods suitable to the different terrains. The Creek terrain used soil burial method by shovelling soil, ditching or trenching along the river bank or near the waterline, combined with spraying of drug to control the snails. The methods of opening a new channel, filling the old ditch, changing sunlight conditions on culverts and hardening channels were used in the ditch terrain. Soil burial or low-toxicity drugs spraying methods were used in the farmland terrain. All in all, environmental transformation and agricultural farm construction, such as flattening land, irrigation of ditches, river building by laying bricks or stones, were the effective measures of snail control in the waterway-network areas (MOH, 2000; Yang et al., 2016).

4. CONTROL PROGRESS AND ITS EFFECT ON THE WATERWAY-NETWORK REGIONS

For schistosomiasis, the epidemic is complex, and the control work was very difficult, especially in the early days after foundation of the programme, due to seriousness of the schistosomiasis epidemic, large population distribution and low development level of national economy. It was a big problem to adopt the appropriate kind of control strategy and measures, in the waterway-network—type endemic areas. According to the epidemic characteristics of schistosomiasis and the prevailing circumstances of the country, on the basis of the research and practice of prevention and cure, the government proposed an action of relying on the masses — the combination of prevention and cure, integrated prevention and control policy and giving priority to chemotherapy to control infection. Sixty years of the prevention and treatment practices showed that this policy is in conformity with the specific conditions of the country. According to the endemic feature, control strategy and control experiences of schistosomiasis in different areas of the waterway-network region (Cheng and Song, 1997; Jinli et al., 1982; Xu, 1994; Zheng et al., 1997), the progress of the control processes were generally divided into four stages (Fig. 10) as discussed in the following subsections.

4.1 Investigation and preparation stage

Before liberation, schistosomiasis seriously affected the lives of the people, it caused substantial morbidity, including wasting, weakness, ascites and growth retardation. Mortality was considerably high. Few years after the founding of The People's Republic of China, during the mid-1950s, the Government of The People's Republic of China recognized the social and economic importance and implication of schistosomiasis. It became a major public health concern. Hence, professional institutions and a national control and research programmes were established as early as the mid-1950s. This programme has been implemented until 2015, including periodic policy reviews to keep the control strategy in line with field realities and to adapt the approaches to the changing economic, epidemiological and socio-political conditions.

During the early 1950s, when the Chinese population was about 600 million, an estimated 11.612 million people were infected with *Schitosoma japonicum* (United Nations, 2002). Among the waterway-network endemic region, the highest proportion of people infected was recorded in the Jiangsu Province. Here, an estimated 371,700 people were infected, which comprised 21.3% of the total population. Large number of infected people and hence a high infection prevalence were also found in Shanghai (number of people infected: 33,016; infection prevalence: 26.3%) and Zhejiang Province (number of people infected: 2.037 million; infection prevalence: 17.5%). The average density of the intediate host snails during mid-1950s was 45.6/0.1 m^2 in Shanghai (Jinli et al., 1982).

4.2 Transmission control stage

In order to effectively control waterway-network region of schistosomiasis, and in the light of the characteristics of the region, integrated control measures targeted on schistosomiasis were carried out with emphasis on environmental management from 1956 to 1980s. It consisted of snail elimination, primarily by environmental management (Fig. 5), followed by diagnostic screening, chemotherapy, provision of clean water and improved sanitation and hygiene. In combination with agricultural engineering and water conservancy projects, large areas were environmentally modified to make them unsuitable

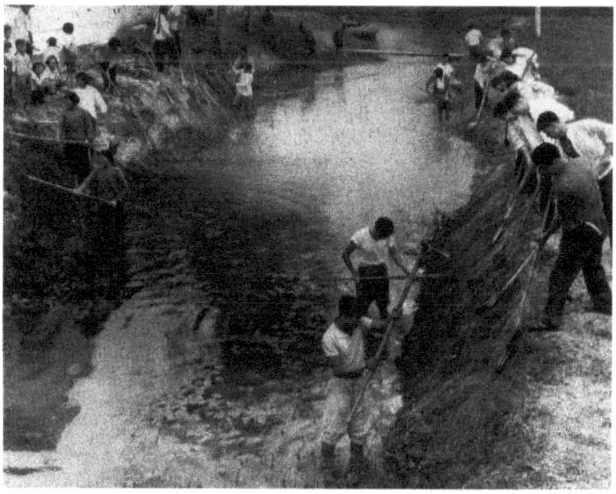

Figure 5 Snail control method by shovelling soil and distributing drugs in Shanghai city.

as habitats for the amphibious snails. Many of the approaches included methods with distinctive Chinese features which were applied in the waterway-network endemic areas.

Shanghai is a typical waterway-network endemic area. In the 1950s, because of the lack of understanding of snail ecology, only single shovel soil method was used as the control measure. Snail density was reduced, but it was difficult to compress the snail-affected area. Snails remained, and hence the snail breeding started again in the same region. For this reason, snail control measures were readjusted in 1958. To this effect, a series of integrated measures including damming, pumping, furrowing and soil burial were implemented near the river systems (Fig. 4).

Apart from People's Liberation Army (PLA), more than 20,000 people including a large number of middle school students and urban residents worked together with the local populace. Professional snail control teams were organized, and drug was used as a supplement to improve and consolidate the control effect. At the same time, active water sanitation management was carried out in the region. Family toilets near rivers were discouraged, and wells were dug in the village areas. In 1958, improved centralized sanitary management was reached at 78.62% in the endemic area. As a result, integrated control measures played an important role in the control of schistosomiasis infection. Regrettably, due to the 3 years of natural disasters and the resulting inadequate work control, there was a rebound of the snail situation and the snails resurfaced once more. With this endemic background, the control scheme in Shanghai region was adjusted again in 1964. In order to focus aggressive efforts to eliminate key environmental snails, the control area was moved from all the districts to key environmental snail districts; control teams were reconstituted as professional teams rather than from the masses. An integrated rapid drug control method (drug soaking, spaying, land filling) was carried out combined with construction for irrigation and water conservancy, which greatly reduced the density of snails, and the snail distribution was compressed from flakes to points in the map. At the same time, snail investigation of paddy fields was intensified and a large area of land snail was discovered (Fig. 6). A similar method was used in this area which gave good results. Up to 1968, aquatic snails in the whole region decreased by 85.8% and the land snails decreased by 96% compared with 1965 (Fig. 5). As there was a steady decline in the number of snail-infected areas and the number of patients, screening and treatment measures were strengthened again in the Shanghai region. Similar control strategy was used in other waterway-network regions, such as

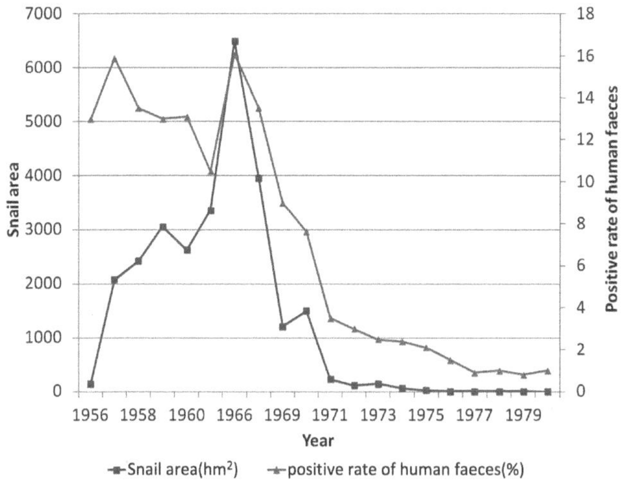

Figure 6 Percentage of snail area and pollution of infection rate in Shanghai (1956–80).

Kunshan County in Jiangsu Province and Jiashan County in Zhejiang Province (Zheng et al., 1997).

As a result, great success was achieved in these areas. In Shanghai, during this period, a total of 29.34 million people were examined and 1.86 million were treated in nine endemic areas. A total of 556,000 domestic cattle were investigated and 25,000 were treated. No acute cases of schistosomiasis and infected cattle were found in all the districts for more than 11 years by the end of 1975 (Table 3). No infected snail was found in the examined 126,176 snails by the end of 1980 (Jinli et al., 1982).

In Kunshan County of Jiangsu Province, according to the field surveillance carried out in 1980, among the 2206 cases of *S. japonicum*–infected persons and in comparison with the data at the early 1950, the number of infected people decreased by 80.4%. Among 19,245 examined cattle, 87 were found infected in 1980. The positive rate of stool examination was

Table 3 Cattle infection from year 1958 to 1978 in Shanghai

Cattle	1958	1963	1970	1971	1972	1973	1974	1975–78
Number of examination	2455	182	368	3729	553	1102	870	1835
Infection number	548	34	3	2	2	1	0	0
Infection rates (%)	22.3	18.68	0.82	0.05	0.36	0.09	0	0

0.45%; a decrease of 0.6% as compared to the early 1950s. Snail control also achieved great progress.

In 1980, intermediate host snails were found on a total surface area of 76.6 km^2. This translates to a decrease of 92.6% compared to the corresponding surface area of 1,000,321 km^2 during the early 1950s. More importantly, the control strategy not only decreased the patients and snail area, but also promoted agricultural production and economic development (Fig. 7). The experience gained proved that most snail habitats can be eliminated by snail control through environmental management as the main strategy (Fig. 8).

4.3 Transmission interruption stage

Great success was achieved in waterway-network endemic area in the early 30 years. Schistosomiasis control campaigns focused on transmission control had eliminated large areas of snail habitats and the number of schistosomiasis cases reduced remarkably. Schistosomiasis was then circumscribed to certain core regions that have been demonstrated to be more difficult to sustain control, such as the low endemic area and the area by the lake or marshland of the Yangtze River. Morbidity remained a serious problem with more than 10,000 cases of advanced schistosomiasis.

With the advent of praziquantel and the development of improved diagnostic techniques, the expert committee of the World Health Organization (WHO) replaced the strong emphasis on transmission control by morbidity control during the mid-1980s (WHO, 1985). The introduction of praziquantel, a highly effective, low-cost anti-schistosomiasis drug, led to the national schistosomiasis control strategy to shift from transmission control to

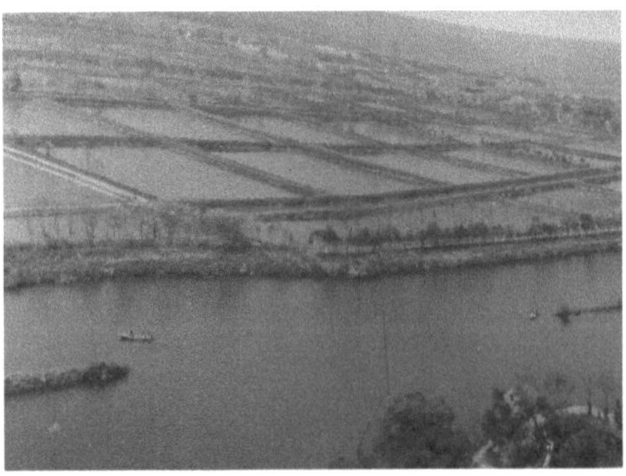

Figure 7 Snail fields changed into fish ponds by environmental transformation in Jiangsu Province.

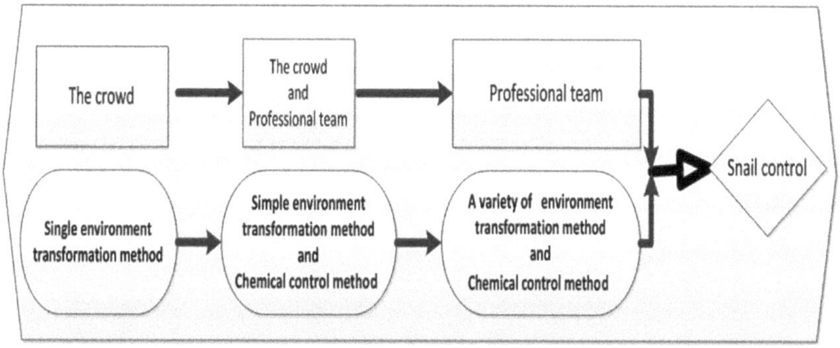

Figure 8 Evolution of snail control method in waterway-network region.

morbidity control in accordance with the new WHO global strategy of Tambo et al. (2015) with considerable success. For instance, in Kunshan County, no new infections were found in five consecutive years (1986–90), and only one reinfected case was found by the end of 1990 (Fig. 9).

Consequently, a stepwise control strategy was employed for controlling schistosomiasis in these core regions (Collins et al., 2012). The first step was to control morbidity through mass chemotherapy in the severely endemic areas and selective chemotherapy in less severely endemic areas. Further steps included snail control through mollusciciding and/or environmental modification, as well as health education and sanitation. For example, in

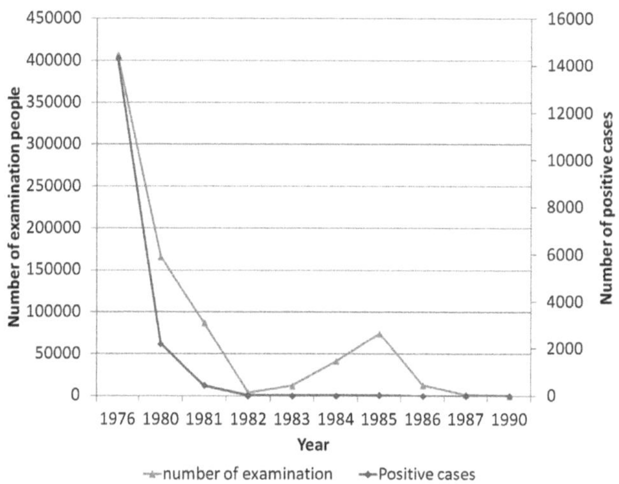

Figure 9 Number of examined and positive-tested people in Kunshan County of Jiangsu Province (1976–90).

1992 a joint project supported by the World Bank, which was also an important component of National Schistosomiasis Control Program, was initiated. The primary objectives were to control morbidity due to schistosomiasis and in some areas to interrupt the transmission. With the introduction of the anti-schistosomal drug praziquantel, the strong reliance on praziquantel-based morbidity control during the 10-year World Bank Loan Project (WBLP) for Schistosomiasis Control in The People's Republic of China, complemented with health education and continued to yield rich dividend in snail control (Xianyi et al., 2005; Zhou et al., 2005).

By the end of the year 1995, the endemic townships gradually reached transmission interruption criteria and schistosomiasis in the waterway-network regions had been eliminated in Shanghai, Jiangsu, Zhejiang and Guangdong provinces (Wu et al., 2005; Zheng, 1988).

4.4 Consolidation and surveillance (1990s to present)

Since 1990s, after the elimination of schistosomiasis, an overall surveillance and consolidation work has been unfolded in the water-network regions. When the program is focussed on the surveillance of the snail and the disease, it must be combined with the urbanization and economic development in rural areas, integrated with the improvement of ecological environment of rural areas and change of people's unhealthy living habits, through the establishment of modern, hygienic facilities in villages and towns so as to guarantee the real implementation of integrated control and management approaches. As a result, by the end of 1994 in Shanghai, among the 5.5 million rural residents the availability of running water supply had reached 98.7%, and Shanghai become the first city in the The People's Republic of China to realize running water supply in rural areas. This was endorsed by the National Patriotic Health Campaign Committee through an assessment. By the end of the year 2000, a total of 1234 million new sanitary toilets had been built up in peasants' households, 92.6% of the 1.33 million peasants' households had their own sanitary toilets and human night soil is now mostly sanitized (Handing et al., 2002). The total amount of original snail habitats along the rivers was found to be 46,261 million m^2 and among these habitat areas, 13,991 million m^2 have been thoroughly modified and the snails eliminated. There were 120,211 million m^2 original snail-ridden ditches, canals and mud flats of which 25,342 million m^2 have been thoroughly modified, with a modification rate of 21.1%. Many areas which have undergone environmental management have been kept free from snails for about 10–20 years. By the end of 2011, no new local infection case has been found in both human and livestock in the waterway-network regions in the whole country. Achievement of schistosomiasis eradication has been effectively consolidated. The time taken by the waterway-network region to reach the criteria was over 15 years and the programme has now entered a long-term surveillance phase. However, due to the fact that the prevalence and spread of schistosomiasis is influenced by many factors, the outbreaks appear repeatedly in some waterway-network regions. Some of these main factors include:

(1) *Biological factors*: Though the living snail density achieved the acceptance criteria, which was difficult to seize, by strengthening control measures such as molluscicide, detection and treatment of livestock, if surveillance and consolidation are weakened, the remaining snails easily breed into a large population and can cause an epidemic rebound. For instance, certain waterway-network regions found high density of snails' areas which accounted for more than 20% of the total snail area in Zhejiang Province in 2000 which had reached transmission interruption criteria in 1995. After 10 years of transmission interruption, 57.38 km^2 snail area have been found in 6 counties and 134 villages in Shanghai (Gao et al., 1998).

(2) *Natural factors*: Due to the changes in ecological impacts of floods (Zhou et al., 2002), returning farmland for lake and large water conservancy construction, an exogenous source of infection of input snails appeared in waterway-network area which caused an epidemic. Research has shown that input snails can reproduce in waterway-network region and can cause a high prevalence of schistosomiasis. Surveillance result showed that in Songjiang and Jinshan districts in Shanghai, 23 river-ways were found to have snails which occurred on the flotage between 1997 and 2002 (Jiang et al., 2003). Gaochun County of Jiangsu Province reached transition interruption in 1985, but in 1999 large infected snails area were discovered again in this county after the floods in 1998 (Fig. 11) (Shi et al., 2004). Moreover, climate change has been proven to be a factor of the transmission of vector-borne diseases (Githeko et al., 2000; Kilpatrick and Randolph, 2012; Medlock and Leach, 2015), and it has also been demonstrated that schistosomiasis, being snail-borne, is affected by the climate change (Mas-Coma et al., 2009; McCreesh and Booth, 2013). The rise in temperature may cause snail survival and reproduction in currently nonbreeding sites, resulting in the potential transmission of schistosomiasis (McCreesh et al., 2015). It is therefore considered that climate change may affect, in a long term, the progress of schistosomiasis elimination in The People's Republic of China (Butler, 2012; Mayala et al., 2015).

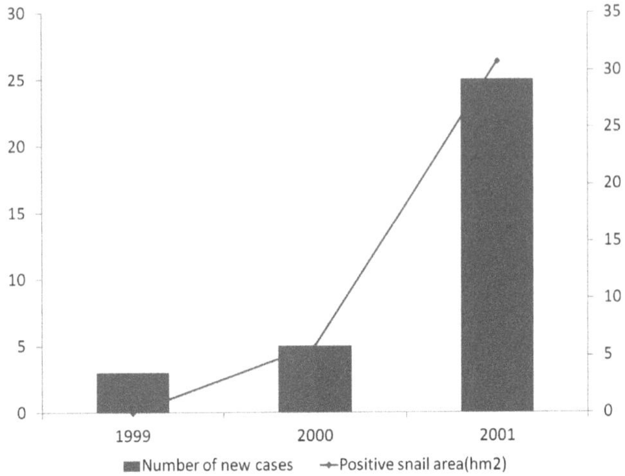

Figure 10 Schistosoma epidemics monitoring results in Gaochun County from 1999 to 2001.

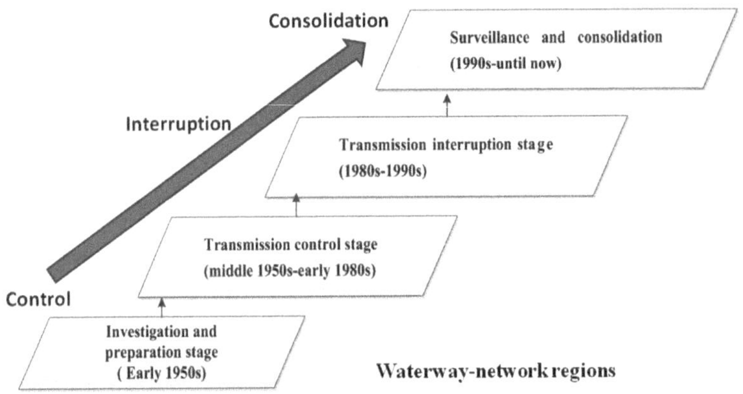

Figure 11 Control status of schistosomiasis in waterway-network regions in The People's Republic of China at different stages.

(3) *Social factors*: The diminished funding after the WBLP in The People's Republic of China in the early 2000s, in conjunction with wider demographic, environmental and socioeconomic transformations and changes in the health sector and professional control teams, including cost escalation and declining quality and availability of primary health care and preventive care, contributed to the reemergence of schistosomiasis in certain parts of the country. From the history of schistosomiasis control in The People's Republic of China, it is considered that reduced political will and financial support may pose a great threat to the progress of schistosomiasis elimination

(Fan, 2012). Moreover, with the progress of urbanization and the increasing mobility of the population imported schistosomiasis cases in some areas also showed an increase of trend (Wen et al., 2004). Between 1996 and 2005 in Shanghai, 31 input cases were found and among them 14 cases were acute (Jiang et al., 2007). Between 1996 and 2009 in Zhejiang Province, 174 imported cases were found which included 36 acute cases (Liyong et al., 2010). These emergent new circumstances have become potential risk factors to influence the achievements of prevention and consolidation and have become the main issues and priorities in transmission interrupted areas (Zheng et al., 2013).

5. FUTURE CHALLENGE

In future work, based on the Schistosomiasis Prevention Act, the surveillance and consolidation in waterway-network regions should be strengthened to eliminate the potential risk factors and prevent the spread of schistosomiasis (Lin et al., 1996; Liu et al., 2014):

1. In waterway-network areas which still have potential risk factors, risk evaluation should be carefully carried out in the areas which still have the possibility of snail habitats proliferation and infection input. At the same time, passive and active surveillance of snails and patients should be carried out steadily.
2. The strategy 'wipe out the remnants of snails with prevention of the input snails as supplement' should be adopted in the snail surveillance and control work. The history of snail habitats and snail-suitable environment should be taken into account, especially focussing on production and living areas of the population. Timely investigation should be carried out when infection of snails is found; the drug and environment change can be used to control the snails in agriculture and fishing industry.
3. During the disease surveillance and control work, 'control on the exogenous source of infection with clean endogenous source of infection as supplement' strategy should be adopted. The movement of people and livestock from uncontrolled or epidemic county is vital to the population. Suspected cases of schistosomiasis should be reported by medical institutions promptly, diagnosed cases should be reported through the disease surveillance information report management system timely through the internet and then epidemiological investigation process should be implemented timely as well (Feng et al., 2016; Wang et al., 2016).

4. From the history of schistosomiasis control in The People's Republic of China, the long-term and complex work on schistosomiasis should be fully understood (Cao et al., 2016; Zhang et al., 2016). The waterway-network area should remain stable and controlled by a professional team that should ensure funds for surveillance and consolidation. In addition, to ensure that prevention and treatment course to be effective, The People's Republic of China should also establish sensitive and efficient surveillance and early warning mechanisms to effectively cope with the possible outbreak of schistosomiasis thus preventing the resurgence of an epidemic (Zhou, 2009; Zhu et al., 2011).

Although remarkable progress has been made in the control of waterway-network regions of schistosomiasis during the past 60 years, the disease remains endemic in 124 counties in the other types of regions. To consolidate the achievements made to date and to ultimately eliminate the disease, The People's Republic of China still has a long way to go. However, the prospects are bright and the tasks ahead can be achieved alongside the social and economic development of the country. The experiences gained in The People's Republic of China are likely to stimulate schistosomiasis control and guide integrated and sustainable control elsewhere in the world (Tambo et al., 2014; Xu et al., 2016a,b).

ACKNOWLEDGEMENTS

This project was supported by the National S & T Major Program (grant no. 2012ZX10004220), Project of Health Department of Jiangsu Province (No. RC2011094) and Science Foundation of Jiangsu Province (BS20105024).

REFERENCES

Butler, C.D., 2012. Infectious disease emergence and global change: thinking systemically in a shrinking world. Infect. Dis. Poverty 1, 5.

Cao, Z.G., Zhao, Y.E., Willingham, A.L., Wang, T.P., 2016. Towards the elimination of schistosomiasis japonica through control of the disease in domestic animals in the People's Republic of China: a tale of over 60 years. Adv. Parasitol. 92.

Chen, M.G., Zheng, F., 1999. Schistosomiasis control in China. Parasitol. Int. 48, 11–19.

Chen, M.G., 2014. Assessment of morbidity due to *Schistosoma japonicum* infection in China. Infect. Dis. Poverty 3, 6.

Cheng, J., Song, W., 1997. Elimination and surveillance schistosomiasis in Qingpu county. Zhongguo Xue Xi Chong Bing Fang. Zhi Za Zhi (Chin J. Schisto Control.) (in Chinese).

Collins, C., Xu, J., Tang, S., 2012. Schistosomiasis control and the health system in P.R. China. Infect. Dis. Poverty 1, 8.

Fan, K.W., 2012. Central-provincial relations for anti-schistosomiasis policy in china. Iran. J. Public Health 41, 1–11.

Feng, Y., Liu, L., Xia, S., Xu, J.F., Bergquist, R., Yang, G.J., 2016. Reaching the surveillance-response stage of schistosomiasis control in the People's Republic of China: a modelling approach. Adv. Parasitol. 92.

Gao, Z., Xijun, J., Zhenrong, C., Lixin, W., Zhenggeng, Z., Desheng, H., 1998. 10 years monitoring report after eradication of schistosomiasis in Shanghai. In: Zhongguo Xue Xi Chong Bing Fang Zhi Za Zhi (Chin J Schisto Control), pp. 159–161 (in Chinese).
Githeko, A.K., Lindsay, S.W., Confalonieri, U.E., Patz, J.A., 2000. Climate change and vector-borne diseases: a regional analysis. Bull. WHO 78, 1136–1147.
Handing, P., Desheng, H., Ketai, W., 2002. Approach to surveillance and consolidation during past 15 years after elimination of schistosomiasis in Shanghai. Acta Trop. 82, 301–303.
Jiang, X., Wang, K., Jin, F., He, T., Huang, D., 2003. Investigations on snails's distribution and ecology in rivers of shanghai suburbs. Zhongguo Xue Xi Chong Bing Fang. Zhi Za Zhi (Chin J. Schisto Control.) 15, 456–458 (in Chinese).
Jiang, X., Jin, Y., Cai, L., 2007. Analysis of imported schistosomiasis cases in Shanghai city, 1996–2005. Zhongguo Xue Xi Chong Bing Fang. Zhi Za Zhi (Chin J. Schisto Control.) 390–400 (in Chinese).
Jinli, C., Deyu, H., Gongyong, S., 1982. Schistosomiasis has been eliminated in Shanghai. Acta Acad. Med. Primae Shanghai.
Kilpatrick, A.M., Randolph, S.E., 2012. Drivers, dynamics, and control of emerging vector-borne zoonotic diseases. Lancet 380, 1946–1955.
Li, Z.J., Ge, J., Dai, J.R., Wen, L.Y., Lin, D.D., Madsen, H., et al., 2016. Biology and control of snail intermediate host of *Schistosoma japonicum* in the People's Republic of China. Adv. Parasitol. 92.
Lin, J., Du, W., Li, Y., Chen, B., 1996. Situation of schistosomiasis eliminated region and proposals for consolidating the outcome of schistosomiasis in China Strait. J. Prev. Med.
Liu, L., Yang, G.J., Zhu, H.R., Yang, K., Ai, L., 2014. Knowledge of, attitudes towards, and practice relating to schistosomiasis in two subtypes of a mountainous region of the People's Republic of China. Infect. Dis. Poverty 3, 16.
Liyong, W., Wei, Z., Xiaolan, Y., Shaobin, L., Mingdong, Z., Lulu, G., et al., 2010. Longitudinal surveillance and control strategy of schistosomiasis in Zhejiang province. Acta Parasitol. Med. Entomol. Sin. 17, 135–139 (in Chinese).
Mas-Coma, S., Valero, M.A., Bargues, M.D., 2009. Climate change effects on trematodiases, with emphasis on zoonotic fascioliasis and schistosomiasis. Vet. Parasitol. 163, 264–280.
Mayala, B.K., Fahey, C.A., Wei, D., Zinga, M.M., Bwana, V.M., Mlacha, T., et al., 2015. Knowledge, perception and practices about malaria, climate change, livelihoods and food security among rural communities of central Tanzania. Infect. Dis. Poverty 4, 21.
McCreesh, N., Booth, M., 2013. Challenges in predicting the effects of climate change on *Schistosoma mansoni* and *Schistosoma haematobium* transmission potential. Trends Parasitol. 29, 548–555.
McCreesh, N., Nikulin, G., Booth, M., 2015. Predicting the effects of climate change on *Schistosoma mansoni* transmission in eastern Africa. Parasites Vectors 8, 4.
Medlock, J.M., Leach, S.A., 2015. Effect of climate change on vector-borne disease risk in the UK. Lancet Infect. Dis. 15, 721–730.
MOH, 2000. *Schistosoma Japonicum* Control of Manual, third ed. Shanghai Scientific and Technical Shanghai.
Shi, Z., Fu, H., Tang, Y., 2004. Surveillance of re-prevalent factors of schistosomiasis after its transmission has been interruption in Gaochun county. Zhongguo Xue Xi Chong Bing Fang. Zhi Za Zhi (Chin J. Schisto Control.) 471–472 (in Chinese).
Tambo, E., Ai, L., Zhou, X., Chen, J.H., Hu, W., Bergquist, R., et al., 2014. Surveillance-response systems: the key to elimination of tropical diseases. Infect. Dis. Poverty 3, 17.
Tambo, E., Khater, E.I., Chen, J.H., Bergquist, R., Zhou, X.N., 2015. Nobel prize for the artemisinin and ivermectin discoveries: a great boost towards elimination of the global infectious diseases of poverty. Infect. Dis. Poverty 4, 58.
United Nations, 2002. World Urbanization Prospects: The 2001 Revisions. Population Division Department of Economics and Social Affairs of the United Nations, New York.

Wang, X.Y., He, J., Yang, K., Liang, S., 2016. Applications of spatial technology in schistosomiasis control programme in the People's Republic of China. Adv. Parasitol. 92.

Wen, L., Cai, L., Zhang, R., Zhou, X.-N., 2004. Analysis of 37 city imported schistosomiasis cases. Zhongguo Xue Xi Chong Bing Fang. Zhi Za Zhi (Chin J. Schisto Control.) 31–33 (in Chinese).

WHO, 1985. The Control of Schistosomiasis: Report of a WHO Expert Committee. Technical Report Series.

Wu, X.H., Chen, M.G., Zheng, J., 2005. Surveillance of schistosomiasis in five provinces of China which have reached the national criteria for elimination of the disease. Acta Trop. 96, 276–281.

Xianyi, C., Liying, W., Jiming, C., Xiaonong, Z., Jiang, Z., Jiagang, G., et al., 2005. Schistosomiasis control in China: the impact of a 10-year World Bank Loan Project (1992–2001). Bull. WHO 83, 43–48.

Xu, J., 1994. Four years snail reproduction investigation and analysis in gaoyou lake. Zhongguo Xue Xi Chong Bing Fang. Zhi Za Zhi (Chin J. Schisto Control.) 104–105 (in Chinese).

Xu, J., Bergquist, R., Qian, Y.J., Wang, Q., Yu, Q., Peeling, R., et al., 2016a. China-Africa and China-Asia collaboration on schistosomiasis control: a SWOT analysis. Adv. Parasitol. 92.

Xu, J., Steinman, P., Maybe, D., Zhou, X.N., Lv, S., Li, S.Z., et al., 2016b. Evolution of the national schistosomiasis control programmes in the People's Republic of China. Adv. Parasitol. 92.

Xu, S., 1985. Relationship between control, elimination of lakes schistosomiasis and livestock schistosomiasis. Chin. J. Vet. Sci. Tech. 31–35 (in Chinese).

Yang, Y., Zhou, Y.B., Song, X.X., Li, S.Z., Zhong, B., Wang, T.P., et al., 2016. Integrated control strategy of schistosomiasis in the People's Republic of China: projects involving agriculture, water-conservancy, forestry, sanitation and environmental modification. Adv. Parasitol. 92.

Zhang, L.J., Li, S.Z., Wen, L.Y., Lin, D.D., Abe, E.M., Zhu, R., et al., 2016. Establishment and function of schistosomiasis surveillance system towards elimination in the People's Republic of China. Adv. Parasitol. 92.

Zheng, G., 1988. The Historical Experiences on Preventive Medicine in New China, Vol. III, Disease Control. People's Health Press, Beijing.

Zheng, J., Chen, Y., Xue, M., 1997. Review of schistosomiasis epidemic and control situation in Jiashan county. Zhongguo Xue Xi Chong Bing Fang. Zhi Za Zhi (Chin J. Schisto Control.) 357–358 (in Chinese).

Zheng, Q., Vanderslott, S., Jiang, B., Xu, L.L., Liu, C.S., Huo, L.L., et al., 2013. Research gaps for three main tropical diseases in the People's Republic of China. Infect. Dis. Poverty 2, 15.

Zhou, D., Li, Y., Yang, X., 1994. Schistosomiasis control in China. World Health Forum 15, 387–389.

Zhou, X.-N., 2009. Surveillance and forecast of schistosomiasis transmission in China. Zhongguo Xue Xi Chong Bing Fang. Zhi Za Zhi (Chin J. Schisto Control.) 341–344 (in Chinese).

Zhou, X., Dandan, L., Huiming, Y., Honggen, C., Leping, S., Guojing, Y., et al., 2002. Use of landsat TM satellite surveillance data to measure the impact of the 1998 flood on snail intermediate host dispersal in the lower Yangtze river basin. Acta Trop. 82, 199–205.

Zhou, X.N., Wang, L.Y., Chen, M.G., Wu, X.H., Jiang, Q.W., Chen, X.Y., et al., 2005. The public health significance and control of schistosomiasis in China—then and now. Acta Trop. 96, 97–105.

Zhu, R., Zhao, G., Li, H., Guo, J., 2011. Development and prospect of surveillance network of schistosomiasis in China. Zhongguo Xue Xi Chong Bing Fang. Zhi Za Zhi (Chin J. Schisto Control.) 14–17 (in Chinese).

CHAPTER FIVE

The Establishment and Function of Schistosomiasis Surveillance System Towards Elimination in The People's Republic of China

L.-J. Zhang[*,§,¶], S.-Z. Li[*,§,¶,1], L.-Y. Wen[||,¶¶], D.-D. Lin[#], E.M. Abe[*,§,¶,**], R. Zhu[*,§,¶], Y. Du[*,§,¶], S. Lv[*,§,¶], J. Xu[*,§,¶], B.L. Webster[§§], D. Rollinson[§§], X.-N. Zhou[*,§,¶]

[*]Key Laboratory of Parasite and Vector Biology of the Chinese Ministry of Health, Shanghai, The People's Republic of China
[§]WHO Collaborating Center for Tropical Diseases, Shanghai, The People's Republic of China
[¶]National Institute of Parasitic Diseases, Chinese Center for Disease Control and Prevention, Shanghai, The People's Republic of China
[||]Institute of Parasitic Diseases, Zhejiang Academy of Medical Sciences, Hangzhou, The People's Republic of China
[#]Jiangxi Provincial Institute of Parasitic Diseases, Nanchang, Jiangxi, The People's Republic of China
[**]Federal University Lafia, Lafia, Nasarawa, Nigeria
[§§]Wolfson Wellcome Biomedical Laboratories, Life Sciences, The Natural History Museum, London, United Kingdom
[¶¶]Zhejiang Academy of Medical Sciences, Hangzhou, Zhejiang, The People's Republic of China
[1]Corresponding author: E-mail: stoneli1130@126.com

Contents

Advances in Parasitology, Volume 92
ISSN 0065-308X
http://dx.doi.org/10.1016/bs.apar.2016.03.003

Abstract

Schistosoma japonicum is the main schistosome species in The People's Republic of China, causing intestinal schistosomiasis, a debilitating disease of public health importance. The People's Republic of China used to be heavily endemic with schistosomiasis, but great progress has been made through the vigorous efforts of the national control programmes in the last six decades. Presently, efforts are geared towards eliminating schistosomiasis from The People's Republic of China by the end of 2025 through effective schistosomiasis surveillance, an important component in the drive towards schistosomiasis elimination. Therefore, this article explicitly outlines the development and progress made in schistosomiasis surveillance since 1990 with a special focus on the new surveillance system in use. Although the surveillance system has steadily improved over the years, it is faced with many challenges. Hence, more efforts are needed to establish an effective and sensitive evaluation system for the national schistosomiasis elimination programme in The People's Republic of China.

1. INTRODUCTION

Schistosomiasis, caused by infection with parasitic trematodes, continues to be a public health problem in developing countries, mainly found in Africa, Asia and Latin America. Besides causing serious health problems to humans, schistosomiasis also greatly hinders social and economic development of affected areas (Zheng, 2009). Historically, schistosomiasis was endemic in 12 provinces with 11,600,000 patients and 1,200,000 infected cattle in the 1950s in The People's Republic of China (Chen and Feng, 1999). However, with the strong political commitment and efficient control efforts, great progress has been made in controlling the continued transmission of schistosomiasis in The People's Republic of China (Collins et al., 2012). Disease transmission has been interrupted in five provinces; these include Shanghai (1985), Guangdong (1985), Guangxi (1988), Fujian (1987) and Zhejiang (1995) (Utzinger et al., 2005; Wang et al., 2008). Also, with the implementation of the national medium- and long-term schistosomiasis prevention and control plan (2004–2015) and two rounds of the national programme for schistosomiasis control, the endemic areas have greatly reduced (Wang et al., 2009a,). At the end of 2014, five provinces, including Sichuan, Yunnan, Jiangsu, Hubei and Anhui, attained the status of schistosomiasis transmission control (the infection rates of both residents and domestic animals were less than 1%). Moreover, the lowest levels of infection in both humans and cattle in history have been recorded in the last decade (Xu et al., 2016a). A total of 115, 614 schistosomiasis cases including 30,880 advanced cases were reported at the end of 2014 in The People's Republic of China. In addition, of the 919,579 cattle raised in endemic regions, only 666 were confirmed positive by stool examination (Fig. 1).

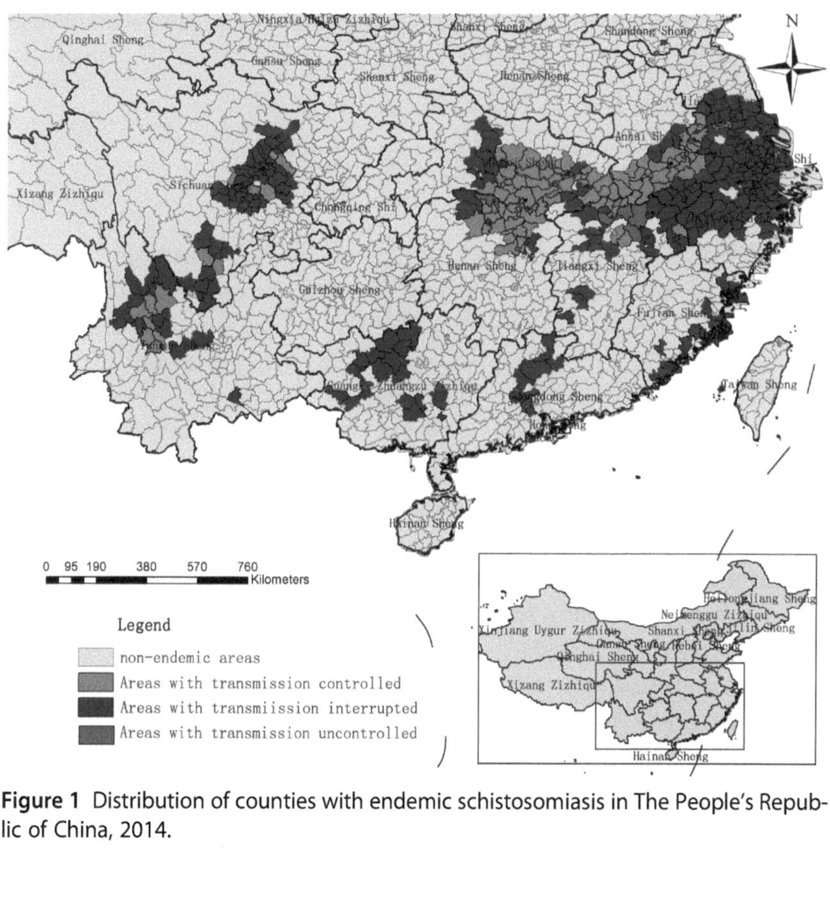

Figure 1 Distribution of counties with endemic schistosomiasis in The People's Republic of China, 2014.

Although schistosomiasis distribution is focal, transmission is complex and difficulties include identifying and managing the infection source, high number of patients and livestock and controlling intermediate host snails. The potential infection or reinfection risk in controlled areas has been recognized for a long time due to the multiple infection sources, frequent floods and human behavioural factors (Utzinger et al., 2005). New cases of cattle or human infection and the re-emergence and distribution of infected snail hosts have been reported in regions where transmission has previously been interrupted or controlled (Wang et al., 2004; Wu et al., 2004). Therefore, it is important to improve and strengthen the surveillance and monitoring system. Since 2010, studies on the construction of sensitive monitoring networks and early warning systems have become a priority in the field of schistosomiasis control in The People's Republic of China (Xu et al., 2014; Yang et al., 2014).

This article systematically reviews the history of the establishment and development of the schistosomiasis surveillance system in The People's Republic of China. The different prevention and control stages, as well as the endemic areas in The People's Republic of China are described. In addition, problems associated with the current Chinese schistosomiasis surveillance systems are also discussed and analyzed.

2. SURVEILLANCE OF SCHISTOSOMIASIS

2.1 Purposes and framework

The definition of surveillance in epidemiology is "the monitoring of activities with an approach that include some characteristics for long-term, continuous, systematic information collection and analysis on the dynamic distribution of disease and its impact factors, to provide scientific basis for implementation of the diseases control programme and intervention measures" (Jiang, 2003).

The main purpose of schistosomiasis surveillance is to better understand the changing patterns of epidemiological characteristics of schistosomiasis and its related impact factors, elucidate the transmission patterns and potential transmission risk of schistosomiasis and adopt the intervention measures for schistosomiasis control in response (Yang et al., 2006). In addition, it helps provide results for effective evaluation of schistosomiasis control strategies and measures.

However, the frame of schistosomiasis surveillance in transmission-controlled areas is different from transmission-interrupted areas. In transmission-controlled areas, the major tasks are to identify and treat patients with schistosomiasis and infected livestock, as well as application of molluscicides for vector snail control in areas where transmission still persists (Zhou et al., 2005). Furthermore, factors associated with schistosomiasis epidemiology are also monitored in these areas (Cao et al., 2016; Liu et al., 2016; Shi et al., 2016; Zhang et al., 2016). In transmission-interrupted areas, there are no patients with schistosomiasis or infected livestock but vector snails inhabit the areas. The major surveillance tasks in transmission-interrupted areas are snail detection, molluscicidal application, monitoring imported infection sources and control of other potential risk factors (Wen et al., 2011; Wu et al., 2005; Zhu et al., 2009).

2.2 Contents and indicators

The surveillance indicators for schistosomiasis mainly included schistosomiasis cases, infected domestic animals, vector snails and the related epidemic factors (Xu et al., 2014).

2.2.1 Schistosomiasis cases

According to the diagnostic criteria issued in 2006, schistosomiasis cases are classified into the following categories: acute schistosomiasis, chronic schistosomiasis and advanced schistosomiasis. Acute schistosomiasis is one of the important indexes to measure the severity of the schistosomiasis epidemic situation in a certain area (Lin et al., 2007). Therefore, surveillance is focused on acute cases where uncontrolled transmission occurs.

2.2.2 Domestic animals

Livestock are a major reservoir host. The surveillance on domestic animals mainly includes cattle, sheep, pigs and horses (Dang et al., 2006), with cattle being the main surveillance focus, as they play a major role in schistosomiasis transmission (Guo et al., 2001).

2.2.3 Snail intermediate hosts

Oncomelania hupensis is the only intermediate host involved in the transmission of *Schistosoma japonicum*, which plays a key role in schistosomiasis transmission (Yang et al., 2009; Zhou et al., 2010). The snail's geographic distribution is consistent with that of schistosomiasis strictly (Li et al., 2016). Therefore, snail monitoring is an important component of the surveillance system including the snail-ridden areas, density and infection rate of snail hosts.

2.2.4 Related epidemic factors

The surveillance on related epidemic factors mainly included surveillance on water level, rainfall, temperature (Wang et al., 2015b; Zhou et al., 2008), the residents' occupational activities and lifestyle and the implementation of schistosomiasis prevention and control measures (Liu et al., 2014; Salam et al., 2014).

3. IMPLEMENTATION AND ACHIEVEMENTS OF SCHISTOSOMIASIS SURVEILLANCE

In general, surveillance can be classified into passive surveillance and active surveillance. In passive surveillance, the subordinate unit routinely reports to the superior unit with surveillance data and information, and the superior unit passively accepts those data. In The People's Republic of China, routine statutory infectious disease reports belong to passive surveillance. Schistosomiasis is categorized as a Class B infectious disease in The People's Republic of China, and the statutory report of schistosomiasis began in 2004 (Jin et al., 2006). So far, most of the reported cases are acute schistosomiasis. In active surveillance, the superior unit conducts special investigations or the subordinate unit collects information in strict accordance to meet special needs. In line with different monitoring purposes, the active surveillance for schistosomiasis in The People's Republic of China can be divided into three categories: (1) repetitive cross-sectional sampling survey, ie, national surveys on schistosomiasis endemicity; (2) longitudinal monitoring of fixed sentinel surveillance, ie, surveillance on sentinel sites. The narrow sense of surveillance usually refers to sentinel surveillance (3) risk surveillance, ie, consolidated surveillance in areas where schistosomiasis transmission has been interrupted.

Specific to the surveillance on schistosomiasis, it usually includes the following types.

3.1 Routine surveillance and emergency endemic surveillance

In The People's Republic of China, the routine surveillance and emergency endemic surveillance on schistosomiasis began in 2005. The routine surveillance of schistosomiasis covers 32 provinces/autonomous regions/municipalities (P/A/M) (excluding Hong Kong, Macao and Taiwan), with main efforts in areas endemic with schistosomiasis, this includes 12 southern P/A/M. The routine surveillance mainly included case reports, case surveys and acute schistosomiasis warnings.

3.1.1 Case report

All levels of medical institutions, disease prevention and control centres, health quarantine institutions and other medical-related institutions are required to report within 24 h after a schistosomiasis case is diagnosed according to the Law of The People's Republic of China on the prevention and treatment of infectious diseases. Schistosomiasis cases are reported through the Web-based Information System of Diseases Prevention and Control. Contents of this report system include name, gender, age, address, contact information, occupation and case classification coded as acute schistosomiasis, chronic schistosomiasis and not classified.

From 2004 to 2014, a total of 1874 acute schistosomiasis cases were reported (Fig. 2). With the significant decrease in acute schistosomiasis cases resulting from the effective schistosomiasis control programme in The People's Republic of China, more attention has been paid to chronic cases.

3.1.2 Case survey

Case surveying investigates the detailed information of the schistosomiasis cases. The focus of case surveying differs at the different control stages of schistosomiasis and with The People's Republic of China's approaches to schistosomiasis control goal of elimination, every schistosomiasis case, including acute, chronic and advanced schistosomiasis cases, was investigated. Information collected in the case survey mainly included name, gender, age, address, contact information, occupation, history of schistosomiasis, history of schistosomiasis treatment, time of diagnosis, diagnostic results, clinical symptoms, results from sera test and stool examination and characteristics of infection sites.

3.1.3 Emergency epidemic surveillance

In 2003, the emergency disposal plan for schistosomiasis (trial) was issued, which defined emergency epidemics that require emergency disposal.

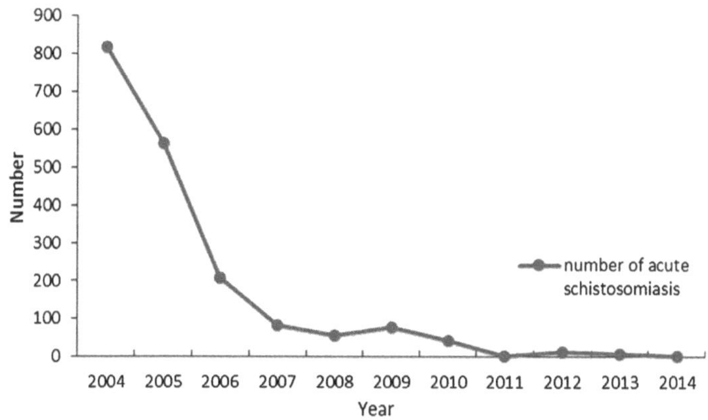

Figure 2 Annual reported cases of acute schistosomiasis from 2004 to 2014, The People's Republic of China (excluding Hong Kong, Macao and Taiwan).

In areas where schistosomiasis transmission is not controlled, detection of 10 or more acute cases in one village within 2 weeks, or five or more acute cases in the same environment within 1 week are considered as emergency epidemic. In areas where schistosomiasis transmission is controlled, detection of five or more acute schistosomiasis cases in one village within 2 weeks, or three or more acute schistosomiasis cases in the same environment within 1 week are considered as emergency epidemic. In areas where schistosomiasis transmission has been interrupted, detected schistosomiasis infection in local residents, livestock or vector snails is considered as an emergency epidemic. However, it is considered as emergency epidemic too if the snail, local infected patients or livestock are detected in areas without schistosomiasis.

Once an emergency epidemic is confirmed, all acute cases were investigated, and the people who had contact with the same infected water were followed up within 2 weeks. The scope of the infection sites can be determined using information collected by the case surveys. In those areas, surveys were conducted to collect data on vector snails, as well as other related natural and social factors including water level, rainfall, temperature, natural disasters, movement of humans and livestock, activities and lifestyle of residents. There were 18 emergency epidemics since the plan was initiated, with 6 emergency epidemics in 2004 and 12 emergency epidemics in 2005 (Hao et al., 2006; Xiao et al., 2004).

3.2 Cross-sectional sampling survey

Three rounds of national sampling surveys on the prevalence of schistosomiasis were successively organized and conducted in 1989, 1995 and 2004. The results not only showed the national dynamic situation of schistosomiasis but also provided an important scientific basis for developing strategies for schistosomiasis control at different stages.

The results from the 1989 survey revealed that there were 1,638,000 patients and 200,000 infected cattle in uncontrolled areas, with infection rates at 10.20% and 13.29%, respectively. This survey provided a scientific basis for the formulation of the eighth "five-year plan" on schistosomiasis control, and also provided systematic and reliable data for the approval of the World Bank Loan Programme for Schistosomiasis Control (WBLPSC) project.

The second national sampling survey of schistosomiasis was conducted in 1995 after the conclusion of the WBLPSC (Zhu et al., 2016). Results from this survey showed 865,084 patients with schistosomiasis and 100,251 infected cattle, and the infection rates were 4.89% and 9.06%, respectively. There were reductions of 47.19% and 49.87% in case numbers compared with that of the first round survey. This survey comprehensively evaluated the effect of the eighth "five-year plan" on schistosomiasis control and the WBLPSC with the results providing guidance for the ninth "five-year control plan" on schistosomiasis in The People's Republic of China.

In 2004, the third national sampling survey of schistosomiasis was conducted in seven P/A/M where schistosomiasis transmission was still uncontrolled. Survey results suggested that the infection rate of residents and cattle were 2.50% and 4.36%, respectively, and there were 726,112 patients from the seven P/A/M. The results of this survey highlighted the important role of livestock as an infection source in the transmission of schistosomiasis in The People's Republic of China. In addition, this survey exposed the challenges in schistosomiasis control: (1) apparent diffusion of *Oncomelania* snails; (2) the relatively high number of schistosomiasis cases and the rising number of acute cases; (3) new or re-emerging endemic foci rising in areas where transmission has already been controlled or interrupted. These observations supported the development of new comprehensive schistosomiasis control strategies with emphasis on infection source control, and the issuing of the National Medium and Long Term Plan on Schistosomiasis Control from 2004 to 2015.

3.3 Sentinel surveillance

Sentinel surveillance is the core of the schistosomiasis surveillance system. It is an encompassing component of schistosomiasis surveillance and it simply implies that, surveillance on schistosomiasis mainly means sentinel surveillance. Generally, sentinel surveillance on schistosomiasis in The People's Republic of China has experienced four stages.

3.3.1 First stage (from 1990 to 1998)

In the eighties, efforts on schistosomiasis control were faced with severe challenges: schistosomiasis epidemics seriously rebounded in some areas, the number of patients with schistosomiasis was high and outbreaks of acute schistosomiasis occurred from time to time (Mao, 1986). Therefore, the Chinese Ministry of Health decided to set up sentinels for schistosomiasis surveillance. A total of 14 surveillance sentinels were established in eight provinces. Sentinel surveillance was designated in each administrative village (county) and the chosen sites represented different endemic types and levels during that period. The sentinel sites were distributed as follows: three sentinel sites in Hunan and Hubei provinces, two sites in Jiangxi and Sichuan provinces and one site in Anhui, Yunnan, Jiangsu provinces and Shanghai municipality. The main contents of the systematic surveillance included collecting schistosomiasis infection rates of permanent residents and livestock, and surveying snails during spring and autumn. Results from the surveillance indicated schistosomiasis endemicity status and the implementation of the systematic surveillance improved the quality of the schistosomiasis control programme. In addition, the surveillance system also provided information that helped in evaluating the performance of WBLPSC.

Taking into account the four counties in Jiangxi (Duchang and Xinjian counties) and Sichuan province (Xichang and Lushan counties) for instance, which belong to the lake and marshland type (Jiangxi province) and hilly/mountainous type (Sichuan province), respectively. The infection rate of populations in Duchang county had declined significantly, while the infection rate in the other three counties fluctuated during the nine surveillance years, especially in Lushan county with signs of re-emergence (Fig. 3).

3.3.2 Second stage (from 2000 to 2004)

The scope of surveillance for schistosomiasis during the first stage was narrow; however, the surveillance contents were simple. In 2000, the Chinese Ministry of Health made adjustment to the national surveillance programme and set up a total of 21 sentinel sites in eight P/A/M. In addition to the epidemiological information, the surveillance contents also included local control measures and implementation intensity. After 5 years of surveillance, the infection rate of residents decreased yearly in six sites,

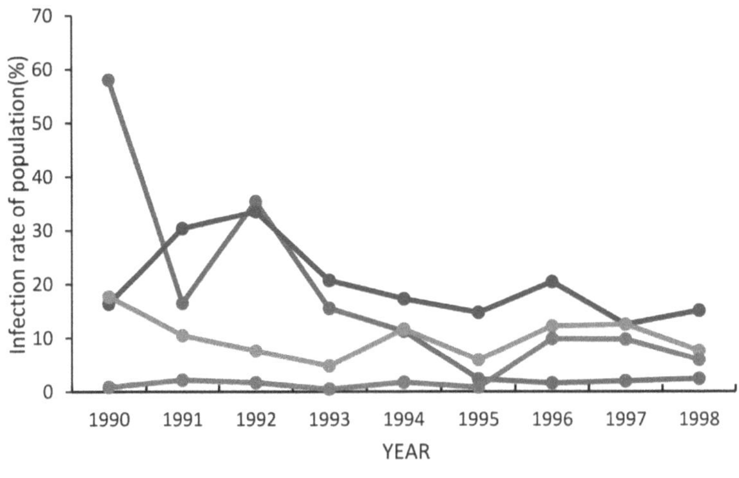

Figure 3 Infection rates of four surveillance sites from 1990 to 1998.

increased yearly in one site and fluctuated in the rest of the sites (Zhao et al., 2006).

The first two stages lasted 15 years, with focus on epidemic information of schistosomiasis. The surveillance results reflected the changes of schistosomiasis endemicity, and provided a basis for the evaluation of schistosomiasis prevention and control measures in The People's Republic of China. Data collected during these 15 years also exposed certain problems, such as limitations of implementing simple chemotherapy measures, difficulties in controlling schistosomiasis reinfection, the inadequate knowledge on the role of cattle in schistosomiasis transmission and the increasing number of imported cases in transmission-controlled or transmission-interrupted areas. Those analyses provided guidance for future improvement of schistosomiasis prevention and control strategies.

However, the sentinel surveillance during the first two stages covered only eight P/A/M that are endemic with schistosomiasis, the number of the surveillance sites in each P/A/M were not more than three and there was no sentinel surveillance in areas with potential transmission risk of schistosomiasis.

3.3.3 Third stage (from 2005 to 2014)

In 2005, 81 national schistosomiasis surveillance sites were established in 11 P/A/M where schistosomiasis transmission was ongoing (Fig. 4). Of particular interest is the surveillance site in Chongqing around the Three Gorges Dam (TGD) to monitor the potential risk for schistosomiasis transmission after the construction of TGD. The contents of the surveillance included usual infection rates of humans, livestock and snails, and natural and social factors such as economic, meteorological and hydrological data were added compared with the first two stages.

This stage lasted 10 years and the scope of the sentinel surveillance covered all P/A/M endemic areas with schistosomiasis except Fujian province. The number of surveillance sites in each province increased; there were 16 surveillance sites in the Hunan and Hubei provinces. The results of the surveillance reflected the epidemic situation at that time. The infection rates of residents and livestock declined significantly during the 10 years (Fig. 5).

3.3.4 Fourth stage (from 2015 to present)

With schistosomiasis control in The People's Republic of China gradually approaching the stage of transmission control, the control work in The People's Republic of China is focused on surveillance. The number of

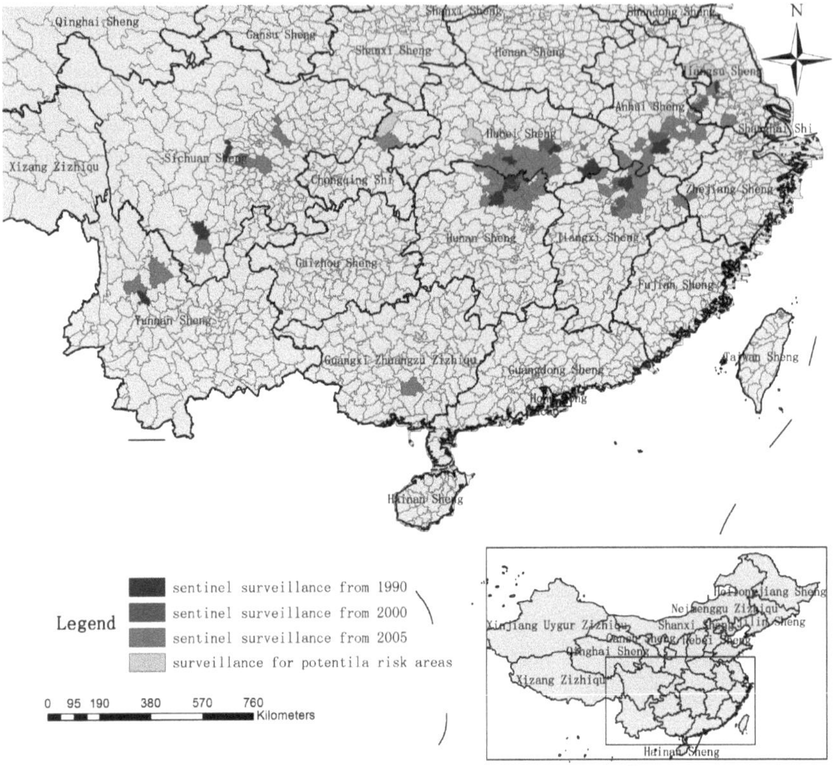

Figure 4 Distribution of the surveillance sites at the first three stages.

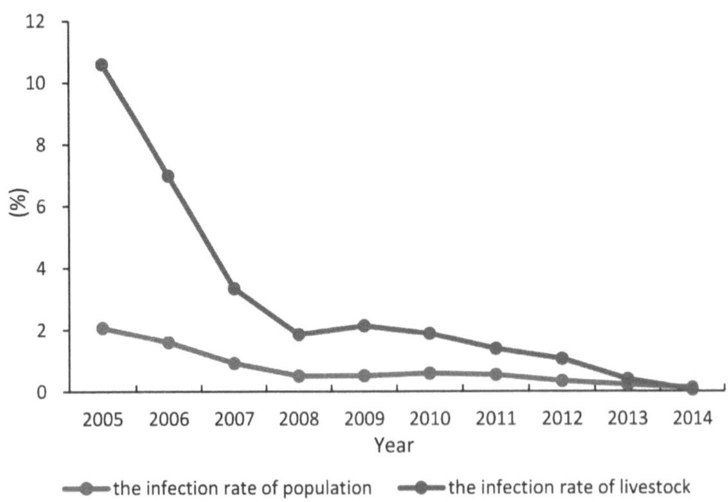

Figure 5 Infection rates of residents and livestock from 2005 to 2014.

surveillance sites falls short of the surveillance needs, and especially in counties with transmission interruption, surveillance work requires strengthening to prevent the rebound of schistosomiasis epidemic. In 2014, 458 national surveillance sites were established in 13 P/A/M, with complete coverage of counties endemic with schistosomiasis and extension to areas with potential transmission risk around TGD.

The development of schistosomiasis sentinel surveillance especially the surveillance from 2015 has presented several characteristics of the changing trend on schistosomiasis sentinel surveillance in The People's Republic of China.

3.3.4.1 Scope of schistosomiasis sentinel surveillance

The scope of schistosomiasis sentinel surveillance has been continuously expanding. The coverage of the surveillance programme has extended from 6 P/A/M in 1990 to 13 P/A/M in 2015 and the number of surveillance sites has increased from 14 to 458, covering all schistosomiasis endemic counties. In addition, four surveillance sites with potential schistosomiasis transmission risk have been added around TGD areas (Fig. 6).

3.3.4.2 Contents of schistosomiasis sentinel surveillance

The protocol of schistosomiasis sentinel surveillance has been constantly improved and adjusted based on the demands of schistosomiasis control; these include case investigation, early warning, serological examination, adoption of the loop-mediated isothermal amplification (LAMP) technology and examination of wildlife faeces.

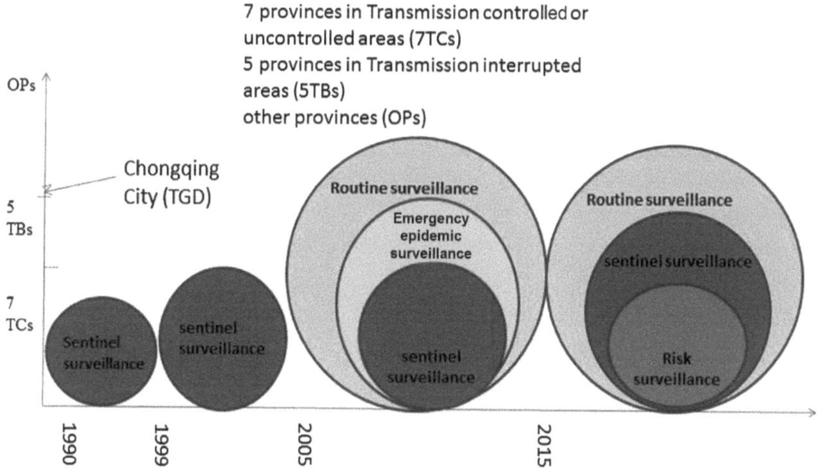

Figure 6 Scope of the schistosomiasis surveillance system at different stages in The People's Republic of China.

At the fourth stage of the sentinel surveillance, case investigation has been extended to cover those confirmed schistosomiasis cases, so as to trace the infection source aiding the gradual elimination of infection sources. This measurement of case management is very important during the process of transiting from transmission control to schistosomiasis elimination in The People's Republic of China. The early warning system has been strengthened to monitor acute schistosomiasis cases, which could feature sudden onset and possible mass outbreak. The early warning system can also help identify, investigate and respond to the epidemics as well as ensure early treatment. In the new surveillance programme the measurements of antibody titre has become much stricter. Antibody level reflects the level of population exposure during a certain period of time, and dynamic changes of the geometric mean and positive antibody titre are important to analyze the changes of local schistosomiasis prevalence (Xie et al., 2012). Traditional methods such as dissection and microscopic examination can only find sporocysts and cercariae in snails. However, it usually takes more than 2 months for miracidia-infected snails to shed cercariae. To solve this issue, LAMP technology targeting nucleic acid has been adopted for snail testing. Moreover, the LAMP technology can also detect DNA markers during the early developmental stages of schistosome parasites in snails, in addition to detecting the biological information of sporocysts and cercariae in snails, thus helping to improve the detection rate of infected snails (Tong et al., 2015). Wildlife faeces investigations can detect environmental infection risks and improve the sensitivity of the surveillance system.

3.3.4.3 Surveillance methods

At the new surveillance stage, based upon different epidemic levels and characteristics, the surveillance areas are divided into areas with transmission control, areas with transmission interruption and potential risk areas around the Three Gorge Reservoir. The transmission-interrupted areas are further divided into areas with and without snails. Different areas can adapt different surveillance items and methods to meet their specific prevention and control needs.

At the fourth stage of surveillance, the floating population is monitored by both active and passive surveillance. Active surveillance is developed in chosen villages to obtain epidemiological information. However, active surveillance has limited ranges and effectiveness, especially when the infection rate is low. Establishing a proper passive surveillance system and setting up sentinel hospitals and institutions are necessary to supplement the active surveillance system. Fixed and mobile surveillance sites have been set up in different areas that are endemic with schistosomiasis. For transmission-interrupted areas without snails, surveillance is focused on detecting cases especially imported cases and identifying potential transmission risk. The mobile surveillance sites can increase surveillance range and relatively improve sensitivity. Table 1 summarizes the surveillance coverage, items and methods used in the national schistosomiasis surveillance system at the four different stages.

3.4 Risk surveillance

Risk surveillance enables early warning and prevention. The choice of risk surveillance sites mainly relies on the results from routine surveillance. Risk surveillance mainly covers the following areas: areas with epidemic rebound and areas with environmental changes due to natural disasters, water conservancy or transportation. Risk surveillance focuses on imported snails, infected wildlife faeces survey and infected water detection using sentinel mice, which were left in the cell cages on the water surface from 10:00 am to 2:00 pm for two consecutive days in each month during the period May to September, and 17 and 6 infected foci in 2010 and 2012 were detected by this way, respectively (Zheng et al., 2012a, 2013a). In a broad sense, risk surveillance can also include schistosomiasis surveillance in potential endemic areas. In order to avoid the spread of possible schistosomiasis transmission that may arise through climate warming and/or water conservancy, the Chinese Ministry of Health in 2008 established 10 fixed surveillance sites and 30 mobile sentinel sites across 10 counties that are not endemic with schistosomiasis in Jiangsu, Shandong, Anhui and Hubei provinces and Chongqing municipality (Dang et al., 2014). The surveillance in potential endemic areas was mainly implemented by investigating susceptible cases, monitoring the floating population and livestock.

4. CHALLENGES AND FUTURE DIRECTIONS

4.1 Challenges

4.1.1 Low sensitivity of schistosomiasis diagnostics

Before 2005, the Kato-Katz technique was used to identify schistosome eggs in human stool samples and stool hatching methods were carried out to identify infected cattle during the national surveillance programme (Zhao et al., 2005). After 2005, populations were first screened using sera

Table 1 Surveillance coverage, items and methods listed in the national schistosomiasis surveillance system at the four different stages

	First stage	Second stage	Third stage		Fourth stage			
						Counties with transmission interrupted		
Surveillance items	Areas with severe endemic	Areas with severe endemic	Counties with transmission not interrupted	Counties with transmission interrupted (including the Three Gorged Reservoir)	Counties with transmission not interrupted	With snails	Without snails	The Three Gorged Reservoir
Number of sites	14	21	80–81		458			
Number of P/A/M	6	7	12		13			
Setting	Fixed village	Fixed village	Fixed village		Fixed village	Fixed village	Flow village	Fixed village
Examination methods for local residents	Stool examination with Kato-Katz	Screening by sera examination and stool examination with Kato-Katz or only stool examination	Screening by sera examination and stool examination with Kato-Katz	Screening by sera examination and stool examination with Kato-Katz (every other year)	Screening by sera examination and stool examination with Kato-Katz and stool hatching method	Screening by sera examination and stool examination with Kato-katz and stool hatching method	—	—
Examination methods for floating population	None	None	Active surveillance: ≥30 persons	Active surveillance: ≥100 persons	Active and passive surveillance:≥200 persons			Active and passive surveillance: ≥200 persons
Examination methods for livestock	Stool examination	Stool examination	Stool examination	—	Stool examination	Stool examination on imported livestock		

Snail survey	Environment with snails	Environment with snails	Environment with snails or suspected	Environment with snails in history or suspected	Environment with snails or suspected	Environment with snails or suspected	Environment with snails in history or with imported risk	Environment with snails imported risk, more than 5 environments and flotage examination (more than five water areas)
	Microscopic examination	Microscopic examination	Microscopic examination	Microscopic examination	Microscopic examination and LAMP	Microscopic examination and LAMP (if possible)	Microscopic examination and LAMP (if possible)	
Wild faeces investigation	None	None	None	None	Area with snails and human or livestock	None		
Related factors	None	None	Natural and social factors	Natural and social factors	None	None	None	None
	Control measures	Control measures	Control measures	Control measures	Control measures	Control measures	Control measures	Control measures

LAMP, Loop-mediated isothermal amplification; *P/A/M*, provinces/autonomous regions/municipalities.

examination and positive cases were confirmed by Kato-Katz examination (Dang et al., 2008). Some studies showed that the false-negative rate of the Kato-Katz technique was 5.56–89.47%; especially in areas with infection rates less than 3%, the false-negative rate was as high as 30% (Zhu et al., 2005). Effective evaluation of the field application for four serological diagnosis methods showed that the sensitivity of the four methods were all significantly higher than that of the pathogen-detecting methods, but the specificity of serological test was low and this method cannot exclude previous infections (Xu et al., 2007). However, because of the effective schistosomiasis control in The People's Republic of China, the infection rate in most villages was less than 1% (Lei et al., 2014); therefore, using serological diagnostic methods for screening and then Kato-Katz technique for clarification was still unable to avoid the problems of false-positive and false-negative results, which decreased the reliability of surveillance results. Therefore, both stool hatching and Kato-Katz techniques should be used for screening positive results to increase the sensitivity of the results.

4.1.2 Traditional snail survey technology

At present, snail surveys are conducted manually, and the survey quality can be influenced by many factors such as season, climate, light and vegetation (Huang et al., 2010). Therefore the traditional method of snail surveying is unable to meet the requirements of current monitoring work (Zheng et al., 2013b); new technologies such as Geographic Information System and remote sensing, and special analysis methods, can be applied on snail surveillance (Hu et al., 2015; Qiu et al., 2014; Yang et al., 2005; Zhou et al., 2015). Furthermore, easy and rapid detection methods for infected snails should be developed for epidemics and outbreaks of acute schistosomiasis.

4.1.3 Deficiency in the surveillance technology on imported schistosomiasis cases

With the increase in trade and communication between The People's Republic of China and Africa, returning travellers or workers with African schistosomiasis have been frequently reported in The People's Republic of China (Xu et al., 2016a,b). Reports of imported cases of urogenital schistosomiasis, caused by infection with *Schistosoma haematobium,* to The People's Republic of China can be traced back to the 1970s, when The People's Republic of China sent technicians and workers to support infrastructure construction in African countries (Lu et al., 2014). Major clinical manifestations of *S. haematobium* include hematuresis, bladder irritation and urinary tract obstruction. Those cases are often erroneously diagnosed as sexually transmitted diseases, cystitis, tuberculosis or tumours because the symptoms of *S. haematobium* infection are quite different from that of *S. japonicum*. Due to the lack of diagnostic tools and related knowledge of *S. haematobium*, it is difficult for hospitals or institutions to diagnose and control *S. haematobium* in The People's Republic of China. The current surveillance system mainly focuses on *S. japonicum* (Clerinx and Van Gompel, 2011; Hua et al., 2013). Reports of the imported cases were included in the routine case report surveillance; however, most cases were missed.

4.1.4 Lack of effective monitoring network evaluation system

The main function of the current surveillance network largely relies on data collection, which determines the sensitivity, functionality, effectiveness, quality control and cost-effectiveness of the surveillance system. However, there is no systematic evaluation system in place to monitor the surveillance network.

4.2 Future directions

4.2.1 Effective evaluation of schistosomiasis surveillance

The implementation of schistosomiasis surveillance systems is helpful for schistosomiasis control. In areas with schistosomiasis interrupted status, the improvement of surveillance capacity is helpful to detect imported cases and potential outbreaks. For instance, there were imported acute and chronic schistosomiasis cases reported from Shanghai municipality and Zhejiang province, although these two areas reached the level of transmission interruption in 1984 and 1995, respectively (Lei et al., 2014; Wang et al., 2015a; Zheng et al., 2012a,b, 2013b) (Fig. 7).

4.2.2 Sensitivity indexes of schistosomiasis surveillance

The transmission of schistosomiasis is influenced by many factors, including biological, natural and social factors, which reflect the occurrence and development of schistosomiasis epidemics. The indicators for schistosomiasis epidemics include infection rate of humans and livestock, and density/infection rates of vector snails. These indexes are traditional indicators for schistosomiasis surveillance, which can directly reflect the epidemic status. Natural factors mainly refer to factors related to the environment, such as water level, vegetation and rainfall. Survival and reproduction of vector snails are closely related to environmental factors; these include temperature, rainfall,

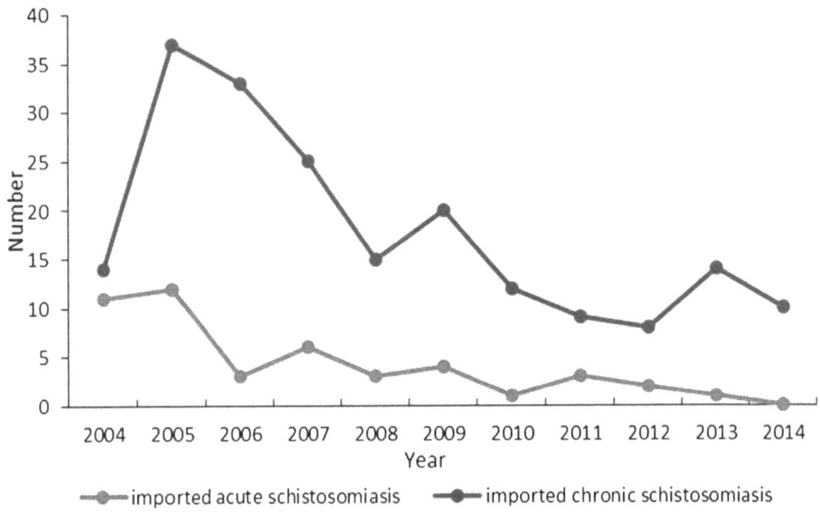

Figure 7 Reported cases from provinces with schistosomiasis transmission interrupted or nonendemic.

vegetation and soil moisture (Bavia et al., 2001; Gomes et al., 2012; Guimaraes et al., 2008; Hu et al., 2013). Social and economic indicators usually include lifestyle factors, population production activities and population mobility.

5. CONCLUSIONS AND RECOMMENDATIONS

At present, The People's Republic of China has established a nationwide schistosomiasis surveillance system and the sentinel surveillance covers all the counties that are endemic with schistosomiasis, as well as potential risk areas (Feng et al., 2016). All the schistosomiasis cases should be reported through the web-based information system including acute, chronic and imported schistosomiasis cases. The design is set up to ensure timely detection, monitoring and treatment of every schistosomiasis case, as well as determine its infection source and transmission route, to prevent potential transmission.

However, with the fast development of economy and technology sectors in The People's Republic of China, improving schistosomiasis surveillance systems is quickly becoming an important task for effective schistosomiasis prevention and control. Since the disease surveillance is gradually transiting from epidemic surveillance to public health surveillance, more attention should be paid to the factors related to schistosomiasis epidemics. Currently, related factor surveillance is still a supplement to epidemic surveillance with uneven surveillance quality; hence, it is difficult to use the data collected effectively. In the future, quantitative data collection of natural, social and behavioural factors will be improved upon the comprehensive related factor surveillance, so as to achieve accurate prediction and detect early warning signs of schistosomiasis transmission or resurgence.

Although the current schistosomiasis surveillance is mainly focused on collecting and summarizing data from previous epidemics, in the future, a schistosomiasis monitoring network is required to enable epidemic forecast, and provide evidence for targeted preventive and control measures (Tambo et al., 2014; Zhou et al., 2011).

COMPETING INTERESTS

The authors declare that they do not have competing interests.

AUTHORS' CONTRIBUTIONS

L.-J. Zhang, S.-Z. Li and X.-N. Zhou conceived the study; L.-J. Zhang, S.-Z. Li wrote the manuscript; L.-Y. Wen, D.-D. Lin, R. Zhu, Y. Du, S. Lv, J. Xu, E.M. Abe, B. L. Webster, D. Rollinson and X.-N. Zhou revised the manuscript and gave approval of the version to be published. All the authors read and approved the final version of the manuscript.

ACKNOWLEDGEMENTS

This study was supported by the National Natural Science Foundation of China (No. 81101280), the National Special Science and Technology Project for Major Infectious Diseases of China (Grant No. 2012ZX10004-220, 2012ZX10004-201 and 2016ZX10004222-006), China–UK Global Health Support Programme(Grant No.: GHSP-CS-OP1-01), The fourth round of Three-Year Public Health Action Plan (GWIV-29).

REFERENCES

Bavia, M.E., Malone, J.B., Hale, L., Dantas, A., Marroni, L., Reis, R., 2001. Use of thermal and vegetation index data from earth observing satellites to evaluate the risk of schistosomiasis in Bahia, Brazil. Acta Trop. 79, 79–85.

Cao, Z.G., Zhao, Y.E., Willingham, A.L., Wang, T.P., 2016. Towards the elimination of schistosomiasis japonica through control of the disease in domestic animals in the People's Republic of China: a tale of over 60 years. Adv. Parasitol. 92.

Chen, M.G., Feng, Z., 1999. Schistosomiasis control in China. Parasitol. Int. 48, 11–19.

Clerinx, J., Van Gompel, A., 2011. Schistosomiasis in travellers and migrants. Travel Med. Infect. Dis. 9, 6–24.

Collins, C., Xu, J., Tang, S., 2012. Schistosomiasis control and the health system in P.R. China. Infect. Dis. Poverty 1, 8.

Dang, H., Zhu, R., Guo, J.G., 2006. Report of the result of national surveillance for schistosomiasis in China, 2005. J. Trop. Dis. Parasitol. 4, 189–193 (in Chinese).

Dang, H., Zhu, R., Guo, J.G., 2008. Surveillance of schistosomiasis in China from 2005~2007. Chin. J. Schistosomiasis Control 20, 241–244 (in Chinese).

Dang, H., Xu, J., Li, S.Z., Cao, Z.G., Huang, Y.X., Wu, C.G., et al., 2014. Monitoring the transmission of *Schistosoma japonicum* in potential risk regions of China, 2008–2012. Int. J. Environ. Res. Public Health 11, 2278–2287.

Feng, Y., Liu, L., Xia, S., Xu, J.F., Bergquist, R., Yang, G.J., 2016. Reaching the surveillance-response stage of schistosomiasis control in the People's Republic of China: a modelling approach. Adv. Parasitol. 92.

Gomes, E.C.S., Leal-Neto, O.B., Albuquerque, J., Silva, H.P., Barbosa, C.S., 2012. Schistosomiasis transmission and environmental change: a spatio-temporal analysis in Porto de Galinhas, Pernambuco – Brazil. Int. J. Health Geogr. 11, 51.

Guimaraes, R.J., Freitas, C.C., Dutra, L.V., Moura, A.C., Amaral, R.S., Drummond, S.C., et al., 2008. Schistosomiasis risk estimation in Minas Gerais State, Brazil, using environmental data and GIS techniques. Acta Trop. 108, 234–241.

Guo, J.G., Ross, A.G., Lin, D.D., Williams, G.M., Chen, H.G., Li, Y., et al., 2001. A baseline study on the importance of bovines for human *Schistosoma japonicum* infection around Poyang Lake, China. Am. J. Trop. Med. Hyg. 65, 272–278.

Hao, Y., Wu, X.H., Xia, G., Zheng, H., Guo, J.G., Wang, L.Y., et al., 2006. Schistosomiasis situation in People's Republic of China in 2005. Chin. J. Schistosomiasis Control 18, 321–324 (in Chinese).

Hu, Y., Zhang, Z.J., Chen, Y., Wang, Z.L., Gao, J., Tao, B., et al., 2013. Spatial pattern of schistosomiasis in Xingzi, Jiangxi province, China: the effects of environmental factors. Parasites Vectors 6, 214.

Hu, Y., Li, R., Bergquist, R., Lynn, H., Gao, F.H., Wang, Q.Z., et al., 2015. Spatio-temporal transmission and environmental determinants of schistosomiasis japonica in Anhui province, China. PLoS Neglected Trop. Dis. 9, e0003470.

Hua, H.Y., Wang, W., Cao, G.Q., Tang, F., Liang, Y.S., 2013. Improving the management of imported schistosomiasis haematobia in China: lessons from a case with multiple misdiagnoses. Parasites Vectors 6, 260.

Huang, S.Y., Zhang, Q.M., Lin, R.X., Deng, Z.H., Zhang, X.C., Huo, l.c, et al., 2010. Establishment and evaluation of quality control methods of *Oncomelania hupensis* snail investigation in transmission interrupted areas of schistosomiasis. Chin. J. Schistosomiasis Control 22, 355–359 (in Chinese).

Jiang, Q.W., 2003. Epidemiology. Science Press, Beijing (in Chinese).

Jin, S.G., Jiang, T., Ma, J.Q., 2006. Brief introduction of Chinese infectious disease detection report information system. China Digit. Med. 1, 20–22 (in Chinese).

Lei, Z.L., Zheng, H., Zhang, L.J., Zhu, R., Xu, Z.M., Xu, J., et al., 2014. Endemic status of schitosomiasis in People's Republic of China in 2013. Chin. J. Schistosomiasis Control 26, 591–597 (in Chinese).

Li, Z.J., Ge, J., Dai, J.R., Wen, L.Y., Lin, D.D., Madsen, H., et al., 2016. Biology and control of snail intermediate host of *Schistosoma japonicum* in the People's Republic of China. Adv. Parasitol. 92.

Lin, D.D., Wang, S.P., Jiang, Q.W., Zhang, S.Q., Xu, J., Fang, J.C., et al., 2007. Technical indexes of the criteria for infection control of schistosomiasis in China. Chin. J. Schistosomiasis Control 19, 5–8 (in Chinese).

Liu, L., Yang, G.J., Zhu, H.R., Yang, K., Ai, L., 2014. Knowledge of attitudes towards, and practice relating to schistosomiasis in two subtypes of a mountainous region of the People's Republic of China. Infect. Dis. Poverty 3, 16.

Liu, Y., Zhou, Y.B., Li, R.Z., Wan, J.J., Yang, Y., Qiu, D.C., et al., 2016. Epidemiological features and control effectiveness of schistosomiasis in mountainous and hilly region of the People's Republic of China. Adv. Parasitol. 92.

Lu, P., Wang, W., Dai, J., Liang, Y., 2014. Imported African schistosomiasis: is it an emerging public health concern in China? J. Travel Med. 21, 72–73.

Mao, S.B., 1986. Recent progress in the control of schistosomiasis in China. Chin. Med. J. 99, 439–443.
Qiu, J., Li, R.D., Xu, X.J., Yu, C.H., Xia, X., Hong, X.C., et al., 2014. Identifying determinants of *Oncomelania hupensis* habitats and assessing the effects of environmental control strategies in the plain regions with the waterway network of China at the microscale. Int. J. Environ. Res. Public Health 11, 6571–6585.
Salam, R.A., Maredia, H., Das, J.K., Lassi, Z.S., Bhutta, Z.A., 2014. Community-based interventions for the prevention and control of helmintic neglected tropical diseases. Infect. Dis. Poverty 3, 23.
Shi, L., Li, W., Wu, F., Zhang, J.F., Yang, K., Zhou, X.N., 2016. Epidemiological features and control progress of schistosomiasis in waterway-network region in P.R. China. Adv. Parasitol. 92.
Tambo, E., Ai, L., Zhou, X., Chen, J.H., Hu, W., Bergquist, R., et al., 2014. Surveillance-response systems: the key to elimination of tropical diseases. Infect. Dis. Poverty 3, 17.
Tong, Q., Chen, R., Zhang, Y., Yang, G., Kumagaid, T., Shimogawarad, R., et al., 2015. A new surveillance and response tool: risk map of infected *Oncomelania hupensis* detected by loop-mediated isothermal amplification (LAMP) from pooled samples. Acta Trop. 141, 170–177.
Utzinger, J., Zhou, X.N., Chen, M.G., Bergquist, R., 2005. Conquering schistosomiasis in China: the long march. Acta Trop. 96, 69–96.
Wang, R.B., Wang, T.P., Wang, L.Y., Guo, J.G., Yu, Q., Xu, J., et al., 2004. Study on the re-emerging situation of schistosomiasis epidemics in areas already under control and interruption. Chin. J. Epidemiol. 25, 564–567 (in Chinese).
Wang, L.D., Utzinger, J., Zhou, X.N., 2008. Schistosomiasis control: experiences and lessons from China. Lancet 372, 1793–1795.
Wang, L.D., Chen, H.G., Guo, J.G., Zeng, X.J., Hong, X.L., Xiong, J.J., et al., 2009a. A strategy to control transmission of *Schistosoma japonicum* in China. N. Engl. J. Med. 360, 121–128.
Wang, L.D., Guo, J.G., Wu, X.H., Chen, H.G., Wang, T.P., Zhu, S.P., et al., 2009b. China's new strategy to block *Schistosoma japonicum* transmission: experiences and impact beyond schistosomiasis. Trop. Med. Int. Health TM IH 14, 1475–1483.
Wang, Q., Xu, J., Zhang, L.J., Zheng, H., Ruan, Y., Hao, Y.W., et al., 2015a. Analysis of endemic changes of schistosomiasis in China from 2002 to 2010. Chin. J. Schistosomiasis Control 27, 229–234 (in Chinese).
Wang, Y.J., Rao, Y.H., Wu, X.X., Zhao, H.N., Chen, J., 2015b. A method for screening climate change-sensitive infectious diseases. Int. J. Environ. Res. Public Health 12, 767–783.
Wen, L.Y., Yan, X.L., Zhang, J.F., Li, L.S., Lin, L.J., Huang, S.Y., et al., 2011. Strategy of solidification and surveillance for schistosomiasis in transmission interrupted provinces in China. Chin. J. Schistosomiasis Control 23, 18–21 (in Chinese).
Wu, X.H., Xu, J., Zheng, J., Guo, J.G., 2004. Challenges and control strategies in areas of schistosomiasis transmission controlled and interrupted in China. Chin. J. Schistosomiasis Control 16, 1–3 (in Chinese).
Wu, X.H., Chen, M.G., Zheng, J., 2005. Surveillance of schistosomiasis in five provinces of China which have reached the national criteria for elimination of the disease. Acta Trop. 96, 276–281.
Xiao, D.L., Yu, Q., Dang, H., Guo, J.G., Zhou, X.N., Wang, L.Y., 2004. Schistosomiasis situation in People's Republic of China. Chin. J. Schistosomiasis Control 16, 401–404 (in Chinese).
Xie, S.Y., Yuan, M., Hu, F., Liu, Y.M., Zeng, X.J., Tao, B., et al., 2012. Study on immune status of patients with schistosomiasis japonica in Poyang Lake region I characterization of

antigen-specific antibody isotype responses to *Schistosoma japonicum*. Chin. J. Schistosomiasis Control 24, 510–513 (in Chinese).

Xu, J., Chen, N.G., Feng, T., Wang, E.M., Wu, X.H., Chen, H.G., et al., 2007. Effectiveness of routinely used assays for the diagnosis of schistosomiasis japonica in the field. Chin. J. Parasitol. Parasit. Dis. 25, 175–179 (in Chinese).

Xu, J., Yang, K., Li, S.Z., Zhou, X.N., 2014. Surveillance system after transmission control of schistosomiasis in P.R.China. Chin. J. Schistosomiasis Control 26, 1–5 (in Chinese).

Xu, J., Steinman, P., Maybe, D., Zhou, X.N., Lv, S., Li, S.Z., et al., 2016a. Evolution of the national schistosomiasis control programmes in the People's Republic of China. Adv. Parasitol. 92.

Xu, J., Yu, Q., Tchuem-Tchuenté, L.A., Bergquist, R., Sacko, M., Utzinger, J., et al., 2016b. Enhancing collaboration between China and African countries for schistosomiasis control. Lancet Infect. Dis. http://dx.doi.org/10.1016/S1473-3099(1015)00360-00366. Published Online: 03 February 2016.

Yang, G.J., Vounatsou, P., Zhou, X.N., Utzinger, J., Tanner, M., 2005. A review of geographic information system and remote sensing with applications to the epidemiology and control of schistosomiasis in China. Acta Trop. 96, 117–129.

Yang, Y., Nie, S.F., Zhou, D.J., 2006. Current status and progress of research on surveillance of schistosomiasis. Chin. J. Schistosomiasis Control 18, 477–479 (in Chinese).

Yang, K., Zhou, X.N., Wu, X.H., Steinmann, P., Wang, X.H., Yang, G.J., et al., 2009. Landscape pattern analysis and Bayesian modeling for predicting *Oncomelania hupensis* distribution in Eryuan county, People's Republic of China. Am. J. Trop. Med. Hyg. 81, 416–423.

Yang, G.J., Liu, L., Zhu, H.R., Griffiths, S.M., Tanner, M., Bergquist, R., et al., 2014. China's sustained drive to eliminate neglected tropical diseases. Lancet Infect. Dis. 14, 881–892.

Zhang, S.Q., Sun, C.S., Wang, M., Lin, D.D., Zhou, X.N., Wang, T.P., 2016. Epidemiological features and control effectiveness of schistosomiasis in lake and marshland region in the People's Republic of China. Adv. Parasitol. 92.

Zhao, G.M., Zhao, Q., Jiang, Q.W., Chen, X.Y., Wang, L.Y., Yuan, H.C., 2005. Surveillance for schistosomiasis japonica in China from 2000 to 2003. Acta Trop. 96, 288–295.

Zhao, G.M., Wang, L.Y., Zhao, Q., Chen, X.Y., Xiao, D.L., He, N., et al., 2006. National surveillance of schistosomiasis in China from 2000 to 2004. Chin. J. Parasitol. Parasit. Dis. 24, 4–9 (in Chinese).

Zheng, H., Sun, L.P., Zhu, R., Tu, Z.W., Li, Y.Y., Yang, W.P., et al., 2012a. Surveillance and forecast of *Schistosoma japonicum*-infected sentinel mice in key water regions of China in 2010. Chin. J. Schistosomiasis Control 24, 5–9 (in Chinese).

Zheng, H., Zhang, L.J., Zhu, R., Xu, J., Li, S.Z., Guo, J.G., et al., 2012b. Schistosomiasis situation in People's Republic of China in 2011. Chin. J. Schistosomiasis Control 24, 621–626 (in Chinese).

Zheng, H., Li, S.Z., Cao, C.L., Zhang, L.J., Sun, L.P., Yang, K., et al., 2013a. Surveillance and response for schistosomiasis japonica based on sentinel mice examination for cercariae-infested water in risk region, 2012. Chin. J. Parasitol. Parasit. Dis. 31, 428–432 (in Chinese).

Zheng, Q., Vanderslott, S., Jiang, B., Xu, L.L., Liu, C.S., Huo, L.L., et al., 2013b. Research gaps for three main tropical diseases in the People's Republic of China. Infect. Dis. Poverty 2, 15.

Zheng, J., 2009. Achievements and challenges in schistosomiasis control in China. Chin. J. Parasitol. Parasit. Dis. 27, 398–401 (in Chinese).

Zhou, X.N., Jiang, Q.W., Sun, L.P., Wang, T.P., Hong, Q.B., Zhao, G.M., et al., 2005. Schistosomiasis control and surveillance in China. Chin. J. Schistosomiasis Control 17, 161–165 (in Chinese).

Zhou, X.N., Yang, G.J., Yang, K., Wang, X.H., Hong, Q.B., Sun, L.P., et al., 2008. Potential impact of climate change on schistosomiasis transmission in China. Am. J. Trop. Med. Hyg. 78, 188–194.

Zhou, X.N., Bergquist, R., Leonardo, L., Yang, G.J., Yang, K., Sudomo, M., et al., 2010. Schistosomiasis japonica control and research needs. Adv. Parasitol. 72, 145–178.

Zhou, X.N., Xu, J., Chen, H.G., Wang, T.P., Huang, X.B., Lin, D.D., et al., 2011. Tools to support policy decisions related to treatment strategies and surveillance of schistosomiasis japonica towards elimination. PLoS Neglected Trop. Dis. 5, e1408.

Zhou, X.N., Olveda, R., Sripa, B., Yang, G.J., Leonardo, L., Bergquist, R., 2015. From gap analysis to solution and action: the RNAS(+) model. Acta Trop. 141, 146–149.

Zhu, H.Q., Cao, C.L., Gao, F.H., Guo, J.G., Bao, Z.P., Wang, X.H., et al., 2005. Evaluation of effectiveness of modified Kato-Katz technique for diagnosis of schistosomiasis japonica. Chin. J. Schistosomiasis Control 17, 273–277 (in Chinese).

Zhu, Y.F., Gao, J.B., Kuang, R.X., He, Y., Wan, Z., Jin, W., et al., 2009. Surveillance methods on infectious source in schistosomiasis transmission interrupted areas. Chin. J. Schistosomiasis Control 21, 428–429 (in Chinese).

Zhu, H., Yap, P., Utzinger, J., Jia, T.W., Li, S.Z., Huang, X.B., et al., 2016. Policy support and resources mobilization for the national schistosomiasis control programme in the People's Republic of China. Adv. Parasitol. 92.

CHAPTER SIX

Applications of Spatial Technology in Schistosomiasis Control Programme in The People's Republic of China

X.-Y. Wang*,§, J. He*,§, K. Yang*,§,1, S. Liang¶,1

*Jiangsu Institute of Parasitic Diseases, Key Laboratory of Parasitic Disease Control and Prevention (Ministry of Health), Jiangsu Provincial Key Laboratory of Parasite Molecular Biology, Wuxi, The People's Republic of China

§Public Health Research Center, Jiangnan University, Wuxi, The People's Republic of China

¶University of Florida, Gainesville, FL, United States

[1]Corresponding authors: E-mail: jipdyk@163.com; songliang@ufl.edu

Contents

Abstract

Schistosomiasis, as the important parasitic disease, has caused serious threats to human health globally. The People's Republic of China has acquired significant achievements

Advances in Parasitology, Volume 92
ISSN 0065-308X
http://dx.doi.org/10.1016/bs.apar.2016.02.020

based on large-scale interventions and innovational technology. The spatial technology was introduced in 1980s and widely used in the study and control of schistosomiasis in The People's Republic of China. This chapter reviews the progress and application of spatial technology in schistosomiasis control by analysing the spatiotemporal pattern of and the impact of ecological changes on schistosomiasis transmission, which have provided the information to design and select the control strategy, and assisted the establishment of the monitoring and early warning system in The People's Republic of China, especially in the marshland and mountainous regions.

1. INTRODUCTION

Spatial epidemiology, a subfield of health geography, focuses on the study of the spatial distribution of health outcomes, and it is the description and analysis of geographically indexed health data with respect to demographic, environmental, behavioural, socioeconomic, genetic and infectious risk factors (Bi and Tong, 2014; Elliott and Wartenberg, 2004; Stoltzfus et al., 2014). Spatial technology, as the important tool of spatial epidemiology, is concerned with the description and examination of disease and its geographical variations (Abbas et al., 2015). The spatial technology can be applied in fields of disease mapping, geographical correlation, clustering, disease clusters and surveillance (Liu et al., 2012; Wiwanitkit et al., 2013; Zhou et al., 2015).

Schistosomiasis remains a major public health issue in tropical and subtropical regions of the world, putting about 800 million people at risk of schistosomiasis infection and more than 200 million infections (Collins et al., 2012; Dam et al., 2015). The schistosomiasis endemic areas can be divided into three types based the environmental characteristics of snail habitats, namely, lake and marshland region, mountainous and hilly region, and water network region (Chen, 2014; Xu et al., 2016; Zhu et al., 2009). Since 1990s, Zhou et al. (1998) firstly applied spatial technology to study the transmission of schistosomiasis in the southern part of The People's Republic of China, and to build a serial conceptual model based on the interaction of the parasite and its intermediate host, the snail and parameters required for the development of both *Schistosoma japonicum* and *Oncomelania hupensis* so as to predict the distribution of schisotosmiasis in The People's Republic of China. This technology has played an important role in the procedure of schisotosmiasis control and elimination in The People's Republic of China.

2. INTRODUCTION OF SPATIAL TECHNOLOGY

Spatial technology includes any of the formal techniques which study entities using their topological, geometrical, or geographical properties, and many are still in their early development, using different analytical approaches and applied in fields as diverse as astronomy. In a more restricted sense, spatial analysis involves the use of techniques applied to structures at the human scale, most notably in the analysis of geographical data (Efron, 1994; Wheatley and Gillings, 2003; Zhou et al., 2015). In the field of disease study, this technology mainly includes geographical information systems (GIS), remote sensing (RS), global positioning system (GPS), Google Earth (GE) and spatiotemporal statistics and models (Feng et al., 2016).

2.1 Geographic information systems

The GIS techniques rely on a computer system to manage and analyse the spatial data. With the support of computer software and hardware, GIS uses the theory of systems engineering and information science, the spatial data according to the geographical coordinates or space for various processing, to complete functions of data input, storage, processing, management, analysis and output, and study all kinds of spatial entity and their mutual relations (Bonham-Carter, 2014; Fotheringham and Rogerson, 2013). It has been adopted as a useful tool by a wide range of disciplines such as environmental planning, property management, emergence planning, automobile navigation systems, urban studies and market analyses. Among others the GIS can provide comprehensive access to the database, query features, and create themes, layouts and reports (Abbas et al., 2015; Chen, 2007).

Spatial query and analysis is the core of GIS functions, which are the essential characteristics different from other information systems. Data query retrieval involves finding and selecting the required data from the data files, databases or storage devices. The spatial query mainly includes address, location, region matching, hierarchical conditions and spatial relation identification. Spatial analysis include buffer analysis, overlay analysis, network analysis, spatial interpolation, spatial classification analysis, spatial statistical analysis, and digital elevation model and terrain analysis. Furthermore, GIS is used to draw maps, which can provide various ways to digital express, operate and display of map features. For example, Fig. 1 shows the distribution of schistosomiasis in The People's Republic of China in 2011 (Li et al., 2014).

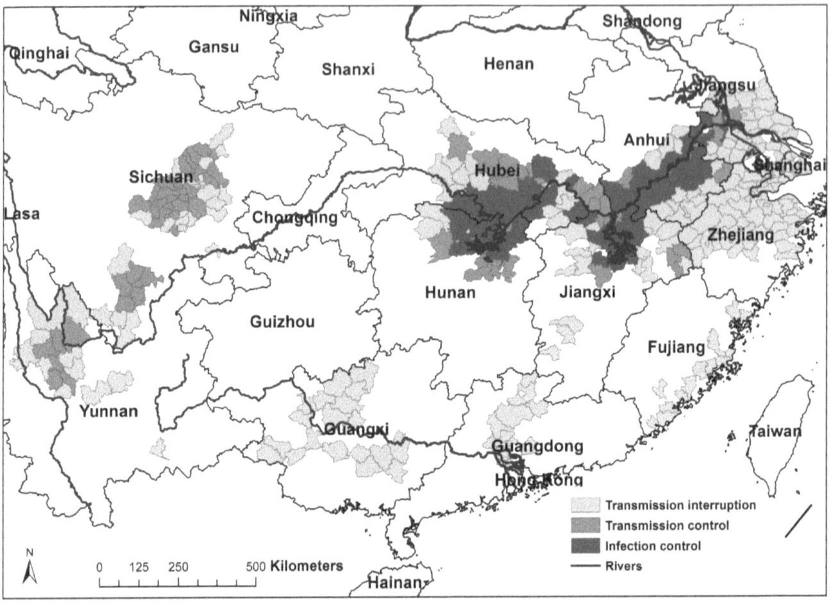

Figure 1 Schistosomiasis distribution in The People's Republic of China in 2011.

In general, the cost of GIS software, such as ArcGIS from ERSI Company, is very expensive, and the operation of the software is also complicated. The usage of GIS is always confined to a relatively small number of trained experts (Thoen, 1995). In view of the fast development of Internet, the combination of GIS can be deployed on the Internet and established intranets of interested user groups, such as the Internet GIS (Web GIS) to extend the considerable functionality of GIS by Internet. The users will be able to access GIS services without purchasing proprietary GIS software (Foote et al., 1997). Once user-friendly Web GIS becomes widely available on the Internet, it could be readily applied to guide schistosomiasis control and disease surveillance in The People's Republic of China and other schistosome-endemic areas (Yang et al., 2005).

2.2 Remote sensing

The technology of RS, emerged in the 1960s, refers to the high-altitude and outer-space platforms, using various sensors (eg, camera, scanner and radar) to obtain the land surface information, through the data transmission and processing, and to realize the relationship between ground object shape, size, location, nature and environment (Jensen and Lulla, 1987; Matthews,

2011). At present, RS technology has entered a fast and timely new stage of offering a variety of the ground observation data, and widely used in military reconnaissance, public health, agriculture and many other fields.

The characteristics of all kinds of spectral reflectance of ground objects are different, thus characteristic curve of spectral reflectance is also different. Up to now, the world has launched more than 200 RS satellites (except for the reconnaissance satellite) to provide scientific research, production and all kinds of social and economic activities (Lillesand et al., 2014). At present, the common RS data come from the resources satellite of United States, France, Canada and China–Brazil. They have different resolution, bandwidth, access time and application fields (Table 1).

With the development of RS technology and interdisciplinary study, RS technology has become a common means of disease control and surveillance, particularly for vector-borne diseases control and monitoring. Prevalence of vector-borne diseases is largely dependent on certain geographical features, and RS technology offers a powerful way as a large, fast and effective means of obtaining surface information. It can be used to obtain the distribution of vector habitats. However, RS cannot directly identify disease-endemic regions. It only indirectly reflects an endemic area or vector breeding grounds through certain RS index, such as vegetation index, humidity, soil type and surface temperature. In The People's Republic of China, many studies also showed that it was economic and effective to monitor the snail habitats in Dongting Lake, Poyang Lake and Yangtze River using medium- and high-resolution RS images. For example, MSS image for photos of Poyang Lake and standard false colour composite interpretation was used to identify the snail habitats after flood in 1983 (Jia et al., 2001). Zhou et al. (1999a) used the RS image and meteorological data to predict the potential schistosomiasis endemic areas, and found that the distribution of schistosomiasis was closely related to factors such as altitude and rainfall. A study also applied RS image and the method of expert agent in Poyang lake area to monitor and simulate the distribution of schistosomiasis (Long et al., 2011).

In The People's Republic of China, the main analysis procedure includes the following. Firstly, the images can be classified according to the typical land cover and vegetation, and categories representing water and land which were separated from the other classes. Flooded areas were determined by subtracting the dry season image from the wet season image. Secondly, more information can be extracted from RS image (Guo et al., 2005), including the following points: (1) The normalized difference vegetation

Table 1 The characteristics of all kinds of satellite RS

Satellite	Spatial resolution	Waveband	Breadth	Access period	Archiving date	Application fields
China–Brazil earth resource satellite	20–256 m	11 Multi	690 km	26 days	1999	Forestry, water conservancy, environmental monitoring, desertification, and so on
NOAA-AVHRR	1.1 km	5 Multi	2800 km	101.2 min	1972	Agriculture, ocean, geology, environment, disaster and so on
LANDSAT MSS	80 m	4 Multi	185 km	16 days	1973	Land resources exploration, environment monitoring
LANDSAT TM	30 m	7 Multi	185 km	16 days	1984	Coastal environment
LANDSAT ETM	30 m 15 m	7 Multi 1 Pan	185 km	16 days	1999	Agriculture, forestry and water resources and land use mapping
EOS	250, 500 or 1000 m	36 Multi	2330 m × 10 km	4 t/d	1999	Atmosphere, ocean and surface features
SPOT 1–4	10 m 20 m	1 Pan 3 Multi	60 km	26 days	1986	Map production, levelling and so on
SPOT 5	2.5 m 5.0 m	1 Pan 4 Multi	60 km	26 days	2002	Map production, levelling and so on
RADARSAT	8–100 m	7 model 25 wave velocity	50–500 km	24 days	1996	The global environment and land use, natural resource monitoring
IKONOS	1 m 4 m	1 Pan 4 Multi	11 km	2.9 days 1.5 days	1999	City, port, land, forest, the environment, disaster investigation
Quick Bird	0.61 m 2.44 m	1 Pan 4 Multi	16.5 × 16.5 km	1–3.5 days	2001	Agriculture, forestry, environmental monitoring, urban management, and evaluation and so on

Multi, multi-spectral; Pan, panchromatic.

index (NDVI) which is calculated as the ratio between measured reflectivity in the red and near-infrared bands of the electromagnetic spectrum normalized by the sum of those bands. (2) The soil moisture can be extracted from apparent thermal inertia (ATI) which is a hot soil characteristic, and it is an internal factor of soil surface. Temperature changes and has a close relationship with soil moisture, but controls the size of soil temperature daily. According to RS method, as long as the highest and lowest temperatures within a day can be gotten soil moisture can be calculated using effective model (Ya et al., 2000). (3) Near-surface temperatures and land surface temperatures (LST) for the study area are derived from the Landsat TM band 7 brightness. (4) The 'wetness' or 'moistness' image was obtained by the tasselled-cap transformation, which allows the extraction of three new brands, namely, brightness, greenness and wetness from Landsat TM images (Crist and Kauth, 1986). Thirdly, large amounts of data from RS will be converted to useful information for further RS model for analysis: for example, finding analysis, indexing analysis, inductive analysis, regional characteristics analysis, change detection analysis, terrain analysis and spatial modelling analysis (Bhatta, 2013).

2.3 Global positioning system

The technology of GPS is a space-based satellite navigation system that provides location and time information in all weather conditions, anywhere on or near the earth where there is an unobstructed line of sight to four or more GPS satellites. It was developed by the US department of defense in the 1970s, as a new generation of satellite navigation and positioning system. The system could provide high-precision navigation, positioning and timing services, and the GPS system has replaced conventional geodetic and engineering surveying (Hofmann-Wellenhof et al., 2013; Yi et al., 2013).

GPS can provide precision navigation within 10 m, it can be used in any weather conditions and any place in the world. Its precision and maintenance is the complete responsibility of the US government. We do not need to pay fees or installation fee when using GPS. If we carry out a small-scale study, it was not suitable for the normal GPS method, then the differential GPS (DGPS) and the application of the phase difference GPS (RTK) technology to realize the high-precision real-time dynamic navigation and positioning, and metre magnitude or centimetre-level accuracy can be obtained in a flash of station coordinates (Lee, 2009).

Therefore, in the collection of public health events or disease status and its influencing factors such as information, we need to use GPS technology to get the spatial location information, related to complete space epidemiological field research work. Application of GPS can obtain a large number of real-time accurate geographical data, realizes the disease data and other related data visualization. It provides the advanced operation platform for further data processing and analysis, and thus better able to study the link between the disease and environment (Zhou et al., 2009).

2.4 Google Earth

GE is a virtual globe, map and geographical information program, and it maps the Earth by the superimposition of images obtained from satellite imagery, aerial photography and 3D globe. It can be calculated from 3D map, the highest accuracy reached military level 5 years ago, low precision is equivalent to 5000 m above the Earth, and can see clearly each road. For some reasons (such as a military secret), GE released satellite images usually 1–3 years ago, but it has matched true geophysical information that its topography, altitude, latitude and longitude information is completely overlapped with outputting GPS information. It therefore has a high practical value for civil use. We can get interior points, lines and surfaces of spatial information through GE, and save it as KML or KMZ file (Williams et al., 2012).

GE software is simple, convenient and suitable for most of the common people. For example, we can use the combination function of pointing, track record and data export by GE map function and a handheld GPS to detect timely and correctly the intermediate host snail in the field (Zheng et al., 2014).

2.5 Spatiotemporal statistics and models

The advent of GIS and RS techniques provided important advances to understand the key environmental factors for the transmission of infectious diseases. Incorporation of these new technologies is increasingly used for the prediction of the prevalence of schistosoma infection (Abbas et al., 2015; Guo et al., 2005; Yang et al., 2005; Zhou et al., 2001). The technology of GIS is related to the geographical spatial data for effective management and comprehensive analysis. However real-world data is not only related to the space but also related with time. In order to study temporal changes, it is necessary to introduce time information in the GIS, namely, spatiotemporal statistics and models. The development history of statistics for spatiotemporal went through classical statistics (long history, on the basis of probability theory, widely applied) and spatial statistics (as an object in space, a single observation). Statistics for spatiotemporal is exploratory spatiotemporal data analysis on the basis of spatial statistics and time series analysis. Basic statistics for spatiotemporal model includes space–time covariance function of temporal and spatial to build, space–time kriging, stochastic differential equations, spatial process of time series analysis and process analysis of spatiotemporal. Kriging is a widely used geostatistical technique for the analysis of spatial correlations and for constructing prediction maps in the field of public health (Goovaerts, 2006; Jerrett et al., 2005; Waller and Gotway, 2004). For example, some authors were to present kriging based on data from a few sites as a solution to the problem of predicting the spatial distribution of *Schistosoma japonicum* infection over a whole region. These methods usually are very difficult to calculate, but we can use some statistical software to solve these problems. For example, SatScan, ArcView and WinBUGS software can be used to solve the problem of space–time scan, Moran's I and spatiotemporal analysis, respectively.

In The People's Republic of China, many studies used space–time scan, Moran's I and other method to solve spatiotemporal problems. Scan statistic can be applied in epidemiology, public health and astronomy to find unusual clusters of events. It is scanning the maximum number of cases through the observation period obtained by using preselected time interval: compared with traditional methods, scan statistics eliminates subjectivity by year, month caused by people, and is without inherent geographical restrictions. Higher test performance (Kulldorff et al., 2005; Kulldorff, 2013) in the epidemiology of the disease has been widely used to analyse space, time or space aggregation of disease and media (Chen et al., 2013; Wang et al., 2008b). Moran's I is a measure of spatial autocorrelation developed by Patrick Alfred Pierce Moran. Spatial autocorrelation is characterized by a correlation in a signal among nearby locations in space. It is more complex than 1D autocorrelation, because spatial correlation is multidimensional (ie, 2D or 3D of space) and multidirectional.

During 2010s, the Bayesian model has been used in the field of epidemiological studies increasingly. It can also analyse the effect of risk factors and disease of space or time distribution, and can be incorporated into the result variables (dependent variable) and explain the uncertainty variables (independent variables) (Ashby, 2006; Liu et al., 2012; Macnab, 2003; Zhang et al., 2015). Some authors used epidemiological data of schistosomiasis and environmental data extracted from high-resolution RS at the village level to build schistosomiasis Bayesian spatiotemporal model to assess the effect of schistosoma epidemics by returning farmland to the lake (Yang et al., 2012b).

3. APPLICATION IN THE SCHISTOSOMIASIS STUDY

In The People's Republic of China, the area of snail habitats was about 372,263.11 hm^2, the area of lake and marshland regions, mountainous and hilly region and water network region was 357,917.57, 14,087 and 197.85 hm^2, accounting for 96.15%, 3.78% and 0.05%, respectively (Hao et al., 2009). Hence, most studies focused on the study in marshland regions and mountainous region.

3.1 Application in lake and marshland regions

The schistosomiasis endemic of lake and marshland regions is wide, and the habitats area of *O. hupensi* snail is complex, mainly distributed in Hubei, Hunan, Anhui, Jiangxi, Jiangsu provinces along the Yangtze River and lakes around. There is a large marshland without water in winter and covered with water in summer. It is difficult to control schistosomiasis in the current lake and marshland regions. The development of spatial technology provides convenient tools to monitor and predict the distribution and spread of the snail and schistosomiasis (Yang et al., 2009).

Satellite RS technology in the application of schistosomiasis monitoring and prediction are mainly concerned with the following aspects: (1) Combination with the surveillance data of snail detection in the field to determine unknown snail habitats. (2) Combination with the history data of snail distribution to anticipate potential schistosomiasis epidemic area. (3) Quantitative or qualitative monitoring the change of the environmental factors to predict corresponding changes of snail habitats. (4) Compare the differences between intermediate host snails in high-density area and low-density area, to identify risk factors affecting the distribution, and so guide the prevention and control of schistosomiasis (Zhang, 2006).

The development of spatial technology provides useful tools to identify environmental factors related to the distribution of intermediate host snails of schistosomiasis, and map and predict disease transmission (Brooker and Michael, 2000). Successful applications of RS and GIS techniques have been reported in the field of different ecological, epidemiological and socio-cultural settings for schistosomiasis in The People's Republic of China (Zhou et al., 2001). For example, an annual mean temperature of 16–20°C, annual precipitation of 1300–2000 mm and 1400–2100 h of total annual daylight were key environmental features for the presence of *O. hupensis* snail habitats (Zheng et al., 1998). The NDVI extracted from multitemporal Landsat TM satellite images from dry and wet seasons, has been used to identify potential snail habitats (Zhou et al., 2002). The snail habitats in the Poyang Lake area were identified by unsupervised classification of Landsat TM images, and the extracted land cover types correlated with snail habitats from historical surveys (Wu et al., 2002). An unsupervised classification employing Landsat ETM + images, and established different vegetation types were closely correlated with snail habitats (Zhang et al., 2003).

3.1.1 Application of spatial and temporal pattern analysis

There were many studies using spatial and temporal pattern analysis to study the distribution of acute case of schistosomiasis and snail. The general analysis procedure about acute cases distribution included the following. Firstly, data of cases and outbreaks were extracted from database of Infectious Diseases Reporting Information System (Wang et al., 2008a). Secondly, the chi-square test can be used to explore associations between the infection status and factors (Shek and Ma, 2011). Thirdly, the secondary space—time database can be established with the county's centre-of-mass coordinate extracted from the national county electronic map using ArcGIS software. The space—time clustering can be performed by retrospective space—time analysis using discrete Poisson model in SaTScan software (Kulldorff, 2006). The time aggregation was specified as 7 days, which was same as the period of weekly report of acute infection with *S. japonicum*, followed by Monte Carlo reiteration statistics 999 times. ArcGIS was used to visualize the space—time cluster regions in map. For example, nine clusters of acute cases were detected by spatiotemporal analysis between June and November in the lake and marshland region (Li et al., 2014).

The analysis procedure about snail distribution included the following information. Firstly, field data about snail, digitized maps with topographical sheets and satellite image should be collected. Secondly, environmental indices can be extracted from the satellite image for example, Landsat 7 ETM + image using the ERDAS Imagine software, including the second modified soil-adjusted vegetation index (MSAVI2), the land surface temperature (LST) and surrogate indices of environmental factors from the tasselled-cap transformed ETM + scene. Thirdly, linear regression and spatial analysis methods can be used for model development to predict the cluster distribution of snails in space according to the theory of mathematical statistics (Johnston and Ver Hoef, 1999; Wang, 1999). The mapping and prediction of schistosomiasis japonica using remotely sensed environmental indices and spatial statistical analyses in The People's Republic of China will henceforth be incorporated in the national control programmers (Zhang et al., 2005).

3.1.2 Impact of ecological environment change on schistosomiasis transmission

During 2000s, climate change has become the common feature with the human society. A climate simulation predicts an increase in the mean global temperature of 2.4–5.4°C from 1990 to 2100 (Allen and Ingram, 2002; Milly et al., 2005; Murphy et al., 2004). Thus, predicted risk profiles of climate-sensitive diseases tend to worsen for most parts of the world, and hence require adaptation and mitigation strategies (Haines et al., 2006; Patz et al., 2005). For example, time-series analysis and predictions suggest that the population at risk of malaria in Africa will slightly increase due to climate change, primarily through expansion of the disease into higher altitudes and lengthened malaria transmission seasons (Haines et al., 2006).

In The People's Republic of China, some studies also predict the spatial distribution of schistosomiasis transmission from an early model about the possibility of schistosomiasis transmission spread, to later models about predicting the potential epidemic area of schistosomiasis, including the study of Zhou et al. (2008) on the impact of climate change on the future transmission of schistosomiasis by biology-based model in The People's Republic of China. Firstly, digital map and temperature data of average daily temperature were collected. Secondly, a biologic model of the parasite and its intermediate host was established based on the relationship between the temperature and different critical stages of the life cycle of *S. japonicum*. Thirdly, a probity analysis was used to establish the relationship between temperature and the hibernation rate of *O. hupensis*. A time-series analytical approach was used to predict the geographical distribution of the freezing line at 2030 and 2050. Fourthly, risk maps were developed by a kriging approach of the spatial analyst model of ArcGIS software. Yang et al. (2010) furthermore, introduced PRECIS regional climate model simulations for A2, B2 greenhouse gas emission scenarios to predict the transmission range and intensity of schistosomiasis in 2050s and 2070s (Fig. 2).

3.1.3 Selection of prevention and control strategy

The suitable and useful control measures and strategy are very important to schistosomiasis control. In 2000s, a study attempted formulating a schistosomiasis control strategy based on predictions for different environmental settings at different scales in The People's Republic of China. Firstly, the geographical coordinates (latitude/longitude) of the centre of each endemic village were recorded using GPS, and GIS database was established using ArcGIS to record the coordinates and the infection rates for each village during the study period. Following, the directional trend of the infection data

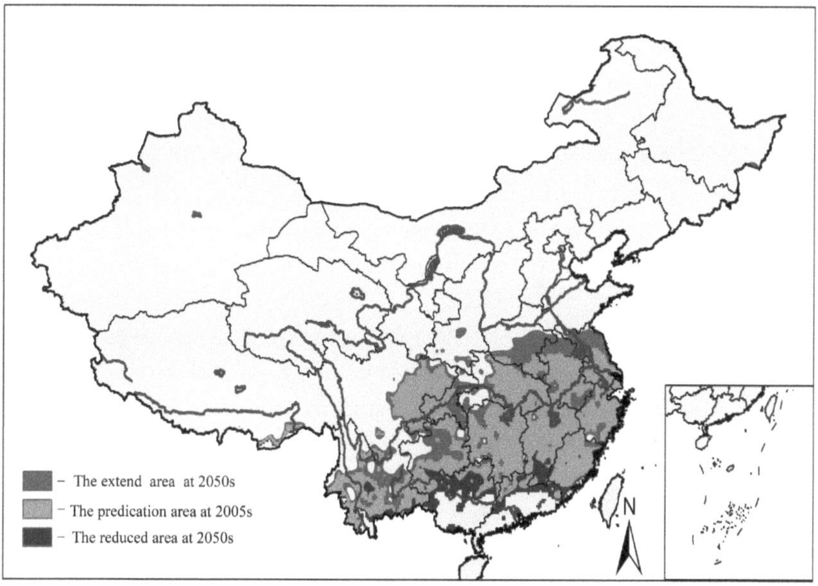

Figure 2 Transmission scale of schistosomiasis in The People's Republic of China under the IPCC B2 scenarios.

can be investigated to identify the presence or absence of trends at a certain direction and selected the suitable order for the ordinary kriging analysis. Next, a prediction map was created to illustrate the spatial pattern of infection rate by the kriging method. Thereafter, endemic levels were classified based on the prediction maps. Suitable control strategy and measure were designed for the different regions based on the local environmental settings as well as epidemic strata. In some villages that were sorted into the second stratum were mainly found in the lake and marshland regions in the northwest near the Yangtze River, and the strategy was to reduce the human infection rate and lighten the morbidity by chemotherapy for villages in the second stratum. The spatial analysis can also be used to improve the formulation of strategies for schistosomiasis control in different environmental settings (Chen et al., 2007).

3.1.4 Establishment of the monitoring and early warning system

Transmission of *S. japonicum* is complicated, involving a variety of biological and social factors. The risk of *S. japonicum* infection is thus related to many different factors, not only environmental but also social (Bergquist and Whittaker, 2012; Tambo et al., 2014). The application of spatial technology in the field of monitoring and early warning mainly include the following: (1) To build the release platform of risk and control information from spatial analysis or from government official to the general public in time, and avoid the risk of infection or to receive the useful control resources. The combination of various technologies into the Web GIS format strengthens overall public health capacity and facilitates decision support system approaches for prevention and control of diseases in resource-poor environments. This platform enables real-time surveillance and risk monitoring with users quickly and intuitively locating any early high-risk area, retrieving detailed performance information and the decision makers are given the possibility of prompt action (Yang et al., 2012a). (2) To carry out any further analysis for the general surveillance, for example, the risk for *S. japonicum* infection in Jiangsu Province, The People's Republic of China, was investigated by a mouse bioassay. Directional distribution analysis and scan statistics were used to explore the spatiotemporal risk pattern. Four statistically significant clusters were detected between 2009 and 2011. Temporal windows for infection risk were seen in June and September (Shi et al., 2013). (3) The combination of the GIS, RS and GE technologies can offer new opportunities for rapid assessment of endemic areas, provision of reliable estimates of populations at risk, prediction of disease and its attributions in remote areas that lack baseline data, and guidance of intervention strategies so that scarce resources are allocated in a cost-effective manner (Sun et al., 2011).

3.2 Application in mountainous and hilly regions

The endemic areas of mountainous and hilly regions are mainly distributed in Sichuan and Yunnan provinces at present. The snail distribution is very wide in strict accordance with the water distribution, and its environment is extremely complex (Zhong et al., 2011). The infection intensity is generally low, and acute cases are mostly scattered. Many studies showed that spatial technology plays a huge role to study the epidemic situation and the distribution of schistosomiasis in the regions. For example, Dong et al. (2006) used sampling survey data from 1995 to 2003 to study infection status between human and cattle by spatial contours method in Yunnan Province, and found that synchronal chemotherapy in human and cattle was very important to control schistosomiasis in Yunan Province. Zhou et al. (1999b) used spatial technology of buffer zone determination, network analysis and CART regressive tree analysis to identify the high-risk area and focus of infection, and successfully provided reference to design control strategy in Sichuan Province. RS technology was also applied to provide environmental data and determine the potential snail habitats in these regions since 1980s (Zhong and Dong, 2008).

3.2.1 Application of spatial and temporal pattern analysis

In The People's Republic of China, many studies used this technology to explore the spatial and temporal pattern of acute case and snail. Habitats of snail in mountainous areas are usually small and often isolated from each other. The precision of spatial analyses is usually determined by the resolution of the underlying data (eg, pixel size and time interval). High-resolution environmental data that can be readily obtained from new satellites facilitate the development of landscape ecology. Yang et al. (2008) used high-resolution SPOT 5 image and Bayesian integrated modelling of indicators from landscape ecology to study the relationship between village-scale variations in landscape composition and snail density, and identify risk factors that govern the density of snail in a mountainous area. This integrated analysis was a powerful and statistically robust approach to identify high-risk areas within a heterogeneous complex and not easily accessed environment. Spatial clustering model was also used to analysis the acute cases of schistosomiasis in this regions (Li, 2010).

3.2.2 Selection of prevention and control strategy

In the various stages of social development and the change of schistosoma epidemics, different control strategies were developed in mountainous regions, for example, from integrated control strategy giving priority to snails elimination to infection source of schistosomiasis control. Spatial technology can also help people decide which control measure is suitable or best according the different settings. Zhang et al. (2012) selected a Bayesian regression model taking into account all the potential risk factors simultaneously through two latent components of random effects: spatially correlated heterogeneities (CH) and spatially uncorrelated heterogeneities (UH) to evaluate the long-term effect of the 10-year World Bank Loan Project (WBLP). The overall prevalence of schistosomiasis was decreasing in 2007–2008 compared with that in 1999–2001, but the spatial distribution of risk remained similar. The analysis showed that the chemotherapy-based, integrated control strategy has been shown to be unable to break the transmission cycle, novel approaches are therefore urgently needed.

4. PROSPECTIVE OF THE SPACE NEW TECHNOLOGY

The distribution of schistosomiasis is closely related to environmental factors, and applying the spatial new technology such as RS and GIS can be more rapidly and easily reveal the distribution of schistosomiasis, to monitor and predict snail habitats and endemic areas of schistosomiasis (Niu et al., 2006). Technical progress in the field of GIS and RS techniques, including geospatial statistics, have provided a new epidemiological approach which is particularly well suited to the study of climate change and ecological transformations. In 2010, time-series analyses, advanced modelling and Bayesian geostatistics are widely employed to deepen our understanding of the epidemiology and control of schistosomiasis, including the use of random-effect models and transmission dynamics. For these kinds of investigations, in particular, the geospatial tools can provide early warning techniques for preemptive planning in order to mitigate future risk and impact.

In general, the prevalence of schistosomiasis is not only decided by natural geographical factors, but also by social, economic, preventive and control work. It was significant using the GIS technology to study the distribution of snail and impact of environmental changes on snail and schistosomiasis diffusion. Principally, with the new technology development of satellite RS spaces, we can obtain more accurate ground hydrology, meteorology, vegetation, soil and other data. It will be our direction to use GIS and RS techniques to guide the schistosomiasis control (Hu, 2010). With the development of future space science and technology, spatial technology will get reuse role in prevention and control of schistosomiasis. However, the spatial technology of epidemiology still faces some problems to be solved: (1) The development of space-based epidemiological research involving multidisciplinary requires a lot of coordination between the various disciplines to develop a more mature and convenient software. (2) The high-quality spatial and temporal epidemiological data are scanty and need more collection with big databases. (3) The spatial epidemiology in schistosomiasis applications was initially started, and spatial model and spatial statistical methods are too simple without systematic thinking.

Future directions of spatial epidemiology in the of schistosomiasis could be developed in the following areas: (1) To improve the quality and timeliness of data collection. (2) To introduce high-resolution RS data including high spatial resolution to achieve get the detailed information about the small snail habitats. (3) To develop the integrated technology of multisource data fusion and classification to meet the demand for the different spatial and spectral resolution in schistosomiasis. (4) To build composite model based on geostatistical and multifactor spatial analysis.

5. CONCLUSION

The People's Republic of China has achieved significantly towards elimination of schistosomiasis transmission, with sustained large-scale interventions (Chen, 2014). The spatial technology has been used in the research and control programme of schistosomiasis in the country in the following aspects: (1) in analysis of the spatiotemporal pattern and the impact of ecological changes on the transmission of schistosomiasis, (2) provide the information to design and optimize the control strategy and (3) the monitoring and early warning system to the national control programme in lake and mountainous regions. Therefore, spatial technology as a new scientific method and means can offer powerful capabilities of spatial data management and analysis, and improve the capacity to control and eliminate schistosomiasis (Xia et al., 2013). It is expected for the spatial technology to produce higher impact to the national schistosomiasis elimination programme in the future (Zheng et al., 2013).

ACKNOWLEDGEMENTS

This project was supported by the National S & T Major Program (grant no. 2012ZX10004220), Project of Health Department of Jiangsu Province (No. RC2011094) and Science Foundation of Jiangsu Province (BS2015024).

REFERENCES

Abbas, T., Younus, M., Muhammad, S.A., 2015. Spatial cluster analysis of human cases of Crimean Congo hemorrhagic fever reported in Pakistan. Infect. Dis. Poverty 4, 9.

Allen, M.R., Ingram, W.J., 2002. Constraints on future changes in climate and the hydrologic cycle. Nature 419, 224–232.

Ashby, D., 2006. Bayesian statistics in medicine: a 25 year review. Stat. Med. 25, 3589–3631.

Bergquist, R., Whittaker, M., 2012. Control of neglected tropical diseases in Asia Pacific: implications for health information priorities. Infect. Dis. Poverty 1, 3.

Bhatta, B., 2013. Analysis of data. In: Research Methods in Remote Sensing. Springer, pp. 61–75.

Bi, Y., Tong, S., 2014. Poverty and malaria in the Yunnan province, China. Infect. Dis. Poverty 3, 32.

Bonham-Carter, G.F., 2014. Geographic Information Systems for Geoscientists: Modelling with GIS. Elsevier.

Brooker, S., Michael, E., 2000. The potential of geographical information systems and remote sensing in the epidemiology and control of human helminth infections. Adv. Parasitol. 47, 245–288.

Chen, Z., Zhou, X.N., Yang, K., Wang, X.H., Yao, Z.Q., Wang, T.P., et al., 2007. Strategy formulation for schistosomiasis japonica control in different environmental settings supported by spatial analysis: a case study from China. Geospat. Health 1, 223–231.

Chen, H.G., Gu, X.N., Zeng, X.J., Lin, D.D., Hang, C.Q., Lu, S.B., et al., 2013. Schistosomiasis epidemic dynamic and prevention and control of the situation Jiangxi province, 2002-2012. Chin. J. Parasitol. Parasit. Dis. 31, 458–463.

Chen, R.J.C., 2007. Geographic information systems (GIS) applications in retail tourism and teaching curriculum. J. Retail. Consum. Serv. 14, 289–295.

Chen, M.G., 2014. Assessment of morbidity due to *Schistosoma japonicum* infection in China. Infect. Dis. Poverty 3, 6.

Collins, C., Xu, J., Tang, S., 2012. Schistosomiasis control and the health system in P.R. China. Infect. Dis. Poverty 1, 8.

Crist, E.P., Kauth, R.J., 1986. The tasseled cap de-mystified. Photogramm. Eng. Remote Sens. 52, 81–86.

Dam, G.J.V., Xu, J., Bergquist, R., Dood, C.J.D., Utzinger, J., Qin, Z.Q., et al., 2015. An ultra-sensitive assay targeting the circulating anodic antigen for the diagnosis of *Schistosoma japonicum* in a low-endemic area, People's Republic of China. Acta Trop. 141, 190–197.

Dong, Y., Feng, X.G., Yang, C.G., Dong, X.Q., 2006. Analysis of geographic information system on transmission of schistosomiasis in Yunnan Province. Chin. J. Schistosomiasis Control 18, 109–111.

Efron, U., 1994. Spatial Light Modulator Technology: Materials, Devices, and Applications. CRC Press.

Elliott, P., Wartenberg, D., 2004. Spatial epidemiology: current approaches and future challenges. Environ. Health Perspect. 112, 998–1006.

Feng, Y., Liu, L., Xia, S., Xu, J.F., Bergquist, R., Yang, G.J., 2016. Reaching the surveillance-response stage of schistosomiasis control in the People's Republic of China: a modelling approach. Adv. Parasitol. 92.

Foote, Kenneth, E., Anthony, P.K., 1997. WebGIS. NCGIA Core Curriculum in GIScience. http://www.ncgia.ucsb.edu/giscc/units/u133/u133.html.

Fotheringham, S., Rogerson, P., 2013. Spatial Analysis and GIS. CRC Press.

Goovaerts, P., 2006. Geostatistical analysis of disease data: visualization and propagation of spatial uncertainty in cancer mortality risk using Poisson kriging and p-field simulation. Int. J. Health Geogr. 5, 7.

Guo, J.G., Penelope, V., Cao, C.L., Jürg, U., Zhu, H.Q., Daniel, A., et al., 2005. A geographic information and remote sensing based model for prediction of *Oncomelania hupensis* habitats in the Poyang Lake area, China. Acta Trop. 96, 213–222.

Haines, A., Kovats, R.S., Campbell-Lendrum, D., Corvalan, C., 2006. Climate change and human health: impacts, vulnerability, and mitigation. Lancet 367, 2101–2109.

Hao, Y., Zheng, H., Zhu, R., Guo, J.G., Wu, X.H., Wang, L.Y., et al., 2009. Schistosomiasis status in People's Republic of China in 2008. Chin. J. Schistosomiasis Control 21, 451–456.

Hofmann-Wellenhof, B., Lichtenegger, H., Collins, J., 2013. Global Positioning System: Theory and Practice. Springer Science & Business Media.

Hu, M.Q., 2010. Application of Spatial Analysis Technology in the Study of Schistosomiasis Epidemic Trend in Hubei Province. Guangxi Medical University.

Jensen, J.R., Lulla, K., 1987. Introductory Digital Image Processing: A Remote Sensing Perspective.

Jerrett, M., Burnett, R.T., Ma, R., Krewski, D., Newbold, K.B., Thurston, G., et al., 2005. Spatial analysis of air pollution and mortality in Los Angeles. Epidemiology 16, 727–736.

Jia, T.W., Jiang, Q.W., Liu, J.L., Lin, T., Wei, J.G., Zhao, G.M., 2001. The study on the identification of the water body from marshland schistosomiasis endemic areas using TM remote sensing data (in Chinese). China Public Health 17, 289–290.

Johnston, K., Ver Hoef, J.M., 1999. Using ArcGIS: Geostatistical Analysis, pp. 49–79.

Kulldorff, M., Heffernan, R., Hartman, J., Mostashari, O., 2005. A space–time permutation scan statistic for disease outbreak detection. PLoS Med. e59.

Kulldorff, M., 2006. SaTScan64 v. 7.0: software for the spatial and space–time scan statistics. In: Spatial Disease Clusters Detection & Inference Statistics in Medicine.

Kulldorff, M., 2013. SaTScan User Guide for Version 9.2.
Lee, J., 2009. Global Positioning/GPS. International Encyclopedia of Human Geography, pp. 548–555.
Li, S.Z., Zheng, H., Abe, E.M., Yang, K., Bergquist, R., Qian, Y.J., et al., 2014. Reduction patterns of acute schistosomiasis in the People's Republic of China. PLoS Negl. Trop. Dis. 8, 141–150.
Li, C.H., 2010. The Application of SPatial Epidemiology on Schistosomiasis Prevention in Hill and Mountain Region. Dali university.
Lillesand, T., Kiefer, R.W., Chipman, J., 2014. Remote Sensing and Image Interpretation. John Wiley & Sons.
Liu, J., Yang, B., Cheung, W.K., Yang, G., 2012. Malaria transmission modelling: a network perspective. Infect. Dis. Poverty 1, 11.
Long, F., Yin, X.K., He, Z.Y., Zuo, J., Li, S.S., 2011. Based on the RS/GIS retrospect and prospect of schistosomiasis research. Chin. J. Urban Econ. 309.
Macnab, Y.C., 2003. Hierarchical Bayesian spatial modelling of small-area rates of non-rare disease. Stat. Med. 22, 1761–1773.
Matthews, M.W., 2011. A current review of empirical procedures of remote sensing in inland and near-coastal transitional waters. Int. J. Remote Sens. 32, 6855–6899.
Milly, P.C.D., Dunne, K.A., Vecchia, A.V., 2005. Global pattern of trends in streamflow and water availability in a changing climate. Nature 438, 347–350.
Murphy, J.M., Sexton, D.M.H., Barnett, D.N., Jones, G.S., Webb, M.J., Matthew, C., et al., 2004. Quantification of modelling uncertainties in a large ensemble of climate change simulations. Nature 430, 768–772.
Niu, H.F., Qing, Y.U., Bao, Z.P., Zhu, R., Yang, D.P., Zhang, H.J., et al., 2006. Application of global positioning system and geographic information system in surveillance of schistosomiasis. Chin. J. Prev. Med. 40, 229–233.
Patz, J.A., Campbell-Lendrum, D., Holloway, T., Foley, J.A., 2005. Impact of regional climate change on human health. Nature 438, 310–317.
Shek, D.T.L., Ma, C.M.S., 2011. Longitudinal data analyses using linear mixed models in SPSS: concepts, procedures and illustrations. Sci. World J. 11, 42–76.
Shi, B., Xia, S., Yang, G.J., Zhou, X.N., Liu, J., 2013. Inferring the potential risks of H7N9 infection by spatiotemporally characterizing bird migration and poultry distribution in eastern China. Infect. Dis. Poverty 2, 8.
Stoltzfus, J.D., Carter, J.Y., Akpinar-Elci, M., Matu, M., Kimotho, V., Giganti, M.J., et al., 2014. Interaction between climatic, environmental, and demographic factors on cholera outbreaks in Kenya. Infect. Dis. Poverty 3, 37.
Sun, L.P., Liang, Y.S., Wu, H.H., Tian, Z.X., Dai, J.R., Yang, K., et al., 2011. A Google Earth-based surveillance system for schistosomiasis japonica implemented in the lower reaches of the Yangtze River, China. Parasit. Vectors 4, 223.
Tambo, E., Ai, L., Zhou, X., Chen, J.H., Hu, W., Bergquist, R., et al., 2014. Surveillance-response systems: the key to elimination of tropical diseases. Infect. Dis. Poverty 3, 17.
Thoen, B., 1995. Interactive Mapping and GIS Thrive on the Web. GIS World 8 (10).
Waller, L.A., Gotway, C.A., 2004. Applied Spatial Statistics for Public Health Data, vol. xviii. Wiley-Interscience [John Wiley & Sons], Hoboken, NJ, p. 494.
Wang, L., Wang, Y., Jin, S., Wu, Z., Chin, D.P., Koplan, J.P., et al., 2008a. Emergence and control of infectious diseases in China. Lancet 372, 1598–1605.
Wang, X.H., Zhou, X.N., Wu, X.H., Yang, K., Lu, S., 2008b. *Schistosoma japonicum* serology positive rate : the preliminary study of time and space distribution pattern. Chin. J. Parasitol. Parasit. Dis. 290–294+298.
Wang, Z.Q., 1999. Geostatistics and its Application to the Ecology. Science Press.
Wheatley, D., Gillings, M., 2003. Spatial Technology and Archaeology: The Archaeological Applications of GIS. CRC Press.

Williams, C.M., Baker, G.S., Ault, B.A., 2012. Enhancing usability of near-surface geophysical data in archaeological surveys via Google Earth. Geol. Soc. Am. Spec. Pap. 492, 49–62.
Wiwanitkit, V., Shi, B., Xia, S., Yang, G.J., Zhou, X.N., Liu, J., 2013. Research priorities in modeling the transmission risks of H7N9 bird flu. Infect. Dis. Poverty 2, 17.
Wu, W.P., Davis, G., Liu, H.Y., Seto, E., Lu, S.B., Zhang, J., et al., 2002. Application of remote sensing for surveillance of snail habitats in Poyang Lake, China. Chin. J. Parasitol. Parasit. Dis. 20, 205–208.
Xia, S., Allotey, P., Reidpath, D.D., Yang, P., Sheng, H.F., Zhou, X.N., 2013. Combating infectious diseases of poverty: a year on. Infect. Dis. Poverty 2, 27.
Xu, J., Steinman, P., Maybe, D., Zhou, X.N., Lv, S., Li, S.Z., et al., 2016. Evolution of the national schistosomiasis control programmes in the People's Republic of China. Adv. Parasitol. 92.
Ya, L.I., Meng, X.U., Tang, Y., 2000. The status and advances of thermal inertia models in measuring soil moisture by remote sensing in China. Chin. J. Agric. Meteorol. 21, 40–43.
Yang, G.J., Vounatsou, P., Zhou, X.N., Utzinger, J., Tanner, M., 2005. A review of geographic information system and remote sensing with applications to the epidemiology and control of schistosomiasis in China. Acta Trop. 96, 117–129.
Yang, K., Wang, X.H., Yang, G.J., Wu, X.H., Qi, Y., Li, H., Zhou, X., 2008. An integrated approach to identify distribution of *Oncomelania hupensis*, the intermediate host of *Schistosoma japonicum*, in a mountainous region in China. Int. J. Parasitol. 38, 1007–1016.
Yang, K., Zhou, X.N., Wu, X.H., Steinmann, P., Wang, X.H., Yang, G.J., et al., 2009. Landscape pattern analysis and Bayesian modeling for predicting *Oncomelania hupensis* distribution in Eryuan County, People's Republic of China. Am. J. Trop. Med. Hyg. 81, 416–423.
Yang, K., Pan, J., Yang, G.J., Li, S.Z., Xu, Y.L., Zhou, X.N., 2010. Projection of the transmission scale and intensity of schistosomiasis in China under A2 and B2 climate change scenario (in Chinese). Adv. Clim. Change Res. 6, 248–253.
Yang, K., Sun, L.P., Huang, Y.X., Yang, G.J., Wu, F., Hang, D.R., et al., 2012a. A real-time platform for monitoring schistosomiasis transmission supported by Google Earth and a web-based geographical information system. Geospat. Health 6, 195–203.
Yang, K., Zhou, X.N., Wang, X.H., Yang, G.J., Jia, T.W., He, W.L., 2012b. Construction and application spatial-temporal model of schistosomiasis japonica in some lake district county. Chin. J. Schistosomiasis Control 24, 14–20.
Yi, T.H., Li, H.N., Gu, M., 2013. Recent research and applications of GPS-based monitoring technology for high-rise structures. Struct. Control Health Monit. 20, 649–670.
Zhang, Z.Y., De zhong, X.U., Zhou, X.N., Zhou, Y., Sun, Z.D., Zhang, B., et al., 2003. Application of satellite image for surveillance of vegetation landscapes of Oncomelenia-snail habitats in marshland using unsupervised classification. Chin. J. Epidemiol. 24, 261–264.
Zhang, Z.Y., Xu, D.Z., Zhou, X.N., Yun, Z., Liu, S.J., 2005. Remote sensing and spatial statistical analysis to predict the distribution of *Oncomelania hupensis* in the marshlands of China. Acta Trop. 96, 205–212.
Zhang, Z.J., Zhu, R., Bergquist, N.R., Chen, D.M., Chen, Y., Zhang, L.J., et al., 2012. Spatial comparison of areas at risk for schistosomiasis in the hilly and mountainous regions in the People's Republic of China: evaluation of the long-term effect of the 10-year World Bank loan project. Geospat. Health 6, 205–214.
Zhang, Z.W., Liu, T., Zeng, J., Chen, Y.E., Yuan, M., Zhang, D.W., et al., 2015. Prediction of the next highly pathogenic avian influenza pandemic that can cause illness in humans. Infect. Dis. Poverty 4, 50.
Zhang, J.Q., 2006. Based on Remote Sensing and Simulation to Monitor and Research the Poyang Lake Area of Schistosomiasis. Remote Sensing Application Research Institute.

Zheng, Y.J., Jang, Q.W., Zhao, G.M., Zhong, J.H., Zhang, S.J., 1998. The function of the overlaying climate data in analysis of Oncomelania snail distribution. Chin. J. Public Health 21–22.

Zheng, Q., Vanderslott, S., Jiang, B., Xu, L.L., Liu, C.S., Huo, L.L., et al., 2013. Research gaps for three main tropical diseases in the People's Republic of China. Infect. Dis. Poverty 2, 15.

Zheng, Z.W., Tan, X.D., Pi, W.L., Liu, Y.Z., Xu, M.X., Zhang, J., et al., 2014. Application of schistosomiasis prevention and checking the snails with GPS and Google Earth. Chin. Trop. Med. 14, 64–65.

Zhong, H.X., Dong, X.Q., 2008. Research progress of remote sensing monitoring distribution of hill type snail. Endem. Dis. Bull. 23, 73–75.

Zhong, B., Wu, Z.S., Chen, L., Liang, S., Dong, X.Q., 2011. Strengthening the achievements of schistosomiasis control in hilly regions of China. Chin. J. Schistosomiasis Control 23, 10–13.

Zhou, X.N., Hong, Q.B., Sun, L.P., Hu, S.S., Sun, N.S., Fuetes, M., et al., 1998. Application of geographic information systems on schistosomiasis surveillance. I Application possibility of Prediction model (in Chinese). Chin. J. Schistosomiasis Control 10, 321–324.

Zhou, X.N., Hu, X.S., Sun, N.S., Hong, Q.B., Sun, L.P., Lu, G.N., et al., 1999a. Application of geographic information systems on schistosomiasis surveillance. II predicting transmission intensity (in Chinese). Chin. J. Schistosomiasis Control 11, 66–70.

Zhou, Y., Maszle, D., Cspear, R., Gong, P., Gu, X.G., Qiu, D.C., et al., 1999b. The applicotion of geographic information system(GIS) and spatial analysis in anti-schistosomiasis in mountainous region. Chin. J. Schistosomiasis Control 263–266.

Zhou, X.N., Malone, J.B., Kristensen, T.K., Bergquist, N.R., 2001. Application of geographic information systems and remote sensing to schistosomiasis control in China. Acta Trop. 79, 97–106.

Zhou, X., Dandan, L., Huiming, Y., Honggen, C., Leping, S., Guojing, Y., et al., 2002. Use of landsat TM satellite surveillance data to measure the impact of the 1998 flood on snail intermediate host dispersal in the lower Yangtze River Basin. Acta Trop. 82, 199–205.

Zhou, X.N., Yang, G.J., Yang, K., Wang, X.H., Hong, Q.B., Sun, L.P., et al., 2008. Potential impact of climate change on schistosomiasis transmission in China. Am. J. Trop. Med. Hyg. 78, 188–194.

Zhou, S.F., Yu, L.X., Wang, S.P., 2009. Research progress on the detection and diagnosis of schistosomiasis. J. Trop. Med. 9, 335–340 (in Chinese).

Zhou, Y.B., Wang, Q.X., Liang, S., Gong, Y.H., Yang, M.X., Chen, Y., et al., 2015. Geographical variations in risk factors associated with HIV infection among drug users in a prefecture in Southwest China. Infect. Dis. Poverty 4, 38.

Zhu, R., Dang, H., Zhang, L.J., Li, H.Z., Zheng, C.J., Wu, X.H., et al., 2009. National surveillance of schistosomiasis in China, 2005-2008. Chin. J. Schistosomiasis Control 358–362.

CHAPTER SEVEN

Reaching the Surveillance-Response Stage of Schistosomiasis Control in The People's Republic of China: A Modelling Approach

Y. Feng[*,§,¶,##,a], L. Liu[*,§,¶,##,a], S. Xia[||,#,***], J.-F. Xu[**], R. Bergquist[§§], G.-J. Yang[*,§,¶,¶¶,||||,1]

[*]Key Laboratory of National Health and Family Planning Commission on Parasitic Disease Control and Prevention, Jiangsu Provincial Key Laboratory on Parasite and Vector Control Technology, Wuxi, The People's Republic of China
[§]Jiangsu Institute of Parasitic Diseases, Wuxi, Jiangsu Province, The People's Republic of China
[¶]Jiangsu Provincial Key Laboratory of Parasite Molecular Biology, Wuxi, The People's Republic of China
[||]National Institute of Parasitic Diseases, Chinese Center for Disease Control and Prevention, Shanghai, The People's Republic of China
[#]Key Laboratory of Parasite and Vector Biology, Ministry of Health, Shanghai, The People's Republic of China
[**]Hubei University for Nationalities, The People's Republic of China
[§§]Geospatial Health, University of Naples Federico II, Naples, Italy
[¶¶]Swiss Tropical and Public Health Institute, Basel, Switzerland
[||||]University of Basel, Basel, Switzerland
[##]Public Health Research Center, Jiangnan University, Wuxi, Jiangsu Province, The People's Republic of China
[***]WHO Collaborating Center for Tropical Diseases, Shanghai, The People's Republic of China
[1]Corresponding author: E-mail: guojingyang@hotmail.com

Contents

[a] These authors contributed equally to this study and share first authorship.

Advances in Parasitology, Volume 92
ISSN 0065-308X
http://dx.doi.org/10.1016/bs.apar.2016.02.006

Abstract

With the goal set to eliminate schistosomiasis nationwide by 2020, The People's Republic of China has initiated the surveillance-response stage to identify remaining sources of infection and potential pockets from where the disease could reemerge. Shifting the focus from classical monitoring and evaluation to rapid detection and immediate response, this approach requires modelling to bridge the surveillance and response components. We review here studies relevant to schistosomiasis modelling in a Chinese surveillance-response system with the expectation to achieve a practically useful understanding of the current situation and potential future study directions. We also present useful experience that could tentatively be applied in other endemic regions in the world. Modelling is discussed at length as it plays an essential role, both with regard to the intermediate snail host and in the definitive, mammal hosts. Research gaps with respect to snail infection, animal hosts and sectoral research cooperation are identified and examined against the prevailing background of ecosystem and socioeconomic changes with a focus on coexisting challenges and opportunities in a situation with increasing financial constraints.

1. INTRODUCTION

The first confirmed Chinese schistosomiasis patient was diagnosed in Hunan Province more than 100 years ago (Logan, 1905). However, schistosomiasis japonica has existed in The People's Republic of China for at least 2100 years and probably much longer (Bergquist and Tanner, 2010; Chen, 2014; Xu et al., 2016a,b; Zhou et al., 2005). In the 1940s, schistosomiasis was a major health risk threatening more than 100 million people, with an estimated 10 million of them infected (Hsu and Wu, 1941), a figure that increased to 11.8 million in the early 1950s (Chen and Feng, 1999).

After 65 years of subsequent controlling efforts, the Chinese Government has succeeded in interrupting schistosomiasis transmission in 313 out of 453 previously endemic counties and controlled the transmission in 135 counties, leaving only 5 counties where it is still difficult to control the disease (Bergquist and Tanner, 2010; Lei and Zhou, 2015; Xu et al., 2016a,b). Based on this remarkable progress, the current goal of the State Council's strategic plan 'Health The People's Republic of China 2020' is to achieve interruption of schistosomiasis transmission nationwide by 2020 (Zhou et al., 2012). In this situation, identification of the remaining sources of infection is essential. At this stage, a shift of the focus from classical monitoring and evaluation to rapid detection and immediate response is of critical importance (Bergquist et al., 2015; Tambo et al., 2014). Such a strategy conducts integrated and streamlined detection of remaining hotspots together with reporting, analysis and interpretation of surveillance data followed by optimized public health response packages (Lier et al., 2009; Wang et al., 2009; Zhou et al., 2013a,b). This is particularly important for the Chinese schistosomiasis control programme due to the high recurrence risk of the disease (Utzinger et al., 2015; Zhou et al., 2005). Wang et al. (2004) reported that resurgence of schistosomiasis was noted in 21 out of 64 areas (33.3%) with transmission interrupted in 16 out of 260 areas under control (6.2%). The fact that the intermediate snail host *Oncomelania hupensis* and cases of locally acquired schistosomiasis were found in six previously nonendemic counties (three in Zhuzhou City, two in Changsha City and one in Taoyuan County) (Zhou et al., 2004) makes it urgent to intensify disease surveillance-response (Zhou et al., 2013a,b). Moreover, as learnt from the eradication of smallpox and the progress on polio, surveillance-response is also the most cost-effective and efficient way to achieve disease elimination (Gao et al., 2013; Liu et al., 2014; Zhou et al., 2011, 2013a,b). A minimal, essential dataset and optimized public health response packages are two major features of this system (Zhang et al., 2016b; Zhou et al., 2013a,b), the key of which is the design of appropriate response packages based on first-hand data. An important component of surveillance-response consists of modelling, an approach capable of predicting ongoing transmission or reemergence of the disease (Wiwanitkit et al., 2015; Zheng et al., 2013; Zhou et al., 2013a,b). Modelling has been successfully applied in assisting the national malaria elimination programme in The People's Republic of China by designing and refining surveillance-response strategies for different transmission zones (Seto et al., 2011; Yang et al., 2012a,b). We aim here at a systematic review emphasizing the following three main components of modelling suitable for the schistosomiasis surveillance-response stage: (1) search for schistosomiasis surveillance-response applications in The People's Republic of China; (2) categorize the models identified according to their fitness; and (3) analyse the discovered and potential applicable fields of modelling. Through the review, we expect to achieve a practically useful understanding of the role of modelling, finding directions for future study and further accelerate the process of schistosomiasis elimination, an experience that should also be of use in other endemic regions in the world.

2. METHODS

International databases (PubMed, ISI Web of Science) and Chinese datasets (China National Knowledge Infrastructure (CNKI) and the Chinese Scientific Journal Database) were searched by medical subject headings (MeSH)/Title/Abstract/Keywords. Searching strategies included the following terms with no restrictions to date or language of publication: 'China', 'model*', 'schistosom*', in combination with 'surveillance' or 'prediction' or 'dynamics' or 'forecasting' or 'statistical' or 'mathematical'. This approach initially produced 352 articles. After screening titles and abstracts by two researchers working jointly, 299 articles were included according to the following criteria: (1) articles targeting The People's Republic of China; (2) articles focussing on schistosomiasis; (3) work using models relevant to surveillance-response systems; and (4) work with models using computational or statistical analyses or simulation of transmission under various conditions.

We extracted information such as model type, input and output data of the model from each article, in some cases by scrutinizing the full text or reviewing the reference lists of important articles. In this process, four extra articles complying with the inclusion criteria were found and included.

Based on the type of output data of the models, we classified them into two major categories, namely (1) the definitive, mammal hosts (mainly humans and bovines) and (2) the *Oncomelania* intermediate host snail. Within each category, the models were further studied, compared and summarized into groups in a target-driven manner. For human and bovine infections, indices like 'infection rate' and 'risk level' were estimated as important parameters and measured at the spatial or temporal level. For snail surveillance, on the other hand, geographical classification was applied due to the varying growth characteristics of *O. hupensis* in different environmental settings. Therefore, as shown in Fig. 1, we divided the models into three groups related to human and bovine infections: temporal forecasting, spatial mapping and parameter estimation via modelling (Xu et al., 2015; Yang, 2016a,b). For snail surveillance-responses, we focused on habitat issues selecting the following three groups: (1) the lake and marshland regions; (2) the hilly and mountainous areas; and (3) the plains with waterway networks (Liu, 2016b; Yang, 2016a,b; Zhang, 2016).

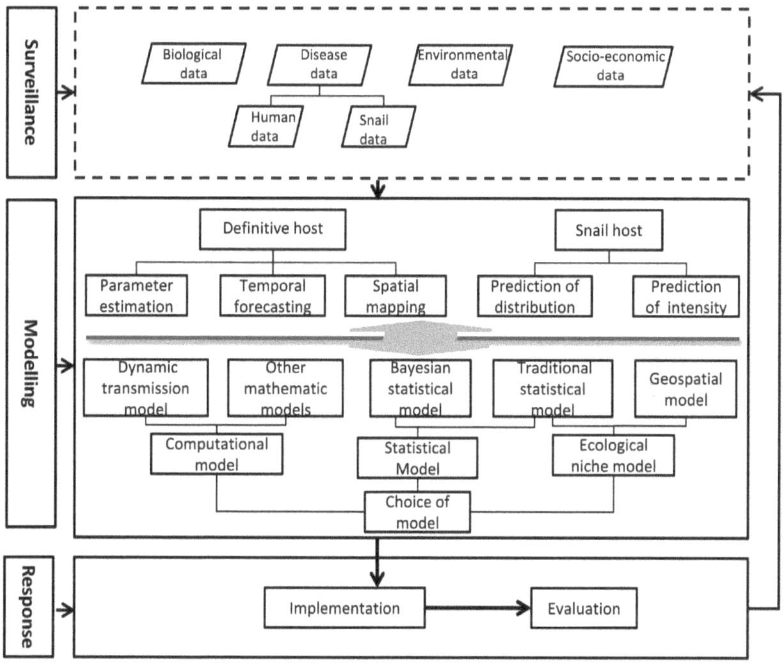

Figure 1 Model categories in a surveillance-response system.

3. MODEL APPLICATIONS IN SURVEILLANCE-RESPONSE SYSTEMS

Modelling integrates surveillance with response and is thus a major element of this process approach. It analyses and interprets the surveillance data and chooses the optimal, appropriate response package, the effectiveness of which is reflected in the new surveillance data obtained after implementation of the package. The information captured by running the model is used to adjust the response package to the situation at hand, a process that can be repeated several times to optimize the response. Surveillance shall be seen as a part of intervention as the response is adjusted according to modelling results (Fig. 1).

3.1 Humans and bovines

3.1.1 Temporal forecasting

We demonstrate that two major types of models, namely those based on time series and those based on a transmission process, function successfully.

Models based on time series predict future prevalence rates based on historical time series data and do so by extracting relevant information on historical indices, summarize the internal patterns and provide a forecast of future indices. The three major types within this group are 'grey models', 'time series models' and 'machine-learning models'.

The grey model is one of the earliest approaches. The name refers to the vague structure of information with incomplete data availability, dynamic randomization and general uncertainty (Deng, 1985), where the work will turn from a less clear or 'grey' perception to a 'white' one, ie, producing a constructive pattern when subjected to mathematical processing of the accumulating generation operator. Predictions are based on the type of pattern that emerges (Gan, 2011). Mei (1989) successfully validated the grey model by forecasting the prevalence of advanced schistosomiasis for 1986 in Wujiang, Jiangsu Province, based on a time series from 1979 to 1985. This model has also been successfully applied to the forecasting of the infection rate, both in humans and bovines (Gan, 2011; Sai et al., 2005; Zhang et al., 2007).

The time series model is based on various mathematical approaches, such as autoregression, exponential smoothing, etc. Autoregressive integrated moving average (ARIMA) is a well-known and an often applied approach that considers time series data as a randomized time-dependent variable. Its internal correlation is useful for temporal prediction (Gan, 2011). Chen et al. (2014b,c) used ARIMA to estimate the human *Schistosoma japonicum* infection rates for the period 2014–18 based on the observed prevalence in the past 25 years. The results indicated that short-term prediction by ARIMA is more accurate than long-term prediction, as accuracy is compromised by increasing numbers of unknown future factors (Chen et al., 2014b,c).

The more recent machine-learning methods provide a useful tool for empirically estimating variables when instructive observations are available rather than a complete theoretical process description. These models encompass a broad range of algorithms (eg, neural networks, support vector machines (SVM), Gaussian processes, decision trees, random forests (RF), etc.) that can provide multivariants, nonlinear, nonparametric regression or classifications that are based on training datasets. In contrast to time series models, they extract nonlinear information from historical data in a 'black box' (Zhou et al., 2014). Zhang et al. (2014) compared the SVM approach with two decomposition methods (regression and exponential smoothing) as well as with the ARIMA model for forecasting accuracy based on prevalence

data of nine typical infectious diseases in the time period 2005–12. SVM was the most accurate method based on three indices for the differences between estimated and observed prevalence of schistosomiasis (Zhang et al., 2014).

To extract both linear and nonlinear information from historical data, hybrid models of the approaches described above were developed. Zhou et al. (2014) integrated the ARIMA model together with a non-linear autoregressive neural network (NARNN) that was compared with using single ARIMA or single NARNN modelling for forecasting schistosomiasis prevalence during 4 years. The resulting upward-directed prevalence trend was closer to reality when the integrated ARIMA-NARNN was applied than with either of the single models (Zhou et al., 2014).

Models based on the transmission mechanism project the simulation in a 'white box', ie, an already known mechanism of schistosomiasis transmission. They are composed of mathematical transmission dynamic (MTD) models and catalytic models.

MTD models express transmission cycles through several mathematical equations embracing various important parameters reflecting each process. In the case of different intervention assumptions, they could project the probable impact for proposed strategies, which facilitates the choice between different options (Williams et al., 2002), thus making these models very useful as decision-making tools in surveillance-response.

Williams et al. (2002) were among the first to apply Barbour (1996) two-host model in schistosomiasis transmission in The People's Republic of China. They extended the model by allowing mammalian host heterogeneity adding field-collected Chinese data for better specification. Human and bovine morbidity was projected with regard to different chemotherapy strategies, including combinations with bovine vaccination schemes for a 10-year period in the lake and marshland region (Williams et al., 2002). All chemotherapy schemes appeared to produce only short-term effects with infection rates swiftly reverting to preintervention levels at interruption of chemotherapy (Williams et al., 2002). These authors also suggested that antifecundity bovine vaccination would be a potential choice to maintain long-term reduction of prevalence and morbidity, something that has been shown by later bovine vaccination experiments (Da'dara et al., 2008; Gray et al., 2014). By extending Barbour's model for allowing heterogeneous mixing between definitive host species, Rudge et al. (2013) compared the importance of various definitive hosts with regard to schistosome transmission in both the lake regions and the mountainous endemic areas. The removal of bovines in the lake and marshland region and rodents from the mountainous areas generated the lowest, basic reproductive number (R_0), indicating that they are the most important intervention strategy targets in the respective regions (Rudge et al., 2013). The decrease of simulated prevalence of other definitive hosts, including humans, after removal of the bovine hosts further agreed with this conclusion (Rudge et al., 2013). Barbour's two-host model was also used to project impact for other strategies (Wu, 2005). These studies contributed to the formulation of a comprehensive strategy focussing on the hosts, which demonstrated excellent effects with a R_0 index of less than one, and reduced snail infections as well (Gao et al., 2013).

Catalytic models, derived from the work by Muench (1959), describe the transmission of schistosomiasis by a catalytic power expressed in one of its equations. With time functioning as an important parameter, the model further demonstrates that the age distribution of the prevalence reflects the severity level of the endemic situation, ie, the more infected young people, the more severe situation (Wu et al., 1995). A variation of catalytic models applied to schistosomiasis data both from the lake and marshland region and the mountainous areas have demonstrated good performance as assessed by the comparison of estimated prevalence with observed data (Wang, 1990; Wu et al., 1995). Yu et al. (1997) used the catalytic model to project the impact of different interventions and then compare their cost-effectiveness. It was suggested that, chemotherapy remains the most cost-effective choice (Yu et al., 1997) despite the quick relapse at interrupted interventions.

Comparisons of different temporal forecasting models are listed in Table 1. Models based on time series provide a forecast of prevalence trends, thus producing an early warning system (EWS) from available data, while models based on transmission dynamics assist decision-making with regard to potential intervention strategies.

3.1.2 Spatial mapping of the schistosomiasis distribution

The spatial distribution of schistosomiasis can be visualized thanks to the development of geospatial technologies, such as geographical information systems (GIS) and remote sensing (RS), applied alone or in combination with statistical or mathematical modelling (Fig. 1). The spatial mapping of schistosomiasis infection could thus help allocate scarce budget resources cost-effectively (Xu et al., 2015; Yang et al., 2005a,b,c, 2015; Yang, 2016a,b).

Table 1 Comparison of temporal forecasting models

Model category	Model type	Comparison items					References
		Historical information capture	Required data	Forecast period	Explicability	Adaptability	
Based on time series	Grey model	Linear function	Simple	Short	Yes	Low adaptability due to strong model hypothesis for the epidemic situation Environmental or social factors rarely included	Zhang et al. (2007, 2014), Gan (2011), Chen et al. (2014b,c), Zhou et al. (2014)
	Time series model	Linear function	Simple	Short	Yes		
	Machine-learning	Nonlinear function	Simple	Flexible[a]	No		
	Hybrid model	Linear + nonlinear functions	Simple	Flexible[a]	No		
Based on transmission process	Dynamic mathematical model	Parameters and equations based on known transmission mechanism	Complex	Long	No	High adaptability with regard to different environmental settings Risk factors can be combined into a framework of mechanisms	Williams et al. (2002), Wang (1990), Wu et al. (1995)
	Catalytic model	Parameters and equations expressing catalytic power in transmission process	Complex	Long	No	High adaptability with regard to different environmental settings	

[a]Depends on original data.

Simple GIS applications provide decision-makers with visualized information on the spread of diseases, including continuous risk maps, prevalence estimates and worm burdens of disease, together with spatial analysis. Zhou et al. (1999a,b,c) mapped the seasonal transmission risk in Jiangsu Province providing different colours corresponding to the level of schistosome transmission risk index. The risk index was calculated by the modified Malone model (Malone et al., 1997) composed of growing degree days, monthly average precipitation and potential evapotranspiration (Zhou et al., 1998). It was based on the fact that schistosome sporocysts in the snail host need 60 days to grow at the optimal temperatures between 18°C and 28°C and that the spread of the next parasite stage, the cercaria, is closely associated with surface water (Zhou et al., 1999a,b,c). Zhao et al. (2009) later improved the modified Malone model by creating a readapted Malone schistosome transmission index model (RMSI) that considered snail survival rates under extreme temperatures, which is essential for schistosome development (Zhao et al., 2009). Zhou et al. (1999a,b,c) and Zhao et al. (2009) both found the coincidence of the risk isoline with the −4°C or −2°C isotherm in January, which is the current boundary of endemic and nonendemic areas of schistosomiasis in The People's Republic of China.

Chen et al. (2007) explored the application of spatial analysis using GIS for a schistosomiasis control project. The second-order ordinary Kriging approach was selected by directional trend analysis as the most suitable way to predict schistosomiasis prevalence in a spatial manner. Schistosomiasis prevalence data were obtained at the village level in Dangtu County, Anhui Province, from 2001 to 2004. Spatial distribution of the whole county was estimated and further classified into four strata from high to low. The stratification provided a chance to discover that the four strata each had different environmental settings. Thus different strategies were formulated for each of them. Prevalence area stratification could also be used for risk factor identification (Chen et al., 2007). Peng et al. (2010) mapped spatial clusters of schistosomiasis-infected cases in the village of Ximiao in Jiangxi Province, using spatial scan statistics in GIS. They were further classified into high-, low- and non-clusters to support risk factors identifications (Peng et al., 2010).

To further assess risk factors of schistosomiasis, the combined application of GIS and RS together with Bayesian statistical models could be of value. Yang et al. (2015b) adopted Bayesian multilevel models with spatial random effects to identify eco-social determinants of schistosomiasis. Demographic data at the individual level, economic/lifestyle data at the household level and human/snail data at the village level were collected. The results showed that the key risk factors were the absence of separate stall housings for livestock breeding and the sanitary status of the households as well as the density of infected snails in the villages (Yang et al., 2015).

From a spatio-temporal perspective, simulation with Bayesian statistical models or mathematical models functions both in relevant factor identification and in facilitating spatial decisions as well (Lai et al., 2013; Xu et al., 2013; Zhou et al., 2010).

Yang et al. (2005a,b,c) employed Bayesian spatio-temporal models to explore the association between climate factors and schistosomiasis infection, as well as the spatial correlation of infection risk between counties in Jiangsu Province for each year between 1990 and 1998. Bayesian smoothed annual *S. japonicum* infection maps were produced. The normalized difference vegetation index (NDVI) was found to be negatively associated with infection risk, while the land surface temperature (LST) was positively associated (Yang et al., 2005a,b,c). In a further step, Zhang et al. (2012) mapped not only the relative risk, but also the ratios of different risk groups of schistosomiasis calculated by Bayesian random-effect model. This model decomposed area-specific random effects into correlated heterogeneity (CH) and uncorrelated heterogeneity (UH). The former encompassed the combined effects of all unmeasured spatially structured risk factors such as rainfall, income and biological factors, ie, those pertaining to *O. hupensis*, while the latter encompassed spatially unstructured factors like age, gender and human behavioural factors. Simulating from county level data in five provinces over a 10-year study period, the chemotherapy-based World Bank Loan Project was evaluated (Zhang et al., 2012). The predicted distribution of relative risk and its posterior probability showed that the most severely affected areas were mainly located along Yangtze River and the great lakes. The change and distribution of various ratios (of UH to CH) showed that CH had gradually turned to be the major risk component for most endemic areas, indicating the need for a further strategy focus on snail control (Li and Lin, 2016; Liu, 2016a; Yang et al., 2016; Zhang et al., 2012).

Xu et al. (2006) employed a spatial-temporal mathematical model to assess the effects of intervillage connectivity in schistosomiasis transmission. It was found that increased connectivity based on neighbourhood relationships and hydrologic connectivity led to geographic clustering of schistosomiasis with higher loads of worm burdens (Xu et al., 2006; Zhu et al., 2015). Gong et al. (2006) proposed a schistosomiasis transmission model capable of simulating the worm load reduction after years of intervention. The projected worm load reduction was vividly illustrated on a map according to different village selection plans for treatment intervention. It further proved that spatial connectivity, estimated by area and slope of villages, as well as water flow directions, is warranted to be considered in the final intervention strategy (Gong et al., 2006).

3.1.3 Parameter estimation via modelling

Schistosomiasis surveillance-response systems rely heavily on the results of the diagnostic methods used. However, the widely used Kato-Katz method has low sensitivity compared with antibody-detection, which instead has a specificity deficit (Xu et al., 2014). Since a proper 'gold standard' diagnostic method is not yet available, modelling plays an important role.

Assuming that the worm counts among different subjects are negatively binomially distributed, Yu et al. (1999) established a mathematical model for variations in faecal *S. japonicum* egg count. It was applied to prevalence data based on the Kato-Katz method in both the lake and mountainous areas in The People's Republic of China, where it achieved good fitness (Xiu et al., 2008; Yu et al., 2000). Using this model, a pocket chart to estimate the true prevalence using observed eggs per gram (EPG) data from single stool samples was created. This type of approach could greatly assist practical use in the field and contribute to rapid responses following surveillance results (Yu et al., 2000).

Zhang et al. (2009) estimated the true prevalence of schistosomiasis by Bayesian modelling based on prevalence data collected by the Kato-Katz method in three low-endemic areas. Superior to costly repeated Kato-Katz smears and the pocket chart mentioned above, Bayesian modelling could be of particular use in areas with low prevalence or low infection intensity (Zhang et al., 2009). Wang et al. (2006) applied a Bayesian hierarchical model to estimate the true prevalence based on the data from the third nationwide sampling survey in all seven endemic provinces in The People's Republic of China. The modelling results from antibody detection alone and a combined method using antibody detection + Kato-Katz applied as confirmatory test indicated that antibody detection alone would be an easier, still feasible diagnostic option to use in practice as part of a surveillance-response system (Wang et al., 2006).

3.2 The *Oncomelania* snail host

As the unique intermediate snail host of *S. japonicum*, the ecology of *O. hupensis* is essential (Li et al., 2016; Mao, 1990). Su (1995) claimed that the geographical distribution of *O. hupensis* is an essential part of its ecology. Back in the 1990s, it was thought that the negative binomial distribution (NBD) was a kind of discrete distribution that could be successfully fitted to *O. hupensis* survey data (Zhou et al., 2012). However, Zhang improved the NBD to generalized negative binomial distribution (GNBD), which could integrate many discrete distributions and which was more flexible in modelling of *O. hupensis* (Zhang et al., 2008b). Hu et al. (2013) compared Gaussian, binomial and Poisson models for schistosomiasis risk prediction, and showed that the Poisson model fitted the data of *O. hupensis* best (Hu et al., 2013). Traditionally, field investigation, as a main method for direct surveillance of snail habitats, has been widely used historically in endemic areas and suspected new areas (Wu et al., 2005). As widely reported, the distribution of *O. hupensis* is closely related to environmental factors, such as dynamic agricultural, ecological and hydrological factors (Remais et al., 2007, 2008; Spear et al., 2004). Benefits contributed by the rapid development of GIS, RS and global positioning systems (GPS) in the past decades have provided ideal tools for the mapping, prediction and monitoring of disease trends. Table 2 summarizes the studies published to date with an emphasis on GIS/RS modelling to predict *O. hupensis* habitats. These models go through multinode information transmission, which projects snail habitat information via the combination of image information and environmental factor information.

3.2.1 Snail habitats in the lake and marshland regions

According to the information in Table 2, most of the studies have focused on the prediction of potential habitats of *O. hupensis* in the lake and marshland regions. Due to the characteristics of snail habitats there, the special rules used in detecting snail habitats can be summarized by the sayings 'land in winter – water in summer' and 'no grass – no snails' (Zhang et al., 2013; Zhang, 2016). Li et al. (1990) first employed the Landsat Thematic Mapper (TM) (https://lta.cr.usgs.gov/) images from the National Oceanic and Atmospheric Administration (NOAA) satellite to identify snail habitats in Xichang and Chengdu and then in the prospected Three Gorges Dam (TGD) area (Zhou et al., 2008; Zhu et al., 2008). The study area was classified into several ecological zones based on soil types and vegetation coverage and then compared with historical records of snail investigation. Interestingly, the authors found places suitable for *O. hupensis* breeding coinciding with local residence areas in terraced fields consisting of old mud sediment. Tu and Wang (1995), Lin and Lin (2001) and Zhou et al. (1999a,b,c) mapped *O. hupensis* distributions using a principal component model on the basis of land utilization and wetlands in different seasons.

Table 2 GIS/RS model application to research on *Oncomelania hupensis*, the intermediate host snail of *Schistosoma japonicum*

Type of endemic area	Study aim	Method	RS images (spatial resolution)	Environmental factors	References
Lake and marshland regions (I)	Create a land cover map of *O. hupensis* habitats	RS image interpretation based on principal component analysis	Landsat MSS (30 m), NOAA (1.1 km)	Land cover and land use type, soil type, wetland vegetation cover type	Li et al. (1990), Tu and Wang (1995), Zhou et al. (1999), Lin and Lin (2001)
	Explore the vegetation landscapes in marshland snail habitats	RS image interpretation based on unsupervised classification	Landsat 7 ETM+ (30 m)	NDVI, tasselled-cap wetness soil chemistry, soil saturation, pH, humidity, temperature, land use, GVI and BI	Yang et al. (2000, 2006), Guo et al. (2002, 2005), Davis et al. (2002), Zhang et al. (2003b,c,d)
	Identify snail habitats	RS image interpretation based on supervised classification	Landsat 7 ETM+ (30 m) and Landsat 5 TM (30 m)	NDVI, land use type, tasselled-cap wetness DEM, waterbody	Xiao et al. (2009), Zhang et al. (2008b), Yuan et al. (2014)
	Explore the relationship between distribution of snails and environmental factors and predict snail habitats	RS images overlaid in ArcGIS	Landsat TM (30 m), CBERS-02B (19.5 m) and ENVISAT RA-2 (80 km)	NDVI, flooding zones, DEM, NDWI, MNDWI, EVI, SR	Zhang et al. (2004a,b, 2013), Yao et al. (2012), Wang et al. (2012), Tseng et al. (2014)
	Explore the relationship between circumstance elements and snails	Spatial analysis together with linear regression analysis	Landsat TM (30 m), Landsat 7 ETM+ (30 m) and Terra-MODIS (250 −1000 m)	NDVISAVI2, LST, tasselled-cap wetness, NDVI, GVI, GEMI, PVI, MSAVI2, soil wet, soil type, pH of soil, elevation	Zhang et al. (2003b, 2005), Qin et al. (2008), Gao et al. (2008), Wu et al. (2014)

Hilly and mountainous region (II)	Predict snail density	Spatial analysis, unsupervised classification	ASTER (30 m) and IKONOS (4 m)	DEM, land cover and land use type	Xu et al. (2004)
	Predict the spatial distribution of *O. hupensis*	Spatial-temporal analysis, Bayesian model	SPOT 5 (5 m) and Landsat 5 TM (30 m)	Land cover and land use type, distance from ditches to village, NDVI, slope	Yang et al. (2008, 2009)
	Monitor snail habitats	Supervised classification	Landsat TM in 2007 (30 m)	NDVI, slope, wetness at ditch	He et al. (2010)
Plain with waterway networks (III)	Predict the potential snail habitats	RS images overlaid in ArcGIS	Landsat ETM+ (30 m)	Water level, NDVI, DEM	Yang et al. (2010)
	Map the high risk of *O. hupensis* habitats	Landscape pattern analysis, multiple logistic regression	Landsat 5 TM (30 m)	Patch FD, paddy farm land proportion, wetness index, NDVI, DEM	Qiu et al. (2014)
Type I, II, III	Determine the relationships between the distribution of *O. hupensis* and snail population genetics	RS images overlaid in ArcGIS	AVHRR (1.1 km)	NDVI	Zhou et al. (1999a,b,c)

Note: *RS*, remote sensing; *MSS*, multispectral scanner; *NOAA*, national oceanic and atmospheric administration; *TM*, thematic mapper; *ETM+*, enhanced thematic mapper plus); *NDVI*, normalized difference vegetation index); *MODIS*, moderate resolution imaging spectroradiometer); *LST*, land surface temperature; *CBERS*, China-Brazil earth resources satellite; *ASTER*, advanced spaceborne thermal emission and reflection radiometer); *AVHRR*, advanced very high resolution radiometer; *GVI*, green vegetation index; *BI*, bright index; *DEM*, digital elevation model; *MSAVI2*, the second modified SAVI; *GEMI*, global environment monitoring index; *PVI*, perpendicular vegetation index; *NDWI*, normalized difference water index; *MNDWI*, the modified normalized difference water index; *EVI*, enhanced vegetation index; *SR*, sun reflectance; *FD*, fractal dimension.

In the early 2000s, an unsupervised classification model mainly based on extracted land cover features was widely used to predict potential *O. hupensis* habitats. For example, two researchers in Jiangsu Province applied unsupervised classification to predict the potential snail habitats affected by the flooding in 1998 (Yang et al., 2000, 2006). The NDVI measurements and waterbody expanses in the dry and wet seasons were extracted by unsupervised classification methods, then these two kinds of images were overlaid to detect the potential snail habitats. Validation with ground truth data both showed a high correlation with the prediction of potential snail habitats. In Poyang Lake, it was found that *O. hupensis* was mainly distributed in the areas where NDVI was relatively higher and tasselled-cap wetness varied between −10 and 3 (Guo et al., 2002). In Jiangning County along the Yangtze River, the land cover of the marshland was classified into 10 types by means of unsupervised classification of images from the Enhanced Thematic Mapper Plus (ETM+) on-board Landsat 7, and further validated by spot checks to determine the snail habitats (Qin et al., 2008).

To increase the classification accuracy of remotely sensed images, decision tree methods and supervised classification methods were applied to study land cover and land use types in *O. hupensis* habitats. Compared with unsupervised classification without prior knowledge, both decision tree and supervised classification require knowledge of the study area. Xiao et al. (2009) used the decision tree threshold segmentation method and GIS spatial analysis to extract environmental factors in the Honghu Lake, including NDVI and tasselled-cap wetness. Meanwhile, by supervised classification, the wetlands were classified into six types: lake, river, paddy, flood plain, pool and ditch. After overlaying all these related factors in ArcGIS (ESRI, Redlands, CA, USA), suspicious snail habitats were identified where the NDVI threshold was in the range of 0.2–0.3 and tasselled-cap wetness threshold between 7 and 13. The accuracy of this prediction model reached as high as 86.2%. In Poyang Lake, Landsat 5 TM images were classified into six land cover types based on different values of NDVI by knowledge decision tree classification. *Oncomelania* snails in Poyang Lake were detected by comparison with historical snail investigation records reaching a classification accuracy of 91.4% (Zhang et al., 2008a). Yuan et al. (2014) employed NDVI and elevation data as environmental factors related to snail habitats. The area of 'land in winter – water in summer' was determined by supervised classification from RS images taken in a flood and dry seasons in Poyang Lake. The overlays with these data showed in suitable areas for snail habitats, which were intersected with an elevation between 13 m and 18 m and NDVI >0.17.

To better reflect the complexity and dynamics of snail distribution, researchers began combining spatial analysis with other modelling technologies. In 2003, Zhang et al. (2003a) extracted NDVI data and images from the moderate resolution imaging spectroradiometer (MODIS) (http://modis.gsfc.nasa.gov/) on-board the Terra satellite in ArcGIS software and used bivariate correlations and stepwise linear regression to study the relationship between NDVI and snail distribution. It was found that the snail density in the marshlands was positively correlated with the mean and maximum NDVI. In a study performed in 2005, the relationship between snail density and the environmental indices (MSAVI2, LST, surrogate indices) extracted from Landsat 7 ETM+ were analysed comparatively by stepwise regression analysis and semivariogram methods (Zhang et al., 2005). Finally, the respective correlation coefficient was calculated as 0.282 and 0.852 (Zhang et al., 2005). In the marshlands of Dongting Lake area, the spatial pattern of snail density and correlation between environmental factors (NDVI, pH, soil humility and vegetation type) and snail distribution were analysed by spatial analysing technology and curvilinear regression analysis (Qin et al., 2008). The results from the correlation analyses indicated that there were positive correlations between the density of *Oncomelania* snails and the NDVI/type of sedgy (one of the major types of local vegetation) while there were negative correlations between that and the PH value/organic content of the soil (Qin et al., 2008). Gao et al. (2008) found that the different values of NDVI, GVI, GEMI, PVI and MSAVI2 could differentiate between areas suitable for snail breeding and those not suitable by spatial analysis and backward multiple regression. Besides, local indicators of spatial association (LISA) statistic and geographically weighted regression (GWR) modelled together with multivariate analyses were applied to explore the possible optimum scopes of the following environmental factors for snails: moisture content, pH, temperature of the soil and elevation. The results were 36.58–61.08%, 6.541–6.89, 24.3–25.7% and 23.5–29.44 m, respectively (Wu et al., 2014).

The ETM-generated data are the most widely used source for the prediction of potential snail habitats, but their broader use is limited by high cost. Comparatively, images from the China–Brazil Earth Resources Satellite (CBERS) provide a better opportunity to detect snail habitats with the advantage of higher resolution (20 m) and free availability. Yao et al. (2012) extracted waterbody information by the NDWI model from multitemporal CBERS-02 images. In ArcGIS software, the areas of waterbody were calculated to determine images from dry season and flooding season and further determine the presence of snail habitats. In Anxiang County, CBERS images were obtained to extract NDWI and NDVI as key environmental factors for *O. hupensis* survival. Then, a model based on knowledge tree of 'land in winter — water in summer', 'no snails — no grass' and 'pattern of vegetation growth (suitable for snail survival)' was developed to identify snail habitats. It showed a sensitivity and specificity of 63.44% and 78.09%, respectively (Zhang et al., 2013).

3.2.2 Snail habitats in the hilly and mountainous regions

In the hilly and mountainous regions, snails are distributed along the valleys, on grassy hill slopes, on the vertical sides of terraced fields and in irrigation ditches (Liu, 2016b; Yang et al., 2008). These snail habitats are normally isolated from each other, which makes it necessary to work at the micro-scale. To obtain remotely sensed images with high spatial resolutions and high accuracy requires more effort in the mountainous regions. In Puge County, Sichuan Province, Landsat TM images were classified into five categories: snail habitats, rivers, residential districts, shadow and other ground objects by supervised classification with the overall classification accuracy reaching 80.2%. The study found that snail habitats were mainly distributed in croplands and grassed hillsides (He et al., 2010). Xu et al. (2004) extracted land cover and land use type from 4-m resolution IKONOS images (http://global.digitalglobe.com/sites/default/files/DG_IKONOS_DS.pdf). Based on 30-m resolution elevation map, snail density was predicted combining field survey data with land cover and land use fractions. In Eryuan County, a mountainous region of snail habitats, SPOT-5 5-m resolution images (https://directory.eoportal.org/web/eoportal/satellite-missions/s/spot-5) were applied to extract land cover and land use categories, NDVI, slope of each ditch and distance from ditches to villages. A two-pronged approach, consisting of landscape pattern analysis and Bayesian spatial modelling approaches, was used to predict the spatial distribution of snails at the local scale (Yang et al., 2008; Yang, 2009). By validation with the deviance information criterion (DIC), the Bayesian spatial model was found to be the best-fitting model in Eryuan County.

3.2.3 Snail habitats in the plains with waterway networks

In the plains with waterway networks, the snail distribution was linear along the ditches evolving from patchy distribution along the river and lakes (Peng et al., 2007; Yang, 2016a,b). Only a few studies have focused on prediction of snail habitats in this type of endemic areas, partly because schistosomiasis has been interrupted in most of these areas. However, *O. hupensis* can reemerge if the local environment changes. In Qianjiang County, land use information was extracted from ZiYuan 1 02c (ZY-102C, The People's Republic of China Center for Resource Satellite Data and Application) satellite images with 2.36-m resolution. Landscape metrics including FD, median patch size (MedPS), patch size coefficient of variance (PSCOV), mean patch fractal dimension (MPFD) and area-weighted mean shape index (AWMSI), NDVI, wetness index (WI), soil texture and topological data were extracted from TM images and carried out at a spatial resolution of 5 m. An integrated approach of landscape pattern analysis coupled with multiple logistic regression models was applied to the data above to predict snail habitats (Qiu et al., 2014). In Chongqing segment of the Three Gorges Reservoir, hydrological data of the main channel and NDVI were extracted from ETM+ data. Potential snail breeding regions in the Three Gorges area were detected and two focus regions of Qukou in Kaixian and Dachang in Wushan were identified for further monitoring.

Most research on snail habitat prediction have focused on micro- or mesoscale. However, Zhou et al. (1999a,b,c) described an innovative application of GIS at the country level. In this study, a potential spatial relationship between the observed distribution of *O. hupensis* and snail population genetics was investigated. The existence of subspecies of *Oncomelania* spp. in The People's Republic of China was supported by the confirmation of a discrete subpopulation model in the snail population structure (Davis et al., 2002).

4. DISCUSSION

4.1 Model classification

Many categorization methods have been proposed for modelling infectious diseases. A majority of them come from a methodological perspective, eg, models could be classified into qualitative estimation, quantitative prediction and/or a combination of the two based on their methodological nature. They could also be divided into stochastic models or nonstochastic models due to the mechanism used for modelling (Zhai, 2012). To better classify the models, our review restricts modelling to those using mathematical or statistical methods. Our classification scheme is based on a target-driven perspective adapted to the requirement of schistosomiasis surveillance-response system in The People's Republic of China, as it might help us better understand the role of modelling in this system.

4.2 Modelling in the schistosomiasis surveillance-response system

Modelling constitutes a powerful approach to data analysis and various applications play an important role in surveillance-response systems. In the system featured by a set of minimized essential dataset (Tambo et al., 2014; Zhou et al., 2013a,b), models, such as 'grey' models, ARIMA and the like, could predict future endemic intensity based on just a series of historical infection rate. After integrating biological, environmental and socioeconomic data, modelling can establish a spatio-temporal comparison system capable of providing outcomes with high predictive power in surveillance-response systems. Compared to conventional statistical methods, models applied in surveillance-response system are useful at different spatial and temporal levels. Liang et al. (2007) reviewed in detail the mechanistic basis of time-varying modifiers of transmission of schistosomiasis, estimated the values for two regions in western China and explored their dynamic influence using a mathematical transmission model. The term 'time-varying' is used to describe risk factors, because some of them are periodic in nature (seasonal) and some are nonseasonal, such as complex patterns of human behaviour (eg, anthropogenic intervention to achieve disease control). Remais et al. (2009) revealed that transmission processes of *S. japonicum* in western China are time-varying and determined what is colloquially referred to as the transmission season, a period between March and October. Scaling is another important issue, which has been developed with regard to the Chinese schistosomiasis situation by Malone et al. (2010), and applied to the study of transmission risk factors by several researchers exploring the Yangtze River Valley at provincial as well as county levels (Liu, 2014; Xu et al., 1999; Yang et al., 2006).

Models are cost-effective approaches when designing intervention packages responsive to warnings coming out of data analysis. One of the particular advantages of models is that they can theoretically estimate the development. In a temporal sense. Some of them can virtually mimic the dynamics of disease transmission in different types of scenarios in a mathematical way, making it possible to estimate possible response strategies in advance. By changing key parameters with the time line, such as prevalence or R_0, it can discriminate between options and tell what would be the optimal strategies. Compared with traditional evaluation methods, model virtualization provides advantages (Williams et al., 2002, see Table 3) that make modelling a very useful tool in the design of response strategy. From a spatial dimension, a variety of models can help predict the potential endemic areas. In turn this also strengthens the surveillance aspect of the strategy.

Table 3 Comparison of preventive intervention evaluation methods

	Methods to compare	
Dimensions to compare	**Traditional evaluation methods**	**Dynamic transmission models**
Evaluation timing	After intervention completed	Before intervention implemented
Evaluation period selection	Single time point evaluation	Flexible (any period of time can be simulated)
Length of evaluation period	Long-term evaluation rarely feasible	Both short- and long-term evaluation feasible
Environmental influence	Environmental confounders	Environmental effects can be controlled
Evaluation efficiency	Time-consuming	Relatively more efficient
Budget demand	Expensive	Budget saving

4.3 Research gaps

To achieve the goal of schistosomiasis elemination by the end of this decade at the country level, The People's Republic of China has made great efforts and set its own Control and Elimination Criteria (Cao et al., 2016). A recently approved official version (GB 15976-2015) sets a requirement of a sensitive and effective county-level surveillance system for the transmission interruption stage (Zhou et al., 2013a,b). The requirement for this stage is now 'no infected snails for five years', instead of 'no snails for two years' as it was in the last version. These criteria not only provide a better chance of data availability, but also indicate notable modelling research gaps.

First, studies generally focus on snail density rather than the proportion of infected snails, which would have been a more useful index. However, it is difficult in practice to completely eradicate all snail hosts in the natural environment (Zhou et al., 2012). Recent studies reveal that *Oncomelania* snails have a trend to grow exponentially when reduced to low densities (Yang et al., 2011, 2012a,b). Therefore, more studies and modelling practices emphasis on infected snails are needed.

Second, important reservoir hosts, such as bovine and rodents, still require more attention. Not many models with regard to surveillance-response focus on these reservoirs, particularly not in the mountainous areas, where it could be an important transmission component (Rudge et al., 2013). As the infected domestic animals are easier to control, wild animals like rodents will most probably remain the infection source in the future (Yang et al., 2016; Zhang et al., 2016a).

Third, the abundance of surveillance data and data varieties reveals a gap of intersectional research cooperation. Modelling technology has the potential to integrate all five major schistosomiasis research directions raised by Feng et al. (2016) and Lei and Zhou (2015) for the current stage in The People's Republic of China, namely, information systems and warning, epidemiology and surveillance technology, intervention and evaluation, biological study as well as ecological study (Lei and Zhou, 2015). Biological study and ecological study, as well as epidemiology and surveillance technology, provide models with scenario, data or parameter values. Information systems and warning could be the connected platform for modelling. Modelling further provides intervention design and could be validated by evaluation. The integration of these researches into a modelling platform should greatly benefit schistosomiasis surveillance-response activities in The People's Republic of China. However, gaps exist with respect to their integration. For example, few biological studies provide sufficient parameter estimation for model building to simulate schistosomiasis transmission. Moreover, the quality of data collected from epidemiological and surveillance activities must be further improved to satisfy the requirement of model use. Besides, knowledge translation restricts in depth integration and constitutes therefore another gap that needs to be closed. The most updated modelling technology contains huge amount of mathematical and computational knowledge. It is too sophisticated for policy makers and public health workers to understand and accept at a glance. The application of GIS technology to visually demonstrate complicated data relieves the situation to some extent, but the need for training and more vivid expression of modelling technology calls for further study.

4.4 Challenges and opportunities

The environmental alterations have led to changes in schistosomiasis transmission (Yang et al., 2016). Global warming, as an example, was found to have shifted the line of potential schistosomiasis endemicity northwards in The People's Republic of China, adding an area with over 20 million people (Yang et al., 2005a,b,c; Zhou et al., 2008). With respect to hydro-electrical power generation, Dai et al. (1995) reported a case study of enlarged schistosomiasis endemic area due to dam construction in the 1990s in Anhui Province (Dai, 1995). Two other major concerns are the TGD and the South-to-North Water Diversion Project (SNWDP). Although studies have shown that the lower water levels and droughts brought by TGD reduce snail density and thus schistosomiasis prevalence (Chen et al.,

2013, 2014a,b,c), snail control in these areas will remain a challenge with regard to surveillance (Wu et al., 2015). The ongoing SNWDP carries the risk of transporting host snails to reproduce in schistosomiasis nonendemic areas with changed ecology as more water will be supplied (Liang et al., 2012; Wang and Zhang, 2002). Although not many schistosomiasis cases have been reported in the nonendemic areas, the potential is there and a reliable surveillance-response system based on modelling technology needs to be put in place without delay.

Second, socioeconomic transformation may also result in increased transmission of schistosomiasis (Liu et al., 2014; Salam et al., 2014; Zhang et al., 2016c). For example, population migration has been a common phenomenon particularly in the rural parts of the country due to the booming economy. According to Cao et al. (2015), migrant populations have the same lifestyles and water contact behaviour as those of the local permanent residents. However, migration was not a feature of the national control programme, and due to administrative delays, this issue is still not covered by the programme, which has resulted in higher schistosome infection rates (Cao et al., 2015). Response packages are to be adjusted to this new situation with surveillance-response assisted with modelling based on the latest information. Besides, new agricultural technology and even lifestyle changes in the new generation are also things occurring in The People's Republic of China, and this brings new unforeseen influences, good or bad, particularly to the rural endemic areas. As we rapidly move towards the era of schistosomiasis elimination, modelling could serve as a powerful tool to identify these growing elements by a sensitive surveillance system and prevent them through a quick response.

Finally, budget shortages might be one of the most significant challenges to schistosomiasis control as financial resources may not be preferentially allocated to the diseases with low prevalence. On the other hand, this might not be a direct threat to modelling, since this is one of the more cost-effective tools in the surveillance-response system. In resource-limited circumstances, modelling may function better in epidemic forecasting and response estimation than evaluations based on traditional field investigations. In this regard, modelling also presents a good approach for the introduction of Chinese experiences to other countries or regions. As the elimination of schistosomiasis at the regional level by 2020 is a common goal for many endemic countries, it is of value to share Chinese experience. Besides capacity building and collaborative research, sharing experiences with respect to modelling and surveillance-response systems is a key choice, particularly for resource-limited countries (Tambo et al., 2014). The real-time GIS Web-based platform (WebGIS) for schistosomiasis surveillance is a good example. It models spatial data, field data and laboratory data and interacts with users, providing evidence-based disease status. It is user-friendly and easy to adapt to any geographical area (Yang et al., 2012c). In these cases, the sharing of modelling technology is less restrained by geographical change but will also contribute to capacity building.

5. CONCLUSIONS

Shifting from monitoring and evaluation to rapid detection and immediate response requires modelling to bridge the two latter components. Modelling thus plays an essential role in schistosomiasis surveillance-response, but more research is required to achieve a practically useful understanding of the current endemic situation and the potential future directions of control (Yang et al., 2005a,b,c; Zhang et al., 2013; Zhou et al., 2010, 2013a,b). The acquired experience has the potential to be shared between control units not only within The People's Republic of China but also with research institutions and control programmes in other endemic areas in the world.

ACKNOWLEDGEMENTS

We appreciate Leping Sun's constructive comments. This work was supported by International Development Research Centre (IDRC), Canada (grant no. 105509-00001002-024 and grant no.108100-001), and grants from the National Nature Science Foundation (grant no. 81102173, 81273192 and 81573261). This work was partially supported by Jiangsu Science and Technology Department (BM2015024). GJY also acknowledges the Program for National S & T Program (grant no. 2008ZX10004-011 and 2012ZX10004-220).

REFERENCES

Barbour, A.D., 1996. Modeling the transmission of schistosomiasis: an introductory view. Am. J. Trop. Med. Hyg. 55 (Suppl.), 135−143.

Bergquist, R., Tanner, M., 2010. Controlling schistosomiasis in Southeast Asia: a tale of two countries. Adv. Parasitol. 72, 109−144.

Bergquist, R., Yang, G.J., Knopp, S., Utzinger, J., Tanner, M., 2015. Surveillance and response: tools and approaches for the elimination stage of neglected tropical diseases. Acta Trop. 141, 229−234.

Cao, C.L., Bao, Z.P., Li, S.Z., Wei, W.Y., Yi, P., Yu, Q., et al., 2015. Schistosomiasis in a migrating population in the lake region of China and its potential impact on control operation. Acta Trop. 145, 88−92.

Cao, Z.G., Zhao, Y.E., Willingham, A.L., Wang, T.P., 2016. Towards the elimination of schistosomiasis japonica through control of the disease in domestic animals in the People's Republic of China: a tale of over 60 years. Adv. Parasitol. 92.

Chen, H.G., Zeng, X.J., Lin, D.D., Lv, S.B., Gu, X.N., Hang, C.Q., et al., 2013. The changes of hydrological regime in Poyang lake after runs of three Gorges project and its impact on prevalence of schistosomiasis in the lake region. Chin. J. Schisto. Control 25, 444–450.

Chen, L., Lu, D., Xu, J., Duan, B., Zhong, B., 2014a. Changes of schistosomiasis endemic situation in Sichuan province and impact on schistosomiasis transmission in three Gorges reservoir area after construction of three Gorges reservoir. Chin. J. Schisto. Control 26, 494–497.

Chen, M., Feng, Z., 1999. Schistosomiasis control in China. Parasitology 48, 11–19.

Chen, M.G., 2014. Assessment of morbidity due to *Schistosoma japonicum* infection in China. Infect. Dis. Poverty 3, 6.

Chen, Y.Y., Cai, S.X., Xiao, Y., Jiang, Y., Shan, X.W., Zhang, J., et al., 2014b. Prediction of epidemic tendency of schistosomiasis with time series model in Hubei province. Chin. J. Schisto. Control 26, 613–617.

Chen, Y.Y., Cai, S.X., Xiao, Y., Shan, X.W., Zhang, J., Liu, J.B., 2014c. Impact of implementation of three Gorges project on schistosomiasis endemic situation in Hubei province. Chin. J. Schisto. Control 26, 498–503.

Chen, Z., Zhou, X.-N., Yang, K., Wang, X.-H., Yao, Z.-Q., Wang, T.-P., et al., 2007. Strategy formulation for schistosomiasis japonica control in different environmental settings supported by spatial analysis: a case study from China. Geospat. Health 1, 223–231.

Da'dara, A.A., Li, Y.S., Xiong, T., Zhou, J., Williams, G.M., McManus, D.P., et al., 2008. DNA-based vaccines protect against zoonotic schistosomiasis in water buffalo. Vaccine 26, 3617–3625.

Dai, S.J., 1995. Investigation of *Oncomelania hupensis* dissemination and schistosomiasis endemic change caused by Chencun hydrological project. Chin. J. Schisto. Control 7, 355–356.

Davis, G.M., Wu, W.P., Liu, H.Y., Williams, G., Lu, S.B., Chen, H.G., et al., 2002. Applying geographic information system and remote sensing to the epidemiology of schistosomiasis in Poyang lake, Jiangxi province, China. Geogr. Inf. Sci. 8, 67–77.

Deng, J.L., 1985. Grey System. National Defense Industry Press, Beijing.

Feng, Y., Liu, L., Xia, S., Xu, J.F., Bergquist, R., Yang, G.J., 2016. Reaching the surveillance-response stage of schistosomiasis control in the People's Republic of China: a modelling approach. Adv. Parasitol. 92.

Gan, X.M., 2011. Study on the Evaluation of Epidemic Situation and Forecasting and Early Warning for Schistosomiasis. Huazhong University of Science and Technology, Wuhan.

Gao, B., Hu, F., Fang, Y., Lin, Y.M., Lu, S.B., Le, X.H., et al., 2008. Studies on rapid determination of susceptible environments with *Schistosomiasis japonicum* in Poyang lake region by remote sensing technology. J. Trop. Dis. Parasitol. 6, 187–190.

Gao, S.J., He, Y.Y., Liu, Y.J., Yang, G.J., Zhou, X.N., 2013. Field transmission intensity of *Schistosoma japonicum* measured by basic reproduction ratio from modified Barbour's model. Parasit. Vectors 6.

Gong, P., Xu, B., Liang, S., 2006. Remote sensing and geographic information systems in the spatial temporal dynamics modeling of infectious diseases. Sci. China Ser. C Life Sci. Chin. Acad. Sci. 49, 573–582.

Gray, D.J., Li, Y.S., Williams, G.M., Zhao, Z.Y., Harn, D.A., Li, S.M., et al., 2014. A multicomponent integrated approach for the elimination of schistosomiasis in the People's Republic of China: design and baseline results of a 4-year cluster-randomised intervention trial. Int. J. Parasitol. 44, 659–668.

Guo, J.G., Chen, H., Lin, D.D., Hu, G., Wu, X., Li, D., et al., 2002. A method of rapid identification snail habitat in marshland of Poyang lake region by remote sensing. Chin. J. Parasitol. Parasit. Dis. 15, 291–296.

Guo, J.G., Vounatsou, P., Cao, C.L., Utzinger, J., Zhu, H.Q., Anderegg, D., et al., 2005. A geographic information and remote sensing based model for prediction of *Oncomelania hupensis* habitats in the Poyang lake area, China. Acta Trop. 96, 213–222.
He, M.Z., Peng, W.X., Zhou, Y.B., Yiao, W.L., Liu, G.M., Jiang, Q.W., 2010. Application of landsat TM images on the snail habitats monitoring in mountainous region. Fudan Univ. J. Med. Sci. 37, 510–513.
Hsu, H.P.H., Wu, K., 1941. Schistosomiasis in China II. Distribution. Nat. Med. J. China 27, 553–564.
Hu, Y., Xiong, C.L., Zhang, Z.J., Bergquist, R., Wang, Z.L., Gao, J., et al., 2013. Comparison of data-fitting models for schistosomiasis: a case study in Xiangzi, China. Geospat. Health 8, 125–132.
Lai, Y.S., Zhou, X.N., Utzinger, J., Vounatsou, P., 2013. Bayesian geostatistical modelling of soil-transmitted helminth survey data in the People's Republic of China. Parasit. Vectors 6, 359.
Lei, Z.L., Zhou, X.N., 2015. Eradication of schistosomiasis: a new target and a new task for the National Schistosomiasis Control Porgramme in the People's Republic of China. Chin. J. Schisto. Control 27, 1–4.
Li, Z.J., Ge, J., Dai, J.R., Wen, L.Y., Lin, D.D., Madsen, H., et al., 2016. Biology and control of snail intermediate host of *Schistosoma japonicum* in the People's Republic of China. Adv. Parasitol. 92.
Li, Z.J., Lin, D.D., 2016. Biology and control of snail intermediate hosts of *Schistosoma japonicum* in China. Adv. Parasitol. 92.
Li, Z.W., Yuan, P., Yin, R., He, S., Gu, X., Zhao, W., et al., 1990. Identification of distribution area of *Oncomelania* by remote sensing technique. Acta Sci. Circum. 10, 217–225.
Liang, S., Seto, E.Y., Remais, J.V., Zhong, B., Yang, C., Hubbard, A., et al., 2007. Environmental effects on parasitic disease transmission exemplified by schistosomiasis in Western China. Proc. Natl. Acad. Sci. U.S.A. 104, 7110–7115.
Liang, Y.S., Wang, W., Li, H.J., Shen, X.H., Xu, Y.L., Dai, J.R., 2012. The South-to-North water diversion project: effect of the water diversion pattern on transmission of *Oncomelania hupensis*, the intermediate host of *Schistosoma japonicum* in China. Parasit. Vectors 5, 52.
Lier, T., Simonsen, G.S., Wang, T., Lu, D., Haukland, H.H., Vennervald, B.J., et al., 2009. Real-time polymerase chain reaction for detection of low-intensity *Schistosoma japonicum* infections in China. Am. J. Trop. Med. Hyg. 81, 428–432.
Lin, T., Lin, D.D., 2001. Classification study on the marshland in endemic area of *Schistosoma japonicum* using satellite TM images data. Chin. J. Prev. Med. 35, 312–314.
Liu, J.B., 2016a. Effectiveness of schistosomiasis control through water-conservancy projects. Adv. Parasitol. 92.
Liu, L., 2014. Multi-scale Investigation on Distribution and Influencing Factors of Schistosomiasis. Master thesis. Jiangsu Institute of Parasitic Diseases, Wuxi.
Liu, L., Yang, G.J., Zhu, H.R., Yang, K., Ai, L., 2014. Knowledge of, attitudes towards, and practice relating to schistosomiasis in two subtypes of a mountainous region of the People's Republic of China. Infect. Dis. Poverty 3, 16.
Liu, Y., 2016b. Epidemiological features and control effectiveness of schistosomiasis in mountainous and hilly region in China. Adv. Parasitol. 92.
Logan, O.T., 1905. A case of dysentery in Hunan province, cause by the trematoda, *schistosoma japonicum*. China Med. Missionary J. 19, 243–245.
Malone, J.B., Yilma, J.M., Hlbahy, M.M., 1997. Geographic information systems and snail born disease in Africa. In: Proceedings of "Workshop on Medical Malacology in Africa": 1997; Harare, Zimbabwe, pp. 22–26.
Malone, J.B., Yang, G.J., Leonardo, L., Zhou, X.N., 2010. Implementing a geospatial health data infrastructure for control of Asian schistosomiasis in the People's Republic of China

and the Philippines. In: Zhou, X.N., Bergquist, R., Olveda, R., Utzinger, J. (Eds.), Advances in Parasitology, Important Helminth Infections in Southeast Asia: Diversity and Potential for Control and Elimination, Pt B, Vol. 73, pp. 71–100.

Mao, S.B., 1990. Biology and Prevention and Control of Shistosomiasis. People's Medical Publishing House, Beijing.

Mei, H.G., 1989. Application of grey model in advanced schistosomiasis. Chin. J. Schisto. Control 1, 55–56.

Muench, H., 1959. Catalytic Models in Epidemiology. Harvard University Press, Cambridge, MA.

Peng, W.X., Wang, J.S., Rong, X.B., Wang, S.H., He, L.C., Fu, Z.Y., 2007. Schistosomiasis prevalence characteristic and epidemic factors in four-lake basin of Jianghan plain, Hubei province. J. Public Health Prev. Med. 18, 66–68, 70.

Peng, W.X., Tao, B., Clements, A., Jiang, Q.L., Zhang, Z.J., Zhou, Y.B., et al., 2010. Identifying high-risk areas of schistosomiasis and associated risk factors in the Poyang lake region, China. Parasitology 137, 1099–1107.

Qin, J.X., Tian, Z.F., Zhang, C., 2008. Environment factors and spatial characters of distribution of *Oncomcelania* snails in islet and beach of Dongting lake area. J. Natur. Dis. 17, 20–27.

Qiu, J., Li, R., Xu, X., Yu, C., Xia, X., Hong, X., et al., 2014. Identifying determinants of *Oncomelania hupensis* habitats and assessing the effects of environmental control strategies in the plain regions with the waterway network of China at the microscale. Int. J. Environ. Res. Public Health 11 (65), 71–85.

Remais, J., Hubbard, A., Wu, Z., Spear, R.C., 2007. Weather-driven dynamics of an intermediate host: mechanistic and statistical population modelling of *Oncomelania hupensis*. J. Appl. Ecol. 44, 781–791.

Remais, J., Liang, S., Spear, R.C., 2008. Coupling hydrologic and infectious disease models to explain regional differences in schistosomiasis transmission in southwestern China. Environ. Sci. Technol. 42, 2643–2649.

Remais, J., Zhong, B., Carlton, E.J., Spear, R.C., 2009. Model approaches for estimating the influence of time-varying socio-environmental factors on macroparasite transmission in two endemic regions. Epidemics 1, 213–220.

Rudge, J.W., Webster, J.P., Lu, D.-B., Wang, T.-P., Fang, G.-R., Basanez, M.-G., 2013. Identifying host species driving transmission of schistosomiasis japonica, a multihost parasite system, in China. Proc. Natl. Acad. Sci. U.S.A. 110, 11457–11462.

Sai, X.Y., Yan, Y.P., Zhang, Z.Y., Cai, K.P., Li, Y.S., Zhou, X.N., et al., 2005. Application of grey model(1,1) in the prediction of schistosomiasis prevalence in Haokou village of Dongting lake. Chin. J. Dis. Control Prev. 9, 29–31.

Salam, R.A., Maredia, H., Das, J.K., Lassi, Z.S., Bhutta, Z.A., 2014. Community-based interventions for the prevention and control of helminthic neglected tropical diseases. Infect. Dis. Poverty 3, 23.

Seto, E.Y., Remais, J.V., Carlton, E.J., Wang, S., Liang, S., Brindley, P.J., et al., 2011. Toward sustainable and comprehensive control of schistosomiasis in China: lessons from Sichuan. PLoS Negl. Trop. Dis. 5, e1372.

Spear, R.C., Seto, E., Liang, S., Birkner, M., Hubbard, A., Qiu, D., et al., 2004. Factors influencing the transmission of *Schistosoma japonicum* in the mountains of Sichuan province of China. Am. J. Trop. Med. Hyg. 70, 48–56.

Su, D.L., 1995. In: Selected Papers of Professor Delong Su. Tianjin Science and Technology Press, Tianjin, China.

Tambo, E., Ai, L., Zhou, X., Chen, J.H., Hu, W., Bergquist, R., et al., 2014. Surveillance-response systems: the key to elimination of tropical diseases. Infect. Dis. Poverty 3, 17.

Tseng, K.H., Liang, S., Ibaraki, M., Lee, H., Shum, C.K., 2014. Study of the variation of schistosomiasis risk in lake Poyang in the People's Republic of China using multiple space-borne sensors for the monitoring and modelling. Geospat. Health 8, 353–364.

Tu, M., Wang, Q., 1995. Identification of the distribution area of *Oncomelania hupensis* by remote sensing. Resour. Environ. Yangtze Val. 4, 81–85.
Utzinger, J., Brattig, N.W., Leonardo, L., Zhou, X.N., Bergquist, R., 2015. Progress in research, control and elimination of helminth infections in Asia. Acta Trop. 141, 135–145.
Wang, L.D., Guo, J.G., Wu, X.H., Chen, H.G., Wang, T.P., Zhu, S.P., et al., 2009. China's new strategy to block *Schistosoma japonicum* transmission: experiences and impact beyond schistosomiasis. Trop. Med. Int. Health 14, 1475–1483.
Wang, R.B., Wang, T.P., Wang, L.Y., Guo, J.G., Yu, Q., Xu, J., et al., 2004. Study on the re-emerging situation of schistosomiasis epidemics in areas already under control and interruption. Chin. J. Epidemiol. 25, 564–567.
Wang, T.P., Zhang, S.Q., 2002. South-to-North water diversion project and *Oncomelania hupensis* dissemination and schistosomiasis transmission. Chin. J. Schisto. Control 23.
Wang, W.F., 1990. Two-stage catalytic model and its application in bovine schistosomiasis epidemiological study. Chin. Vet. Technol. 42–44.
Wang, X.H., Wu, X.H., Zhou, X.N., 2006. Bayesian estimation of community prevalences of *Schistosoma japonicum* infection in China. Int. J. Parasitol. 36, 895–902.
Wang, Z.L., Gao, J., Tao, B., Jiang, Q.L., Zhai, M.L., Zhang, Z.J., et al., 2012. Preliminary study on applying high resolution CBERS images to identify *Oncomelania* snail habitats in lake and marshland regions. Chin. J. Schisto. Control 24.
Williams, G.M., Sleigh, A.C., Li, Y., Feng, Z., Davis, G.M., Chen, H., et al., 2002. Mathematical modelling of schistosomiasis japonica: comparison of control strategies in the People's Republic of China. Acta Trop. 82, 253–262.
Wiwanitkit, V., Tambo, E., Ugwu, E.C., Ngogang, J.Y., Zhou, X.N., 2015. Are surveillance response systems enough to effectively combat and contain the Ebola outbreak? Infect. Dis. Poverty 4, 7.
Wu, J.Y., Zhou, Y.B., Li, L.H., Zheng, S.B., Liang, S., Coatsworth, A., et al., 2014. Identification of optimum scopes of environmental factors for snails using spatial analysis techniques in Dongting lake region, China. Parasit. Vectors 7, 216–228.
Wu, J.Y., Zhou, Y.B., Chen, Y., Liang, S., Li, L.H., Zheng, S.B., et al., 2015. Three Gorges dam: impact of water level changes on the density of schistosome-transmitting snail *Oncomelania hupensis* in Dongting lake area, China. PLoS Negl. Trop. Dis. 9, e0003882.
Wu, K., 2005. Mathematical model for the prediction and evaluation of the effects of control measures for schistosomiasis. Chin. J. Parasitol. Parasit. Dis. 23, 408–414.
Wu, X.H., Chen, M.G., Zheng, J., 2005. Surveillance of schistosomiasis in five provinces of China which have reached the national criteria for elimination of the disease. Acta Trop. 96, 289–293.
Wu, Z.L., Zhang, W.C., Tan, G.T., 1995. Application of catalytic model in sero-epidemiology of schistosomiasis. Chin. J. Epidemiol. 16, 270–273.
Xiao, R., Wang, X.L., Wang, H.L., 2009. The application of remote sensing and geographic information system technology on the study of snail distribution in Honghu wetland. Wetl. Sci. 7, 175–180.
Xiu, L.C., Zhang, Q., Yin, Z.C., Gu, X.G., 2008. Estimation of the true prevalence of schistosomiasis japonica. Mod. Prev. Med. 35, 1216–1218.
Xu, B., Gong, P., Biging, G., Liang, S., Seto, E., Spear, R., 2004. Snail density prediction for schistosomiasis control using Ikonos and ASTER images. Photogrammetric Eng. Remote Sens. 70, 1285–1294.
Xu, B., Gong, P., Seto, E., Liang, S., Yang, C.H., Wen, S., et al., 2006. A spatial-temporal model for assessing the effects of intervillage connectivity in schistosomiasis transmission. Ann. Assoc. Am. Geogr. 96, 31–46.
Xu, J., et al., 2016a. Historical progress of the national schistosomiasis control programme in China. Adv. Parasitol. 92.

Xu, J., Steinman, P., Maybe, D., Zhou, X.N., Lv, S., Li, S.Z., et al., 2016b. Evolution of the national schistosomiasis control programmes in the People's Republic of China. Adv. Parasitol. 92.

Xu, J.F., Xu, J., Li, S.Z., Jia, T.W., Huang, X.B., Zhang, H.M., et al., 2013. Transmission risks of schistosomiasis japonica: extraction from back-propagation artificial neural network and logistic regression model. PLoS Negl. Trop. Dis. 7, e2123.

Xu, J.F., Lv, S., Wang, Q.Y., Qian, M.B., Liu, Q., Bergquist, R., et al., 2015. Schistosomiasis japonica: modelling as a tool to explore transmission patterns. Acta Trop. 141, 213–222.

Xu, X., Zhang, Y., Lin, D., Zhang, J., Xu, J., Liu, Y.M., et al., 2014. Serodiagnosis of *Schistosoma japonicum* infection: genome-wide identification of a protein marker, and assessment of its diagnostic validity in a field study in China. Lancet Infect. Dis. 14, 489–497.

Xu, X.J., Yang, X.X., Dai, Y.H., Yu, G.Y., Chen, L.Y., Su, Z.M., 1999. Impact of environmental change and schistosomiasis transmission in the middle reaches of the Yangtze river following the three Gorges construction project. Southeast Asian J. Trop. Med. Public Health 30, 549–555.

Yang, G.J., Vounatsou, P., Zhou, X.N., Tanner, M., Utzinger, J., 2005a. A Bayesian-based approach for spatio-temporal modeling of county level prevalence of *Schistosoma japonicum* infection in Jiangsu province, China. Int. J. Parasitol. 35, 155–162.

Yang, G.J., Vounatsou, P., Zhou, X.N., Tanner, M., Utzinger, J., 2005b. A potential impact of climate change and water resource development on the transmission of *Schistosoma japonicum* in China. Parassitologia 47, 127–134.

Yang, G.J., Vounatsou, P., Zhou, X.N., Utzinger, J., Tanner, M., 2005c. A review of geographic information system and remote sensing with applications to the epidemiology and control of schistosomiasis in China. Acta Trop. 96, 117–129.

Yang, G.J., Vounatsou, P., Tanner, M., Zhou, X.N., Utzinger, J., 2006. Remote sensing for predicting potential habitats of *Oncomelania hupensis* in Hongze, Baima and Gaoyou lakes in Jiangsu province, China. Geospat. Health 1, 85–92.

Yang, G.J., Zhou, X.N., Sun, L.P., Wu, F., Zhong, B., Qiu, D.C., et al., 2011. Compensatory density feedback of *Oncomelania hupensis* populations in two different environmental settings in China. Parasit. Vectors 4, 133.

Yang, G.J., Sun, L.P., Hong, Q.B., Zhu, H.R., Yang, K., Gao, Q., et al., 2012a. Optimizing molluscicide treatment strategies in different control stages of schistosomiasis in the People's Republic of China. Parasit. Vectors 5, 260.

Yang, G.J., Tanner, M., Utzinger, J., Malone, J.B., Bergquist, R., Chan, E.Y., et al., 2012b. Malaria surveillance-response strategies in different transmission zones of the People's Republic of China: preparing for climate change. Malar. J. 11, 426.

Yang, H.M., Peng, H., Hu, H.B., Xie, Z.Y., Qiu, L., Huang, J.Z., et al., 2000. Prediction of snail habitats in the marshland along the Yangtze river affected by flood in 1998 by remote sensing. Chin. J. Schisto. Control 12, 337–339.

Yang, K., Wang, X.H., Yang, G.J., Wu, X.H., Qi, Y.L., Li, H.J., et al., 2008. An integrated approach to identify distribution of *Oncomelania hupensis*, the intermediate host of *Schistosoma japonicum*, in a mountainous region in China. Int. J. Parasitol. 38, 1007–1016.

Yang, K., 2009. Integrated control strategies of schistosomiasis transmission informed by Bayesian multilevel model at a local scale. Am. J. Trop. Med. Hyg. 81, 203.

Yang, K., Zhou, X.N., Wu, X.H., Steinmann, P., Wang, X.H., Yang, G.J., et al., 2009. Landscape pattern analysis and Bayesian modeling for predicting *Oncomelania hupensis* distribution in Eryuan County, People's Republic of China. Am. J. Trop. Med. Hyg. 81, 416–423.

Yang, K., Sun, L.P., Huang, Y.X., Yang, G.J., Wu, F., Hang, D.R., et al., 2012c. A real-time platform for monitoring schistosomiasis transmission supported by Google Earth and a web-based geographical information system. Geospat. Health 6, 195–203.

Yang, K., Zhou, X.-N., Jia, T.-W., Yang, G.-J., Wu, X.-H., Shi, X.-W., et al., 2015. Eco-social determinants of *Schistosoma japonicum* infection supported by multi-level modelling in Eryuan county, People's Republic of China. Acta Trop. 141, 391–398.

Yang, K., 2016a. Epidemiological features and control effectiveness of schistosomiasis in water-network region in China. Adv. Parasitol. 92.

Yang, K., 2016b. Research and application of spatial technology in schistosomiasis control in China. Adv. Parasitol. 92.

Yang, S.Q., Gao, Y.H., Mei, Y., Tang, Y.H., Chen, Z.J., Wu, C.G., 2010. Detecting potential survival regions of *Oncomelania* based on GIS and RS technique in Chongqing segment of the Three-Gorges reservoir. Resour. Environ. Yangtze Basin 19, 1290–1293.

Yang, Y., Zhou, Y.B., Song, X.X., Li, S.Z., Zhong, B., Wang, T.P., et al., 2016. Integrated control strategy of schistosomiasis in China: projects involving agriculture, water-conservancy, forestry, sanitation and environmental modification. Adv. Parasitol. 92.

Yao, B.D., Wang, Z.L., Zhang, Z.J., Tian, A.P., Zhu, S.P., Hu, B.J., et al., 2012. Application of multitemporal China-Brazil Earth Recourses Satellite-02 data on surveillance of dynamic changes of water body of rivers and *Oncomelania* snail habitats in Anxiang County. Chin. J. Schisto. Control 24, 160–167.

Yu, J.M., Yuan, H.C., Chen, Q.M., Yang, Q.J., 1997. Application of schistosomiasis transmission module in lake and marshland areas. Chin. Public Health 722–724.

Yu, J.M., Yuan, C.H., Chen, Q.M., Yang, Q.J., 1999. Establishment of a stochastic model for variation in fecal *Schistosoma japonicum* egg count and estimation of its parameters. Chin. J. Prev. Med. 33, 38–40.

Yu, J.M., Yuan, H.C., Chen, Q.M., Yang, Q.J., Jiang, Q.W., Vlas, S., et al., 2000. A mathematical model for variations in *Schistosoma japonicum* egg count and application. Chin. J. Dis. Control Prev. 294–298.

Yuan, Y., Zhao, A., Huang, C.Q., 2014. An improved RS/GIS method to obtain snail habitats in the Poyang lake region. J. Jiangxi Norm. Univ. 38, 212–216.

Zhai, Z.G., 2012. Review of the methods and application of infectious disease surveillance response. Chin. Med. Mod. Distance Educ. China 10, 159–162.

Zhang, B., Zhang, Z.Y., Xu, D.Z., Sun, Z.D., Zhou, X.N., Gong, Z.L., et al., 2003a. Study on the relationship between Terra-MODIS image and the snail distribution in marshland of Jiangning county, Jiangsu province. Chin. J. Epidemiol. 24, 257–261.

Zhang, J.F., Xu, J., Bergquist, R., Yu, L.L., Yan, X.L., Zhu, H.Q., et al., 2016a. Development and application of diagnostics in the national schistosomiasis control programme in the People's Republic of China. Adv. Parasitol. 92.

Zhang, J.Q., Gong, J.H., Huang, M.X., Lin, W.P., 2008a. Application of remote sensing image based on knowledge decision tree classification in identifying the habitat of *Oncomelania* snails in Poyang lake region. Chin. J. Schisto. Control 20, 70–74.

Zhang, L.J., Li, S.Z., Wen, L.Y., Lin, D.D., Abe, E.M., Zhu, R., et al., 2016b. Establishment and function of schistosomiasis surveillance system towards elimination in the People's Republic of China. Adv. Parasitol. 92.

Zhang, S., Zhang, Q., Yin, Z.C., 2007. The application of Grey model (1,1) in the prediction of schistosomiasis infection rate. Mod. Prev. Med. 34, 1291–1293.

Zhang, S.J., 2016. Epidemiological features and control effectiveness of schistosomiasis in lake and marshland region in China. Adv. Parasitol. 92.

Zhang, S.Q., Jiang, Q.W., Wang, T.P., Zhao, G.M., Ge, J.H., 2003b. Ecological surveillance on breeding ground for *Oncomelania hupensis* snails in the areas prevalent with islet-type schistosomiasis using remote sensing technology. Chin. J. Prev. Med. 37, 331–334.

Zhang, S.Q., Sun, C.S., Wang, M., Lin, D.D., Zhou, X.N., Wang, T.P., 2016c. Epidemiological features and control effectiveness of schistosomiasis in lake and marshland region in the People's Republic of China. Adv. Parasitol. 92.

Zhang, X.G., Zhang, T., Young, A.A., Li, X.S., 2014. Applications and comparisons of four time series models in epidemiological surveillance data. PLoS One 9, 1–16.
Zhang, Y.Y., Luo, J.P., Liu, Y.M., Wang, Q.Z., Chen, J.H., Xu, M.X., et al., 2009. Evaluation of Kato-Katz examination method in three areas with low-level endemicity of schistosomiasis japonica in China: a Bayesian modeling approach. Acta Trop. 112, 16–22.
Zhang, Z.J., Ong, S.H., Lynn, H.S., Peng, W.X., Zhou, Y.B., Zhao, G.M., et al., 2008b. Generalized negative binomial distribution: a promising statistical distribution for *Oncomelania hupensis* in the lake- and marsh-land regions of China. Ann. Trop. Med. Parasitol. 102, 541–552.
Zhang, Z.J., Zhu, R., Ward, M.P., Xu, W.H., Zhang, L.J., Guo, J.G., et al., 2012. Long-term impact of the world bank loan project for schistosomiasis control: a comparison of the spatial distribution of schistosomiasis risk in China. PLoS Negl. Trop. Dis. 6.
Zhang, Z.J., Bergquist, R., Chen, D.M., Yao, B.D., Wang, Z.L., Gao, J., et al., 2013. Identification of parasite-host habitats in Anxiang county, Hunan province, China based on multi-temporal China-Brazil earth resources satellite (CBERS) images. PLoS One 8.
Zhang, Z.Y., Xu, D.Z., Zhou, X.N., Zhou, Y., Sun, Z.D., Zhang, B., et al., 2003c. Application of satellite image for surveillance of vegetation landscapes of *Oncomelania*-snail habitats in marshland using unsupervised classification. Chin. J. Epidemiol. 23, 261–264.
Zhang, Z.Y., Xu, D.Z., Zhou, X.N., Zhou, Y., Sun, Z.D., Zhang, B., et al., 2003d. Application of Landsat ETM+ images in the surveillance of marshland habitat of *Oncomelania* snails in Jiangning county. J. Fourth Mil. Med. Univ. 24, 139–142.
Zhang, Z.Y., Sun, Z.D., Xu, D.Z., Zhou, Y., Liu, S.J., Gong, Z.L., 2004a. Relationship between distribution of snails and location of water pools in Jiangning county using geographic information system. Chin. J. End. 23, 157–159.
Zhang, Z.Y., Xu, D.Z., Peng, H., Zhou, Y., Zhang, B., Liu, S.J., et al., 2004b. Prediction of the spatial distribution of *Oncomelania* snails in marshland of Jiangning county using the Ordinary Kriging. Chin. J. Parasitol. Parasit. Dis. 22, 170–172.
Zhang, Z.Y., Xu, D.Z., Zhou, X.N., Zhou, Y., Liu, S.J., 2005. Remote sensing and spatial statistical analysis to predict the distribution of *Oncomelania hupensis* in the marshlands of China. Acta Trop. 96, 205–212.
Zhao, A., Gong, P., Bao, S.M., 2009. A readapted Malone schistosome transmission index model. Acta Trop. 109, 98–102.
Zheng, Q., Vanderslott, S., Jiang, B., Xu, L.L., Liu, C.S., Huo, L.L., et al., 2013. Research gaps for three main tropical diseases in the People's Republic of China. Infect. Dis. Poverty 2, 15.
Zhou, L.L., Yu, L.J., Wang, Y., Lu, Z.P., Tian, L.H., Tan, L., et al., 2014. A hybrid model for predicting the prevalence of schistosomiasis in humans of Qianjiang city, China. PLoS One 9.
Zhou, X.N., Hong, Q.B., Sun, L.P., Hu, X.S., Sun, N.S., Fuetes, M., et al., 1998. Application of geographic information systems on schistosomiasis surveillance. I. Application possibility of prediction model. Chin. J. Schisto. Control 10, 321–324.
Zhou, X.N., Hu, X.S., Sun, N.S., Hong, Q.B., Sun, L.P., Lu, G.N., et al., 1999a. Application of geographical information systems on schistosomiasis surveillance II. Predicting transmission intensity. Chin. J. Schisto. Control 11, 66–70.
Zhou, X.N., Kristensen, T.K., Hong, Q.B., Sun, L.P., Fuentes, M., Malone, J.B., 1999b. Analysis for spatial distribution of *Oncomelania* snail in mainland China by geographic information system (GIS) database. Chin. J. Prev. Med. 23, 343–346.
Zhou, X.N., Sun, N.S., Hu, X.S., Sun, L.P., Hong, Q.B., Fuentes, M., et al., 1999c. Application of geographic information systems on schistosomiasis surveillance III. Snail habitats in marshland. Chin. J. Schisto. Control 11, 199–202.

Zhou, X.N., Wang, T.P., Wang, L.Y., Guo, J.G., Yu, Q., Xu, J., et al., 2004. The current status of schistosomiasis epidemics in China. Chin. J. Epidemiol. 25, 555–558.
Zhou, X.N., Wang, L.Y., Chen, M.G., Wu, X.H., Jiang, Q.W., Chen, X.Y., et al., 2005. The public health significance and control of schistosomiasis in China–then and now. Acta Trop. 96, 97–105.
Zhou, X.N., Yang, G.J., Yang, K., Wang, X.H., Hong, Q.B., Sun, L.P., et al., 2008. Potential impact of climate change on schistosomiasis transmission in China. Am. J. Trop. Med. Hyg. 78, 188–194.
Zhou, X.N., Bergquist, R., Leonardo, L., Yang, G.J., Yang, K., Sudomo, M., et al., 2010. Schistosomiasis japonica control and research needs. Adv. Parasitol. 72, 145–178.
Zhou, X.N., Xu, J., Chen, H.G., Wang, T.P., Huang, X.B., Lin, D.D., et al., 2011. Tools to support policy decisions related to treatment strategies and surveillance of schistosomiasis japonica towards elimination. PLoS Negl. Trop. Dis. 5, e1408.
Zhou, X.N., Jiang, Q.W., Guo, J.G., Lin, D.D., Zhu, R., Yang, G.J., et al., 2012. Road map for transmission interruption of schistosomiasis in China. Chin. J. Schisto. Control 24, 1–4.
Zhou, X.N., Bergquist, R., Tanner, M., 2013a. Elimination of tropical disease through surveillance and response. Infect. Dis. Poverty 2.
Zhou, X.N., Xu, J., Lin, D.D., Wang, T.P., Liang, Y.S., Zhong, B., et al., 2013b. Role of the new version of the control and elimination criteria for schistosomiasis in acceleration of the schistosomiasis elimination program in China. Zhongguo Xue Xi Chong Bing Fang. Zhi Za Zhi Chin. J. Schisto. Control. 25, 1–4 (in Chinese).
Zhu, H.M., Xiang, S., Yang, K., Wu, X.H., Zhou, X.N., 2008. Three Gorges dam and its impact on the potential transmission of schistosomiasis in regions along the Yangtze river. Ecohealth 5, 137–148.
Zhu, H.R., Liu, L., Zhou, X.N., Yang, G.J., 2015. Ecological model to predict potential habitats of *Oncomelania hupensis*, the intermediate host of *Schistosoma japonicum* in the mountainous regions, China. PLoS Negl. Trop. Dis. 9, e0004028.

CHAPTER EIGHT

Biology and Control of Snail Intermediate Host of *Schistosoma japonicum* in The People's Republic of China

Z.-J. Li*, J. Ge*, J.-R. Dai[§], L.-Y. Wen[¶,**], D.-D. Lin*, H. Madsen[||], X.-N. Zhou[#,§§,¶¶], S. Lv[#,§§,¶¶,1]

*Jiangxi Provincial Institute of Schistosomiasis Control, Nanchang, The People's Republic of China
[§]Jiangsu Institute of Parasitic Diseases, Wuxi, Jiangsu, The People's Republic of China
[¶]Zhejiang Academy of Medical Science, Hangzhou, Zhejiang, The People's Republic of China
[||]University of Copenhagen, Copenhagen, Denmark
[#]National Institute of Parasitic Diseases, Chinese Center for Disease Control and Prevention, Shanghai, The People's Republic of China
**Institute of Parasitic Diseases, Zhejiang Academy of Medical Sciences, Hangzhou, The People's Republic of China
[§§]WHO Collaborating Center for Tropical Diseases, Shanghai, The People's Republic of China
[¶¶]Key Laboratory of Parasite and Vector Biology of the Chinese Ministry of Health, Shanghai, The People's Republic of China
[1]Corresponding author: E-mail: lvshan000@126.com

Contents

Advances in Parasitology, Volume 92
ISSN 0065-308X
http://dx.doi.org/10.1016/bs.apar.2016.02.003

Abstract

Schistosomiasis caused by *Schistosoma japonicum* is a severe parasitic disease in The People's Republic of China and imposed considerable burden on human and domestic animal health and socioeconomic development. The significant achievement in schistosomiasis control has been made in last 60 years. *Oncomelania hupensis* as the only intermediate host of *S. japonicum* plays a key role in disease transmission. The habitat complexity of the snails challenges to effective control. In this review we share the experiences in control and research of *O. hupensis*.

1. INTRODUCTION

Schistosomiasis is a severe parasitic disease that imposes considerable burden on human and domestic animal health and socioeconomic development (Chen, 2014; Gryseels et al., 2006). Of the six *Schistosoma* species known to infect humans, namely *Schistosoma japonicum*, *Schistosoma mansoni*, *Schistosoma haematobium*, *Schistosoma intercalatum*, *Schistosoma mekongi* and *Schistosoma malayensis*, the former three are of primary importance. The feature and geographical distribution of intermediate snail host exhibits differences in line with different species of schistosomes (Mao, 1990; Zhou, 2005). *Oncomelania hupensis* is the only intermediate host of *S. japonicum*, distributed in The People's Republic of China, Japan, the Philippines and Indonesia (Attwood et al., 2015).

The geographical distribution of *O. hupensis* in The People's Republic of China coincides with the endemic areas of schistosomiasis in 12 southern provinces (municipalities, autonomous regions). A great achievement in schistosomiasis control has been made after national control programmes were implemented since mid-1950s (Collins et al., 2012; Xu et al., 2016). Snail control has played a key role in the achievements. According to national statistics, the total area of snail habitats in The People's Republic of China has decreased by 74.48%, from 14,321 km^2 in 1956 to 3654.68 km^2 in 2013. In this paper, we review the current status of *O. hupensis* research and control in The People's Republic of China.

2. BIOLOGY OF *ONCOMELANIA* SNAILS

2.1 Taxonomy

Oncomelania hupensis (Gredler, 1881) was first discovered in Hubei Province, The People's Republic of China in 1981 and not considered as the intermediate host of *S. japonicum* until 1913. The taxonomy of *O. hupensis* has been a subject of debate due to its wide distribution, complex habitat environment and variable morphological characters (Kang et al., 1958; Mao and Li, 1954). *Oncomelania hupensis* was usually classified into eight subspecies (Zhou, 2005) (Table 1). However, this classification was questioned by some authors. For example, subspecies *O. h. quadrasi* and *O. h. lindoensis* were considered as the same species (Zhou et al., 2009). A 2014 study showed that geographical distance contributes more to genetic divergence than environmental isolation, and among all variables that were

Table 1 Geographical distribution of *Oncomelania* spp. in the World.

Subspecies	Distribution region
Oncomelania (Gredler, 1881)	
O. minima (Bartsch, 1936)	Japan
O. hupensis (Gredler, 1881)	The People's Republic of China
O. h. hupensis (Gredler)	Middle and lower reach of Yangtze River (MLY)
O. h. hupensis fausti strain	Mountains and hills along MLY
O. h. hupensis hupensis strain	Marshlands and lakes along MLY
O. h. tangi (Bartsch)	Southeast coast areas in The People's Republic of China
O. h. hupensis tangi strain	Fujian
O. h. hupensis guangxi strain	Guangxi
O. h. hupensis subei strain	North Jiangsu
O. h. robertsoni (Bartsch)	Southwest China
O. h. hupensis yunnan strain	Yunnan
O. h. hupensis sichuan strain	Sichuan
O. h. formosana (Pilsbry and Hirase, 1905)	Taiwan
O. h. chiui (Habe and Miyazaki, 1962)	Taiwan
O. h. nosophora (Robson, 1915)	Japan
O. h. quadrasi (Mollendorff, 1895)	The Philippines
O. h. lindoensis (Davis and Carney, 1973)	Sulawesi island in Indonesia

analysed, wetland showed the strongest correlation with the genetic pairwise distances, in The People's Republic of China (Liang et al., 2014). *Oncomelania hupensis* distribution is strongly linked to the presence of wetlands, and the distribution pattern of both *O. hupensis* and schistosomiasis might be altered due to the changed wetland resulting from water development projects such as the Three Gorges Dam and the South-to-North water transfer project (Liang et al., 2014; Yang et al., 2016).

Since the 1990s, the numerical taxonomy technique has been applied to morphology of *O. hupensis* from different areas in The People's Republic of China. The studies, however, showed that the classification of *O. hupensis* only based on epigenetic characteristics was unsound, and hence *O. hupensis* in The People's Republic of China can be classified into three geographical strains at genetic level, namely the Hunan, Hubei and Anhui/Jiangxi strains (Zhou, 2005). Furthermore, there was a geographical strain in Sichuan and Yunnan and another in Fujian and Taiwan (Zhou, 2005).

New progress of *Oncomelania* classification has been made with the development and application of molecular biology. SSR-PCR technique was used to analyse 19 populations of *O. hupensis* from eight provinces in mainland The People's Republic of China and found that the average genetic distance of population was 0.22 (Zhou et al., 2007). The study divided those specimens into four groups by applying cluster analysis; 16 populations along the middle-lower Yangzi River basin in five provinces (ie, Hunan, Hubei, Jiangxi, Anhui and Jiangsu) constituted one group and the remaining three groups were from Guangxi, Fujian and Yunnan, respectively. Therefore, *O. hupensis* in mainland The People's Republic of China probably can be accordingly divided into four subspecies, that is, *O. h. hupensis, O. h. robertsoni, O. h. tangi* and *O. h. formosana*. In addition, landscape genetic analysis based on ITS1, ITS2 and 16s genes also indicated four groups that located in four different landscapes, namely the middle and lower reach of Yangtze River, the mountainous areas of Yunnan and Sichuan, the inland hill areas of Guangxi and the inshore hill areas of Fujian (Li et al., 2009).

2.2 Susceptibility to different geographical strains of *S. japonicum*

The susceptibility of *O. hupensis* to schistosomes from different endemic areas and even different habitats within the same area may be variable considerably (Hong et al., 1995; Lin et al., 1994). When exposed to a strain of *S. japonicum*, the infection rate of local snails is much higher than that of snails from other areas. For example, the infection rate of snail from Guichi,

Anhui Province was 84% when infected with local strain, while it was only 32% and 28% for snails from Bixian, Sichuan Province and Dali, Yunnan Province, respectively, when exposed to the same strain (Huang et al., 2002; Xu and Ni, 1987). Resistance to nonlocal strains of schistosomes was also observed (Cao et al., 2009). *Oncomelania hupensis* from marshland areas was found highly susceptible to schistosome strains from hilly areas, while *O. hupensis* from hilly areas showed the low susceptibility even when exposed to local strains of schistosome (Wang et al., 2014) (Table 2).

Interestingly, infectivity of miracidia hatched from eggs isolated from various hosts may be variable. In a study where *O. hupensis* was exposed to miracidia obtained from rabbit, buffalo and mouse, the infection rates were 1.42%, 8.67% and 19.87%, respectively (Tian et al., 2011). There was a significant difference between invisibility of miracidiae; *O. hupensis* was more susceptible to miracidia from mice.

2.3 Factors influencing infection

Experiments indicated that the number of miracidia, distance from the release point, temperature, frequency, time, sex and age of snail may influence infection. The infection rate of snails increase with the number of miracidia in a proper range; excess exposure leads to mortality of snails (He et al., 1989, 1994; Xu et al., 1993).

The infection rate of snails is inversely proportional to the distance from the release point of miracidia, the volume and depth of water (He et al., 1989; Jiang et al., 1989; Wang et al., 2011). The optimum temperature for infection is 10–20°C; the infection rate of snails declined greatly below 10°C and above 20°C (Sun et al., 2004; Yang et al., 2007). In another study where snails were exposed to miracidia of various release time, the infection rate was highest for miracidia 1–4 h post release, while infection rates of snails exposed to miracidia 8 or 12 h post-release were lower (He et al., 1994).

Table 2 Compatibility between *Oncomelania hupensis* and *Schistosoma japonicum*

Strains of *S. japonicum*	Infection rate of snails (No. snails shedding cercariae/No. snails survived)					
	Anhui	**Hubei**	**Guangxi**	**Sichuan**	**Yunnan**	**Fujian**
Anhui	42.9(249/580)	43.8(56/128)	20.0(36/180)	1.5(4/270)	0(0/173)	25.0(1/4)
Hubei	40.9(110/269)	33.1(47/142)	–	0(0/126)	0(0/71)	–
Guangxi	30.7(59/192)	–	9.4(12/128)	0(0/67)	0(0/12)	0(0/66)
Sichuan	4.5(40/881)	10.2(25/244)	–	1.4(5/360)	0.4(1/229)	–
Yunnan	10.8(43/397)	33.6(46/137)	14.9(7/47)	1.0(2/198)	8.3(8/96)	4.0(1/25)

He et al., 1990.

Female snails aged between 3 and 4 months are more susceptible to infection than male snails of the same age (He et al., 1994). However, the male and female snails above 5 months showed the similar susceptibility and duration of cercariae release. Susceptibility of adult snails was higher than that of immature snails (He et al., 1994).

2.4 Factors influencing release of cercariae from snails

Many factors may influence the development and release of cercariae from infected snails, of which temperature is the most notable (Mao, 1990). According to the degree-day model, the accumulative temperature for development of cercariae in snail is 1793.93 ± 232.45 degree-days (Sun et al., 2001). The temperature range 20–35°C is optimal for cercariae release, but 13% of infected snails still can release cercariae at the water temperature of 1°C, which implies that people can become infected during winter months. In addition, pH of the water may influence cercariae release; pH in the range 6.6–7.8 seems optimal for cercariae release (Liang et al., 2004). The lifetime of cercariae is not affected by pH in the range 4.6–9.8 (Liang et al., 2004).

Cercariae release is closely related to light. A circadian rhythm can be observed; the release of cercariae from infected snails mainly occurs in day time (Mao, 1990). Observation of cercariae release from naturally infected snails showed that the peak time is at 7–10 am in marshland areas where cattle were the main infection source, and at 5–9 pm in hilly areas where field rats were the main infection source (Lu et al., 2009; Su et al., 2013).

3. DISTRIBUTION AND SURVEY OF *O. HUPENSIS* IN THE PEOPLE'S REPUBLIC OF CHINA

3.1 Distribution characteristics

Oncomelania hupensis is distributed in 12 southern provinces with an accumulated snail infested area of 14.32 billion m^2 (Fig. 1). The range meets an annual average temperature of over 14°C and an annual average precipitation of over 750mm, which indicates that mild climate and abundant rainfall are necessary for snail (Zhou, 2005). The geographical distribution of *O. hupensis* is consistent with that of schistosomiasis endemic areas in The People's Republic of China (Liu et al., 2016; Shi et al., 2016; Wang et al., 2016). It is possible that potential snail habitats can extend further

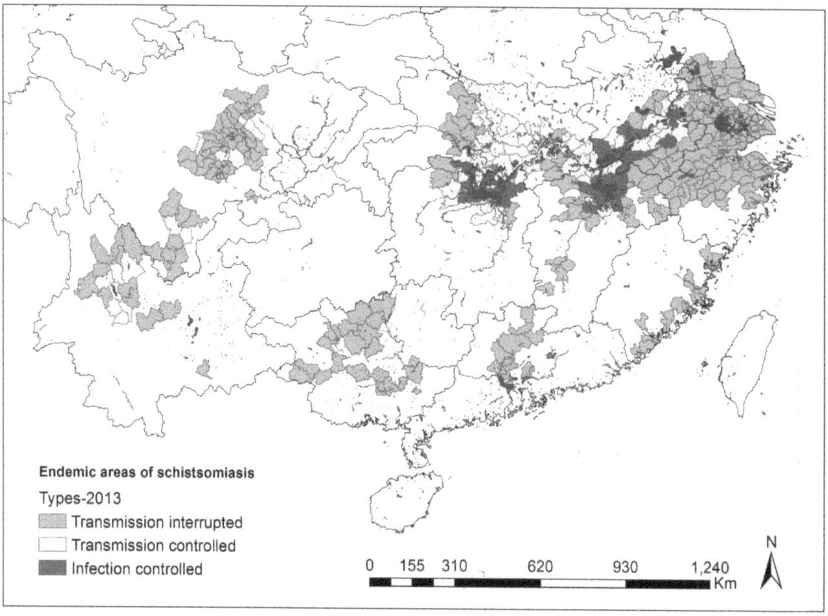

Figure 1 Distribution map of *Oncomelania hupensis* and schistosomiasis in The People's Republic of China, 2013.

to the north in the context of global warming and hence cause the expansion of endemic areas of schistosomiasis (Zhou et al., 2004).

Based on geomorphological features, the snail habitats are classified into three types, namely, marshland and lake area, mountain and hill area and plain water network area (Mao, 1990). These types of snail habitats can be commonly observed in a single county (Mao, 1990).

3.1.1 Marshland and lake areas

A large number of marshlands are formed on both sides of the middle-to-lower reaches of the Yangtze River and around the large lakes connected to the river, which are mainly located in four provinces, namely, Hunan, Hubei, Jiangxi and Anhui (Zhang et al., 2016b). Currently, *O. hupensis* is mainly distributed in these areas, accounting for 96.49% in the whole country (Table 3) (Lei et al., 2014). Marshland is characterized by a large seasonal fluctuation of water level and hence is flooded during summer and re-emerges during winter. Mild climate, abundant rainfall, fertile and humid soil and overgrown grassy vegetation contribute to favourable conditions for snail breeding (Mao, 1990). Snails in these areas generally grow larger than those in mountainous and hilly areas as well as the plain water

Table 3 Snail habitats area and mollusciciding area in The People's Republic of China, 2013

Province	No. township with snails	No. village with snails	Total area (hm^2)	Marshland endemic area (hm^2)		Plain water network endemic area(hm^2)	Mountain and hill endemic area (hm^2)
				Inside embankment	Outside embankment		
Shanghai	8	17	0.93	0.00	0.00	0.93	0.00
Jiangsu	69	190	3293.74	0.00	3056.57	202.97	34.20
Zhejiang	98	369	94.21	0.00	0.00	12.48	81.73
Anhui	211	962	27,396.49	0.00	24,480.08	0.00	2916.41
Fujian	9	14	1.51	0.00	0.00	0.00	1.51
Jiangxi	140	601	78,794.33	3.87	76,952.04	0.00	1838.42
Hubei	352	2604	76,485.70	19,231.60	54,818.65	0.00	2435.45
Hunan	199	922	175,116.23	854.50	173,230.07	0.00	1031.65
Guangdong	0	0	0.00	0.00	0.00	0.00	0.00
Guangxi	5	5	4.96	0.00	0.00	0.00	4.96
Sichuan	361	1850	2600.39	0.00	0.00	0.00	2600.39
Yunnan	56	248	1679.51	0.00	0.00	0.00	1679.51
Total	1508	7782	365,468.00	20,089.98	332,537.41	216.38	12,624.23

network areas, usually over 7.5 mm in height and 3.2 mm in width, with thick and ribbed shell.

Depending on the water level control system, marshlands and lake areas can be classified into four subtypes, namely, 'island', 'marsh', 'embankment' (area from dike towards the marsh/lake) and 'inside embankment' (area protected from flooding by the dike) (Chen, 1980). The distribution of snails exhibit high spatial heterogeneity in these vast marshlands. Two distribution features of snails can be observed, that is, 'two lines' (the highest and lowest elevation lines where snails can be found), thus defining 'three zones' (upper and lower zones with few snails, middle zone with high density) (Li et al., 2006b; Zhou, 2005).

The distribution of snails in marshland is related to micro-ecological factors, such as submerging time in flooding season, groundwater level, soil moisture, vegetation and light intensity (Cao et al., 2015). Prolonged submerging, high groundwater level and moist soil lead to increase in the snail density. Of these factors, the groundwater level had the dominant effect on the snail intensity (Wang et al., 2007). A study revealed that snail density and the percent of frames with snail was highest when the groundwater level was around 32 cm, and soil moisture content of 28–38% was optimal for snail breeding (Zhang et al., 1999). Water-level fluctuation can affect the macro- and micro-environment of snail habitats as well as snail's life activity and distribution status, which in turn, affect schistosomiasis transmission (Li et al., 2010a; Ma et al., 2011). Snails are few in low-elevation marshlands that are submerged over 8 months, or high-elevation marshlands that are submerged less than 3 months. Snail habitat is often characterized by the dominant plant species, such as *Cyperus rotundus*, *Carex tristachya* and *Phragmites communis*.

More than 93% of infected snails in marshland are found in irrigation ditches or marshes within 500 m from residential areas. Density of infected snail shows negative correlation with distance to residential areas (Su et al., 2011). Owing to frequent activities of humans and livestock in snail-occupied ditches and marshlands near the residential areas, the snail habitats were contaminated with faeces, and this led to schistosomiasis transmission (Peng et al., 2007). Although the density of snails in large ditches (width 1–3 m) might be lower than in small ditches (width < 1 m), the prevalence of schistosome in snails in big ditches could be higher than small ones (Guan et al., 1999). It was explained that more frequent activities of humans and livestock occurred around or in the big ditches than in the small ones. In a different location, however, the density of infected snails was not positively correlated with the density of snail, but was related with frequency water contact activity (Wei et al., 2001). In another similar environment, there was the positive correlation between the mean density of snails and the prevalence of infection in snails (Wei et al., 2001).

3.1.2 Mountain and hill areas

This kind of snail habitat can be found in all endemic provinces except Shanghai, but it only accounted for 3.45% in the whole country (Lei et al., 2014; Liu et al., 2016) (Table 3). Complex landscapes due to diverse elevation lead to many small fragments of snail habitat (Mao, 1990). In hill area, the distribution of snails is restrained in specific zones and is strikingly variable. For example, snails can be found at one side of a mountain while none at the other side (Qiu et al., 2014). In the same water system, snails can live both in ditches and farmlands along the entire length of water courses (Qiu et al., 2014). In mountain area, snails usually live in the undergrowth with patchy distribution or along water course with linear distribution. Some snails can inhabit the mountain side and foot. A few snails can survive in spring water on the top of mountain and form the source of the snail distribution (Mao, 1990). In the basins in mountain area, *O. hupensis* is distributed mainly in ditches and farmlands, similar to plain network areas (Mao, 1990).

Less rainfall and lower temperature in mountain and hill areas are the factors affecting the development and breeding of snail, resulting in the snail's smaller size in these areas than in marshland and plain areas with the height of 5.8–6.9 mm and width under 2.85 mm (Zhou, 2005; Zhou et al., 2006). The snail shell is smooth without ribs or with only thin rib lines (Zhou, 2005; Zhou et al., 2006).

In the mountain and hill areas, the highest density of snails is found along river banks, followed by irrigation ditches, farmlands and wild grass ground, where it is the lowest (Xu et al., 2010; Zhang et al., 2007b). The sand content and humidity in soil are the most important factors determining snail presence and survival (Xu et al., 2010; Zhang et al., 2007b). Infected snails are mainly found in ditches, followed by river shore land, pond and river course successively (Xu et al., 2010; Zhang et al., 2007b).

3.1.3 Plain water network area

Plain water network area is mainly located in the Yangtze River delta, covering Shanghai and the part of Jiangsu and Zhejiang provinces (Shi et al., 2016). In this area water courses are well developed and form network with slow water currency, stable water level, weeds in the shore. By the end of 2013, plain water network area with snail only accounted for 0.06% of the national total area (Lei et al., 2014). The snail is medium sized with a height of 6.5–7.5 mm and transverse ribs. *Oncomelania* snails are often distributed along irrigation canals and the density varies among locations (Wang, 2006a). Ponds connected to river or canals, dikes of ridge field, bridge pillars, gap between stone or bricks can be also occupied by *Oncomelania* snails (Mao, 1990).

3.2 Methods for survey of *O. hupensis*

The purpose of snail survey is to obtain information of snail distribution and density as well as characteristics of habitats, and hence help to develop snail control plan, choose control methods and evaluate control effect (Mao, 1990). The targeted areas normally include known snail habitats where snail occurs at present or historically, suspected environments adjoining known snail habitats and potential environments which facilitate the spread of snails. The timing and frequency of survey is determined according to the habitat characteristics and the aim of the survey. Four methods can be selected, namely (1) systematic sampling, (2) environmental sampling, (3) systematic sampling combined with environmental sampling method and (4) thorough investigation (Mao, 1990; Zhou, 2005) (Table 4). Snail sampling is performed using a square frame of 0.1 m^2 and all snails within the frame are collected manually. In systematic sampling, the frames are laid out at an interval of 10–20 m along a line. In the survey area one or several parallel lines should be set at an interval of 10–50 m. The interval between frames or lines can be adjusted according to the size of the area surveyed. In environmental sampling, the frames are placed in locations that are most likely to harbour snails. In a thorough sampling, the frames are not used but the entire area is subjected to a careful visual inspection for snails.

3.3 Snail monitoring

In areas where schistosomiasis transmission has been interrupted, it is necessary to monitor the *Oncomelania* snails in existing and historical snail habitats and to prevent snail spread and consolidate achievements of schistosomiasis control (Dang et al., 2014; Wen et al., 2011). In the existing snail habitats, snail survey is conducted in spring or autumn every year. In the historical snail habitat where snail re-emerged within the last 3 years, one snail survey should be carried out during spring and double surveys should be carried out in important environments (eg, close to village). Thorough snail survey is

Table 4 Methods of snail survey in different habitat types

Type of snail habitat	Method of survey	Applicable environment	Timing of survey
Marshland and lake area	Systematic sampling	High snail density and scattered distribution	Mar., Apr., May or Sep., Oct., Nov.
	Environmental sampling	Historical snail habitat where snail cannot be found by systemic sampling method.	Mar., Apr., May or Sep., Oct., Nov.
	Thorough survey	Snail has been eliminated recently and small area with complex environment where the systematic sampling method is difficult to use.	Mar., Apr., May or Sep., Oct., Nov.
Plain water network area	Systematic sampling	River, ditches, pond	Apr. to Oct.
	Environmental sampling	Historical snail habitat where snail cannot be found by systemic sampling method	Apr. to Oct.
	Thorough survey	Suspected habitat to be confirmed, or areas where snails were eliminated and small area with complex environment where the systematic sampling method is difficult to use.	Apr. to Oct.
Mountain and hill area	Systematic sampling	River, ditch, pond	Apr. to Oct.
	Environmental sampling	Special environment such as hill land, grave mound, bamboo forest	Apr. to Oct.
	Thorough survey	Suspected habitat to be confirmed, or areas where snails were eliminated and small area with complex environment where the systematic sampling method is difficult to use	Apr. to Oct.

performed once every 3 years in the historical habitats where snails have not been found in last 3–9 years, and once every 5 years in those habitats where snails have not been found over 10 years. For areas where snail never was recorded, monitoring site should be established in suspected environment and one or two snail surveys each year for successive 2 years (Chen et al., 2012a; Wang et al., 2013).

3.3.1 Monitoring snails in water bodies

Oncomelania snails are prone to stick to floating matters in water bodies. Therefore, the snails can be collected using floating traps. The traps are usually made of a 0.1 m^2-sized curtain woven by rice straw. Such traps are put into water near the bank of rivers or canals equidistantly for 3 days. The retrieved traps are scrubbed twice by clean water and the *Oncomelania* snails are carefully screened in the filtered water. The method shows simple operation, low labour intensity and better performance than systematic sampling (Cao et al., 1990; Zhang et al., 1989). An experiment using two methods, that is, systematic sampling and attracting snail with rice straw, was conducted along 22 rivers from June to August. The results showed 13.48 snails per 0.1 m^2 (trap of rice straw) while 4.67 snails per 0.1 m^2 (frame in systematic sampling) (Mao, 1990). Furthermore, the former method is more sensitive to young snails; the number of young snails on traps (9.41 snails) is 11.2 times higher than that in frame (0.84 snails) in systematic sampling. The results also indicated that traps collected more snails than did systematic sampling during May–August and October, although the counts were similar in September. This seasonal variation of two methods was mainly affected by variation of movement capability of snail (Cao et al., 1990; Zhang et al., 1989).

3.3.2 Monitoring snails carried by travelling animals, plants and transportation vehicles

In areas where schistosomiasis transmission is interrupted or where nonendemic areas connect endemic area by water courses, potential source of infections (eg, aquatic animals and plants, trees, boats) from schistosomiasis endemic areas should be monitored to avoid the spread of snails (Cao et al., 2016). In 2002, acute schistosomiasis cases were reported in two villages around the marshlands of the Gan river basin in Jiangxi Province where *Oncomelania* snails were never recorded (Zeng et al., 2007). A subsequent survey confirmed the presence of *Oncomelania* snail in the marshlands. Furthermore, 177 fishing boats in this area were investigated. The results showed that all boats carried *Oncomelania* snails with an average number of 13.69 per boat (Zeng et al., 2007). In addition, 90.9% crayfish pots and 75.0% fishing nets in those boats also carried snails (Zeng et al., 2007).

In nonendemic areas connecting snail habitat areas by water courses, floating matters on the river water should be monitored during the flood season or after the withdrawal of water (Zhang et al., 2016a). The method may be net—dredge washing, that is using a net to dredge and collect floating matters including aquatic plants to screen for snails (Yin et al., 1993; Zuo et al., 2010).

3.3.3 Remote sensing technology for snail surveillance

Remote sensing provides a new approach for identifying the potential distribution of *Oncomelania* snails by predicting the suitable habitats (Feng et al., 2016; Zhou et al., 1999). It is widely acknowledged that the flooding time is an important factor for the spread and establishment of *Oncomelania* snail in the lake areas, and species and distribution of vegetation is different due to various flooding days of each year (Yang et al., 2013; Zhang et al., 2013). Cluster analysis of TM images can identify and extract vegetation areas that are suitable for snail presence, then two spatial models can be established, that is, distribution of snail habitat and spatial spread of snail, so that the area of snail habitats and the potential spreading area of snail can be predicted directly (Yang et al., 2013; Zhang et al., 2013).

Landset ETM+ images have the potential to identify the snail habitats in marshlands along rivers (Zhang et al., 2005). It was found that the snail habitats in these areas can be classified into four types of landscapes, and the density of snail was higher in two of them, which was confirmed through field survey. Similarly, Landsat TM images were also used to classify the snail habitats in mountain areas (He et al., 2010). The sensitivity and specificity of the classified snail habitats to correctly predict the actual snail habitats was 79.82% and 85.58%, respectively. By using RS techniques, vegetation features and the ground survey data of actual snail distribution can be overlaid on the classified satellite images. Hence, the snail habitats can be identified precisely and quickly, which facilitates snail survey and control (Li et al., 2010b; Yang et al., 2005). GIS and GPS special analysis and map overlap analysis reveals that epidemic scale of schistosomiasis is closely related to climate and environmental factors including temperature, altitude, and precipitation (Wu et al., 2014; Zhou et al., 1999). Therefore it is possible to predict potential schistosomiasis transmission areas by analysing these climate factors (Wu et al., 2014; Zhou et al., 1999). RS technique also provides a feasible way for snail surveillance, and can be applied as a supplementary tool for snail detection (Wang et al., 2016). The predictive accuracy for the distribution of *O. hupensis* was up to 86.2%, and it was identified that 82.77% of suspicious snail habitats were located in ditches (Xiao et al., 2009; Yang et al., 2008a).

3.3.4 Early identification of infection in snails

Loop-mediated isothermal amplification (LAMP) is a relatively new nucleic acid amplification technique (Chen et al., 2016). LAMP has been successfully used for detecting schistosome-infected *O. hupensis* due to its high specificity, sensitivity, convenience and efficiency (Kumagai et al., 2010; Tong et al., 2015; Yu et al., 2011).

It is well known that it takes more than two months from miracidia invasion to cercariae release (Mao, 1990). The conventional microscopic examination by crushing snail can only find daughter sporocyst and cercariae of schistosome in snail. Instead, LAMP technique based on targeting nucleic acid can detect not only daughter sporocyst and cercariae but also DNA targets at even earlier development stage, and hence the detection rate of schistosome-infected snail can be improved (Deng et al., 2009; Wang et al., 2010).

Infections in snail can be detected by LAMP as early as one week after the snails were exposed to miracidia, and the time of detection can be also shortened from 6 h by routine PCR to 2 h (Yu et al., 2011). In addition, LAMP was more sensitive to infections (Deng et al., 2014; Yu et al., 2008). Tong et al. (2015) employed LAMP to examine snails collected from 28 snail habitats in Hunan, Hubei and Anhui provinces, and mapped high risk areas of schistosomiasis transmission by using ArcMap. Those results could provide basic data for schistosomiasis surveillance and intervention strategy.

4. CONTROL OF *O. HUPENSIS*

The People's Republic of China has developed a series of snail control methods in the last 60 years, including environment modification and chemical mollusciciding (Zhou, 2005). Environment modification include burial of surface soil harbouring snails, cement-lining of irrigation ditches, conversion of paddy fields into dry crop farming, utilization of marsh land for vegetables and crops, blocking river branch for aquaculture, reclaiming uncultivated land, weeding for manure collection and so on. Especially, tree planting in *O. hupensis* snail habitats is a novel snail control method (see cross-reference in this volume). Chemical mollusciciding is the primary measure in areas where snail habitat modification cannot be implemented temporarily (Zhou, 2005). Table 5 compares the advantages and disadvantages of these two snail control methods. In 2013, the total area where chemical molluscicide was applied was up to 134,423.49 hm^2 with 71,968.41 hm^2 of actual molluscicide area, and the area of environment modification for snail control was 5852.21 hm^2 (Lei and Zhou, 2015).

4.1 Environment modification for snail control

Snail habitat modification has significant effects on schistosomiasis control in The People's Republic of China (Lei and Zhou, 2015). Lots of snail habitats in various endemic areas have been changed by agricultural practice, water

Table 5 Comparison of two snail control methods

Method	Advantage	Disadvantage
Snail habitat modification	1. More effective than molluscicides and has a long-term effect 2. Saving resources: Reclaiming abandoned fields can improve the local agricultural structure, and make better use of local resources (labour force, materials) 3. Public participation: public awareness on schistosomiasis can be improved by community participation 4. No environmental pollution	1. Large one-time investment is needed when reclaiming land, construction of flood control project and irrigation ditches 2. Effect on snail control is slower than chemical molluscicides and needs to be assessed for a long time 3. Less scope of application
Chemical molluscicides	1. Wide application 2. Easy operation, saving time and labour 3. Immediate effect 4. Can be used repeatedly	1. High price 2. Toxic to nontarget organisms (eg, fish, aquatic animals and plants) 3. Possible environmental pollution 4. Need to be used repeatedly

conservancy and urbanization, which have rendered such environments unsuitable for the snails (Yang et al., 2016).

In marshland and lake areas, environmental modification play an important role in schistosomiasis transmission control, such as building snail retention reservoirs at the entrance of major irrigation canals (water goes to irrigation canal through the reservoir where the snails are retained and sunk), embanking the lowland for aquaculture, and enclosing marshland for planting. A field observation on the effect of a snail retention reservoir in Gongan, Hubei Province showed that the percent of frame with living snails declined from 11.83% in 2004 to 8.81% in 2011 after the reservoir was built in 2005 (Fang et al., 1998). Meanwhile, the mean density of snails dropped from 1.36 per 0.1 m^2 to 0.35 per 0.1 m^2 accordingly. Another comprehensive modification project was carried out in Jixing village in 2003 employing multiple measures, such as cement-lining of irrigation canals, changing production structure, improving water and sanitation, health education and tree planting (Fang et al., 1998). The snail habitat area went down from 41.75 hm^2 in 2003 to 0.83 hm^2 in 2011 and the percentage of frames with living snails and mean density of living snails dropped by 81.52% and 95.03%, respectively. The proportion of infected snails decreased from 0.92% to 0 (Chen et al., 2012b). This study indicated that the comprehensive control strategy with multiple measures has a better effect than the single measure for snail control. In the 1990s, a project of snail habitat modification was implemented in the Dongting Lake area in Hunan Province, which is a typical marshland endemic area with high prevalence of infection in people and high density of snails and infected snails (Fang et al., 1998). Depending on topographical features of specific marshlands, four measures were used, that is embanking the lowland for aquaculture, enclosing marshland for tree, enclosing marshland for reed, reclaiming and cultivation of marshland. Three years later, the density of living snails and infected snails significantly declined. Of these measures, the first one can eliminate snails completely as seen in Table 6 (Fang et al., 1998).

Environmental modification also has significant effect on snail control in plain water network areas. Seven localities in Hubei Province were selected as the observing sites to investigate the effect of 57 previous projects on habitat modification between 1997 and 2001 (Wang et al., 2002). Measures, such as water storage for aquaculture, digging new and filling old small irrigation canals, reclaiming and cultivation, burying soil with sands and cement-lining of irrigation canals, were taken for snail control. Five years later, the area infested with snails, the area potentially suitable as snail habitat,

Table 6 Effect comparison of different measures for snail habitat modification in the Dongting Lake basin

		Density of living snails			Density of infected snails		
Measure	**Location**	**Before (one/0.1 m^2)**	**3 years later (one/0.1 m^2)**	**Rate of decline (%)**	**Before (one/0.1 m^2)**	**3 years later (one/0.1 m^2)**	**Rate of decline (%)**
Water storage for fishing in low lying land	Choutang village, Xiangyin County	1.800	0.000	100.0	0.0190	0.0000	100.0
Enclosing marshlands and not allowing grazing	Junshan Farm	1.505	0.056	96.3	0.0454	0.0026	94.3
Enclosing marshlands for reed planting	Qilihu, Chen County	1.808	1.129	37.6	0.0032	0.0000	100.0
Reclaiming and cultivation without enclosing marshlands	Shangfang village, Zhao County	0.638	0.013	98.0	0.0072	0.0000	100.0

the density of snails and infected snails decreased by 71.7%, 90.5%, 96.5% and 95.9%, respectively (Wang et al., 2002). Of the five measures, burying soil with sands and cement-lining of irrigation canals were particularly effective in controlling snails. In another study, a programme of snail control, combined with comprehensive agriculture development, was implemented in Xichahu village, Hubei Province to establish agricultural, forestry and fishing facilities by changing snail habitat condition (Zhang et al., 2007a). In addition, irrigation canals were expanded and facilities, such as bridges, culverts and snail retention reservoirs were built at the sources of snail populations to reduce the risk of snail spread after floods (Zhang et al., 2007a). The study showed that snails were under effective control after 4 years of the programme. The area infested with snail, the infection rate of residents and cattle dropped by 98.01%, 90.60% and 87.16%, respectively (Zhang et al., 2007a). The local economic development was rapid with a 42% increase in agricultural productivity and a 11.53% increase in rural per capita net income (Zhang et al., 2007a).

A comprehensive snail control project was carried out along Yangtze River in Huangshi, Hubei Province during 1996–2000 (Hu et al., 2001). Measures included reclaiming land for cultivation, covering marshland with sand, tree planting, crop planting in woodland, urban construction and development (building park and wharf along the river) and using chemical molluscicides. Five years later, the total area with snail dropped by 97.18%. The number of infected snail went down to 0. The mean density of living snails declined by 95.19%. The effect of environment modification for snail control was higher than chemical drug (Hu et al., 2001). In Ruizhou, Jiangsu Province, the snail area along Yangtze River accounted for 93.7% of the district's entire snail area. A programme of snail habitat modification was conducted in one of such areas, including building low banks and reclaiming the marsh land for mechanical cultivation (Tao et al., 2012). In the same year, the density of living snails decreased by 99.75%, and living snails were not found in survey in 2010 and 2011 (Tao et al., 2012).

Modification in hilly endemic areas may be cement-lining of irrigation canals, burying snail habitat, digging new canals and burying old ones, dam expansion, reclaiming land and cultivation and returning abandoned land to forestry (Li et al., 2011). Jurong, Jiangsu Province is a typical hilly endemic area, where a project of snail habitat modification was carried out from 2001 to 2010 (Li et al., 2011). After the project, no snails were found in 12 hot spots, and the residual snail area decreased to 1.2 hm^2 in other three hot spots with rapid dropping of snail area and density. Especially, the rates of decline of snail area and density were 100% when measures of digging new ditches and burying old ones and water storage on banks were taken (Table 7) (Li et al., 2011).

Tree planting for snail control is mainly carried out in marshland and lake areas. Planting poplars in marshlands at relatively high altitude can decrease the density of snail by changing vegetation structure of marshland and make it unsuitable for snail habitat. After planting trees on areas with snail, the surviving snails lack nutrition and therefore cannot reproduce primarily due to reduced lactate dehydrogenase and succinic dehydrogenase caused by the decline of glycogen content (Peng, 2001; Zhang et al., 2013). During 1986–2000, 16 projects of tree planting for snail control had been implemented in five provinces located in the middle and lower branches of Yangtze River. As a result of the 15 years of study, the percentage of frames with living snails stably dropped every year, from 19.03% in the fourth year of the project to 3.61% in 2000; the mean density of snail declined from 2.7 per 0.1 m^2 to 0.5 per 0.1 m^2. The established forestry prevented the activities of people and livestock on marshlands and hence decreased the risk of infection transmission. The mean density of infected snail went down to 0 in the 3rd year of the project from 0.004 per 0.1 m^2 at the beginning (Huang et al., 2011; Peng, 2001).

Water conservancy projects for schistosomiasis control aim at changing snail habitats by conducting a series of measures, such as hardening banks of river and lake, constructing isolated canals, culvert and sluice gates, snail retention reservoirs, cement-lining of irrigation ditches and others (Mao et al., 2010; Yang et al., 2016; Zhu et al., 2009). Twenty-eight water conservancy projects were implemented in endemic areas of seven provinces between 2007 and 2011. The systematic evaluation showed that all these projects had effect on snail populations (Table 8). However, the studies also implied that snails could re-inhabit if cement-lined irrigation canals were not continuously maintained and managed. In this case, the cement surface would be damaged by mud deposition and growth of aquatic plants, which may facilitate formation of snail habitats. Once snails were carried by water from noncemented ditches, they can breed. Therefore, its effect in snail control may be compromised, especially in long term (Zhu and Zhang, 2012).

The Three Gorges Dam operating since 2003 had a significant influence on snail habitats (McManus et al., 2010; Seto et al., 2008; Zhu et al., 2008). Monitoring results in recent years showed that the density and area infested by snails were decreasing in Dongting Lake, Poyang Lake and the

Table 7 Comparison of effect of different measures of snail habitat modification in hilly endemic areas

Measure	Project	Before modification		After modification		Rate of decline of snail area (%)	Rate of decline of snail density (%)
		Area with snail (hm^2)	Density of snail (one/0.1 m^2)	Area of snail (hm^2)	Density of snail (one/0.1 m^2)		
Digging new ditches and burying old ones	Changlong Moutain	0.28	0.42	0.00	0.00	100.00	100.00
	Kongqing erdao Basin	0.40	0.35	0.00	0.00	100.00	100.00
	Gaolun Basin	0.48	0.32	0.00	0.00	100.00	100.00
	Shanggan Basin	0.95	0.32	0.00	0.00	100.00	100.00
	Daxi Moutain	4.95	4.20	0.00	0.00	100.00	100.00
	Lutang Basin	0.80	3.60	0.00	0.00	100.00	100.00
Reservoir construction	Pochong Basin	0.70	0.45	0.00	0.00	100.00	100.00
	Kongqing Village	0.07	0.58	0.00	0.00	100.00	100.00
Digging fishpond	Fangshan Basin	7.07	4.50	0.00	0.00	100.00	100.00
	Daxintang marshland	1.44	2.40	0.40	0.36	72.22	85.00
Comprehensive measures in small watershed	Yucheng Basin	2.20	3.20	0.00	0.00	100.00	100.00
	Wuqi Basin	1.65	1.30	0.00	0.00	100.00	100.00
	Dongshanchong, Lutang Basin	0.26	0.80	0.00	0.00	100.00	100.00
	Lita Basin I	3.60	3.40	0.50	0.64	86.11	81.18
	Lita Basin II	4.70	3.20	0.30	0.72	93.62	77.50

Table 8 Comparison of snail control effect before and after water resources projects were implemented, 2007–2011

Type of project	Location of project	Area with snails (hm^2)			Percent of frames with snails(%)			Density of living snails (one/0.1 m^2)		
		Before	After	Rate of decline (%)	Before	After	Rate of decline (%)	Before	After	Rate of decline (%)
Water storage for fishing in low bank										
	Caipeng lake in Duchang county, Jiangxi	496,000	0	100.00	0.00	0.00	–	0.00	0.000	100.00
	Xiwei bank in Xinzi county, Jiangxi	655,000	32,000	95.11	0.20	0.00	100.00	0.00	0.000	100.00
	Nanxin Village in Wuhu city, Anhui	20,000	0	100.00	2.17	0.00	100.00	0.04	0.000	100.00
Retention reservoirs										
	Dongza in Junshan district, Hunan	0	0	100.00	9.40	0.00	100.00	0.11	0.000	100.00
	Majiazui in Gongan county, Hubei	8400	8400	0.00	29.50	21.80	26.10	1.21	0.280	76.86
	Jiuxia Canal in Gongan County, Hubei	16,000	16,000	0.00	18.70	7.50	59.89	1.09	0.910	16.51
	Xiagan Canal in Gongan County, Hubei	12,000	12,000	0.00	18.70	7.00	62.57	1.09	0.290	73.39
	Irrigation ditch in Hujiatan, Jiangxi	–	0	100.00	13.43	0.00	100.00	0.99	0.000	100.00
	Irrigation ditch of Hujiatan, Jiangxi	–	0	100.00	15.76	0.42	97.34	0.76	0.010	98.68
	Irrigation station, Fenghuangjing, Wuwei county, Anhui	0	0	100.00	0.06	0.00	100.00	0.00	0.000	100.00
	Touqiao Floodgate of Xia River, Ganjiang District, Jiangsu	3800	0	100.00	31.17	0.00	100.00	1.20	0.000	100.00
	Xiangyang sluice gate, Xinjiang District, Jiangsu	0	0	100.00	26.42	18.50	29.98	0.91	4.580	−403.30
	Liugong sluice gate, Xingjiang District, Jiangsu	0	0	100.00	0.00	0.00	100.00	0.00	0.000	100.00
Cement lining of canals										
	Trunk canal, Yueyang, Hunan	8100	0	100.00	36.58	0.00	100.00	1.68	0.000	100.00
	Ditches, Junshan District, Hunan	66,300	0	100.00	50.30	19.57	61.09	2.66	1.370	48.50
	Jingyang Village, Xuanzhou District, Anhui	28,400	8500	70.07	22.28	0.00	100.00	0.75	0.000	100.00

Xintao Village, Nanling, Anhui	12,000	12,000	0.00	0.20	0.00	100.00	0.00	0.000	100.00
Bianming River, Jurong, Jaingsu	41,490	0	100.00	0.36	0.00	100.00	0.00	0.000	100.00
Panjia River, Yizheng, Jiangsu	27,398	0	100.00	0.00	0.00	100.00	0.00	0.000	100.00
Irrigation areas Huanglianggen reservoir, Dongpo, Sichuan	1300	32	97.54	0.00	0.00	—	0.00	0.000	100.00
Irrigation areas Meiwan reservoir, Danling, Sichuan	3300	1064	67.76	5.86	0.00	100.00	0.14	0.000	100.00
Dongfeng ditch, Dongpo, Sichuan	1015	306	69.85	22.60	13.20	41.59	1.60	0.280	82.50
Maqiao Village, Meishan, Sichuan	1975	25	98.73	80.30	19.70	75.47	2.30	0.650	71.74
Simen Village, Guanghan, Sichuan	7900	160	97.97	30.00	17.10	43.00	1.63	0.920	43.56
Shajing, Dali, Yunnan	1000	960	4.00	15.80	0.19	98.80	1.00	0.000	100.00
Gaojia Village, Lijiang, Yunnan	988	436	55.87	34.90	9.93	71.55	1.10	0.160	85.45
Pumping station									
Western sluice gate, Chiangjiang Village, Junshan, Hunan	20,000	0	100.00	11.20	0.30	97.32	0.42	0.004	99.05
Lianhu farm, Danyang, Jiangsu	500,000	0	100.00	10.80	1.31	87.87	0.37	0.024	93.51

middle-lower reaches of Yangtze River. For example, out of five monitoring sites set up in Dongting Lake in 2005, two sites became snail-free by 2010 and the other three sites showed decline of 93%, 24% and 34% in the density of living snail, respectively (Zhu et al., 2011). Similarly, according to the 8-year continuous monitoring in 12 sites in the Poyang Lake areas, the mean density of snail and the density of infected snail decreased by 94.21% and 98.97%, respectively (Chen et al., 2013). Operation of the Three Gorges Dam leads to a considerable decline of water level as well as change of fluctuation dynamics in the two lake areas. Such change disturbed the natural breeding rhythm of snails and thereby caused the decline of the snail density (Chen et al., 2013).

Modification of snail habitats, combined with comprehensive development of agriculture, can not only achieve significant effects in snail control but also produce economic benefit (Duan and Ji, 2004). A comprehensive agriculture project in Hunan Province, including excavation of fishponds, embankment of low marshland for aquaculture, conversion of paddy fields into dry crops farm, cultivation of winter crops, was carried out in marshlands of Dongting Lake (Qing et al., 2003). The density of infected snail in these areas decreased by 93.5% five years later, meanwhile the annual economic benefit reached 80.6 million RMB (Qing et al., 2003). Between 1998 and 2002, an agriculture structure adjustment was implemented in Lipu, Hubei Province, a plain water network and marshland area, including conversion of paddy field into dry crop farm, establishment of big vegetable farms, planting Italian poplars in marshlands, excavation of pond for fishing and seeding (Duan and Ji, 2004). The agriculture project led to decrease of about 91% of snail-infested areas and produced favourable socioeconomic benefits with the net income per capita of 800 RMB (Duan and Ji, 2004).

4.2 Molluscicides

Since the 1950s, a variety of chemicals have been used for mollusciciding in The People's Republic of China, for example, nicotinanilide, calcium cyanamide, unslaked lime, trichlorphon, metaldehyde, benzene hexachloride, carbamide, naphthalene, acetbromamide and sodium pentachlorophenate (Table 9). Currently, WHO recommends niclosamide for snail control since its toxicity is lower than others.

4.2.1 Niclosamide

Niclosamide was researched and developed by the Bayer (Germany) Company initially. Gonnert and Schranfstatler first reported the molluscicidal

Table 9 Benefits and side effects of chemicals used in The People's Republic of China for molluscicidin g

Molluscicides	Benefit	Side effects	Reference
NaPCP	High effect on mature and young snails as well as eggs	High toxicity to human, livestock, aquatic animals with teratogenic, carcinogenic and mutagenic effect; serious environmental pollution	Zhao and Gao (1997)
Acetabromamide	High effect on mature and young snails as well as eggs; water soluble; low toxicity to human, fishes and shrimps	Easily deliquescent; unstable to heat, acid and alkali; causing dermatitis	Zhu and Yin (1986)
Nicotinanilide	High effect; lower toxicity to fish and no harmfulness to human and livestock; convenient	Low solubility in water; low effect on eggs and climbing snails; expensive; low output	Chen et al. (1991)
Metaldehyde	High effect	Prone to clot; difficult to spray evenly; toxic to human liver and kidney	Gao et al. (1992)

effects of such chemical compound at the 6th International Tropical Medicine and Malaria Conference in 1959 and named it Bayer-73. Chinese scientists synthesized niclosamide in laboratory in 1960 and developed it into a 50% paste. Because of its agglomeration during storage, niclosamide was not widely used in the field until the initiation of World Bank loan project for schistosomiasis control in The People's Republic of China in 1992. This project designated niclosamide, a 50% wettable powder of niclosamide ethanolamine salt (WPN), as the only chemical molluscicide.

To date, wettable powder and suspension of niclosamide have been developed in The People's Republic of China and applied for large-scale snail control by immersion or spraying methods. The sensitivity of *O. hupensis* to niclosamide remains high even more than two decades of repeated, extensive application for snail control in the main endemic areas of The People's Republic of China (Dai et al., 2014). An experiment of WPN (wettable powder niclosamide) lethal effect on adult snails collected from 37 sites covering all the three types of endemic regions showed that all snails could be killed at 1 mg/L WPN after 24-h immersion or at 0.5 mg/L after 48-h immersion (Dai et al., 2005b). In another study niclosamide also showed high toxicity to eggs and young snails with 100% of mortality at 0.25 mg/L after 24 h (Dai et al., 2005a).

The formulation of niclosamide has been improved according to the environmental features, which makes the application more convenient, effective and cheaper (Table 10) (Yang et al., 2012). WPN shows excellent suspensibility in water and is highly toxic to snails by immersion or spraying methods. Water is normally needed as carrier and hence WPN is used in environments with abundant water. A field study indicated that the mortality rate of snails was 81.1% at 2.0 mg/m^2 using spraying method after 15 days (He et al., 2007). However, WPN is prone to clot during storage and application, which leads to the decline of drug effect and the damage of spraying machine (Dai et al., 2003). Wang (Wang, 2006b) applied WPN at 2 g/m^2 in the field and found that the mortality rates of snails after 3, 5, 7, 15 and 30 days were 71.58%, 62.80%, 69.03%, 90.16% and 95.48%, respectively. Dai et al. (Dai et al., 2003) applied a 25% niclosamide suspension for mollusciciding in the field by spraying method with the concentration of 0.5 mg/m^2, and found the mortality rates of snails to be 95.77%, 99.07% and 97.29% after 3, 7, 15 days, respectively. When the suspension was used with the concentration of 0.5 mg/L by immersion method, the mortality rate of snails in soil was 95% after 24, 48 and 72 h (Dai et al., 2003). In another study, the 4% WPN by powdering method was used in dried snail habitats and at 25 g/m^2, 50 g/m^2 and 75 g/m^2 of this chemical, the mortality rates of snails after 3 days were 84.56%, 93.56% and 98.02%, respectively (Bao et al., 2006).

Dai et al. (2005b) observed in a study that the 25% niclosamide suspension performed better than the 50% WPN; even its active component reduced by half. It was found that the suspension adsorbs on the surface of snail and this improves its lethal effect, and the formulation can be widely used in the complex environments, such as mountain areas or river marshlands, due to its low toxicity, stability, cheap price and convenient operation.

Yang et al. (2012) compared niclosmide suspension emulsion with wettable powder and suspension formulations of niclosamide. When

Table 10 Comparison of different formulations of niclosamide applied in The People's Republic of China for snail control

Formulation	Active component	Application environment	Using method	Advantages	Disadvantages	Reference
Wettable powder	50% niclosamide ethanolamine salt	Areas with abundant water	Immersion, spraying	Better suspension in water; Excellent effect	Prone to clot; inconvenient; High toxicity to nontarget organism	He et al. (2007)
Powder	4% niclosamide ethanolamine salt	Water-deficient areas	Powdering	Convenient application without water limitation	Optimum effect depending on weather (raining); toxicity to nontarget organism	Dai et al. (2003)
Suspension	25% niclosamide	Complex environments (eg, mountains and river marshlands)	Immersion, spraying	High effect; low toxicity, stable; cheap; convenient	Toxicity to nontarget organism	Dai et al. (2008)
Suspension emulsion	50% niclosamide ethanolamine salt	Large-scale spraying in the field	Immersion, spraying	High effect; soluble in water	Organic solvent; expensive; environment pollution; toxicity to nontarget organism	Dai et al. (2005b)
Naro preparation	25% niclosamide	Water-accessible areas	Immersion, spraying	High effect; soluble in water; applicable in cold weather	Toxicity to nontarget organism	Jiang et al. (2007) and Guo et al. (2006)
Slow release preparation	5%, 10%, 50%, 70% niclosamide ethanolamine salt	Water-deficient areas	spraying	Long-term effect; convenient	Environmental pollution due to slow degradation; toxicity to nontarget organism	Kenawy and Rizkel (2004)

suspension emulsion of niclosamide with the concentration of 0.12 mg/L was applied, its effect was higher than that of wettable powder, while there was no difference with that of the suspension. The suspension emulsion of niclosamide is suitable for use in large-scale field spraying due to its excellent mollusciciding effect and water solubility. The effect of niclosamide naro-preparation was similar to WPN, and it can be used without the temperature limitation (Guo et al., 2006; Zhang et al., 2007b). The active time of slow-release preparations of niclosamide was longer to 16 days than that of the common WPN, and the mollusciciding effect went up with the decline of water hardness and rise of water pH value (Kenawy and Rizkel, 2004).

4.2.2 Novel molluscicides for snail control

Although niclosamide shows good molluscicidal efficacy, its toxicity to fish and other aquatic animals as well as environmental pollution is considerable. Therefore, development of environment-friendly, highly effective and low toxic chemical molluscicides is always the priority (Xia et al., 2014). Many plant species have been confirmed to contain components of molluscicidal activity against *O. hupensis* (Chen et al., 2012a; Guo et al., 2011; Xin et al., 2006; Yang et al., 2008b). Plant molluscicides, such as Rongbao and Luowei, show high lethal effect on snails and overcome the disadvantages of niclosamide.

4.2.2.1 Rongbao

'Rongbao' is a kind of alkaline nitrogen waste and appears as black and grey powder. The active component is calcium cyanamide. 'Rongbao' has the similar lethal effect on snails as niclosamide but a better long-term efficacy than niclosamide. Furthermore, the molluscicide shows low toxicity to fish and other aquatic animals (Liu et al., 2007; Lu et al., 2006). A laboratory experiment showed that all *Oncomelania* snails died when immersed in a solution containing 80 mg/L Rongbao for 2 days or sprayed with the molluscicide of 30 g/m^2 for 1 day. Field study also showed good effect; the mortality rate of snails was 97.18% when the snails were immersed with Rongbao of 50 mg/L for seven days, without observing the death of other aquatic animals. When 30 g/m^2 of Rongbao was applied by spraying and powdering in the field, the mortality rates of snails after 15 days were 74.15% and 81.11%, respectively (Li et al., 2006a). Due to the high cost of Rongbao, niclosamide still is the only molluscicide widely used in The People's Republic of China for snail control. However, because of the low toxicity to fish, Rongbao can be applied in small scale in aquaculture areas (Gu et al., 2008).

4.2.3 Luo-wei

'Luo-wei' is a novel plant molluscicide obtained by extracting triterpenoid compound from camellia. A 4% yellow 'Luo-wei' powder (TDS) was developed in The People's Republic of China. The active component is saponins (Tang et al., 2010). The application of the powder in different types of endemic areas by either immersion or spraying is highly toxic to *O. hupensis*, similar with that of niclosamide ethanolamine salt (WPN). After 1, 3, 7, 15 days of TDS application, the mortality rates of snails increased over time, and the density of living snails at 15 days was significantly lower compared with density before the application (Jia et al., 2013; Sun et al., 2010; Tang et al., 2010). Toxicological test indicated that TDS is highly toxic to fish but low to birds. Decapods are highly sensitive to TDS spraying, while the risk of immersion is low. Hence, the mollusciciding methods should be adopted according to the distribution of fish, bird and decapod in snail-occupied areas. The spraying method on dry land is recommended due to its low toxicity (Sun et al., 2010). However, 'Luo-wei' needs more toxicological tests before it can be used for snail control in field in The People's Republic of China.

5. CHALLENGES AND PRIORITIES

A great achievement in schistosomiasis control has been made in The People's Republic of China in the past six decades (Zheng et al., 2013). By the end of 2014, out of a total 453 schistosome-endemic counties, 313 had reached the criteria of transmission interruption, 135 reached transmission control and only five are still at the epidemic control stage (Lei and Zhou, 2015). Around 8000 patients confirmed by stool examination were reported with only two acute cases in 2014 (Lei and Zhou, 2015). However, the snail-infested area is still as large as 3.64 billion m^2 (Lei and Zhou, 2015). During the implementation of a 10-year national programme of schistosomiasis control since 2004, the snail-infested area in The People's Republic of China only decreased by 5.23% from 384,599.97 hm^2 in 2004 to 365,468.00 hm^2 in 2013 (Hao et al., 2005; Lei et al., 2014). Although the decline of snail-infested area is not significant, snail control programmes played an important role to reduce the density of snails in endemic areas and thus significantly lowered the risk of schistosomiasis transmission. According to national statistics in 2013, the area of chemical mollusciciding and environment modification for snail control were 1.344 billion m^2 and 5800 hm^2, respectively.

Wide distribution of snail and low coverage of chemical mollusciciding are the main reasons for the current status, which are the key factors to hinder the process of schistosomiasis elimination in The People's Republic of China. The People's Republic of China still faces big challenges to achieve the goal of schistosomiasis elimination nationally, and the following research and application priorities should be strengthened to provide scientific support for that goal (Lei and Zhou, 2015; Zheng et al., 2013).

5.1 Development of innovative techniques

O. hupensis, the only intermediate host of *S. japonicum*, plays a vital role in schistosomiasis transmission. One key index for schistosomiasis elimination in the newly issued 'criteria for control and elimination of schistosomiasis' is that no infected snail can be found for successive 5 years. Therefore, monitoring snail habitats or high risk zones should be emphasized in the endemic surveillance system towards schistosomiasis elimination in The People's Republic of China. During the last 10 years The People's Republic of China implemented an integrated strategy with a focus on the infection sources control. This strategy successfully reduced patients and ill livestock and thus weakened the role of humans and livestock in the schistosomiasis transmission. However, several dozens of wild animals can serve as reservoirs of *S. japonicum* and their capability in transmission is not yet evaluated in field. Moreover, population migration is more and more frequent in The People's Republic of China. All these factors increase the possibility of snail infection with schistosome (Liu et al., 2013; Xiong et al., 2014). In addition, owing to lack of modern tools, snail survey in The People's Republic of China still relies on manual work with the disadvantages of high labour intensity, high cost and low coverage. Monitoring and warning systems should be based on sensitive early detection and modern information techniques. Therefore, more practical and sensitive techniques of snail survey need to be developed to improve monitoring level on snail habitats, especially simple and rapid methods for detection of infected snails. And a dynamic monitoring and warning system and technique on snail, which can identify, simulate, predict and evaluate influence of environmental factors and infection sources on snail distribution, also need be established to improve the sensitivity and efficiency of snail detection and surveillance in epidemic areas.

5.2 Research on control strategy

Killing of snails is one of the key strategies for schistosomiasis transmission control as well as one of the measures of The People's Republic of China's national antischistosomiasis programme. Environmental modification is the fundamental measure for snail control (Yang et al., 2016). However, it has its shortcomings of huge one-time investment and less scope of application. With the development of social economy and the construction of new rural villages in The People's Republic of China, more and more ecological methods for snail control will appear, for example, the projects of agriculture, forestry, water conservation and tourism for snail control (Zheng et al., 2013). At present, the application of chemical molluscicides is still the main method for snail control in The People's Republic of China, but these chemicals need to be used repeatedly, and have toxicity to aquatic animals causing economic loss and affecting the development of aquaculture industry (Dai et al., 2007; Sun et al., 2010; Tang et al., 2015). Therefore, there is a need to speed up the development of novel molluscicides with high efficiency, low cost, user friendliness and low toxicity to nontarget organisms; or new biological approaches for snail control, especially, environment-friendly and benefit-oriented ecological molluscicid-ing should be developed.

5.3 Theoretical research

Research on biological theory of *S. japonicum* and *Oncomelania* needs to be further strengthened to develop new strategy and technology for snail control. As studies based on morphology, anatomy, protein and DNA tests have shown, certain genetic diversity exists in *Oncomelania* in mainland The People's Republic of China, and *Oncomelania* interspecific differentiation is possible; the susceptibility of *Oncomelania* to schistosome infection may be under control of its genetic materials, which cause significant differences in infection rates of snails from different areas when infected with geographical strain of *S. japonicum* from the same or different areas (He et al., 1990; Huang et al., 2002; Jiang et al., 2007). With the development of genomics, transcriptomics and proteomics, studies on classification of infra-species, different geographical strain, even sex of *Oncomelania* and interspecific difference of *Oncomelania* need to be further pursued. Also, research on host—parasite relationship between *S. japonicum* and *Oncomelania* needs to be strengthened, including genetic difference between *Oncomelania* and *S. japonicum*, molecular basis of gene co-evolution and symbiosis, biological characteristics and immunological mechanism of susceptibility difference of *Oncomelania* for geographical strains of *S. japonicum,* functional gene of *Oncomelania* susceptibility and transmission threshold of *Oncomelania*. These studies would likely contribute to the development of a schistosomiasis vaccine and chemical molluscicides.

6. CONCLUSION

Oncomelania hupensis, the only intermediate host of *S. japonicum*, shows high diversity, which makes it possible to widely distribute and explore complex landscapes in The People's Republic of China. Although routine chemical mollusciciding did lower the density of snails and thus the risk of schistosomiasis transmission, the area of snail habitats did not change as expected in the last 10 years. Along with great achievement in schistosomiasis control in humans and domestic animals, snail control should be highlighted in future control programmes. The next 10-year national plan (2016–2025) towards schistosomiasis elimination has been formulated and snail control is one of the fundamental measures (Liu et al., 2014). Facing the challenges in snail control, it is urgent to develop high-effective, low-toxic, cheap and user-friendly chemical molluscicides, to research novel, long-standing and thoroughgoing methods for snail control, and to establish sensitive and real-time monitoring and warning techniques in low schistosome-endemic areas (Tambo et al., 2014).

REFERENCES

Attwood, S.W., Ibaraki, M., Saitoh, Y., Nihei, N., Janies, D.A., 2015. Comparative phylogenetic studies on *Schistosoma japonicum* and its snail intermediate host Oncomelania hupensis: origins, dispersal and coevolution. PLoS Negl. Trop. Dis. 9, e0003935.

Bao, J.G., Zhang, G.H., Wu, W.D., Zhang, S.Q., Zhang, X.Y., Lv, D.B., Fang, G.R., Wang, F.F., Zhu, L., Dai, Q.J., 2006. Snail control effect of 4% Powder of niclosamide ethanolamine salt in field trial. Parasit. Dis. Infect. Dis. 2, 163–165 (in Chinese).

Cao, C.L., Bao, Z.P., Li, S.Z., Wei, W.Y., Yi, P., Yu, Q., Zhu, H.Q., Xu, J., Guo, J.G., Feng, Z., 2015. Schistosomiasis in a migrating population in the lake region of China and its potential impact on control operation. Acta Trop. 145, 88–92.

Cao, Q., Gu, B.L., Hang, M.D., Wang, D., Du, S.R., Fan, X.N., Ju, S.Y., He, S.Y., 1990. Survey residual *Oncomelania* snails by straw curtain. Chin. J. Schistosomiasis Control 2, 66–68 (in Chinese).

Cao, Z.G., Wang, T.P., Zhang, S.Q., Wang, E.M., Yao, G.X., Fang, R.G., Jiang, L., Zhu, L., Yang, W.P., Guo, J.D., 2009. Compatibility between *Schistosoma japonicum* and their snail hosts from snail-existent non-endemic areas of schistosomiasis. J. Trop. Dis. Parasitol. 7, 1–3 (in Chinese).

Cao, Z.G., Zhao, Y.E., Willingham, A.L., Wang, T.P., 2016. Towards the elimination of schistosomiasis japonica through control of the disease in domestic animals in the People's Republic of China: a tale of over 60 years. Adv. Parasitol. 92.

Chen, G.X., 1980. Subtypes and variable of *Oncomelania hupensis* snails in marshland. Bull. Hunan Med. Coll. 5, 129–130 (in Chinese).

Chen, H.G., Zeng, X.J., Lin, D.D., Lv, S.B., Gu, X.N., Hang, C.Q., Li, Z.J., 2013. The changes of hydrological regime in Poyang Lake after runs of three Gorges project and its impact on prevalence of schistosomiasis in the lake region. Chin. J. Schistosomiasis Control 25, 444–450 (in Chinese).

Chen, M.G., 2014. Assessment of morbidity due to *Schistosoma japonicum* infection in China. Infect. Dis. Poverty 3, 6.

Chen, S.B., Ai, L., Hu, W., Xu, J., Bergquist, R., Qin, Z.Q., Chen, J.H., 2016. New anti-schistosome approaches in the People's Republic of China: development of diagnostics, vaccines and other new techniques belonging to the 'omics' group. Adv. Parasitol. 92.

Chen, Y.Q., Xu, Q.M., Liu, Y.L., Li, X.R., Yang, S.L., Zhuge, H.X., 2012a. Laboratory evaluation of the molluscicidal activity of *Pulsatilla chinensis* (Bunge) Regel saponins against the snail *Oncomelania hupensis*. Biomed. Environ. Sci. 25, 224–229.

Chen, Y.Y., Xu, X.J., Yang, Z.Q., He, Z.W., Wan, D.F., Huang, W.J., Hou, Y.Y., Wei, Q., 2012b. Evaluation of environmental modification project on the control of schistosomiasis transmission in lake and marshland regions. J. Public Health Prev. Med. 23, 23–26 (in Chinese).

Chen, Z.P., Tao, H.Q., Hua, D.S., Shen, B.R., Chan, H.L., 1991. Evaluation of molluscicidal effect of nicotinanilide against *Oncomelania* snails. Chin. J. Parasitol. Parasit. Dis. 9, 216–218 (in Chinese).

Collins, C., Xu, J., Tang, S., 2012. Schistosomiasis control and the health system in P.R. China. Infect. Dis. Poverty 1, 8.

Dai, J.R., Li, Y.Z., Wang, W., Xing, Y.T., Qu, G.L., Liang, Y.S., 2014. Sensitivity of Oncomelania hupensis to niclosamide: a nationwide survey in China. Int. J. Environ. Res. Public Health 11, 3086–3095.

Dai, J.R., Liang, Y.S., Li, H.J., Hua, W.Q., Xi, W.P., Guan, X.H., Zhu, Y.C., 2005a. Molluscicidal effect of suspension concentrate of niclosamide against *Oncomelania* snail eggs and young snails. Chin. J. Schistosomiasis Control 17, 39–41 (in Chinese).

Dai, J.R., Liang, Y.S., Li, H.J., Tong, J.X., Zhu, Y.C., 2007. Evaluation of toxicity of suspension concentrate of niclosamide. Chin. J. Schistosomiasis Control 19, 415–417 (in Chinese).

Dai, J.R., Xu, F.N., Liang, Y.S., Zhang, Y., Zhu, Y.C., 2003. Development of a novel suspension concentrate of niclosamide and its molluscicidal effect against *Oncomelania* snails. Chin. J. Schistosomiasis Control 15, 3–6 (in Chinese).

Dai, J.R., Wang, W., Liang, Y.S., Li, H.J., Guan, X.H., Zhu, Y.C., 2008. A novel molluscicidal formulation of niclosamide. Parasitol. Res. 103, 405–412.

Dai, J.R., Zhu, Y.C., Liang, Y.S., Li, H.J., Gong, M.T., Zhang, J.T., Guan, X.H., 2005b. Development of a novel synergism compound suspension concentrate of niclosamide and chlorphoxim I. Formula and its characteristics. Chin. J. Schistosomiasis Control 17, 413–416 (in Chinese).

Dang, H., Xu, J., Li, S.Z., Cao, Z.G., Huang, Y.X., Wu, C.G., Tu, Z.W., Zhou, X.N., 2014. Monitoring the transmission of *Schistosoma japonicum* in potential risk regions of China, 2008–2012. Int. J. Environ. Res. Public Health 11, 2278–2287.

Deng, P.C., Wang, Q.B., Kuang, M.Y., Xu, S., 2014. Development of a LAMP assay for fast detecting *schistosoma japonicum*-infected *Oncomelania hupensis*. J. Xiangnan Univers. (Medical Sci. 16, 7–11 (in Chinese).

Deng, P.C., Zhang, R.S., Liang, Y., Zhang, Y.K., Yang, Q.L., 2009. Detection of *Schistosoma japonicum*-infected *Oncomelania hupensis* by loop-mediated isothermal amplification. Chin. J. Vet. Sci. 29, 1017–1019 (in Chinese).

Duan, Z.Q., Ji, P., 2004. Agricultural engineering prevention snail control by high-efficiency agriculture base. Chin. J. Vet. Parasit. 12, 23–24 (in Chinese).

Fang, J.C., Yi, M.Y., Wu, Z.W., Zhao, Z.Y., Wang, F.H., 1998. Cost-benefits analysis of environmental modifications projects in shistosome transmission sites of Dongting Lake. Chin. J. Schistosomiasis Control 10, 207–211 (in Chinese).

Feng, Y., Liu, L., Xia, S., Xu, J.F., Bergquist, R., Yang, G.J., 2016. Reaching the surveillance-response stage of schistosomiasis control in the People's Republic of China: a modelling approach. Adv. Parasitol. 92.

Gao, S.N., Liu, J.B., Xiao, Y.L., Liu, J., Hu, J.P., 1992. Enlarged field trials of metaldehyde against *Oncomelania* snails. Hubei Prov. Med. 3, 22–24 (in Chinese).

Gryseels, B., Polman, K., Clerinx, J., Kestens, L., 2006. Human schistosomiasis. Lancet 368, 1106–1118.

Gu, D.A., Zhang, Z.H., Yan, Z.W., Zhou, X.N., Xu, X.W., Ai, S.Y., Zhang, H., 2008. Comparison of molluscicidal effect and cost-effect of Rongbao and niclosamide. Chin. J. Schistosomiasis Control 20, 106–109 (in Chinese).

Guan, W.H., Yuan, H.C., Zhao, G.M., Yu, J.M., Yang, Q.J., 1999. Survey of schistosomiasis epidemic in Dam-Circle Marsh Region. Chin. J. Pub. Health 15, 686–688 (in Chinese).

Guo, D.Z., Chen, J., Liu, Y.D., Yao, H., Han, F.A., Pan, J., 2011. A high-performance molluscicidal ingredient against *Oncomelania hupensis* produced by a rhizospheric strain-from Phytolacca acinosa Roxb. Pharmacogn. Mag. 7, 277–283.

Guo, F., Jiang, L., Li, X.S., Dai, J.R., Zhu, Y.C., 2006. Preparation of niclosamide nanoparticle by the method of Top-down. Chin. J. Schistosomiasis Control 18, 411–415 (in Chinese).

Hao, Y., Wu, X.H., Xia, G., Zheng, H., Guo, J.G., Wang, L.Y., Zhou, X.N., 2005. Schistosomiasis situation in P.R. of China in 2004. Chin. J. Schistosomiasis Control 17, 401–404 (in Chinese).

He, J.C., Wang, H., Wu, M.T., Chen, X.F., Shu, Q.M., Tao, W., Xu, Y.X., Zhang, S.Q., 2007. Observation on the molluscicidal effect of niclosamide ethanolamine salt dustable powder by dusting in fields. J. Trop. Dis. Parasitol. 5, 153–155 (in Chinese).

He, M.Z., Peng, W.X., Zhou, Y.B., Yihuo, W.L., Liu, G.M., 2010. The application of remote sensing image to monitoring of *Oncomelania hupensis* in mountainous areas. Bull. Fudan Univers. 37, 510–513 (in Chinese).

He, S.Y., Liu, H.S., Xu, Z.Y., Leng, X.L., Zhu, Q., Shen, M.X., Dong, M.H., Wu, Y.H., 1989. Quantitative study on the relationship between the number of *Schistosoma japonicum* miracidia and the infection rate of *Oncomelania* snails. Chin. J. Schistosomiasis Control 1, 28–32 (in Chinese).

He, Y.X., Guo, Y.H., Ni, C.H., Xia, F., Liu, H.X., Yu, Q.F., Hu, Y.Q., 1990. Studies on the strain differences of *Schinstosoma Japonicum* in the mainland of China Ⅰ. Compatibility between Schistosomes and their snail hosts. Parasit. Dis. Infect. Dis. 8, 92–95 (in Chinese).

He, Y.X., Ni, C.H., Liu, H.X., Hu, Y.Q., You, Q.F., 1994. Infectivity of different numbers and ages of *Schistosoma japonicum* miracidia to *Oncomelania hupensisi hupensis*. Acta Parasitol. Med. Entomol. Sin. 1, 22–26 (in Chinese).

Hong, Q.B., Zhou, X.N., Sun, L.P., Chen, S.D., Jiang, Y.J., Guo, B.Y., Xu, Q., Wu, Z.X., Lu, A.S., 1995. Susceptibility of *Oncomelania hupensis* to *Schistosoma japonicum*. Chin. J. Schistosomiasis Control 7, 83–86 (in Chinese).

Hu, C.X., Zou, X.S., Chen, B.K., Liu, S.J., Lu, X.Y., Dou, R.Z., Li, H., Lin, C.J., 2001. Interrupting schistosomiasis transmission by comprehensive measures in beach areas of Huangshi region of the Yangtze River. J. Pract. Parasit. Dis. 9, 58–61 (in Chinese).

Huang, X.B., Xia, P.F., Yang, L.H., Jiang, Y., 2002. Susceptibility of *Oncomelanian hupensis* from different areas infected with *Schistosoma japonicum* and generation attack ability to rabbits. Chin. J. Schistosomiasis Control 14, 35–37 (in Chinese).

Huang, Y., Zhang, S.Q., He, J.C., Cao, Z.G., Wang, T.P., Gao, F.H., Zhang, G.H., Lu, D.B., 2011. Effect of project of afforestation for schistosomiasis prevention on snail control in marshland and lake regions. Chin. J. Schistosomiasis Control 23, 138–144 (in Chinese).

Jia, T.W., Sun, L.P., Hong, Q.B., Tao, B., Cai, J.X., Li, Y.S., Lin, D.D., Yu, X.L., Zhou, X.N., 2013. Field evaluation of a novel plant molluscicide "Luo-wei" against *Oncomelania hupensis* Ⅰ. Molluscicidal effect by the spraying method in lake and marshland regions. Chin. J. Schistosomiasis Control 25, 125–128 (in Chinese).

Jiang, D.Y., Liang, Y.S., Jiang, Y.J., Huang, Y.X., 1989. Impact on infected of *Schistosoma japonicum* miracidium to *Oncomelania hupensis* about water depth. Chin. J. Schistosomiasis Control 10, 63 (in Chinese).

Jiang, Y.J., Huang, X.,Y., Hong, Q.B., Xi, W.P., 2007. Observation on number of cercariae hatching from infected snails from different areas. Chin. J. Schistosomiasis Control 19, 376–377 (in Chinese).
Kang, Z.B., Wang, C.K., Zhou, S.L., 1958. Studies on the geographical distribution and morphology of the *Oncomelania* snails, an intermediate host of *Schistosoma Japonicum* in hupeh province, China. Acta Zool. Sin. 10, 225–241 (in Chinese).
Kenawy, e-R., Rizkel, e-S., 2004. Polymeric controlled release formulations of niclosamide for control of Biomphalaria alexandrina, the vector snail of schistosomiasis. Macromol. Biosci. 4, 119–128.
Kumagai, T., Furushima-Shimogawara, R., Ohmae, H., Wang, T.P., Lu, S., Chen, R., 2010. Detection of early and single infections of *Schistosoma japonicum* in the intermediate host snail, *Oncomelania hupensis*, by PCR and Loop-Mediated Isothermal Amplification (LAMP) Assay. Am. J. Trop. Med. Hyg. 83, 542–548.
Lei, Z.L., Zheng, H., Zhang, L.J., Zhu, R., Xu, Z.M., Xu, J., Fu, Q., Wang, Q., Li, S.Z., Zhou, X.N., 2014. Endemic status of schistosomiasis in People's Republic of China in 2013. Chin. J. Schistosomiasis Control 26, 591–597 (in Chinese).
Lei, Z.L., Zhou, X.N., 2015. Eradication of schistosomiasis: a new target and a new task for the national schistosomiasis control porgramme in the People's Republic of China. Chin. J. Schistosomiasis Control 27, 1–4 (in Chinese).
Li, G.P., Wei, W.Y., Lv, G.L., Xia, M., 2006a. Study on molluscicidal effects of Rongbao and Rongya against *Oncomelania hupensis*. Pract. Prev. Med. 13, 871–873 (in Chinese).
Li, S.M., Chen, S.J., Wu, X.J., Chen, X.Q., Zhang, R.P., Zhang, J.R., 2011. Evaluation on cost-effectiveness of snail control project by environmental modification in hilly regions. Chin. J. Schistosomiasis Control 23, 85–88 (in Chinese).
Li, S.Z., Wang, Y.X., Yang, K., Liu, Q., Wang, Q., Zhang, Y., Wu, X.H., Guo, J.G., Bergquist, R., Zhou, X.N., 2009. Landscape genetics: the correlation of spatial and genetic distances of *Oncomelania hupensis*, the intermediate host snail of *Schistosoma japonicum* in mainland China. Geospat. Health 3, 221–231.
Li, Y.P., He, Z., He, M.Z., Jiang, J., Li, J.X., Zhou, Y.B., Zhang, Z.J., Jiang, Q.W., 2010a. Impact of the changing water level on the variance of *Oncomelania hupensis* populations in lake area with general additive model. Chin. J. Epidemiol. 31, 1148–1154 (in Chinese).
Li, Z.J., Chen, H.G., Gong, P., Zeng, X.J., Liu, Y.M., Xie, S.Y., 2010b. Study on relationship between vegetation and spatial distribution of Oncomlania snails in Poyang Lake region. Chin. J. Schistosomiasis Control 22, 132–135 (in Chinese).
Li, Z.J., Chen, H.G., Liu, Y.M., Zeng, X.J., Lin, D.D., Wan, W.H., 2006b. Studies on relationship between vegetation and snail distribution inside and outside embankment of Poyang Lake region. Chin. J. Schistosomiasis Control 18, 406–410 (in Chinese).
Liang, L., Liu, Y., Liao, J., G, P., 2014. Wetlands explain most in the genetic divergence pattern of *Oncomelania hupensis*. Infect. Genet. Evol. 27, 436–444.
Liang, Y.S., Dai, J.R., Li, H.J., Xu, Y.L., Xu, M., Zhu, Y.C., 2004. Impact of water temperature on shedding and infectivity of cercariae of *Schistosoma japonicum*. Chin. J. Schistosomiasis Control 16, 164–167 (in Chinese).
Lin, Z.C., Xu, D.M., Tao, H.Q., Zhu, M.D., Chen, Z.P., 1994. Susceptibility of *Oncomelania* to infection of *schistosoma japonicum* from Zhenjiang and other places. Chin. J. Schistosomiasis Control 6, 140–143 (in Chinese).
Liu, L., Yang, G.J., Zhu, H.R., Yang, K., Ai, L., 2014. Knowledge of, attitudes towards, and practice relating to schistosomiasis in two subtypes of a mountainous region of the People's Republic of China. Infect. Dis. Poverty 3, 16.
Liu, X.P., Wang, T.P., Wang, Q.J., Yin, X.M., Zhou, L., Wang, F.F., Wang, Y., Fang, G.R., 2013. Infection status of schistosomiasis japonica in marshland and regions. Chin. J. Pathog. Bio. 8, 445–447 (in Chinese).

Liu, Y., Zhou, Y.B., Li, R.Z., Wan, J.J., Yang, Y., Qiu, D.C., Zhong, B., 2016. Epidemiological features and control effectiveness of schistosomiasis in mountainous and hilly region of the People's Republic of China. Adv. Parasitol. 92.

Liu, Y.H., Li, B.G., Yin, G.L., Li, Y.L., Luo, B.R., Mu, L.S., Li, W.B., Su, M.Y., Li, G.B., Xiong, K., 2007. Field study on molluscicidal effects of Rongbao and Rongya against *Oncomelania hupensis* in Yunnan. Parasit. Infect. Dis. 5, 41–42 (in Chinese).

Lu, D.B., Wang, T.P., Rudge, J.W., Donnelly, C.A., Fang, G.R., Webster, J.P., 2009. Evolution in a multi-host parasite: chronobiological circadian rhythm and population genetics of *Schistosoma japonicum* cercariae indicates contrasting definitive host reservoirs by habitat. Int. J. Parasitol. 39, 1581–1588.

Lu, G.L., Wei, W.Y., Li, G.P., Xia, M., Yang, G.F., Zhao, Z.Y., 2006. Observation on long-term field molluscicidal effects Rongbao. Pract. Prev. Med. 13, 1462–1464 (in Chinese).

Ma, W., Liao, W.G., Feng, S.X., 2011. Hydrological Effects Mechanism and Risk Assessment Methods of Schistosomiasis Transmission. China Water & Power Press, Beijing.

Mao, S.B., 1990. The Biology of *Schistosoma* and Prevention of Schistosomiasis. People's Medical Publishing House, Beijing.

Mao, S.B., Li, L., 1954. Notes on the classification of the *Oncomelania* snail hosts *Schistosoma japonicum*. Acta Zool. Sin. 6, 1–14 (in Chinese).

Mao, Y., Zhong, B., Yang, Y., Xu, L., Qian, X.H., Chen, L., Wan, X.X., Tan, B.F., Deng, Q.H., Wang, Z.X., et al., 2010. Evaluation of water engineering project for schistosomiasis control in Meishan and Guanghan in Sichuan 2007–2008. Parasit. Dis. Infect. Dis. 8, 22–26 (in Chinese).

McManus, D.P., Gray, D.J., Li, Y., Feng, Z., Williams, G.M., Stewart, D., Rey-Ladino, J., Ross, A.G., 2010. Schistosomiasis in the People's Republic of China: the era of the three Gorges dam. Clin. Microbiol. Rev. 23, 442–466.

Peng, X.W., Wang, J.S., Rong, X.B., Wang, S.H., He, L.C., Fu, Z.Y., 2007. Epidemic characteristics and factors of schistosomiasis in four-lakes region of Hubei province. J. Public Health Prev. Med. 18, 66–69 (in Chinese).

Peng, Z.H., 2001. Study on the beaches snails outwipping forest ecological engineering. Eng. Sci. 3, 12–16 (in Chinese).

Qing, S.T., Hu, S.G., Zhang, Q., Zhu, C.X., Qiu, B.G., Wang, L.P., Guo, Y.X., Liu, G.H., Shi, L.L., 2003. For snail control and schistosomiasis control with the comprehensive agricultural development. Chin. J. Vet. Parasit. 11, 32–34 (in Chinese).

Qiu, J., Li, R.D., Xu, X.J., Yu, C.H., Xia, X., Hong, X.C., Chang, B.R., Yi, F.J., Shi, Y.Y., 2014. Identifying determinants of *Oncomelania hupensis* habitats and assessing the effects of environmental control strategies in the plain regions with the waterway network of China at the microscale. Int. J. Environ. Res. Public Health 11, 6571–6585.

Seto, E.Y., Wu, W., Liu, H.Y., Chen, H.G., Hubbard, A., Holt, A., Davis, G.M., 2008. Impact of changing water levels and weather on *Oncomelania* hupensis hupensis populations, the snail host of *Schistosoma japonicum*, downstream of the Three Gorges Dam. Ecohealth 5, 149–158.

Shi, L., Li, W., Wu, F., Zhang, J.F., Yang, K., Zhou, X.N., 2016. Epidemiological features and control progress of schistosomiasis in waterway-network region in P.R. China. Adv. Parasitol. 92.

Su, J., Zhou, F., Lu, D.B., 2013. A circular analysis of chronobiology of *Schistosoma japonicum* cercarial emergence from hilly areas of Anhui, China. Exp. Parasitol. 135, 421–425.

Su, W., He, L.C., Yuan, M.Z., Peng, X.W., Zhao, Y.S., 2011. Distribution of infected snails in marshland and lake regions. J. Pathog. Biol. 6, 606–608 (in Chinese).

Sun, H.C., Liu, X.L., Liu, R.H., 2010. Research on environmental biosafety of "Luo-wei" powder (TDS) plant molluscicide in 4 percent. J. Yangtze River Sci. Res. Ins. 27, 102–104. +108 (in Chinese).

Sun, L.P., Zhou, X.N., Hong, Q.B., Huang, Y.X., Wu, F., Yang, K., 2004. Effect of *Schistosoma japonicum* infection on *Oncomelania hupensis*. Chin. J. Schistosomiasis Control 16, 265–268 (in Chinese).

Sun, L.P., Zhou, X.N., Hong, Q.B., Yang, G.Q., Xi, W.P., Dai, J.R., Wu, F., 2001. The preliminary study on the crowing degree day (GDD) of *Schistosoma japonicum* developing the intermediate snail host, *Oncomelania hupensis*. Chin. J. Zoonoses 17, 80–82 (in Chinese).

Tambo, E., Ai, L., Zhou, X., Chen, J.H., Hu, W., Bergquist, R., Guo, J.G., Utzinger, J., Tanner, M., Zhou, X.N., 2014. Surveillance-response systems: the key to elimination of tropical diseases. Infect. Dis. Poverty 3, 17.

Tang, M., Xiong, Y., Jia, T.W., Wu, Z.S., Zhou, M.H., 2015. Analysis of controlled trial of fish toxicity on TDS and niclosamide in snail control. Parasit. Dis. Infect. Dis. 13, 1–5 (in Chinese).

Tang, W.J., Sun, H.C., Liu, R.H., 2010. Efficiency trials of Plant molluscicide "Luo-wei" on killing *Oncomelania hupensis*. J. Yangtze River Sci. Res. Ins. 27, 105–108 (in Chinese).

Tao, H.Y., Xia, A., Zhao, Y.M., Jiang, J., 2012. Effect and cost-benefit of *Oncomelania* snail control by plowing and planting in Jiaobei Beach of Zhenjiang City. Chin. J. Schistosomiasis Control 24, 576–578 (in Chinese).

Tian, Y., Wang, T.P., Wang, Q.Z., Lv, D.B., Yin, X.M., Zhou, L., Wang, Z.L., Wang, F.F., Wang, Y., Zhang, L.S., 2011. Susceptibilities of *Oncomelania hupensis* snails to *Schistosoma japonicum* miracidia from different hosts. Chin. J. Schistosomiasis Control 23, 446–448 (in Chinese).

Tong, Q.B., Chen, R., Zhang, Y., Yang, G.J., Kumagai, T., Furushima-Shimogawara, R., Lou, D., Yang, K., Wen, L.Y., Lu, S.H., et al., 2015. A new surveillance and response tool: risk map of infected *Oncomelania hupensis* detected by loop-mediated isothermal amplification (LAMP) from pooled samples. Acta Trop. 141, 170–177.

Wang, C., Yu, C.X., Ji, M.J., Song, L.J., Yin, X.R., Qian, C.Y., Wang, J., Wu, G.L., 2010. Use of loop-mediated isothermal amplification (LAMP) to detect whole blood samples infected with *Schistosoma japonicum*. J. Pathog. Biol. 5, 749–753 (in Chinese).

Wang, C.Z., Lu, D.B., Guo, C.X., Li, Y., Gao, Y.M., Bian, C.R., Su, J., 2014. Compatibility of *Schistosoma japonicum* from the hilly region and *Oncomelania hupensis hupensis* from the marshland region within Anhui, China. Parasitol. Res. 113, 4477–4484.

Wang, J.G., Liao, H.Y., Zhong, G.T., Yu, B.K., Huang, S.S., 2002. Observation on the effect of schistosomiasis through snail control by environmental modification. Chin. J. Schistosomiasis Control 14, 200–202 (in Chinese).

Wang, J.R., Wu, Y.K., Gao, N.X., Zhang, H.F., Zhu, P.H., Ma, Q.Q., Xu, N.H., 2013. Evaluation of schistosomiasis surveillance after blocking of its transmission in Jiaxing, Zhejiang, 1995–2012. Dis. Surveill. 28, 567–569 (in Chinese).

Wang, L.D., 2006a. Process and Prospect of Schistosomiasis Control in China. People's Medical Publishing House, Beijing.

Wang, W., Li, H.J., Li, Y.Z., Xing, Y.T., Wei, J.Y., Dai, J.R., Liang, Y.S., 2011. Impact on susceptibility to miracidium of *Schistosoma japonicum* of *Oncomelania* in different density and at different distance: a simulated field study. Parasit. Infect. Dis. 9, 4–6 (in Chinese).

Wang, X.Y., He, J., Yang, K., Liang, S., 2016. Applications of spatial technology in schistosomiasis control programme in the People's Republic of China. Adv. Parasitol. 92.

Wang, Y.R., Zhou, J.X., Zhou, Z.X., Sun, Q.X., 2007. Time-space changing regularity of dominant water factors and snail distribution density in beaches, Dongting Lake. J. Huazhong Agr. Univers. 26, 859–864 (in Chinese).

Wang, Z.C., 2006b. Cost-effective analysis of eliminating *Oncomelania* with 4% niclosamide ethanolamine salt. J. Public Health Prev. Med. 17, 40–43 (in Chinese).

Wei, F.H., Xu, X.J., Liu, J.B., Yang, X.X., 2001. Study on the distribution of *Oncomelania hupensis* snail in irrigation schemes of Jianghan Plain. Chin. J. Schistosomiasis Control 13, 31–35 (in Chinese).

Wen, L.Y., Yan, X.L., Zhang, J.F., Li, L.S., Lin, L.J., Huang, S.Y., Li, L., Liang, Y.S., 2011. Strategy of solidification and surveillance for schistosomiasis in transmission interrupted provinces in China. Chin. J. Schistosomiasis Control 23, 18–22 (in Chinese).
Wu, J.Y., Zhou, Y.B., Li, L.H., Zheng, S.B., Liang, S., Coatsworth, A., Ren, G.H., Song, X.X., He, Z., Cai, B., et al., 2014. Identification of optimum scopes of environmental factors for snails using spatial analysis techniques in Dongting Lake Region, China. Parasit. Vectors. 7, 216.
Xia, J., Yuan, Y., Xu, X.J., Wei, F.H., Li, G.L., Liu, M., Li, J.Q., Chen, R.J., Zhou, Z.P., Nie, S.F., 2014. Evaluating the effect of a novel molluscicide in the endemic schistosomiasis japonica area of China. Int. J. Environ. Res. Public Health 11, 10406–10418.
Xiao, R., Wang, X.L., Wang, H.L., 2009. The application of remote sensing and geographic information system technology on the study of snail distribution in Honghu Wetland. Wetl. Sci. 7, 175–180 (in Chinese).
Xin, X.F., Zhang, J., Bo, S.Y., Wang, G.Z., Wang, G.Z., 2006. Quality evaluation for immunological diagnosis kits of schistosomiasis. Chin. J. Schistosomiasis Control 18, 119–121 (in Chinese).
Xiong, C.R., Yin, X.R., Song, L.J., Shen, S., Wang, J., Gao, H., Liu, X., Yu, C.X., Yang, K., 2014. Comparison of the effectiveness of loop-mediated DNA amplification (LAMP) and microscopic dissection at detecting snails infected with *Schistotoma japonicum*. Chin. J. Pathog. Bio. 9, 1084–1087 (in Chinese).
Xu, J., Steinman, P., Maybe, D., Zhou, X.N., Lv, S., Li, S.Z., Peeling, R., 2016. Evolution of the national schistosomiasis control programmes in the People's Republic of China. Adv. Parasitol. 92.
Xu, X.J., Ni, C.H., 1987. Observation on the difference in susceptibility of *Oncomelania* snails to different isolates of *Schistosoma japonicum*. Chin. J. Parasitol. Parasit. Dis. 1, 25–28.
Xu, Y.X., Chu, C.Z., Wu, Y.L., Cheng, S.J., Gao, F.H., Zhang, G.H., Cheng, J., Wang, S.W., 2010. Relationship between distribution of infected snails and transmission of acute schistosomiasis in hilly regions. Chin. J. Schistosomiasis Control 22, 72–73 (in Chinese).
Xu, Z.Y., Zhu, Q., Shan, D.C., Wu, Y.H., You, C., Dong, M.H., He, S.Y., 1993. Further study on the relationship between the number of *Schistosoma japonicum* miracidia and the infection rate of *Oncomelania* snails. Chin. J. Schistosomiasis Control 5, 217–219 (in Chinese).
Yang, G.J., Sun, L.P., Hong, Q.B., Zhu, H.R., Yang, K., Gao, Q., Zhou, X.N., 2012. Optimizing molluscicide treatment strategies in different control stages of schistosomiasis in the People's Republic of China. Parasit. Vectors. 5, 260.
Yang, G.J., Utzinger, J., Sun, L.P., Hong, Q.B., Vounatsou, P., Tanner, M., Zhou, X.N., 2007. Effect of temperature on the development of *Schistosoma japonicum* within *Oncomelania hupensis*, and hibernation of *O. hupensis*. Parasitol. Res. 100, 695–700.
Yang, G.J., Vounatsou, P., Zhou, X.N., Tanner, M., Utzinger, J., 2005. A Bayesian-based approach for spatio-temporal modeling of county level prevalence of *Schistosoma japonicum* infection in Jiangsu province, China. Int. J. Parasitol. 35, 155–162.
Yang, K., Li, W., Sun, L.P., Huang, Y.X., Zhang, J.F., Wu, F., Hang, D.R., Steinmann, P., Liang, Y.S., 2013. Spatio-temporal analysis to identify determinants of *Oncomelania hupensis* infection with *Schistosoma japonicum* in Jiangsu province, China. Parasit. Vectors. 6, 138.
Yang, K., Wang, X.H., Yang, G.J., Wu, X.H., Qi, Y.L., Li, H.J., Zhou, X.N., 2008a. An integrated approach to identify distribution of *Oncomelania hupensis*, the intermediate host of *Schistosoma japonicum*, in a mountainous region in China. Int. J. Parasitol. 38, 1007–1016.
Yang, X.M., Chen, S.X., Xia, L., Chen, J., 2008b. Molluscicidal activity against *Oncomelania hupensis* of Ginkgo biloba. Fitoterapia 79, 250–254.

Yang, Y., Zhou, Y.B., Song, X.X., Li, S.Z., Zhong, B., Wang, T.P., Bergquist, R., Zhou, X.N., Jiang, Q.W., 2016. Integrated control strategy of schistosomiasis in the People's Republic of China: projects involving agriculture, water-conservancy, forestry, sanitation and environmental modification. Adv. Parasitol. 92.

Yin, Y.Z., Chen, K.B., Shen, H.Z., 1993. Study on emphases and method of *Oncomelania* snails monitoring after the elimination of schistosomiasis. Shanghai J. Prev. Med. 5, 43–44 (in Chinese).

Yu, C.X., Yin, X.R., Hua, W.Q., Gao, Q., 2008. Establishment of loop mediated isothermal DNA amplification for identifying *Oncomelania* snails infected with *Schistosoma japonicum*. J. Pathog. Biol. 3, 661–664. +669 (in Chinese).

Yu, C.X., Yin, X.R., Wang, J., Song, L.J., Qian, C.Y., Wu, F., He, W., Zhang, W., 2011. Creation and use of a LAMP kit to rapidly detect snails infected with *Schistosoma japonicum*. J. Pathog. Biol. 6, 121–123 (in Chinese).

Zeng, X.J., Chen, H.G., Huang, B.N., Jiang, W.S., Wan, B.P., Xie, F., Ge, J., Liu, Z.H., Hu, W.C., 2007. Causes of spread of *Oncomelania* snails and its control in Ganjiang Valley. Chin. J. Schistosomiasis Control 19, 120–123 (in Chinese).

Zhang, J.S., Wang, Z.F., Zhao, C.Y., Meng, Y., 2007a. Effect of comprehensive measures for schistosomiasis control in marshland and lake regions. Chin. J. Schistosomiasis Control 19, 306–307 (in Chinese).

Zhang, L.J., Li, S.Z., Wen, L.Y., Lin, D.D., Abe, E.M., Zhu, R., Du, Y., Lv, S., Xu, J., Rollinson, D., et al., 2016a. Establishment and function of schistosomiasis surveillance system towards elimination in the People's Republic of China. Adv. Parasitol. 92.

Zhang, S.Q., Sun, C.S., Wang, M., Lin, D.D., Zhou, X.N., Wang, T.P., 2016b. Epidemiological features and control effectiveness of schistosomiasis in lake and marshland region in the People's Republic of China. Adv. Parasitol. 92.

Zhang, X.D., Qi, L.H., Huang, L.L., Fei, S.M., Jiang, J.M., Wang, Z.Y., 2007b. Influences of soil environmental factors on *Oncomelania* Snail distribution in the hilly and mountainous areas. Acta Ecol. Sin. 27, 2460–2467 (in Chinese).

Zhang, X.D., Yang, X.C., Peng, Z.H., 1999. Relationships between the surviving *Oncomelania* and beaches environmental factors. Acta Ecol. Sin. 19, 265–269 (in Chinese).

Zhang, Y.K., Tao, H.Q., Liu, X.T., Shen, B.R., Zheng, J.C., Jiang, Y.M., Xu, F.H., Fan, X.L., 1989. Research on trap underwater young *Oncomelania* snails by the straw. Chin. J. Schistosomiasis Control 1, 37–38. +53 (in Chinese).

Zhang, Z.J., Bergquist, R., Chen, D.M., Yao, B.D., Wang, Z.L., Gao, J., Jiang, Q.W., 2013. Identification of parasite-host habitats in Anxiang county, Hunan Province, China based on multi-temporal China-Brazil earth resources satellite (CBERS) images. PLoS One 8, e69447.

Zhang, Z.Y., Xu, D.Z., Zhou, X.N., Zhou, Y., Liu, S.J., 2005. Remote sensing and spatial statistical analysis to predict the distribution of *Oncomelania hupensis* in the marshlands of China. Acta Trop. 96, 205–212.

Zhao, W.X., Gao, S.F., 1997. Practical Schistosomiasis. People's Medical Publishing House, Beijing.

Zheng, Q., Vanderslott, S., Jiang, B., Xu, L.L., Liu, C.S., Huo, L.L., Duan, L.P., Wu, N.B., Li, S.Z., Xia, Z.G., et al., 2013. Research gaps for three main tropical diseases in the People's Republic of China. Infect. Dis. Poverty 2, 15.

Zhou, X.N., 2005. Science on *Oncomelania* Snail. People's Medical Publishing House, Beijing.

Zhou, X.N., Li, S.Z., Liu, Q., Zhang, Y., 2009. Advances on genetics and biological characteristics of *Oncomelania hupensis*. Chin. J. Parasitol. Parasit. Dis. 27, 412–418 (in Chinese).

Zhou, X.N., Sun, N.S., Hu, X.S., Sun, L.P., Hong, Q.B., Fuentes, M., Malone, J.B., 1999. Application of geographic information systems on schistosomiasis surveillance III. Snail habitats in marshland. Chin. J. Schistosomiasis Control 11, 199–202 (in Chinese).

Zhou, X.N., Yang, K., Hong, Q.B., Sun, L.P., Yang, G.J., Liang, Y.S., Huang, Y.X., 2004. Prediction of the impact of climate warming on transmission of schistosomiasis in China. Chin. J. Parasitol. Parasit. Dis. 22, 262–265 (in Chinese).
Zhou, Y.B., Yang, M.X., Zhao, G.M., 2007. *Oncomelania hupensis* (Gastropoda:Rissooidea): intermediate host of *Schistosoma japonicum* in China: genetics and molecular phylogeny based on amplified fragment length polymorphisms. Malacologia 49, 367–382.
Zhou, Y.B., Zhao, G.M., Peng, W.X., Wei, J.G., Jiang, Q.W., 2006. Study on morphologic quantitative characteristics of *Oncomelania hupensis* III. Morphologic variations and their spatial correlation among snail populations. Chin. J. Schistosomiasis Control 18, 241–246 (in Chinese).
Zhu, C.F., Fang, Y.H., Wang, J.S., 2011. Research on influence of TGP impoundment on schistosomiasis in beach areas of middle Yangtze River and Dongting Lake. Yangtze River 42, 12–15 (in Chinese).
Zhu, C.F., Zhang, S.Q., 2012. Research on quantitative evaluation on snail elimination effect by water conservancy structure measures. Yangtze River 43, 72–75 (in Chinese).
Zhu, C.F., Zhang, S.Q., Cai, K.P., 2009. Research on assessment criteria of schistosomiasis prevention related with water conservancy in the Yangtze River basin. Yangtze River 40, 3–6 (in Chinese).
Zhu, D.P., Yin, J.Y., 1986. Enlarged field trials of bromoacetamide against *Oncomelania* snails. Chin. J. Parasitol. Parasit. Dis. 4, 90–92 (in Chinese).
Zhu, H.M., Xiang, S., Yang, K., Wu, X.H., Zhou, X.N., 2008. Three Gorges Dam and its impact on the potential transmission of schistosomiasis in regions along the Yangtze River. Ecohealth 5, 137–148.
Zuo, Y.P., Sun, D.K., Huang, Y.X., Gao, Y., Guo, J.H., She, G.S., Gao, J.B., Huang, D.R., Ma, Y.C., Zheng, B., et al., 2010. Study on surveillance and early-warning system of schistosomiasis in first phase of east route of the South-to-North Water Diversion ProjectII. Surveillance of *Oncomelania hupensis* and schistosomiasis. Chin. J. Schistosomiasis Control 22, 420–424 (in Chinese).

CHAPTER NINE

Integrated Control Strategy of Schistosomiasis in The People's Republic of China: Projects Involving Agriculture, Water Conservancy, Forestry, Sanitation and Environmental Modification

Y. Yang*[,§,¶], Y.-B. Zhou*[,§,¶,1], X.-X. Song*[,§,¶], S.-Z. Li[§,||,#], B. Zhong**, T.-P. Wang[§§,|||], R. Bergquist[¶¶], X.-N. Zhou[||,#,§], Q.-W. Jiang*[,§,¶]

*Department of Epidemiology, School of Public Health, Fudan University, Shanghai, The People's Republic of China

[§]Key Laboratory of Public Health Safety, Ministry of Education, Shanghai, The People's Republic of China

[¶]Center for Tropical Disease Research, Shanghai, The People's Republic of China

[||]WHO Collaborating Centre for Tropical Diseases, Shanghai, The People's Republic of China

[#]National Institute of Parasitic Diseases, Chinese Center for Disease Control and Prevention, Shanghai, The People's Republic of China

**Sichuan Provincial Center for Disease Control and Prevention, Chengdu, The People's Republic of China

[§§]Anhui Institute of Parasitic Disease, Hefei, The People's Republic of China

[¶¶]Geospatial Health, University of Naples Federico II, Naples, Italy

[|||]Anhui Provincial Institute of Schistosomiasis Control, Hefei, Anhui Province, The People's Republic of China

[1]Corresponding author: E-mail: ybzhou@fudan.edu.cn

Contents

Advances in Parasitology, Volume 92
ISSN 0065-308X
http://dx.doi.org/10.1016/bs.apar.2016.02.004

Abstract

Among the three major schistosome species infecting human beings, *Schistosoma japonicum* is the only endemic species in The People's Republic of China. Schistosomiasis is endemic in 78 countries and regions and poses a severe threat to public health and socioeconomic development. Through more than 60 years of hard work and endeavour, The People's Republic of China has made considerable achievements and reduced the morbidity and prevalence of this disease to the lowest level ever recorded, especially since the introduction of the new integrated control strategy in 2004. This review illustrates the strategies implemented by giving successful examples of schistosomiasis control from the different types of remaining endemic areas. The challenge to control or eliminate *S. japonicum* is analysed in order to provide useful information to policy makers and scientists.

1. INTRODUCTION

Major successes in the control of *Schistosoma japonicum* have been achieved in the last 60 years, yet infections due to this helminth parasite remain an important public health issue in The People's Republic of China (Chen, 2014). The current national control programme involves a comprehensive strategy, which is adapted to different socioecological settings, aiming at multiple transmission pathways. This chapter reviews the components of the integrated control strategy, summarizes our experience and understanding of the complexity of schistosomiasis control and paves the ground for future elimination of this disease, which has been a scourge for many millions of people in The People's Republic of China for thousands of years.

2. BACKGROUND

Schistosomiasis japonica remains a major public health issue and a significant cause of morbidity in The People's Republic of China (Utzinger et al., 2005; Xu et al., 2015; Yang et al., 2014; Zhou et al., 2005). Two features of the *S. japonicum* life cycle distinguish it from other forms of schistosomiasis: first, *Oncomelania hupensis*, the only intermediate host snail of *S. japonicum*, is amphibious (Li et al., 2016). These snails breed in water networks (canals and lakes), marshlands and a variety of microhabitats in hilly and mountainous environments, which complicates control. Second, more than 40 mammalian species, including dogs, pigs and cattle can serve as reservoir hosts, which greatly adds to the complexity of control and elimination (Liu et al., 2016; Wang et al., 2008b).

Although schistosomiasis is generally referred to as a neglected tropical disease, this is not the case in The People's Republic of China. During the past six decades, the control of this disease has been regarded as a top priority and the Chinese Government has launched a series of control programmes (McManus et al., 2010; Utzinger et al., 2005; Yang et al., 2014; Zhou et al., 2005). This sustained effort has resulted in a substantial reduction in the prevalence of human *S. japonicum* infection. By the end of 2004, the estimated human population infected with schistosomes was 726,000, compared to approximately 11.6 million infected in the early 1950s (Zhou et al., 2005, 2007a). The number of provinces in which this disease is still rampant has dropped from 12 to 7, with 5 formerly endemic provinces reaching the national criteria of transmission interruption in the last century (Xu et al., 2016; Zhou et al., 2007a). Despite this achievement and continued strong control effort, progress has stalled (Utzinger et al., 2005; Zhang et al., 2012b). Recent experiences warn that reductions in infection and morbidity may be transient. Resurgence of schistosomiasis infection was noted after the cessation of the World Bank Loan Project (WBLP) on schistosomiasis control in 2002 (Liu et al., 2013a; Seto et al., 2011; Zhang et al., 2012b). National surveys of schistosomiasis in The People's Republic of China show that the prevalence of *S. japonicum* in humans did not substantially change from 1995 (4.9%) to 2004 (5.1%) in the lake and marshland regions. The situation in other endemic areas of southern China is similar (Zhang et al., 2016a; Zhou et al., 2007a). More than 80% of current cases are found in the lake and marshland regions of Hunan, Hubei, Jiangxi, Anhui and Jiangsu Provinces with vast areas of *O. hupensis* habitats, where the control of schistosomiasis transmission has proven particularly challenging (Wang et al., 2009a). In the hilly and mountainous areas of Sichuan and Yunnan Provinces, *S. japonicum* has raged without limit for years (Liu et al., 2016; Spear et al., 2004). Compared to the other endemic provinces of The People's Republic of China, these regions are sparsely populated and underdeveloped. Although they also have lower snail population densities, the variable and intricate topography makes control difficult (Lu et al., 2013). The intractable situation here, in particular, underscores the urgent need to better understand the transmission dynamics following chemotherapy-based control so that re-emergence can be avoided and improvement in human well-being maintained (Zhou et al., 2005).

The past approach to reduce the rate of schistosomiasis infection through the use of simultaneous chemotherapy for humans and domestic cattle has only been temporarily effective as chemotherapy alone will not eliminate schistosomiasis (Bergquist et al., 2005; Colley et al., 2014; Useh, 2013; Zhou et al., 2007b). Reinfection contributes to a high proportion of cases of schistosomiasis in both humans and domestic animals and, besides, long-term repeated chemotherapy has led to poor compliance and decreased efficacy (Liu et al., 2014; Utzinger et al., 2005). In addition, the use of chemical molluscicides or modifications of *O. hupensis* habitats to control snail populations have resulted in environmental pollution and ecological damage (Colley et al., 2014; Lin et al., 2007). Other factors, such as the recent complex changes in the environment due to climate change, frequent flooding and population migration, have compromised recent efforts to control schistosomiasis. As a result, more residents have become infected and the habitats of *Oncomelania* snails have increased (Li et al., 2007; McManus et al., 2010; Zhou et al., 2008).

In 2004, the State Council of The People's Republic of China established two targets for the National Schistosomiasis Control Programme: (1) to reduce human infection prevalence by 2008 in all endemic counties to less than 5%, including 110 counties that had a prevalence exceeding 5%; and (2) to reduce human prevalence to less than 1% by 2015 (Utzinger et al., 2005; Zhou et al., 2007a). The Work Plan for the Mid-and Long-term of National Schistosomiasis Control Programme from 2004 to 2015 was released in the same year (Liu et al., 2013a). On the basis of experience and lessons from past schistosomiasis control practices with respect to the endemic status and zoonotic nature of *S. japonicum* in various and situations and ecologies, a new, comprehensive control strategy was developed aiming at interrupting the transmission pathways (Wang et al., 2009a) (Fig. 1). In line with the introduction of this new control strategy, the first pilot study was implemented in

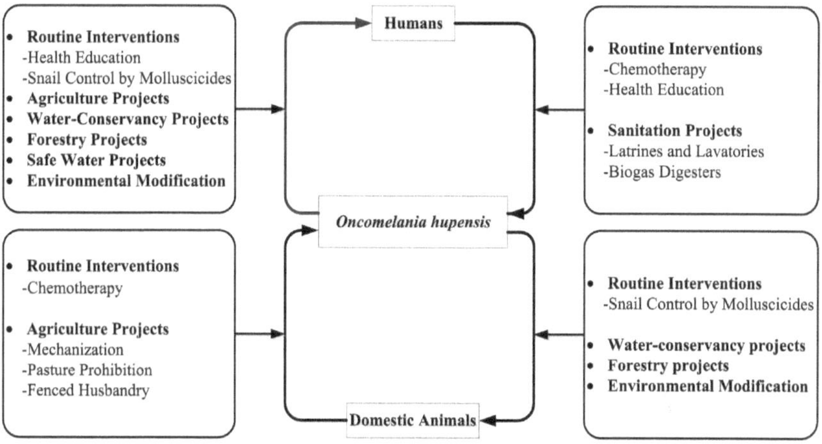

Figure 1 A sketch of *Schistosoma japonicum* transmission pathways and control projects included in the integrated control strategy in The People's Republic of China.

two villages in Jinxian County, Jiangxi Province, in 2005. Subsequently, the strategy was undertaken in another four pilot regions, ie, Anxiang County of Hunan Province, Hanchuan City of Hubei Province, Guichi District of Anhui Province and Puge County of Sichuan Province. After accumulating field-based evidence and further improving the strategy in light of gained experience, the new strategy was scaled up and recognized as the national control approach. It involves a multicomponent approach founded on routine interventions (ie, simultaneous chemotherapy of humans and cattle, snail control by molluscicides and health education). Apart from routine interventions, the comprehensive control strategy covers the following projects: agriculture (ie, removal of bovines and their replacement with mechanized equipment, special rules for pasture and fenced husbandry), water conservancy (ie, building of dam reservoirs, management of lakes, rivers and canals, etc.), sanitation (ie, provision of lavatories, latrines, biogas digesters, piped water/safe wells, etc.), forestry and land management. Successful establishment and implementation of this integrated approach means efficient intersectoral collaboration, especially between departments in charge of agriculture, water conservation, forestry, natural resources, communication, land and education (Utzinger et al., 2005; Wang et al., 2008b).

In this review, we summarize the various approaches on agriculture, water conservancy, forestry, sanitation and safe water and land environmental management describing five national pilot projects. We also provide a discussion about the challenges of the current control strategy of schistosomiasis in The People's Republic of China.

3. COMPONENT PROJECTS OF THE INTEGRATED CONTROL STRATEGY OF SCHISTOSOMIASIS

3.1 Agriculture

Current agriculture projects for schistosomiasis control comprise a battery of interventions, including removal of bovines and their replacement with mechanic equipment, rules for pasture, fenced husbandry and paddy-upland rotation, etc. Bovines are recognized as the main *S. japonicum* infection source in The People's Republic of China and they contribute to an estimated 75–90% of the egg contamination in the endemic areas (Cao et al., 2016; Hong et al., 2013a; Zhang et al., 2016b). Considering the fact that about 80% of snail infections originate from cattle, the reduction of this source of infection plays a key role in any integrated control strategy of *S. japonicum* (Gray et al., 2008; Wang et al., 2008b; Xu et al., 2015). Promotion of rearing livestock in pens, agricultural mechanization (phasing out water buffaloes tilling the earth for motorized equipment) and grazing prohibition in snail-infested grasslands are key ingredients of present schistosomiasis control strategies (Hong et al., 2013a; Wang et al., 2009a). Raising bovines behind fences and preventing domestic animals from grazing in close contact with *O. hupensis* snails would block the transmission from already infected livestock to the snails, thus interrupting the next step of the transmission of *S. japonicum* to humans. The introduction of farm machinery also reduces the human infection risk by lowering the likelihood of water contact. Pengshan County removed 97.6% of their bovines in 2006 and became the first bovine-free county in Sichuan Province. Due to this intervention, the rate of infection with *S. japonicum* in humans decreased from 3.7% in 2005 to 0.4% in 2006 (Min, 2008). Studies have shown that the prevalence rates in both humans and cattle decreased significantly after implementation of the measures described above together with mass drug administration using praziquantel of both villagers and bovines and molluscicide treatment of snail-infested areas (Cao et al., 2014; Chen et al., 2006, 2014; Hong et al., 2013a; Hu et al., 2010; Liu et al., 2013b; Xiang et al., 2013; Zhu et al., 2011). Yet, complete removal of bovines is hardly feasible since they play an important role in agricultural production and are major sources of income in the mountainous regions of the Sichuan and Yunnan Provinces (Zhong et al., 2011). In this situation, emphasis was focused on grazing prohibition in snail-infested grasslands and fenced husbandry. These simpler measures have also resulted in a declining trend of infection rates in humans (Li et al., 2012a; Yang et al., 2009; Yi Huo et al., 2009). To implement these interventions, local governments provide funding and subsidies for farmers to remove cattle from the grasslands and instead purchase mechanized farm equipment such as tractors (Wang et al., 2009a).

Additionally, in rice paddy fields, where *O. hupensis* is widely distributed, farmers cannot avoid contact with water contaminated with schistosome cercariae. Therefore, paddy-upland rotation adjusted to local conditions has been applied to reduce the snail habitats (Wang et al., 1997). Predators and biological competitors have also been used to control snail populations and been used together with construction of dykes and fish ponds (Colley et al., 2014; Rollinson et al., 2013; Yuan et al., 2005).

Increasing crop production through irrigation takes place across the globe at different scales. A close correlation between the distribution of *O. hupensis* and water canal systems has been observed in endemic regions and frequent human water contact occurs along the canals and ditches resulting in increased numbers of schistosomiasis patients (Yuan et al., 2005). If only water resource development and management could be combined with sound snail control measures (Dong et al., 2013; Huang et al., 2012; Xu et al., 2014), schistosomiasis control would yield twice the result with half the effort. Therefore, environmental considerations should be included in discussions at the very beginning when designing irrigation schemes (Xu et al., 2010).

3.2 Water conservancy

The role of water bodies (lakes, rivers of various size, artificial irrigation schemes, water reservoirs and canals) in the transmission of schistosomiasis cannot be overestimated (McManus et al., 2010; Seto et al., 2007; Steinmann et al., 2006). Water not only secures the survival of the intermediate host snails, but provides also the opportunity for *Schistosoma* cercariae to develop and eventually penetrate the human skin at water contact. Water bodies in endemic areas are frequently contaminated by the faeces of humans and other mammalian hosts infected with *S. japonicum* (Colley et al., 2014; Useh, 2013).

Construction of dam reservoirs for the generation of electricity and irrigation systems as well as for provision of drinking water attracts snails and expands their habitats and are therefore potential emerging schistosome transmission sites (Chen et al., 2010, 2013; Li et al., 2012b; McManus et al., 2010; Xu et al., 2010). For this reason, strategies to minimize such negative effects for schistosomiasis control should be integral parts in the planning and implementation of future water projects. The expansion of snail habitats can, to some extent, be controlled by health impact assessment and subsequent health risk management measures during the planning and design phases of water conservancy projects (Steinmann et al., 2006; Xu et al., 2010; Yuan et al., 2005). It is thus possible to manage water resources without increasing snail populations that would exacerbate the schistosomiasis situation.

Modification of rivers banks and lake shores has led to a remarkable improvement in schistosomiasis situation in The People's Republic of China (Chen et al., 2010; McManus et al., 2010). Both the banks of major rivers traversing the Chinese plains and those of the smaller streams of the hilly regions provide breeding spots for *O. hupensis*. The snails are confined to an area located approximately 1 m above and 1 m below the water level. Rivers and canals have been restructured by straightening, deepening and cementing the banks to discourage growth of aquatic vegetation and thus increase the water flow. Construction of small reservoirs and ponds in the hilly and mountainous regions has proved effective in snail control there (Dong et al., 2008b). Burying the snails under a thick layer of soil through hydraulic reclamation is highly effective and even more so when combined with the use of molluscicides. In addition, measures such as changing water levels and raising the land of islets by adding sand from the surrounding bottom reduce snail habitats and populations (Xu et al., 2010; Zhu et al., 2009).

There is no doubt that irrigation canals or ditches play a significant role in snail breeding, but the situation can be improved by concrete lining of ditch and canal banks, digging and dredging, including sinks and other facilities that block snail spread when new water ways are constructed (Huang et al., 2012; Su et al., 2004; Xu et al., 2010) (Fig. 2). Snail sinks slow down water flow and create suitable conditions for the deposition of *Oncomelania* snails so as to prevent their spread into irrigation systems (Ding et al., 2008; Jiang and Wang, 2012; Su et al., 2004; Zhu et al., 2014) (Fig. 3), while chemical molluscicides are used to kill snails that collect in the snail sinks (Jiang and Wang, 2012; Zhu et al., 2014). The use of concrete or tile drains reduces surface water and control snail habitats and populations in the irrigation systems in this way (Wei et al., 2004). Alteration of water levels through intermittent drying out of impoundments and irrigation canals or ditches would probably have an additional, beneficial effect. Although environmental management is useful, a lasting effect requires far-reaching changes and provision for maintenance of snail control facilities and

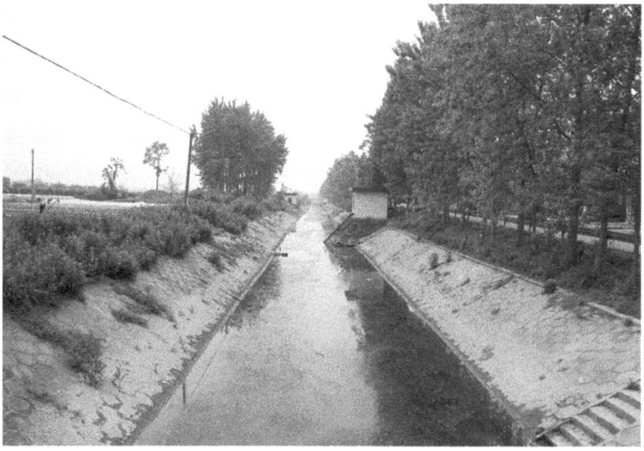

Figure 2 Concrete irrigation systems for environmental management preventing the establishment of *Oncomelania* snail habitats.

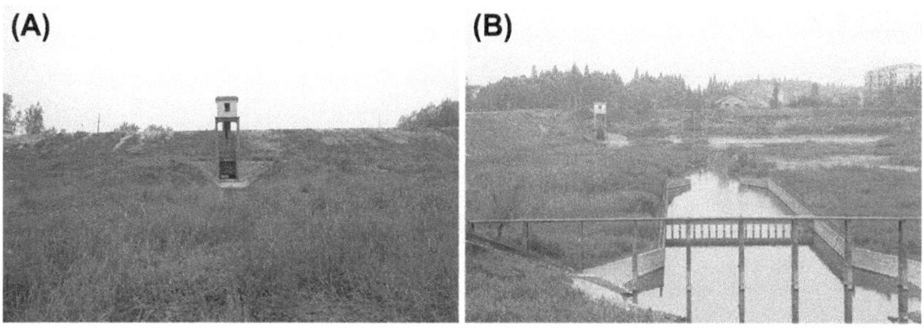

Figure 3 Restructured water connections (A) and pools (B) preventing snails to spread from the outside to the inside of embankments.

equipment (Li et al., 2016). In the absence of maintenance of instituted constructions, the intermediate host snails may reoccur with an increasing density, even in cemented ditches (Ding et al., 2013; Xu et al., 2010).

In general, environmental management does work in most settings, but constructions must be kept in good condition and adjusted to the local situation in order to guarantee permanent effects (Ding et al., 2013; Xu et al., 2010; Zhu et al., 2009).

3.3 Forestry

Snail control combined with forestry projects is an essential component of the integrated control strategy of schistosomiasis, both in the lake and marshland regions and the mountain areas in The People's Republic of China (Jiang et al., 2013; Liu et al., 2011; Zhang et al., 2006, 2012a). Places along lakes and rivers, where effective control of the water edge cannot easily be achieved, have attracted attention as they constitute risk areas. To deal with this situation, ecological engineering for snail control and schistosomiasis prevention has been instituted (Fig. 4). The practice of planting fast growing and adapting trees such as Chinese ash, Chinese tallow, poplar and willow, etc., leads to changes in soil temperature, humidity, pH values and vegetation density, which make the land less susceptible to *O. hupensis* (Zhang et al., 2006, 2013). Moreover, certain chemicals in the fallen leaves of these trees are toxic to *Oncomelania* snails (Sun and Peng, 2013; Yang et al., 2011; Zhang et al., 2006). Agroforestry or intercropping is a land management system in which crops are grown among lines of trees. It combines both agricultural and forestry technologies to create more diverse, productive and sustainable land-use programmes (Hong and Wang, 2012; Liu et al., 2011; Meng et al., 2012; Tang et al., 2011). Through a complex array of carefully selected trees and crops, these environmental management measures forge a forest ecosystem which counteracts the growth of *Oncomelania* snails, thus lowering the risk for schistosomiasis infection (Huang et al., 2011; Tang et al., 2011; Zhang et al., 2006, 2013). However, attention must be paid to the distance between lines of trees to make room for discharge of flood water and intercropping. A distance of approximately 10 m should be kept between the trees and the river banks in case of possible damage (Sun et al., 2006; Zhang et al., 2006) (Fig. 4). Both trees and crops

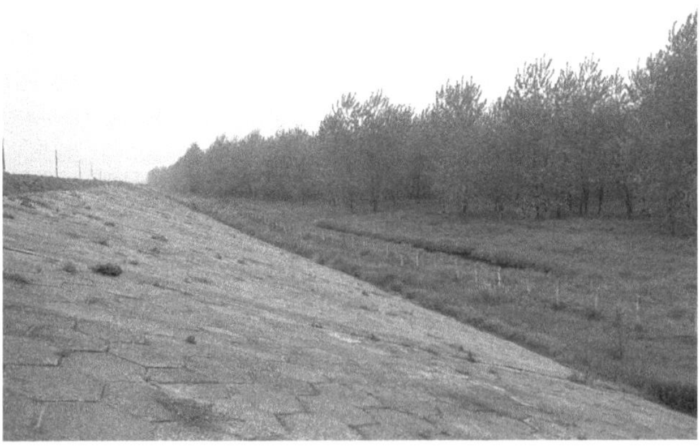

Figure 4 Environmental management involving forestation and cemented river banks reduce snail habitats. Fences have been installed to prevent animals from grazing in grasslands where *Oncomelania* snails are present.

should be chosen carefully according to environmental and climatic conditions. In addition, buffer areas surrounding the planted forests are designed to reduce human activities in heavily endemic areas. This reduces human and bovine water contact and risk for infection (Zhang et al., 2006). As for snail control in wetlands and wildlife as well as nature reserves, epidemic surveillance has been enhanced and facilities constructed to stop the diffusion of snails. Warning signs have been erected to warn people of the danger of schistosomiasis infection in endemic regions.

3.4 Sanitation and safe water

The provision of safe water supply, sanitation and hygiene (WASH) is a critical component of sustainable schistosomiasis control (Campbell et al., 2014). Human excreta are the main source of bacterial and viral agents causing diarrhoea through contamination of natural and artificial water bodies. Given the presence of the intermediate host snails, untreated human waste completes the schistosomiasis transmission cycle (Colley et al., 2014; Wang et al., 2009a). For this reason, an appropriately constructed sanitation infrastructure that ensures safe disposal of human and domestic animal excreta, especially bovine faeces, is vital for schistosomiasis control (Dong et al., 2008a; Gao et al., 2009). Household lavatories, latrines with triple compartment tanks (Fig. 5) and biogas digesters can stem contamination of freshwater sources by infected individuals and are therefore promoted and built in rural and endemic regions (Remais et al., 2009; Wang et al., 2009a) (Fig. 6). Biogas systems produce methane from human and animal waste providing access to clean and renewable energy, and studies have demonstrated that anaerobic biogas digesters can destroy *S. japonicum* eggs through chemical inactivation and removal through sedimentation (Carlton et al., 2012; Remais et al., 2009). Other benefits include reduced greenhouse gas emissions, improved air quality in rural kitchens and increased grain output through improving soil quality by organic fertilization (Lansing et al., 2008; Remais et al., 2009). Fishermen's boats have been equipped with containers for human waste, so that it can be disposed of on land instead of in the water (Gao et al., 2009; Wang et al., 2009a). These measures have received funding by local governments and the provision of improved sanitation by safe water projects and proper treatment of human and animal waste has proven effective in endemic regions in The People's Republic of China (Dong et al., 2008a; Gao et al., 2009; Zhang et al., 2005).

Indisputably, water is irreplaceable in the transmission of schistosomiasis (Useh, 2013). In rural and poor agricultural communities without piped

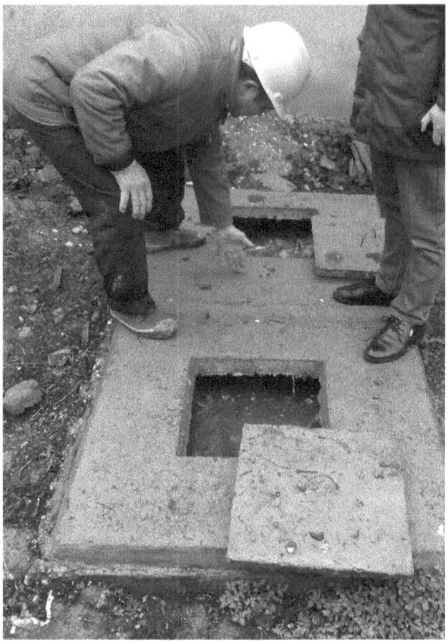

Figure 5 Triple compartment sewage facilities reduce schistosomiasis transmission by inactivating schistosome eggs.

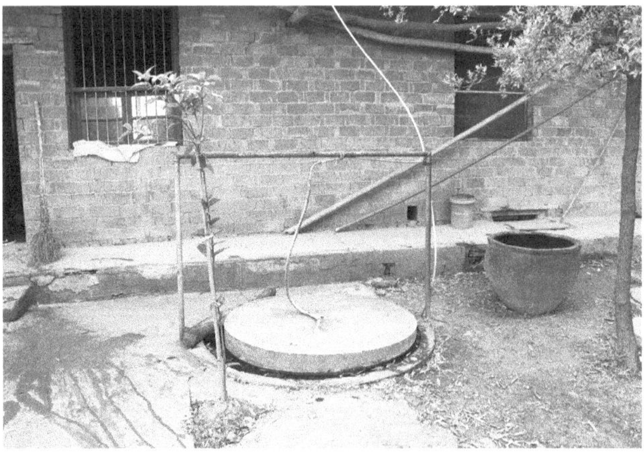

Figure 6 A household biogas digester, an important innovation that prevents water contamination from infected individuals and domestic animals.

water, residents depend on local streams or natural pools for agricultural as well as recreational and sanitary needs, thereby exposing themselves to schistosomiasis infection (McManus et al., 2010; Utzinger et al., 2005). The contamination of natural water resources through untreated disposal of human and animal waste is part of the vicious circle that translates into higher risks for local schistosomiasis infection (Colley et al., 2014). Therefore, access to safe drinking water, especially in rural and endemic areas have received exclusive priority for schistosomiasis control in The People's Republic of China (Carlton et al., 2012). Not surprisingly, studies have shown that the prevalence rates of schistosomiasis are lower where access to safe water is available than in otherwise similar areas (Zhang et al., 2005). Provision of WASH has always been advocated for schistosomiasis control by the World Health organization (WHO), but it should be emphasized that this issue is only one part of a multicomponent control strategy (Campbell et al., 2014).

3.5 Environmental modification

Oncomelania hupensis, the sole intermediate host snail of *S. japonicum*, is vastly distributed in The People's Republic of China (Utzinger et al., 2005; Zhou et al., 2009). These snails can survive and breed in the water networks of lakes and marshlands in the plains as well as in the smaller streams in the endemic areas in the hills and mountains. Reduction of the snail-infected areas through sophisticated land modification projects has always been part of The People's Republic of China's national schistosomiasis control programmes due to the vast distribution of *O. hupensis*, which remains a strong impediment to the control and eventual elimination of *S. japonicum* to this day (Rollinson et al., 2013).

The projects on environmental modification consist of a series of snail control measures, including land management, amelioration of waterlogged fields and ecological land conservation, etc. (Hu et al., 2010; Xu et al., 2013) (Fig. 7). The original aim of these projects is to protect arable farmland and raise grain production to support the increasing population, but they also play an essential part in controlling snail populations in places where *S. japonicum* is still endemic (Utzinger et al., 2005). Chemical molluscicides often fail in waterlogged paddy fields with crisscrossing irrigation canals and ditches. Therefore, the waterlogged fields in these snail-breeding areas are drained by various measures, eg, by raising the land above the water table through construction of concrete ditches and embedded pipe drains. Much of the farmland in the lake and marshland areas has been obtained through construction of dykes and embankments to enclose lakes and rivers and the *O. hupensis* snails cannot survive in this environment (Huang et al., 2012). Another simple, yet very effective practice is to suffocate the snails by filling disused irrigation ditches with the freshly dug-out soil of new ones. Moreover, it is imperative to accept the last resort of relocating villages

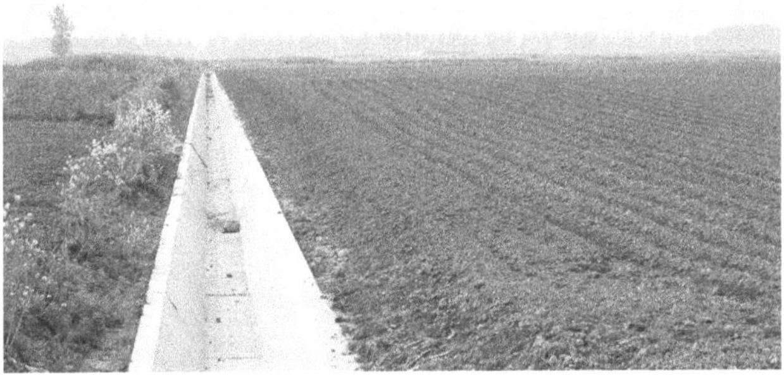

Figure 7 Land modification projects combined with concrete lined irrigation ditches in an endemic area in The People's Republic of China.

where the epidemic situation of schistosomiasis is severe and the snail habitats cannot be controlled.

It has been shown that land modification, eg, filling in natural willow groves and levelling low-lying land has a significant effect on the density of *O. hupensis* snails (reduced from 33.2 per m^2 in 2010 to 0.1 per m^2 in 2012) at the banks and beaches of the Yangtze River after the flood season (Gao et al., 2013). Another longitudinal study in Hubei Province suggests that land consolidation, in conjunction with replacement of water buffaloes for tilling by motorized equipment, effectively reduces the snail-infested areas and interrupts transmission (Xu et al., 2013). In one high-risk region a reduction of the human schistosomiasis infection rate from 78.9% in 2012 to 0.5% in 2008 was recorded (Xu et al., 2013).

4. SUCCESSFUL COMMISSIONS: FIVE NATIONAL PILOT CONTROL PROJECTS

In 2005, five national pilots of integrated control strategy of schistosomiasis were designated to accumulate first-hand experience and evidence regarding the efficiency and feasibility of the strategy within various settings. The following areas were chosen: Guichi District in Anhui Province, Anxiang County in Hunan Province, Hanchuan City in Hubei Province, Jinxian County in Jiangxi Province and Puge County in Sichuan province. The findings are given in the following sections.

4.1 Guichi District, Anhui Province

4.1.1 Study area

Guichi District belongs to the lake and marshland region, is located in the middle and lower reaches of the Yangtze River in Anhui Province and has a population of 0.65 million out of which 0.40 million are at risk for *S. japonicum* infection. The Qiupu River basin, the Jiuhua River, the Yangtze River basin and the Shengjin Lake region comprise the endemic areas, which are moulded by the difficult terrain, fluctuating water levels, crisscrossing rivers and a vast distribution of *Oncomelania* snail habitats. This situation makes Guichi District a representative endemic focus of the lake and marshland regions. Historically, this district stands out as one of the most serious *S. japonicum*–endemic areas in the country. By the end of 2004, the infection rates of human and bovines were 3.9% and 7.7%, respectively, and there were approximately 29.8 km^2 of snail-infested areas (Wang et al., 2009c). Residents live by the rivers or lakes and they farm the grasslands, which are colonized by *Oncomelania* snails and usually also contaminated by human and cattle excreta. Frequent water contact and lack of decent sanitation make the locals vulnerable to schistosomiasis infections (Wang et al., 2006, 2008a; Zhou et al., 2011).

4.1.2 Interventions

In 2005, the Guichi District was designated as a national pilot area for schistosomiasis integrated control. The new strategy was implemented between 2006 and 2008 in 13 villages randomly selected from an original screen of 40 villages. Before initiation, routine measures had been used to control *S. japonicum* infection, including simultaneous chemotherapy with praziquantel for all villagers and cattle, snail control by molluscicides and health education programmes. Intensive health education, focused on the need to avoid snail-infested areas and associated water bodies, was carried out in all 13 villages among more than 90% of the residents.

Complementary efforts were made during the study period. All bovines, being the recognized infection source, were phased out and replaced with mechanized equipment with subsidies from local government. By February 2006, a total of 1131 bovines were removed from the Qiupu River basin and 738 farm machines purchased instead. By March 2007, 896 bovines were replaced with 806 farm machines in the basin of the Jiuhua and Yangtze Rivers. In November 2007, 227 pieces of farm equipment took the place of 1021 bovines in the Shengjin Lake region (Wang et al., 2009c). Other kinds of domestic animals were fenced in and improved sanitation was achieved by supplying piped water and lavatories/latrines, which were also funded by the local government. The number of household lavatories in the Qiupu River basin, the Jiuhua-Yangtze River basin and the Shengjin Lake region amounted to 5343, 1767 and 250, respectively. Safe water access was available for 84.4% of the households in the Qiupu River area and 92.5% in the Jiuhua-Yangtze River basin (Wang et al., 2009c). In addition, environmental management was undertaken to reduce the snail habitats (eg, crop changes to reduce water consumption in the snail-inhabited areas) (Chen et al., 2006; Wang et al., 2009c; Zhou et al., 2011).

4.1.3 Results

In the Qiupu River basin, compared to the situation in 2005, the average infection rate of residents, the density of infected snails and the infection rate of snails decreased by 68.6%, 96.0% and 96.0%, respectively, after the implementation of the integrated control strategy in 2008 (Fig. 8A). In the Jiuhua-Yangtze River basin, compared to 2006, the same parameters decreased by 51.6%, 71.2% and 69.0%, respectively (Fig. 8B), while in the Shengjin Lake region, compared to 2007, they decreased by 49.6%, 73.6% and 51.8%, respectively. In addition, the number of cases of acute schistosomiasis in all the areas investigated decreased significantly after implementing the comprehensive control strategy in 2008. Taken together, these results suggest that the new integrated control strategy can substantially reduce the burden of schistosomiasis, at least in the lake and marshland regions (Wang et al., 2009c).

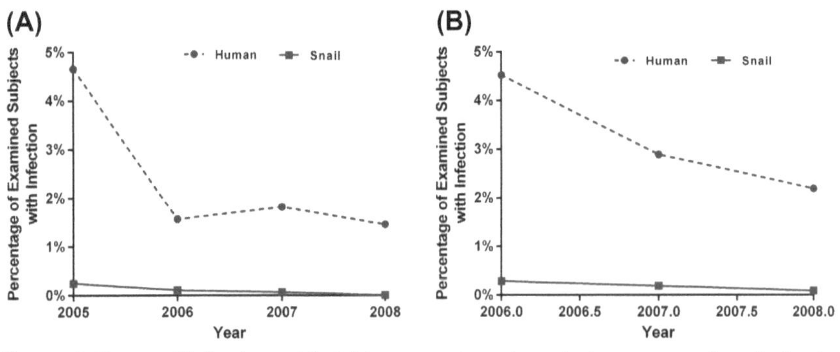

Figure 8 Rates of infection with *Schistosoma japonicum* in humans and snails in the Qiupu River basin (A) and in the Jiuhua-Yangtze River basin (B).

4.2 Anxiang County, Hunan Province

4.2.1 Study area

Anxiang County is located in the northwest of Dongting Lake in Hunan Province. It has a population of about 0.55 million, 0.43 million of whom still depend on farming, and the county's economy relies on animal husbandry. The 34 sluice gates, 172 km of embankments and vast marshlands crisscrossed by canals and rivers make Anxiang County another major *S. japonicum* focus in the lake and marshland regions, where the control of schistosomiasis transmission has proven particularly challenging. In 2005, Anxiang County became one of the national pilot study areas of the integrated control strategy (Zhu et al., 2011).

4.2.2 Interventions

Routine control measures were in force before the initiation of the new, integrated control strategy that has been undertaken since 2005. Chemotherapy with praziquantel has been available for all infected villagers in the autumn every year with selective treatment for high-risk populations including fishermen and herdsmen twice a year. The molluscicide niclosamide was used twice a year, while health education was carried out among residents focussing on provision of a good understanding of this particular disease and the behavioural changes needed to be implemented. These interventions continued in all villages (Li et al., 2013).

Additional interventions were included in parallel with the routine measures. First, 9583 bovines and 9504 sheep were removed from this county to eliminate this source of infection. Activities were carried out in a two-stage process. Removal of cattle and sheep were instituted in 50 villages in the first stage in 2005, a measure that was expanded to include all endemic villages in a subsequent second stage. All sheep were killed and most water buffaloes replaced with farm machinery ($n = 7841$) or transferred to nonendemic regions. Losses caused by the removal of bovines and sheep were well compensated. Second, tap water and lavatories were built to improve sanitation. As a result, access to safe water supply and household lavatories became available to 90% and 80% of all families, respectively. Biogas pools ($n = 11,563$) were constructed covering 80% of all local family residencies. Third, environmental management was implemented, including forestry and agricultural projects. A cumulative 254.3 ha of land were subjected to forestry projects and 32.0 km of ditches and canals were cemented to counteract snail habitats. Fourth, industrial restructuring was promoted to create employment opportunities for local people, who transferred from rural labour to this new environment (Li et al., 2013).

4.2.3 Results

The annual survey data on *S. japonicum* infection in humans, domestic animals and snails from 2004 to 2012 were collected and analysed. After the implementation of the comprehensive strategy to control the source of *S. japonicum* infection and *Oncomenania* snails, the percentage of villagers with schistosomiasis declined to 0.6% from 11.2% within the study period. The infection rate of livestock decreased from 17.1% to zero. The percentage of snails infected with *S. japonicum* fell to zero in 2012 compared with 1.1% in 2004 (Fig. 9). These results show that the comprehensive control measures instituted to reduce the transmission of *S. japonicum* infection from humans and cattle to snails are effective in the marshland and lake region (Li et al., 2013; Zhu et al., 2011).

4.3 Hanchuan City, Hubei Province

4.3.1 Study area

Hanchuan City is located in typical marshland along the lower reach of the Hanjiang River in central Hubei Province, The People's Republic of China. It has a population just above one million, 0.53 million of whom are in the danger of schistosomiasis infection. The Hanjiang River is the largest tributary of the Yangtze River, and vast marshland areas suitable as breeding sites for *Oncomelania* snails emerge each year following the monsoon season

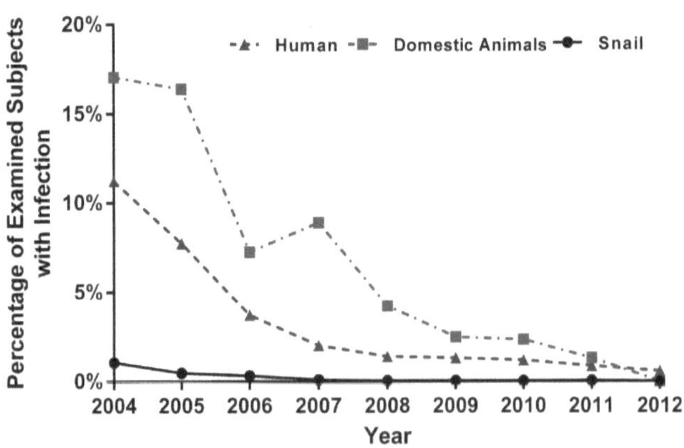

Figure 9 Rates of *Schistosoma japonicum* infection in Anxiang County 2004 through 2012.

flooding. Hanchuan City is highly endemic for schistosomiasis. In 2004, there were 367 endemic villages and approximately 22.1 km^2 of snail-infested area in this region. Ninety-seven cases of new infections and ten cases of acute schistosomiasis occurred in the same year. The prevalence of schistosomiasis in humans and bovines in 2004 was 6.9% and 8.8%, respectively (Xiang et al., 2014). From 2005 to 2013, the new, integrated control strategy was carried out in the marshland areas around this city.

4.3.2 Interventions

Prior to the new, comprehensive control strategy, routine control interventions, comprising simultaneous chemotherapy with praziquantel of villagers and bovines, mollusciciding and health education were implemented. These measures continued in all schistosomiasis-endemic villages with the additional interventions integrated. The pilot stage from 2005 to 2007 involved only five towns along the Hanbei River, a tributary of the Hanjiang River implementing the integrated strategy in all affected villages in Hanchuan. The new interventions included (1) removal of 11,800 bovines from 2005 to 2013 replacing them with 1441 farm machines, which was supported with government subsidies; (2) prohibition of grazing in the snail-infested grasslands coupled with promotion of rearing cattle and sheep inside fences (this approach covered 6377 livestock); (3) human and animal faeces was managed by building lavatories with three-cell septic tanks and biogas pools plus providing toilet containers for the fishermen's boats from 2005 to 2013 (approximately 40,000 lavatories and 24,000 biogas digesters were constructed reaching 85.0% and 80.7% coverage, respectively with another 15 latrines available at the fishermen's docking sites); (4) snail control interventions including agriculture, forestry, water conservancy, land management and infrastructure construction were instituted to reduce the snail habitats (Chen et al., 2014; Hong et al., 2013a; Wang et al., 2009b, 2010; Xiang et al., 2013, 2014).

4.3.3 Results

After the implementation of the comprehensive measures, the infection rates of human and cattle decreased from 6.4% to 8.1% in 2004 to 0.6% and zero in 2013, respectively (Fig. 10). There were no cases of acute schistosomiasis since 2007, no new infections since 2011 and no infected snails found since 2012. Compared with 2004, the average density of living snails dropped by 56.8% and 68.4%, respectively. In 2013, all the 367 endemic villages in 26 townships reached the criteria of transmission control (Xiang et al., 2014).

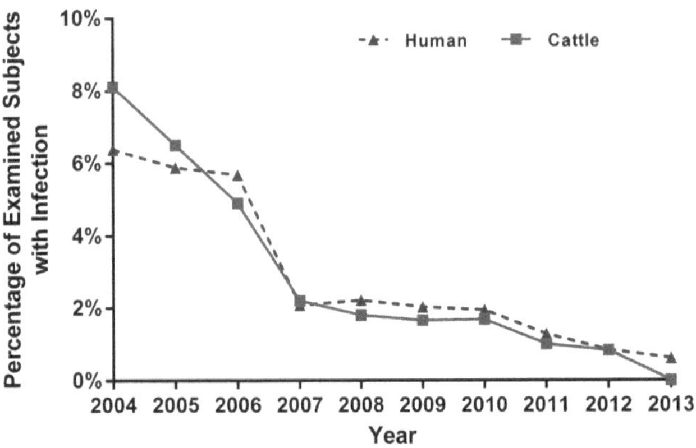

Figure 10 Rates of *Schistosoma japonicum* infection in humans and cattle from 2004 to 2013 in Hanchuan City, Hubei, The People's Republic of China.

Taken together, these results show that the integrated control strategy could control the schistosomiasis transmission effectively in the marshland and lake regions (Xiang et al., 2014).

4.4 Jinxian County, Jiangxi Province

4.4.1 Study area

Poyang Lake, the largest freshwater water body in The People's Republic of China, is located in northern Jiangxi Province. The surface area of the lake fluctuates dramatically between flood and dry seasons. Along with the Dongting Lake in Hunan Province, the Poyang Lake influences the schistosomiasis transmission strongly in the lake and marshland regions. Jinxian County has a population of just under 1 million people and was chosen as a national pilot area for comprehensive control of schistosomiasis in June 2005, involving three villages around Poyang Lake, in which *S. japonicum* is endemic, namely Xinhe, Aiguo and Guanghui (Wang et al., 2009d).

There is 13.3 km^2 of snail-infested grasslands long the embankment around the Poyang Lake where these three villages are situated. The local residents farm the grasslands and fish in lake near these grasslands. Both humans and cattle in this area are often infected with schistosomiasis with humans at particular risk due to frequent water contact through their daily activities such as fishing, cultivating crops, cutting weeds, pasturing and swimming (Hu et al., 2008; Wang et al., 2009a, 2012). In 2004, the prevalence of schistosomiasis in humans and bovines in this pilot was 9.3% and 11.0%, respectively (Wang et al., 2009d).

4.4.2 Interventions

In 2005, the comprehensive control strategy was implemented in the original three villages and expanded to all villages of the Sanli Township in Jiangxi Province the following year. Routine interventions, such as chemotherapy, mollusciciding and health education continued along the new measures. An intensified health education programme was carried out to promote a better understanding of *S. japonicum* with the aim of bringing about behavioural changes that would interrupt transmission. Additional health education sessions were provided to schoolchildren to create a schistosomiasis-free campus. The following new interventions were incorporated into this comprehensive strategy: (1) regulations were implemented to replace water buffaloes with small farm machines, thus eliminating them as an infection source. In all, 2156 bovines were removed and replaced with 489 farm machines in these three villages; (2) cattle grazing in the snail-infested grasslands was prohibited and warning signs were put up. Management staff was employed to ensure the measure was implemented; (3) safe water supply covering 60.3% of the local households was provided and well-designed household lavatories with three-cell septic tanks and methane pools were constructed in 1275 households accounting for 81.2% of the local families. All boats were provided with toilet containers so that human faeces could be brought ashore and treated. Besides, public latrines were installed at schools and docking sites, including four middle-large biogas pools; (4) crop and husbandry structure changes were advocated (eg, promotion of oilseed rape cultivation and poultry farming). To practically implement these comprehensive interventions, the government provided funding and subsidies to remove cattle from the grasslands and build public latrines, public methane pools, piped water and wells (Hong et al., 2013b; Liu et al., 2013b; Wang et al., 2009a,d).

4.4.3 Results

After the implementation of comprehensive interventions to control the source of *S. japonicum* infection, the percentage of infected villagers declined to 1.6% in 2006 from 9.3% in 2004. Compared with 2005, the density of infected snails had decreased by 97.2% 2 years later. In addition, human ascariasis and trichuris infections dropped by 59.1% and 48.2%, respectively. The overall results suggest that a multicomponent comprehensive control strategy of schistosomiasis is effective in the marshland and lake regions, which will remain a problem even after criteria for infection control are attained (Hong et al., 2013b; Wang et al., 2009d).

4.5 Puge County, Sichuan Province

4.5.1 Study area

Covering an area of 50.2 km^2 the town of Tezi is geographically large, but the population is only approximately 4000. However, the number of livestock, including cattle, sheep, horses and pigs, is more the double the human population. Tezi lies in the Northeast of Puge County, Sichuan Province and has a complex topography with mountains and valleys varying in altitude between 1000 and 2500 m above the mean sea level. It is a typical mountainous *S. japonicum*–endemic area. In spite of a snail-infested area of just above 1 km^2, the infection rates of humans and cattle have been recorded at 35.5% and 30.5%, respectively (Yi Huo et al., 2009).

Tezi is an underdeveloped region inhabited by the Yi people, an ethnic minority group in The People's Republic of China. They carve out their existence on the sides of steep mountain slopes far from the cities keeping a primitive way of life and depending on animal husbandry for their livelihood. Soil erosion and high mountains and steep slopes make agricultural production and transportation difficult, so cattle and horses are indispensable. Therefore, removal of cattle to control schistosomiasis might not be an option here as the locals sometimes even live under the same roof together with their livestock. In addition, lavatories, latrines or any other form of sanitation facilities are not only unavailable but also difficult to envisage in this dispersed situation. Both human and domestic animal faeces are left untreated. Residents of Tezi farm the grassland along the mountain streams that also provide pasture for their animals. These streams are colonized by the *Oncomelania* snails and as water contact is frequent, transmission of schistosomiasis involving both humans and livestock is rampant (Yi Huo et al., 2009).

4.5.2 Interventions

In April 2005, Tezi was designated a national pilot study area of the integrated control strategy of schistosomiasis, which was implemented in all villages between 2006 and 2013.

Simultaneous chemotherapy with praziquantel is routinely available for all residents 5–65 years of age and domestic animals in this area to reduce the morbidity due to *S. japonicum* and, in turn, to lower the snail infection rate through reduced faecal contamination of the environment. In addition, pasture in the snail-infested grasslands was prohibited and regulations were implemented to promote raising domestic animals in pens. Fifteen carefully selected, safe grazing pasture areas were established and faeces-treatment pools were built. Management staff was employed to ensure that the animal waste was properly disposed of and the following interventions were implemented to reduce humans as source of infection:

1. Household tap water was installed, 290 simple lavatories were constructed covering 98.7% of the households and 267 gas pools were built so that biogas from the septic tanks could be collected and used as fuel. Treated human and animal waste was used as organic fertilizers.
2. Repeated mollusciciding was used to reduce the snail populations and environmental management aiming at eliminating snail habitats, including paddy-upland rotation, cementing the ditches, etc., were instituted.
3. An intensified health education programme, adjusted to local conditions, was carried out among the residents to promote a good understanding of the *S. japonicum* life cycle and better compliance for chemotherapy as well as awareness of the importance of proper treatment of human and cattle sewage.

To reach all local people, billboards and publicity materials were written bilingually in Chinese and the Yi language (Chen et al., 2016; Liu et al., 2014; Yi Huo et al., 2009).

4.5.3 Results

After the implementation of the comprehensive interventions described above, the percentage of infected villagers decreased by 97.7% to 0.3% in 2013 compared to 2005. The infection rate of livestock dropped by 96.0% to 0.4% in 2013 compared to 2005 (Fig. 11) and the area of snail-infested grasslands shrunk by almost a third. No infected snails were found after 2007. Household lavatories are now available for 98.7% of the local families. In general, the results suggest that the multicomponent comprehensive antischistosomiasis strategy is even effective in the mountainous regions, which are notoriously difficult to control for this disease (Yi Huo et al., 2009).

5. CHALLENGES

Although The People's Republic of China has achieved great success of schistosomiasis control based on a programme that has been active without interruption since the early 1950s, there are still considerable challenges (Zheng et al., 2013). One is the ongoing process of implementing the new, comprehensive control strategy, consolidating the achievements made and reaching the goals set by 'Work Plan for the Mid-and Long-term of

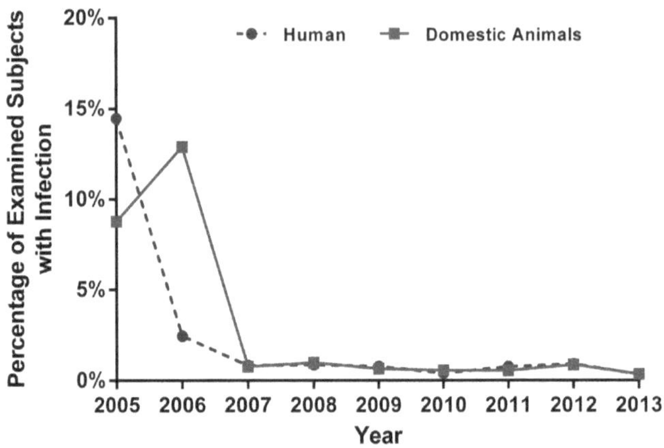

Figure 11 Rates of *Schistosoma japonicum* infection in humans and domestic animals based on data from 2005 to 2013 in Puge County, Sichuan, The People's Republic of China.

National Schistosomiasis Control Programme', which has yet to be finalized (Lei and Zhou, 2014a,b; Zhou et al., 2005, 2012).

Political commitment and provision of finance are critically important in finalizing the work plan and obtain sustainable and effective control of the schistosomiasis (Wang et al., 2008b, 2014). However, local governments may not be able to bear the financial burden of large investments in projects involving the full spectrum of activities that involve agriculture, water conservancy, forestry, sanitation and environmental modification. As for major water resource projects, allocations from The People's Republic of China's Central Government budget cover 30% of total amount of investment, while the remaining 70% must rely on local financial support. Small projects constitute the full responsibility of local governments (Xu et al., 2010; Zhu et al., 2016). Promotion of replacing cattle with mechanized equipment, construction of sanitation facilities, including latrines, biogas systems and forestry programmes are held back by lack of government fiscal subsidies. The full effect of the control efforts is jeopardized by inadequate and inequitable government investments, which contributes to lack of service of agricultural machines and poor operation and maintenance of abovementioned approaches. It is therefore imperative that strong policy programmes and financial support be undertaken by the The People's Republic of China's Government without delay to ensure continued successful and sustainable schistosomiasis control (Lei and Zhou, 2014a,b).

Intersectoral collaboration between the health sector and other governmental sectors, prominently the agriculture, education, water resources and forestry sectors, have a key role in the efforts to reach successful and effective comprehensive control of schistosomiasis (Lei and Zhou, 2014a,b). Although the new control strategy is integrated with other society development efforts, such as rural energy development and construction of a new rural, trans-department communication system, planning and coordination should be enhanced to leverage and direct existing intersectoral funding to the schistosomiasis-endemic areas (Lei and Zhou, 2014a,b; Remais et al., 2009). Also, efforts may be compromised, as the professional teams, especially at the primary level, are greatly weakened by shrinking investment for schistosomiasis control that results in long-term expert staff retiring without adequate replacements, reduced staff mobility, inadequate facilities and lack of training (Lei and Zhou, 2014a,b). Further, the role of each project in the integrated control strategy of schistosomiasis, which is primarily aimed at reducing the source of infection, remains largely ignored without national-scale evaluation. The five national pilot studies summarized here do not necessarily involve all the interventions of the comprehensive control strategy. These combinations are driven by differences in socioecological conditions. In the context of outcome related to the interventions in endemic areas, a scientific and systematic assessment of the effects and benefits of this multicomponent control strategy of schistosomiasis in various settings is currently unavailable. While extensive control efforts in endemic areas have greatly decreased infection intensity and prevalence, current surveillance methods and diagnostic tools would lead to underestimation of the endemic status in areas with low prevalence (Xu et al., 2015; Zhou et al., 2005, 2012). Moreover, there is a strong need to determine what level and/or coverage of this new integrated control strategy are required to have a favourable effect on schistosomiasis transmission and, in the longer perspective, elimination.

6. THE WAY FORWARD

Over the past six decades of endeavour, The People's Republic of China has made remarkable progress in schistosomiasis control with strong reduction of transmission achieved in most endemic areas (Chen, 2014; Collins et al., 2012). The pilot studies presented here show that control of schistosomiasis is an achievable goal, which requires an integrated strategy adapted to different eco-epidemiological settings. To achieve further advances in schistosomiasis control, sustainable financial resources and political commitment need to be assured. Moreover, the comprehensive control strategy requires collective and multidisciplinary efforts. Intersectoral collaboration, especially between the Departments of Health, Finance, Land and

Resources, Water Resources, Agriculture and Forestry, should be strengthened to facilitate the national programme of schistosomiasis control in The People's Republic of China.

ACKNOWLEDGEMENTS

This work was supported by the National S & T Major Programme (Grant No. 2012ZX10004-220 and 2008ZX10004-011), Consulting Service for Center of Excellence in Global Health Policy Development and Governance in The People's Republic of China (GHSP-CS-OP3-02), National Natural Science Foundation of The People's Republic of China (No. 30872159) and Shanghai Leading Academic Discipline Project (Project No. B118).

REFERENCES

Bergquist, N.R., Leonardo, L.R., Mitchell, G.F., 2005. Vaccine-linked chemotherapy: can schistosomiasis control benefit from an integrated approach? Trends Parasitol. 21, 112–117.

Campbell, S.J., Savage, G.B., Gray, D.J., Atkinson, J.A., Soares, M.R., Nery, S.V., et al., 2014. Water, sanitation, and hygiene (WASH): a critical component for sustainable soil-transmitted helminth and schistosomiasis control. PLoS Negl. Trop. Dis. 8, e2651.

Cao, C.L., Bao, Z.P., Yang, P.C., Chen, Z., Yan, J., Ren, G.H., et al., 2014. Schistosomiasis control effect of measures of replacing cattle with machine for cultivation and forbidding depasturage of livestock on marshlands in marshland and lake regions. Chin. J. Schistosomiasis Control 26, 602–607.

Cao, Z.G., Zhao, Y.E., Willingham, A.L., Wang, T.P., 2016. Towards the elimination of *Schistosomiasis japonica* through control of the disease in domestic animals in the People's Republic of China: a tale of over 60 years. Adv. Parasitol. 92.

Carlton, E., Liang, S., McDowell, J., Li, H., Luo, W., Remais, J., 2012. Regional disparities in the burden of disease attributable to unsafe water and poor sanitation in China. Bull. World Health Organ. 90, 578–587.

Chen, G.X., Han, M.S., Wang, M.S., He, Z.G., Ni, Y., 2006. Analysis of the effect on the comprehensive measures of replacing cattle by machine and reconstructing water supply and lavatory to control the schistosomiasis for five years. J. Trop. Dis. Parasitol. 4, 160–163.

Chen, Y.Y., Yuan, Y., Zhou, B., Zhu, Y., Peng, X., Xu, X.J., 2010. Effect evaluation of large water conservancy project on control of schistosomiasis transmission. Chin. J. Schistosomiasis Control 22, 411–414.

Chen, H.G., Zeng, X.J., Lin, D.D., Lv, S.B., Gu, X.N., Hang, C.Q., et al., 2013. The changes of hydrological regime in Poyang Lake after runs of Three Gorges Project and its impact on prevalence of schistosomiasis in the lake region. Chin. J. Schistosomiasis Control 25, 444–450.

Chen, Y.Y., Liu, J.B., Huang, X.B., Cai, S.X., Su, Z.M., Zhong, R., et al., 2014. New integrated strategy emphasizing infection source control to curb *Schistosomiasis japonica* in a marshland area of Hubei Province, China: findings from an eight-year longitudinal survey. PLoS One 9, e89779.

Chen, L., Zhong, B., Xu, J., Li, R.Z., Cao, C.L., 2016. Health education as an important component in the national schistosomiasis control programme in the People's Republic of China. Adv. Parasitol. 92.

Chen, M.G., 2014. Assessment of morbidity due to *Schistosoma japonicum* infection in China. Infect. Dis. Poverty 3, 6.

Colley, D.G., Bustinduy, A.L., Secor, W.E., King, C.H., 2014. Human schistosomiasis. Lancet 383, 2253–2264.

Collins, C., Xu, J., Tang, S., 2012. Schistosomiasis control and the health system in P.R. China. Infect. Dis. Poverty 1, 8.

Ding, Z.J., Li, Z.S., Wang, D.F., Zhang, G.B., 2008. Effect of snail retention tanks for obstructing snails spreading in ditches of hilly regions. Chin. J. Schistosomiasis Control 20, 485.

Ding, Z.J., Wang, D.F., Wei, Z.Y., He, B., He, Y.L., Yu, Y.S., et al., 2013. Causes of re-emergence of Oncomelania snails in hardened ditches. Chin. J. Schistosomiasis Control 25, 213–214+216.

Dong, X.H., Qin, B., Gu, S.L., Wang, X., Piao, Y.Y., Chen, C.H., 2008a. Effect of toilets improvement in reducing snails and residents infected with schistosomiasis. J. Trop. Dis. Parasitol. 6, 191–193.

Dong, X.Q., Feng, X.G., Dong, Y., Xiong, M.T., Jiang, H., Shen, M.F., et al., 2008b. Epidemiological characteristics and control strategies of schistosomiasis in mountainous areas of Yunnan Province. Chin. J. Schistosomiasis Control 20, 135–137.

Dong, Y., Feng, X.G., Huang, P., Dong, X.Q., Shi, X.W., Yang, W.C., 2013. Effect of water-saving irrigation engineering on schistosomiasis control in Eryuan County of Yunnan Province. Chin. J. Schistosomiasis Control 25, 393–395.

Gao, Y., Sun, L.P., Wu, H.H., Yang, J., Hong, Q.B., Xi, T.Z., et al., 2009. Study on schistosomiasis control measures in mobile boat fishermen II effect of comprehensive measures with emphasis on management of boat fishermen feces for schistosomiasis control. Chin. J. Schistosomiasis Control 21, 262–266.

Gao, G.T., Liu, Y.X., Sun, Z., Hu, J.G., Hu, Q., 2013. Effect of land consolidation project on detention of *Oncomelania hupensis* snails in flood at Yangtze River beach. Chin. J. Schistosomiasis Control 25, 545–547.

Gray, D.J., Williams, G.M., Li, Y., McManus, D.P., 2008. Transmission dynamics of *Schistosoma japonicum* in the lakes and marshlands of China. PLoS One 3, e4058.

Hong, X.L., Wang, X.Y., 2012. Effects of reclaiming and cultivation in marshland on Oncomelania snail control. Chin. J. Schistosomiasis Control 24, 364–365.

Hong, X.C., Xu, X.J., Chen, X., Li, Y.S., Yu, C.H., Yuan, Y., et al., 2013a. Assessing the effect of an integrated control strategy for *Schistosomiasis japonica* emphasizing bovines in a marshland area of Hubei Province, China: a cluster randomized trial. PLoS Negl. Trop. Dis. 7, e2122.

Hong, X.L., Wang, X.Y., Li, X.Q., 2013b. Evaluation on effect of schistosomiasis control after attainment of criteria for infection control in Jinxian County. Chin. J. Schistosomiasis Control 25, 98–99.

Hu, Z.H., Hong, X.L., Wang, X.Y., Hu, M.Z., Hu, S.Z., Fan, Y.L., et al., 2008. Surveillance of schistosomiasis in Jinhong village, Jinxian county, 2005–2007. Chin. J. Schistosomiasis Control 20, 465–466.

Hu, H.X., Wang, J., Xiong, Y.Q., Tang, L., Wang, L., Ni, X.M., et al., 2010. Effect of land consolidation project combined with chemotherapy for humans and domestic animals on the transmission of schistosomiasis. J. Pub Health Prev. Med. 21, 75–76.

Huang, Y., Zhang, S.Q., He, J.C., Cao, Z.G., Wang, T.P., Gao, F.H., et al., 2011. Effect of project of afforestation for schistosomiasis prevention on snail control in marshland and lake regions. Chin. J. Schistosomiasis Control 23, 138–144.

Huang, Y.X., Zhu, Z.F., Hang, D.R., Li, W., Chen, S.J., Zhang, K., et al., 2012. Effect of water conservancy schistosomiasis control projects in rivers and estuaries connecting with the Yangtze River on Oncomelania snail control. Chin. J. Schistosomiasis Control 24, 522–526.

Jiang, T., Wang, J.M., 2012. Progress of technology of pumping water at middle level of water body to prevent *Oncomelania* snail spreading. Chin. J. Schistosomiasis Control 24, 491–494.

Jiang, J.M., Yang, L., Fei, S.M., Mo, K.L., Sun, Q.X., 2013. Mollusicidal effects of some species of plants in hilly and mountainous areas. Chin. J. Schistosomiasis Control 25, 255–258.
Lansing, S., Botero, R.B., Martin, J.F., 2008. Waste treatment and biogas quality in small-scale agricultural digesters. Bioresour. Technol. 99, 5881–5890.
Lei, Z.L., Zhou, X.N., 2014a. Progress and challenges of the National Schistosomiasis Control Programme during the period of the 12th Five-year Plan. Chin. J. Parasitol. Parasit. 32, 81–85.
Lei, Z.L., Zhou, X.N., 2014b. Eradication of schistosomiasis:a new target and a new task for the National Schistosomiasis Control Programme in the People's Republic of China. Chin. J. Schistosomiasis Control 27, 1–4, 2015-2004-2029 2023:2025:2000.
Li, Y.S., Raso, G., Zhao, Z.Y., He, Y.K., Ellis, M.K., McManus, D.P., 2007. Large water management projects and schistosomiasis control, Dongting Lake region. China. Emerg. Infect. Dis. 13, 973–979.
Li, B.G., Chen, S.R., Li, W.B., Luo, J.J., Mu, L.X., Tian, S.H., et al., 2012a. Results of schistosomiasis control in plateau and canyon areas in Yunnan province. China Trop. Med. 12, 1483–1487.
Li, F., Min, F.Y., Lu, J.Y., Wang, J.S., 2012b. Problems and improvements of water conservancy projects combined with schistosomiasis control in river beaches. Chin. J. Schistosomiasis Control 24, 339–341.
Li, X.S., Li, F.Y., Zhu, S.P., Zhou, Y.B., Yi, P., Luo, Z.H., et al., 2013. Effect of comprehensive schistosomiasis control measures with focus on buffalo and sheep removal in Anxiang County. Chin. J. Schistosomiasis Control 25, 291–292 +295.
Li, Z.J., Ge, J., Dai, J.R., Wen, L.Y., Lin, D.D., Madsen, H., et al., 2016. Biology and control of snail intermediate host of *Schistosoma japonicum* in the People's Republic of China. Adv. Parasitol. 92.
Lin, D.D., Wu, H.W., Wu, G.L., Zhou, X.N., 2007. Review and evaluation on optimal combined strategies for schistosomiasis control in China. Chin. J. Schistosomiasis Control 19, 234–237.
Liu, G.F., Li, K., Zhang, C.H., 2011. Snail control effect and eco-economical benefit of forest for snail control and schistosomiasis prevention in mountainous regions. Chin. J. Schistosomiasis Control 23, 386–389.
Liu, R., Dong, H.-F., Jiang, M.-S., 2013a. The new national integrated strategy emphasizing infection sources control for schistosomiasis control in China has made remarkable achievements. Parasitol. Res. 112, 1483–1491.
Liu, W., Cao, C.L., Chen, Z., Li, S.Z., Tang, L., Xiao, Y., et al., 2013b. Evaluation of the comprehensive schistosomiasis control measures with emphasis on infection source of replacing cattle with machine. Chin. J. Parasitol. Parasit. 206–211.
Liu, L., Yang, G.J., Zhu, H.R., Yang, K., Ai, L., 2014. Knowledge of, attitudes towards, and practice relating to schistosomiasis in two subtypes of a mountainous region of the People's Republic of China. Infect. Dis. Poverty 3, 16.
Liu, Y., Zhou, Y.B., Li, R.Z., Wan, J.J., Yang, Y., Qiu, D.C., et al., 2016. Epidemiological features and control effectiveness of schistosomiasis in mountainous and hilly region of the People's Republic of China. Adv. Parasitol. 92.
Lu, L.T., Zhu, R., Zhang, L.J., Zhong, B., Feng, X.G., Xu, X.L., et al., 2013. Evolution of schistosomiasis control and prevention strategies in hilly regions with schistosomiasis endemic in China. Chin. J. Schistosomiasis Control 25, 528–532.
McManus, D.P., Gray, D.J., Li, Y., Feng, Z., Williams, G.M., Stewart, D., et al., 2010. Schistosomiasis in the People's Republic of China: the Era of the Three Gorges Dam. Clin. Microbiol. Rev. 23, 442–466.
Meng, C.L., Jiang, J.M., Tang, R.Q., Fei, S.M., Zhou, J.X., Zhang, X.D., et al., 2012. An analysis of agro-forestry management patterns in schistosomiasis prevention of forestry in hilly and mountainous areas of Sichuan. J. Sichuan For. Sci. Technol. 33, 9–19.

Min, L., 2008. Strategy of implementation of the no-cattle county for schistosomiasis control in Pengshan County. Chin. J. Schistosomiasis Control 20, 64–65.

Remais, J., Chen, L., Seto, E., 2009. Leveraging rural energy investment for parasitic disease control: schistosome ova inactivation and energy co-benefits of anaerobic digesters in rural China. PLoS One 4, e4856.

Rollinson, D., Knopp, S., Levitz, S., Stothard, J.R., Tchuem Tchuenté, L.-A., Garba, A., et al., 2013. Time to set the agenda for schistosomiasis elimination. Acta Trop. 128, 423–440.

Seto, E.Y.W., Lee, Y.J., Liang, S., Zhong, B., 2007. Individual and village-level study of water contact patterns and *Schistosoma japonicum* infection in mountainous rural China. Trop. Med. Int. Health 12, 1199–1209.

Seto, E.Y., Remais, J.V., Carlton, E.J., Wang, S., Liang, S., Brindley, P.J., et al., 2011. Toward sustainable and comprehensive control of schistosomiasis in China: lessons from Sichuan. PLoS Negl. Trop. Dis. 5, e1372.

Spear, R.C., Seto, E., Liang, S., Birkner, M., Hubbard, A., Qiu, D., et al., 2004. Factors influencing the transmission of *Schistosoma japonicum* in the mountains of Sichuan Province of China. Am. J. Trop. Med. Hyg. 70, 48–56.

Steinmann, P., Keiser, J., Bos, R., Tanner, M., Utzinger, J., 2006. Schistosomiasis and water resources development: systematic review, meta-analysis, and estimates of people at risk. Lancet Infect. Dis. 6, 411–425.

Su, W.X., Wei, X.W., Li, M., Luo, S.X., 2004. Effects of snail sinks and cement banks in canals for preventing snails form diffusing. Chin. J. Schistosomiasis Control 16, 223–224.

Sun, Q.X., Peng, Z.H., 2013. Screening of biological materials for plantations for snail control and schistosomiasis prevention and research progress in studies on inhibiting mechanism. Wetl. Sci. Manage. 9, 8–11.

Sun, Q.X., Zhang, J.F., Zhou, J.X., 2006. Discussions on forestry ecological programs for schistosomiasis prevention. Wetl. Sci. Manage. 2, 44–46.

Tang, G.Y., Li, K., Zhang, C.H., 2011. Distribution of *Oncomelania hupensis* snails and effect of plantations on snail control under different land uses at a gentle hilly region. Chin. J. Schistosomiasis Control 431–434.

Useh, M.F., 2013. In: El Ridi, R. (Ed.), Schistosomiasis, Parasitic Diseases—Schistosomiasis.

Utzinger, J., Zhou, X.N., Chen, M.G., Bergquist, R., 2005. Conquering schistosomiasis in China: the long march. Acta Trop. 96, 69–96.

Wang, W.L., Fang, T.Q., Pan, D.Z., Cai, Z.D., Tian, Z.H., Shu, B.X., 1997. Effect of crop rotation combined with population and cattle chemotherapy in the control of schistosomiasis in lake regions. Chin. J. Parasitol. Parasit. 15, 87–91.

Wang, T., Zhang, S., Wu, W., Zhang, G., Lu, D., Ornbjerg, N., et al., 2006. Treatment and reinfection of water buffaloes and cattle infected with *Schistosoma japonicum* in Yangtze River Valley, Anhui province, China. J. Parasitol. 92, 1088–1091.

Wang, H.Y., Zhang, Z.J., Peng, W.X., Zhou, Y.B., Zhao, G.M., Chen, G.X., et al., 2008a. Analysis of endemic situation of schistosomiasis in Guichi District of Chizhou City, Anhui Province from 2000 to 2006. Chin. J. Schistosomiasis Control 20, 89–92.

Wang, L., Utzinger, J., Zhou, X.-N., 2008b. Schistosomiasis control: experiences and lessons from China. Lancet 372, 1793–1795.

Wang, L.D., Chen, H.G., Guo, J.G., Zeng, X.J., Hong, X.L., Xiong, J.J., et al., 2009a. A strategy to control transmission of *Schistosoma japonicum* in China. N. Engl. J. Med. 360, 121–128.

Wang, S.R., Xiang, R.D., Zhang, J.M., Zhang, Z.H., Liu, T.H., Yu, B., et al., 2009b. Impact of farming prohibition on schistosomiasis endemic in marshland of Hanbei River, Hanchuan City. Chin. J. Schistosomiasis Control 21, 69–71.

Wang, T.P., Chen, G.X., Cao, Z.G., He, Z.G., Zhang, S.Q., Han, S.M., et al., 2009c. Effect of comprehensive schistosomiasis control strategy with emphasis on infectious source

control in Guichi District, Chizhou City, Anhui Province. Chin. J. Schistosomiasis Control 21, 250–258.
Wang, X.Y., Hong, X.L., Hu, Z.H., 2009d. Effect of comprehensive measures for schistosomiasis control in Jinxian County. Chin. J. Schistosomiasis Control 21, 72–73 +75.
Wang, S.R., Xiang, R.D., Zhang, Z.H., Zhang, J.M., Xu, X.W., Yu, B., et al., 2010. Evaluation on the outcome of 'herd-prohibiting and tractor-ploughing' for schistosomiasis control on river banks. J. Pub Health Prev. Med. 21, 55–59.
Wang, X.Y., Hong, X.L., Fan, Y.L., Hu, S.Z., 2012. Investigation on transmission factors of schistosomiasis after replacement of bovine with machine in Jinxian County. Chin. J. Schistosomiasis Control 24, 716–717.
Wang, W., Dai, J.R., Liang, Y.S., 2014. Apropos: factors impacting on progress towards elimination of transmission of schistosomiasis japonica in China. Parasite Vector 7, 408, 2015-2004-2029 2023:2022:2000.
Wei, W.Y., Zhu, S.H., Gan, M.H., Lu, G.L., Liu, Z.C., Shi, M.Z., et al., 2004. Study on environmental modification in snail habitats by isolated canals in Dongting Lake region. Chin. J. Schistosomiasis Control 16, 338–342 +320.
Xiang, R.D., Zhang, Z.H., Wang, S.R., Yu, B., Xu, X.W., Deng, F., et al., 2013. Effects of different prevention and control measures on schistosomiasis prevalence in different limnetic regions. Chin. J. Schistosomiasis Control 25, 506–509.
Xiang, R.D., Zhang, Z.H., Yu, B., Shan, X.W., Xu, X.W., Fang, R., et al., 2014. Effect of comprehensive schistosomiasis control strategy based on infection source control in Hanchuan City. Chin. J. Schistosomiasis Control 26, 658–661.
Xu, X.J., Lu, J.Y., Peng, X., 2010. Function and significance of water conservancy and anti-schistosomiasis project to control schistosomiasis transmission in China. Chin. J. Schistosomiasis Control 22, 403–406.
Xu, C.M., Xiao, X.L., Zheng, S.L., Lu, J., Zhang, L.P., Fan, Q., et al., 2013. Sequential implementing farmland consolidation and replacing cattle with machine to control schistosomiasis. Chin. J. Schistosomiasis Control 25, 541–542.
Xu, F.M., Zhang, L.H., Lu, H.M., Qin, J.S., Cao, W.M., Xie, G.P., 2014. Effect of schistosomiasis control projects in Hexi Reservoir on Oncomelania snail control. Chin. J. Schistosomiasis Control 26, 59–61.
Xu, J., Xu, J.-F., Li, S.-Z., Zhang, L.-J., Wang, Q., Zhu, H.-H., et al., 2015. Integrated control programmes for schistosomiasis and other helminth infections in P.R. China. Acta Trop. 141, 332–341.
Xu, J., Steinman, P., Maybe, D., Zhou, X.N., Lv, S., Li, S.Z., et al., 2016. Evolution of the national schistosomiasis control programmes in the People's Republic of China. Adv. Parasitol. 92.
Yang, K., Li, H.J., Yang, W.C., Shi, X.W., Qi, Y.L., 2009. Effect of comprehensive schistosomiasis control measures with emphasis on infectious source control in dam areas of mountainous region, Yunnan Province. Chin. J. Schistosomiasis Control 21, 272–275.
Yang, Y.F., Peng, Z.H., Sun, Q.X., Zhou, J.X., 2011. Biochemical mechanism of suppressing schistosomiasis with sapium trees. Wetl. Sci. Manage 7, 4–8.
Yang, G.J., Liu, L., Zhu, H.R., Griffiths, S.M., Tanner, M., Bergquist, R., et al., 2014. China's sustained drive to eliminate neglected tropical diseases. Lancet Infect. Dis. 14, 881–892.
Yi Huo, W.L., Zhou, Y.B., Liu, G.M., Wu, Z.S., Wang, S.A., Xu, L., et al., 2009. Effect of four-year comprehensive schistosomiasis control in Puge County, Sichuan Province. Chin. J. Schistosomiasis Control 21, 276–279.
Yuan, Y., Xu, X.J., Dong, H.F., Jiang, M.S., Zhu, H.G., 2005. Transmission control of schistosomiasis japonica: implementation and evaluation of different snail control interventions. Acta Trop. 96, 191–197.

Zhang, S.Q., Wang, T.P., Tao, C.G., Chen, G.X., Chen, J.S., Xu, H., et al., 2005. Observation on comprehensive measures of safe treatment of night-soil and water supply, replacement of bovine with machine for schistosomiasis control. Chin. J. Schistosomiasis Control 17, 437–442.
Zhang, X.D., Qi, L.H., Zhou, J.X., Liu, G.H., Huang, L.L., 2006. Functions and prospects of forestry ecological engineering on preventing schistosomiasis. World For. Res. 19, 33–37.
Zhang, C.H., Tang, G.Y., Liu, F.Y., Li, K., 2012a. Effect of agroforestry model on inhibition of Oncomelania snails in plateau mountainous area of Yunnan Province. Chin. J. Schistosomiasis Control 24, 514–517.
Zhang, Z., Zhu, R., Ward, M.P., Xu, W., Zhang, L., Guo, J., et al., 2012b. Long-term impact of the World Bank Loan Project for schistosomiasis control: a comparison of the spatial distribution of schistosomiasis risk in China. PLoS Negl. Trop. Dis. 6, e1620.
Zhang, S.Q., Xu, Y.M., Cao, Z.G., Jin, W., Yang, W.P., Wang, T.P., 2013. The effects of a forestation project to control schistosomiasis on environmental factors. J. Pathol. Biol. 8, 986–987+1001.
Zhang, L.J., Li, S.Z., Wen, L.Y., Lin, D.D., Abe, E.M., Zhu, R., et al., 2016a. Establishment and function of schistosomiasis surveillance system towards elimination in the People's Republic of China. Adv. Parasitol. 92.
Zhang, S.Q., Sun, C.S., Wang, M., Lin, D.D., Zhou, X.N., Wang, T.P., 2016b. Epidemiological features and control effectiveness of schistosomiasis in lake and marshland region in the People's Republic of China. Adv. Parasitol. 92.
Zheng, Q., Vanderslott, S., Jiang, B., Xu, L.L., Liu, C.S., Huo, L.L., et al., 2013. Research gaps for three main tropical diseases in the People's Republic of China. Infect. Dis. Poverty 2, 15.
Zhong, B., Wu, Z.S., Chen, L., Liang, S., Dong, X.Q., Qiu, D.C., 2011. Strengthening the achievements of schistosomiasis control in hilly regions of China. Chin. J. Schistosomiasis Control 23, 10–13.
Zhou, X.N., Wang, L.Y., Chen, M.G., Wu, X.H., Jiang, Q.W., Chen, X.Y., et al., 2005. The public health significance and control of schistosomiasis in China-then and now. Acta Trop. 96, 97–105.
Zhou, X.N., Guo, J.G., Wu, X.H., Jiang, Q.W., Zheng, J., Dang, H., et al., 2007a. Epidemiology of schistosomiasis in the People's Republic of China, 2004. Emerg. Infect. Dis. 13, 1470–1476.
Zhou, Y.B., Zhao, G.M., Jiang, Q.W., 2007b. Effects of the praziquantel-based control of schistosomiasis japonica in China. Ann. Trop. Med. Parasitol. 101, 695–703.
Zhou, X.N., Yang, G.J., Yang, K., Wang, X.H., Hong, Q.B., Sun, L.P., et al., 2008. Potential impact of climate change on schistosomiasis transmission in China. Am. J. Trop. Med. Hyg. 78, 188–194.
Zhou, Y.B., Yang, M.X., Zhao, G.M., Wei, J.G., Jiang, Q.W., 2009. *Oncomelania hupensis* (Gastropoda: Rissooidea), intermediate host of *Schistosoma japonicum* in China: genetics and molecular phylogeny based on amplified fragment length polymorphisms. Malacologia 49 (2), 367–382, 2015-08-31 08:55:00.
Zhou, Y.B., Liang, S., Chen, G.X., Rea, C., He, Z.G., Zhang, Z.J., et al., 2011. An integrated strategy for transmission control of *Schistosoma japonicum* in a marshland area of China: findings from a five-year longitudinal survey and mathematical modeling. Am. J. Trop. Med. Hyg. 85, 83–88.
Zhou, Y.B., Liang, S., Jiang, Q.W., 2012. Factors impacting on progress towards elimination of transmission of *Schistosomiasis japonica* in China. Parasite Vector 5, 275.
Zhu, Y., Peng, X., Liang, X.Y., Yuan, X.B., Xiong, X.H., Dong, Y., et al., 2009. Effect of hydraulic schistosomiasis control projects on disease prevention. Chin. J. Schistosomiasis Control 21, 227–229.

Zhu, S.P., Li, S.M., Wei, C.J.Y.Q., Lu, B.K., Liao, Y.Z., Chen, J.A., et al., 2011. Evaluation of schistosomiasis control effect of buffalo removal in Anxiang County. Chin. J. Schistosomiasis Control 23, 546–550.
Zhu, C.F., Zeng, Q.F., Li, Y.Y., Huang, Y.X., Huang, W.J., 2014. Quantitative evaluation on snail control effect of snail settling pool. Yangtze River 45, 97–100.
Zhu, H., Yap, P., Utzinger, J., Jia, T.W., Li, S.Z., Huang, X.B., et al., 2016. Policy support and resources mobilization for the national schistosomiasis control programme in the People's Republic of China. Adv. Parasitol. 92.

CHAPTER TEN

Towards the Elimination of Schistosomiasis japonica through Control of the Disease in Domestic Animals in The People's Republic of China: A Tale of over 60 Years

Z.-G. Cao*,§, Y.-E. Zhao*,1, A. Lee Willingham¶, T.-P. Wang§,||,1

*Department of Pathogenic Biology and Immunology, Xi'an Jiaotong University Health Science Center, Xi'an, Shannxi Province, The People's Republic of China
§Anhui Provincial Institute of Schistosomiasis Control, Hefei, Anhui Province, The People's Republic of China
¶Ross University School of Veterinary Medicine, Basseterre, St Kitts, West Indies
||Anhui Institute of Parasitic Disease, Hefei, The People's Republic of China
[1]Corresponding authors: E-mail: zhaoyae@mail.xjtu.edu.cn; tpwang906@163.com

Contents

Advances in Parasitology, Volume 92
ISSN 0065-308X
http://dx.doi.org/10.1016/bs.apar.2016.03.001

Abstract

Schistosomiasis japonica, an endemic, zoonotic tropical parasitic disease caused by *Schistosoma japonicum*, remains an important public health concern in The People's Republic of China. Unlike other species of *Schistosoma*, over 40 species of wild and domestic animals can act as reservoir hosts of *S. japonicum*, which increases the difficulty for the control of this tropical disease. It is widely recognized that domestic animals, particularly water buffaloes and cattle, play an important role in the transmission of *S. japonicum*. Hence, since the 1950s when The People's Republic of China commenced fight against the disease, the control of animal schistosomiasis has been carried out almost synchronously with that of human schistosomiasis, such that great strides have been made over the past six decades. In this chapter, we review the history and current status of schistosomiasis control in domestic animals in The People's Republic of China. We thoroughly analyse the prevalence of domestic animal schistosomiasis at different stages of schistosomiasis control and the role of different species of domestic animals in transmission of the disease, summarize the control strategies and assess their effectiveness. Furthermore, the challenges ahead are discussed and recommendations for future direction are provided.

1. INTRODUCTION

Schistosomiasis japonica, caused by the blood fluke *Schistosoma japonicum*, is mainly prevalent in The People's Republic of China, the Philippines and small foci of Indonesia, with The People's Republic of China being the most heavily endemic of the three countries (Chen, 2014; Gryseels et al., 2006; Tambo et al., 2014). The eggs of *S. japonicum* identified in two ancient corpses from Hunan and Hubei provinces excavated in 1972 and 1975, respectively, indicate that the disease has been present for over 2100 years in The People's Republic of China (Hunan Medical College, 1979; Wei et al., 1980); however, the first clinical case was not detected until 1905 when typical *S. japonicum* eggs were found in a patient's stool (Logan, 1905). Few scientific records were available concerning the endemic status of schistosomiasis before the founding of The People's Republic of China in 1949. In the 1950s, large-scale epidemiological surveys aimed at investigating the incidence, prevalence and intensity of *S. japonicum* infections revealed that the disease was endemic in 12 provinces (autonomous regions/municipalities), mainly along the south side of the Yangtze River. It was estimated that 11.6 million people were infected with the parasite, with over 100 million more at risk of infection (Li et al., 2016). About 1.2 million cattle were detected to have the disease, and the habitat with an area of 14.3 billion m^2 was found to breed *Oncomelania hupensis*, the intermediate host snail of *S. japonicum* (Chen and Feng, 1999). Hence, a national control programme was launched in the mid-1950s in recognition of the serious threat of the disease. This programme is being implemented until today, and periodic policy reviews are performed to keep the control strategy in line with field realities and to adapt the approaches to the changing economic, epidemiological and sociopolitical conditions.

From the mid-1950s, great strides have been made in the control of schistosomiasis in The People's Republic of China. Between 1985 and 1995, disease transmission was interrupted in five provinces of Guangdong, Shanghai, Fujian, Guangxi and Zhejiang (Shi et al., 2016). By 2014, among the other seven endemic provinces, Sichuan, Yunnan, Jiangsu and Hubei reached the criteria of transmission control (both human and domestic animal infection prevalence less than 1%), while Anhui, Jiangxi and Hunan reached the criteria of infection control (both human and domestic animal infection prevalence less than 5%). The number of infected cases has been reduced by over 99%, reaching the lowest historic level of 115,614 infections in 2014. The area of *O. hupensis* habitats was estimated to be 3.6 billion m^2 which is about 25% of that in 1950s (Shi et al., 2016). However, schistosomiasis is still endemic in 140 counties in the remaining seven provinces, and most of these counties are distributed in the lake and marshland regions along the lower and middle reaches of the Yangtze River and also some mountainous regions of Yunnan and Sichuan provinces (Lei et al., 2015; Liu et al., 2014a; Wang et al., 2008). In these areas, snail elimination is very difficult due to their vast habitats in the lake region and the complicated environment in the mountainous area, and it is also very difficult to further decrease the prevalence of *S. japonicum* among humans and domestic animals by routine control measures. Therefore, schistosomiasis remains a major public health problem in The People's Republic of China (Salam et al., 2014; Zheng et al., 2013).

Unlike other *Schistosoma* species, many mammals can act as infectious sources of *S. japonicum* which increases the difficulty of disease control.

Besides humans, over 40 species of wild and domestic animals have been reported to be the reservoir hosts of *S. japonicum* in The People's Republic of China. Thus, zoonotic transmission is considered very important in transmission of *S. japonicum* (Wang et al., 2005). Mammals were initially determined to be infected percutaneously with *S. japonicum* in 1909 (Fujinami and Nakamura, 1909). Faust and Meleney (1924) were the first to determine that animals in The People's Republic of China were infected with the parasite when they detected *S. japonicum* eggs in faeces of a water buffalo in Fuzhou City, Fujian Province, southern China. It has been theorized that *S. japonicum* originally parasitized animals, and then gradually became a zoonosis eventually infecting humans, even though infections in animals were discovered later than in humans. It is postulated that animals in the order Rodentia may be the earliest final host of *S. japonicum*. There is no evidence of endemic areas where only human infection exists without animal infection (Mao, 1990). In The People's Republic of China, the distribution of human and animal schistosomiasis closely overlaps and is considered to be interdependent. Hence, control of *S. japonicum* infection in reservoir hosts, notably domestic animals, has been deemed essential to achieve effective and sustainable control of human schistosomiasis (Wang et al., 1998; Yin et al., 2003).

2. SPECIES OF ANIMAL HOSTS, THEIR SUSCEPTIBILITY AND PATTERN OF *S. JAPONICUM* INFECTION

2.1 Species of animal hosts and their susceptibility to *S. japonicum*

It is estimated that over 40 species of wild and domestic animals comprising 28 genera and 7 orders can be naturally infected with *S. japonicum* (Table 1).

This multitude of mammals can be infected with *S. japonicum*, but the susceptibility varies among different species. Laboratory studies indicate susceptibility to *S. japonicum* infection in descending order among 13 species of animal reservoirs is mice, rabbits, dogs, goats, cattle, rhesus monkeys, guinea pigs, sheep, white rats (*Rattus norvegicus albus*), brown rats (*Rattus norvegicus socer*), pigs, water buffaloes and horses. Among them, domestic animals including cattle, pigs, goats, sheep and dogs are susceptible to *S. japonicum* infection and develop considerable morbidity, while water buffaloes and horses are less susceptible with minimal health impacts (He et al., 1960). Compared with water buffaloes, cattle tend to be more susceptible, and the infection rate in cattle is usually higher than

Table 1 List of animal hosts naturally infected with *S. japonicum*[a]

Order	Species	Disease in hosts[b]	Egg in stool[b]	Epidemiological importance[b]
Order Insectivora	*Crocidura attenuata*		+	−
	Erinaceus europaeus		+	±
	Suncus suncus murinus	++	+	−
Order Rodentia	*Apodemus agrarius ningpoensis*	++	++	+
	Callosciurus erythraeus ningpoensis		+	−
	Eothenomys melanogaster columus		+	−
	Hystrix subcristata subcristata		+	−
	Microtus mandarinus	+	+	−
	Mus musculus		−	−
	Rattus confucianus socer			
	Rattus flavipectus flavipectus		++	+
	Rattus fulvescens huang			
	Rattus losea exugnus			
	Rattus nitidus			
	Rattus norvegicus	++	++	+
	Rattus rattus	+	+	±
Order Lagomorpha	*Lepus cuniculus*	+++	++	+
	Lepus sinensis	++	+	+
Order Carnivora	*Canis familiaris*	+++	+++	++
	Felis bengalensis chinensis			−
	Felis domestica	+	+	±
	Panthera pardus fusca			−
	Herpestes urva			−
	Meles meles leptorynchus		+	−
	Malogale (Helictis) moschata		+	−
	Mustela sibirica davidiana		−	−

(*Continued*)

Table 1 List of animal hosts naturally infected with *S. japonicum*[a]—cont'd

Order	Species	Disease in hosts[b]	Egg in stool[b]	Epidemiological importance[b]
	Nyctereutes procyanoides			
	Viverricula indica palliada		–	–
	Vulpes vulpes			–
Order Perissodatyla	*Equus asinus*	+	–	–
	Equus equus	+	±	+
Order Artidactyla	*Bos taurus*	+++	+++	+++
	Bos buffelus	++	++	++
	Capra hircus	+++	++	++
	Hydropotes inermis inermis	+	+	–
	Muntiacus reevesi	+	+	–
	Ovis aries	+	+	+
	Sus scrofa	++	++	++
	Sus scrofa chirodonta	+	–	–
Order Primates	*Macaca mulatta*	+	+	

[a]The original version of this table was provided by Ming-gang Chen.
[b]"–" represents negative results, "±" represents controversial results, and "+" represents positive results. "+", "++" and "+++" indicates the degree of positive increased in turn.

that in water buffaloes in the same endemic foci, even though water buffaloes are more frequently in contact with infested water than cattle. Field surveys during the 1950s and 1960s from endemic foci of Jiangsu, Jiangxi, Hunan and Fujian provinces showed that the infection rate ranged from 27.5% to 60% in cattle, whereas it was 9.2% to 20.6% in water buffaloes. Clinical symptoms in cattle schistosomiasis are more severe than in water buffaloes (Ministry of Health, 1998). Water buffaloes have the tendency of self-cure thus the time period they excrete eggs in their faeces is short, as their infection rate decreases as the animals age (Li et al., 2014a). Goats are very susceptible to schistosomiasis japonica developing a severe syndrome with high morbidity and excreting large numbers of eggs in their faeces. Pigs are also susceptible to *S. japonicum* infection; however, the development of juvenile schistosomes to adults is lower in pigs than that in cattle and goats. Like water buffaloes, pigs can self-cure (Liu, 1991). The infection rate in rats is quite high in some endemic areas, especially in *Rattus norvegicus*, *Apodemus agrarius ningpoensis* and *Rattus rattus*. While the amount of faeces produced by rats is relatively small, their intensity of infection is high with large numbers of schistosome eggs excreted.

The ratio of the amount of faeces produced per day by rats compared to humans is about 1:24.9, whereas the ratio of the number of miracidia hatching per gram of faeces between rat and man is 1:0.07. Eggs excreted from *R. norvegicus* are noted to hatch easily. It is suggested that the rat is one of the most important animal reservoirs for schistosomiasis, which cannot be ignored in control efforts (Ministry of Agriculture, 1998). Studies have demonstrated that the susceptibility of rats to *S. japonicum* in decreasing order is *Bandicota indica*, *Rattus rattus hainanicus*, *Rattus flavipectus flavipectus*, *Rattus losea* and *R. norvegicus* (Liu et al., 1992). The reed vole, *Microtus fortis*, a dominant species in the Dongting Lake area where schistosomiasis is highly endemic, can be infected with *S. japonicum* cercaria; however, the schistosomula cannot develop into mature adults (Li et al., 1965).

2.2 Route of *S. japonicum* infection

The major route for animal infection with *S. japonicum* is contact with infested water, and is known to occur in three ways: percutaneously, through mucosal penetration and congenitally. Percutaneous infection occurs when *S. japonicum* cercariae invade an animal's body through penetrating its skin when the animal comes in contact with infested water. Percutaneous infection of cercaria is reported to be not affected by particular body site nor skin thickness. Cutaneous infection is considered the major infection route in animals. The second is mucosal infection whereby cercaria invades an animal's body through the mucosa of the digestive system when the animals drink water or eat grasses containing cercariae. It has been reported that milk cows and rabbits have been infected with schistosomiasis when given wet green grass collected from endemic areas that were contaminated with cercaria (Mao, 1990). The third route is congenital infection whereby *S. japonicum* can transmit from an infected mother to her foetus. Congenital transmission of *S. japonicum* was first reported in animals in the 1950s. In The People's Republic of China, the first report of the presence of adult schistosomes in aborted calves was described in 1959, and schistosome eggs have been detected in newborn bovine faeces (Wang, 1959). In order to observe the congenital transmission of *S. japonicum*, three pigs in middle and later gestational period of pregnancy were infected with 9000 cercariae each, and schistosome eggs were found in all 26 offspring piglet's faeces 5–6 weeks after delivery (Willingham et al., 1999). In addition, an animal model for congenital transmission of *S. japonicum* has been established successfully in rabbits (Qian et al., 2002).

3. PREVALENCE OF *S. JAPONICUM* INFECTION IN DOMESTIC ANIMALS

3.1 Before implementation of Chinese national control programme

Although schistosomiasis is an ancient and important zoonotic disease in The People's Republic of China, there were few scientific records on the prevalence of the disease in domestic animals as well as in humans before the founding of The People's Republic of China in 1949. In the 1950s, many epidemiological surveys on schistosomiasis were conducted, and the results revealed high prevalence in domestic animals (Table 2) (Mao, 1990; Shen, 1992). The available data showed that there were 1.5 million farm cattle suffering from schistosomiasis, with a further 5 million at risk of infection. In a survey in the lake region in Hubei Province, 1051 domestic animals of eight species were examined, and seven species were found to be infected, namely cattle, water buffaloes, pigs, dogs, goats, donkeys and cats, with the highest prevalence (46.4%) seen in cattle (National Research Committee on Schistosomiasis, 1957). Results from Jiangsu, Hunan, Guangdong and other

Table 2 *S. japonicum* prevalence in domestic animals in The People's Republic of China from epidemiological surveys reported during the 1950s (Mao, 1990)

Endemic foci			
Province	**County**	**Domestic animal**	**Prevalence (%)**
Hubei Province	Yangxin County	Cattle	36.8
		Water buffaloes	34.6
Hunan Province	Two counties	Cattle	48.8
		Water buffaloes	5.3
Zhejiang Province	Jiashan County	Cattle	85.9
		Water buffaloes	46.8
	Four counties	Pig	2.5
Yunnan Province	–	Pig	23.4
Jiangxi Province	Yongxiu County	Pig	51.8
	Six counties	Bovine*	31.8
		Pig	17.5
		Dog	49.5
		Goat	1.2
Anhui Province	Guichi County	Cattle	75
		Water buffaloes	40
		Donkey	16.7
		Pig	4

*Bovine = cattle + water buffaloes.

endemic areas also demonstrated infections of *S. japonicum* in domestic animals, with the highest prevalence in bovines (ie, cattle and water buffaloes). The prevalence was highest in cattle followed in descending magnitude by water buffaloes, pigs, dogs and other domestic animals (Mao, 1990; Shen, 1992).

3.2 After implementation of Chinese national control programme

Facing the serious endemic situation, a national schistosomiasis control programme was launched during the mid-1950s and still continues. This national control programme is based on periodic policy reviews to keep the control strategy in line with field realities and to adapt the approaches to the changing economic, epidemiological and sociopolitical conditions (Wang et al., 2008). Data from three nationwide epidemiological surveys conducted in 1989, 1995 and 2004 revealed a continuous decline in the prevalence of *S. japonicum* infection in domestic animals, although it was still relatively high. The latest nationwide survey on animal schistosomiasis in 2012 showed a significant reduction in the prevalence of *S. japonicum* infection in domestic animals as compared with that in 2004.

3.2.1 1989: the first nationwide sampling survey

In order to understand the endemic situation of schistosomiasis and assess the effectiveness of control efforts, a systematic sampling survey on the disease was conducted in endemic provinces in 1989. In the survey, 1786 of a total of 13,437 bovines were found infected with the parasite, as revealed by miracidial hatching technique, with an overall prevalence of 13.29%. The prevalence in cattle was 16.55% (530/3203) while the prevalence in water buffaloes was 12.27% (1256/10,234). The prevalence was higher in water buffaloes than in cattle in the marshland and lake regions, while a higher prevalence was detected in cattle in the hilly and mountainous regions. In addition, prevalence was found to be 3.11% (315/10,115), 10.4% (34/327), 2.62% (68/2600) and 5.64% (87/1543) in pigs, sheep/goats, dogs and other domestic animals, respectively (Table 3) (Ministry of Health, 1993).

3.2.2 1995: the second nationwide sampling survey

In 1995, the second nationwide sampling survey on schistosomiasis was organized covering eight provinces, namely Hunan, Hubei, Jiangxi, Anhui, Jiangsu, Zhejiang, Sichuan and Yunnan where the disease was still endemic. The prevalence of *S. japonicum* infection in domestic animals was

Table 3 Results of miracidial hatching test of domestic animals in endemic provinces of The People's Republic of China in 1989

	Cattle			Water buffaloes			Pigs		
Province	No. examined	No. positive	Prevalence (%)	No. examined	No. positive	Prevalence (%)	No. examined	No. positive	Prevalence (%)
Hunan	50	22	44.00	2113	358	16.94	1656	100	6.04
Hubei	207	8	3.86	2795	523	18.71	3792	108	2.85
Jiangxi	397	43	10.83	1484	113	7.61	201	7	3.48
Anhui	–	–	–	932	77	8.26	461	12	2.60
Sichuan	1205	341	28.30	2016	159	7.89	3024	60	1.98
Yunnan	1344	116	8.63	894	26	2.91	981	28	2.85
Total	3203	530	16.55	10,234	1256	12.27	10,115	315	3.11

determined using miracidial hatching technique in all endemic provinces except Zhejiang. The results showed a 9.09% (1317/14,543) overall prevalence in bovines, with 7.17% (229/3196) and 9.59% (1088/11,347) prevalence for cattle and water buffaloes, respectively. In addition, prevalence was found to be 2.09% (183/8762) and 2.46% (28/1137) in pigs and small ruminants, respectively. In Sichuan Province, the prevalence was 1.87% (25/1340) in dogs, and 3.33% (18/540) infection was observed in equines (ie, horses, donkeys and mules) in Yunnan Province (Table 4). Compared with the data captured from the first nationwide survey, the prevalence of *S. japonicum* infection was reduced by 56.68%, 21.84%, 32.8%, 76.35% and 26.63% in cattle, water buffaloes, pigs, sheep/goats and dogs, respectively.

The survey indicated bovine prevalence of 11.56% (890/7702), 6.27% (427/6808) and 0% (0/33) in the marshland and lake regions, the hilly

Table 4 Results of miracidial hatching test of domestic animals in endemic provinces of The People's Republic of China in 1995

	Cattle			Water buffaloes			Pigs		
Province	No. examined	No. positive	Prevalence (%)	No. examined	No. positive	Prevalence (%)	No. examined	No. positive	Prevalence (%)
Hunan	73	4	5.48	1931	189	9.79	1706	25	1.47
Hubei	131	16	12.21	4006	600	14.98	2322	110	4.74
Jiangxi	497	24	4.83	1504	46	3.06	2259	26	1.15
Anhui	91	3	3.30	891	49	5.50	666	11	1.65
Jiangsu	–	–	–	272	6	2.21	973	3	0.31
Sichuan	329	9	2.74	1888	152	8.05	–	–	–
Yunnan	2075	173	8.34	855	46	5.38	836	8	0.96
Total	3196	229	7.17	11,347	1088	9.59	8762	183	2.09

Goats and sheep			Dogs			Others		
No. examined	No. positive	Prevalence (%)	No. examined	No. positive	Prevalence (%)	No. examined	No. positive	Prevalence (%)
17	15	88.24	31	6	19.35	8	0	0
78	19	24.36	7	7	7/7	–	–	–
–	–	–	–	–	–	–	–	–
–	–	–	–	–	–	–	–	–
–	–	–	2317	50	2.16	622	73	11.74
232	0	0	245	5	2.04	913	14	1.53
327	34	10.40	2600	68	2.62	1543	87	5.64

and mountainous regions and the plain regions with waterway networks, respectively. Separately 11.84% (849/7172), 5.77% (239/4142) and 0% (0/33) prevalence were found in water buffaloes in these three types of endemic regions, respectively, while 7.74% (41/530) and 7.05% (188/2666) of cattle were egg-positive in the lake and mountainous regions, with no cattle examinations having been conducted in the plain regions (Ministry of Health, 1998).

3.2.3 2004: the third nationwide sampling survey

In 2004, the third nationwide sampling survey was conducted in the seven endemic provinces: Hubei, Hunan, Jiangxi, Anhui, Jiangsu, Yunnan and Sichuan. Results from the survey showed 4.37% (404/9274) prevalence in bovines overall, with 3.68% (106/2883) and 4.66% (298/6391) prevalence for cattle and water buffaloes, respectively. In addition, 0.27%

Goats and sheep			Dogs			Others		
No. examined	No. positive	Prevalence (%)	No. examined	No. positive	Prevalence (%)	No. examined	No. positive	Prevalence (%)
6	9	9/16	–	–	–	–	–	–
77	16	9.04	–	–	–	–	–	–
–	–	–	–	–	–	–	–	–
–	–	–	–	–	–	–	–	–
12	1	0.16	–	–	–	–	–	–
			1340	25	1.87	–	–	–
32	2	0.60	–	–	–	540	18	3.33
137	28	2.46						

(5/1839) and 1.44% (17/1179) of pigs and goats/sheep were found egg positives, respectively. In the provinces of Yunnan and Sichuan, 539 domestic animals including horses, donkeys, mules and dogs were examined; however, no positives were detected (Table 5). Compared with the second nationwide survey, the prevalence of *S. japonicum* reduced by 48.68%, 21.46%, 87.08%, 41.46% and 100% in cattle, water buffaloes, pigs, sheep/goats and dogs, respectively, and a decline was also observed in other domestic animals.

The overall prevalence of bovine schistosomiasis was 6.04% (250/4139) and 3.0% (154/5135), cattle schistosomiasis 4.55% (34/747) and 3.37% (72/2136), and water buffalo schistosomiasis 6.37% (216/3392) and 2.73% (82/2999) in the marshland/lake regions and the hilly/mountainous regions, respectively. The testing of *S. japonicum* infection was not performed in bovines in the plain regions with waterway networks in this survey (Ministry of Health, 2006).

Results from the three epidemiological sampling surveys demonstrated a reduction in the prevalence of *S. japonicum* infection in domestic animals during the period from 1989 to 2004 (Fig. 1).

3.2.4 Current prevalence

In 2012, a nationwide survey on the infection of *S. japonicum* in domestic animals in the seven remaining schisotosomiasis endemic provinces of Hunan, Hubei, Jiangxi, Anhui, Jiangsu, Sichuan and Yunnan showed a further significant reduction of *S. japonicum* infection in domestic animals (Li et al., 2014a). A census estimated that there were 1,033,056 bovine, 2,024,512 goats/sheep and 891,301 other domestic animals, including pigs, dogs, horses and so on, in these provinces. The prevalence, determined by conducting the miracidial hatching test on faecal samples, were found to be 0.58% (3961/684,899) in bovines, 0.57% (406/71,473) in sheep/goats, and 0.01% (21/142,976) in other domestic animals. Region-specific prevalence showed that the infection rate of bovines and sheep/goats was much higher in Hunnan and Jiangxi provinces than in the other five provinces, whereas there were no domestic animals found to be infected with *S. japonicum* in Jiangsu Province (Table 6) (Li et al., 2014a). The results suggested that the control of schistosomiasis in bovines and sheep/goats in the Dongting Lake region in Hunan Province and the Poyang Lake region in Jiangxi Province remains a key and difficult issue for the national schistosomiasis control program in The People's Republic of China. In addition, continued epidemiological surveillance conducted in the five provinces of Guangdong,

Table 5 Results of miracidial hatching test of domestic animals in endemic provinces of The People's Republic of China in 2004

	Cattle			Water buffaloes			Pigs			Goats and sheep			Others		
Province	No. examined	No. positive	Prevalence (%)	No. examined	No. positive	Prevalence (%)	No. examined	No. positive	Prevalence (%)	No. examined	No. positive	Prevalence (%)	No. examined	No. positive	Prevalence (%)
Hunan	215	13	6.05	874	83	9.50	116	0	0.00	184	9	4.89	0	0	0.00
Hubei	225	8	3.56	2464	125	5.07	0	0	0.00	0	0	0.00	1	0	0.00
Jiangxi	451	15	3.33	742	33	4.45	0	0	0.00	200	0	0.00	0	0	0.00
Anhui	20	1	5.00	422	21	4.98	910	3	0.33	365	7	1.92	0	0	0.00
Jiangsu	70	0	0.00	31	0	0.00	0	0	0.00	0	0	0.00	0	0	0.00
Sichuan	1151	52	4.52	1389	28	2.02	100	0	0.00	20	0	0.00	137	0	0.00
Yunnan	751	17	2.26	469	8	1.71	713	2	0.28	410	1	0.24	401	0	0.00
Total	2883	106	3.68	6391	298	4.66	1839	5	0.27	1179	17	1.44	539	0	0.00

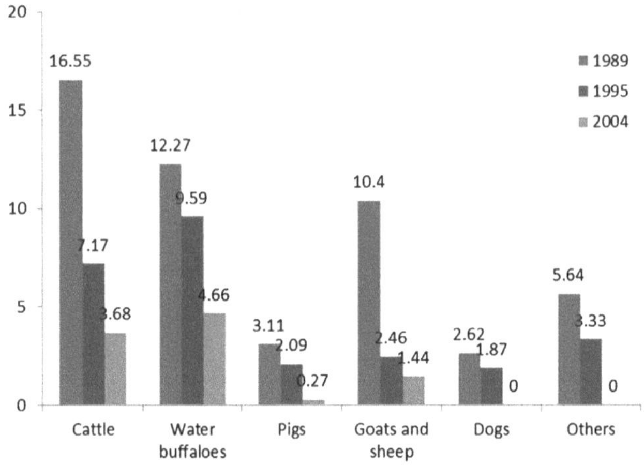

Figure 1 Comparison of *S. japonicum* prevalence (%) in domestic animals among the three nationwide sampling surveys conducted in The People's Republic of China.

Shanghai, Fujian, Guangxi and Zhejiang which achieved the criteria of schistosomiasis elimination between 1985 and 1995, indicated no infected domestic animals in those provinces (Li and Lin, 2007; Tang et al., 2012).

4. EFFECT OF *S. JAPONICUM* INFECTION ON DOMESTIC ANIMALS

Many epidemiological surveys in the 1950s indicated that schistosomiasis greatly threatened the health of domestic animals and caused considerable economic loss in livestock production. In Yeyang Cattle Farm, Anhui Province, 416 of 1292 cattle (32.2%) died from schistosomiasis after 6 months of pasturing on *S. japonicum*-contaminated marshland. In Xiangyin County, Hunan Province, all of the 90 goats imported from nonendemic areas in northern China died shortly after pasturing on contaminated beaches of the Dongting Lake (National Schistosomiasis Research Committee, 1959). In Saihu Lake Farm, Jiujiang City, Jiangxi Province, all of their 50 goats died from schistosomiasis within one year. Experimental study showed that there was no change in the body weight of goats infected with 50 cercariae, whereas the body weight of goats decreased by 24% after infection with over 100 cercariae within 40 days (Liu, 1991).

During the 1990s, several reports showed a large number of deaths due to schistosomiasis in domestic animals. In March 1998, Sujiahepo Domestic Farm of Hanshou County, Hunan Province, imported 43 cattle and 51 goats

Table 6 Results of miracidial hatching test of domestic animals in endemic provinces of The People's Republic of China in 2012

	Bovine				Goats and sheep				Others			
Province	Total no. of animal	No. examined	No. positive	Prevalence (%)	Total no. of animal	No. examined	No. positive	Prevalence (%)	Total no. of animal	No. examined*	No. positive	Prevalence (%)
Hunan	192,527	95,665	1172	1.23	117,416	20,226	182	0.90	–	–	–	–
Hubei	191,645	201,071	499	0.25	119,737	20,407	58	0.28	–	–	–	–
Jiangxi	162,681	119,697	1999	1.67	22,694	6177	124	2.01	–	–	–	–
Anhui	49,030	26,220	144	0.55	72,821	9431	42	0.45	–	–	–	–
Jiangsu	19,052	3410	0	0.00	374,223	8626	0	0.00	199,095	7483	0	0
Sichuan	198,753	120,273	17	0.01	1,143,933	3323	0	0.00	290,848	123,596	17	0.01
Yunnan	219,368	118,563	130	0.11	173,688	3283	0	0.00	401,358	11,897	4	0.03
Total	1,033,056	684,899	3961	0.58	2,024,512	71,473	406	0.57	891,301	142,976	21	0.01

from nonendemic areas, almost all of which suffered from fever, emaciation, loss of appetite and diarrhea after they were grazed for 5 months on an islet inhabited by *Oncomelania* snails. By December of that year 27 of the cattle and 37 of the goats died from schistosomiasis (Jin, 1990). In Qili Lake of Dongzhi County, Anhui Province, 55 (32%) of 172 goats were found positive by the miracidial hatching technique between 1993 and 1995, and two of them were determined to have died from schistosomiasis (Tan, 1997). In 1996, at Shashan village of Tangtian Township, Guichi County, Anhui Province, a domestic farm established close to a river beach with many infested snails, which imported 56 cattle and 500 goats from nonendemic areas in northern Anhui province, experienced 20 cattle and more than 200 goats dying from schistosomiasis after they were pastured on the marshlands for few months (Xu and Wang, 1997).

From these data it can be inferred that schistosomiasis can cause serious economic losses due to death and reduced production of livestock. However, the implementation of the national control programme resulted in fewer and fewer deaths in domestic animals in the 2010s. Domestic animals in endemic areas may suffer from syndromes such as fever, emaciation, poor appetite and diarrhea following infection, but few deaths are recorded. However, the domestic animals without specific immunity from nonendemic areas usually have a higher mortality due to schistosomiasis if they are moved to endemic areas. Only a few reports are available in terms of production losses caused directly by *S. japonicum* infection, such as the reduction of growth, milk production and working capacity as well as impacts on reproduction.

5. THE ROLE OF DOMESTIC ANIMALS IN THE TRANSMISSION OF SCHISTOSOMIASIS

Domestic animals have been proved to play an important role in the transmission of schistosomiasis. Understanding their distribution, prevalence and evaluating their roles in the transmission of *S. japonicum* is of great importance for schistosomiasis control. The major animal reservoir species involved in transmission needed to be determined in order to develop an effective control programme. The contribution of a reservoir host in transmission of the disease cannot be evaluated solely based on *S. japonicum* infection. In addition to prevalence, the following factors should be taken into consideration: (1) species of domestic animals, their susceptibility to *S. japonicum*, daily egg output, and hatching rate of eggs; (2) number of that domestic animal host; and (3) the likelihood of eggs excreted in the faeces of that host contaminating water sources that serve as *Oncomelania* snail habitats.

5.1 Evaluation indicators

Currently, three parameters are employed to evaluate environmental contamination of *S. japonicum* eggs in The People's Republic of China: (1) total egg output from a host per day (EPD), which is estimated using the formula EPD for a host = number of the host × infection rate of the host × eggs per gram (EPG) of the host faeces × weight of faeces excreted per day/100; (2) relative index of transmission (RIT) = total number of the host species (Hi) × infection rate of the host (Pi) × EPD of the host (EPDi) × egg hatching rate of the host (EHRi)/Σ(Hi × Pi × EPDi × EHRi), 'Σ' represents sum, 'i' represents different kinds of hosts; and (3) the actual index of contamination in snail habitat areas, that is, estimated number of eggs from faeces excreted by all kinds of hosts per unit area.

The first indicator represents the potential contamination, the second expresses potential importance of a host's impact on transmission, and the third reflects actual contamination (Ministry of Health, 2000).

5.2 Evaluating the role of various domestic animals in schistosomiasis transmission

Based on EPD and RIT, humans are predominant in the transmission of *S. japonicum*, while other hosts play a lesser role (Su et al., 1999; Wang et al., 2000; Xu et al., 2001). Human's high EPD was probably related to the methods used for faecal egg counts using the Kato–Katz technique (Ministry of Health, 2000), whereas animals' EPG was estimated by counting the number of miracidia per gram faeces. Animal's EPG is always underestimated since not all eggs in their faeces hatch. During the 2000s, the significance of humans as a transmission source appears to be decreasing compared with that of their contribution during the1960s and 1970s. The use of fresh human stools as fertilizer ('night soil') has decreased in importance, and behavioural changes have occurred with regard to the habit of human defection in the fields and water bodies. These two factors, in combination with lower human prevalence rates due to repeated chemotherapy have made the human contribution to transmission of schistosomiasis less important compared to that of domestic animals. Ruminants (ie, cattle, water buffaloes, sheep and goats), in particular, graze during the transmission season in the contaminated areas and often defaecate directly onto the snail habitats (Wang et al., 1998; Zheng et al., 1990a,b,c).

Domestic animals, notably ruminants, graze freely in the marshland and lake regions because of abundant grass pastures. Their activities are wide ranging, thereby resulting in high frequency of contact with infested water and high likelihood of infection. In addition, they graze on grasslands mainly in spring and autumn when rainfall is plentiful, and the temperature and climate suitable for *S. japonicum* egg hatching.

5.2.1 Cattle and water buffaloes

Many investigations have revealed that bovines play the most important role among domestic animals in the transmission of schistosomiasis in The People's Republic of China (Zhang et al., 2016b). This is because they are large animals (water buffaloes often exceed 500 kg in weight), depositing considerable amounts of excreta near or in surface water, and their faeces (manure) in the environment often takes a long time to dry. As a result, the eggs in the manure may remain viable for a long time. Cattle and water buffaloes often live longer than 10–12 years, and they may harbour large numbers of schistosomes and develop hepatointestinal disease.

In the marshland and lake regions, bovines have been found to be the major infectious source of schistosomiasis transmission. Cattle and water buffaloes accounted for 70–90% of the relative egg contamination indices on the marshlands from the 1970s until the 1990s according to different field surveys, with the index much lower for humans (Mao, 1990). One large-scale epidemiological survey conducted in 2001 indicated that more than 90% of schistosome eggs in the flood plains around the Poyang Lake were excreted by cattle and water buffaloes (Guo et al., 2001). A later epidemiological survey on an islet in the Yangtze River in Anhui Province showed that bovines were responsible for 99.7% of the schistosome egg contamination (Liu et al., 2013). An epidemiological survey conducted in five endemic villages in the marshlands and lake regions of Anhui Province from 1992 to 1995 showed that 90%, 8.48% and 0.2% of the RIT was contributed by humans, bovines and other animals, respectively; however, the actual contamination index due to bovines accounted for 99.83% of the total (Shi et al., 1992).

In the mountainous and hilly regions, faeces from bovines and wild rats appear to play a major role in the contamination of fields with schistosome eggs, while human faeces play a less important role. An investigation in Weishan County, Yunnan Province around 1990 showed that the EPD contributions of humans, bovines, and other animals was 32.84%, 60.87%, and less than 6%, respectively (Zheng et al., 1990a,b,c), which was comparable to the results from Leqiu Conuty, Yunnan Province (Yang and Yang, 1996).

Since cattle are more susceptible to *S. japonicum* than water buffaloes, they usually have a higher prevalence. In addition, water buffaloes have the capacity to self-cure (Li et al., 2014b). Therefore at the individual level, the role of cattle in transmission of schistosomiasis is deemed more important than that of water buffaloes. However, water buffaloes are more populous than cattle in the marshlands and lake regions, have much more water contact and are prone to defaecate while in the water resulting in an increased likelihood of infection and contamination.

5.2.2 Pigs

The role of pigs in the transmission of schistosomiasis is disputed with some reports indicating that they are an important reservoir host while others suggest that pigs cannot serve as a major reservoir host since they can recover naturally through self-cure and generally are slaughtered within one year thus limiting their contribution to contamination (Shi et al., 1992). Compared with bovines, the range and frequency of pigs' activities and grazing on the marshlands are limited; however, the prevalence of *S. japonicum* infection remains quite high in pigs. A survey in Anhui Province showed a 21.3% (13/61) prevalence in pigs (Wang et al., 1998). Pigs are considered one of the important reservoirs of schistosomiasis in certain regions since the prevalence of porcine schistosomiasis ranks third after that of cattle and water buffalo, and the total number of pigs remains stable even though their life span is relatively short. However, during the 2000s pigs have been considered of less importance in transmission due to their increasing confinement in pens as a result of government efforts, thus limiting their access to marshland areas (Gray et al., 2008).

5.2.3 Goats and sheep

In the past, goats and sheep were mainly bred in the mountain areas, hence they did not contribute much to overall transmission (Sleigh et al., 1998). However, during the 2010s, goats and sheep have been imported into the marshland and lake regions with a steady increase in their numbers observed every year. Goats and sheep have been found to be highly susceptible to *S. japonicum*. Although their mean daily defaecation volume is 70 times less than that of water buffaloes, they are considered to be emerging important infectious sources of schistosomiasis as they often graze freely in the transmission areas (Xu and Wang, 1997; Zhang et al., 1998).

5.2.4 Dogs and cats

According to a survey conducted in the 1990s in Hubei Province, the prevalence of schistosomiasis in dogs was 75(9/12)%, and they were considered to be of great epidemiological importance in the transmission of schistosomiasis (Su et al., 1994). However, exposure of dogs to infested water is low. Other investigations revealed that dogs and cats were not important infectious sources of schistosomiasis because they had a relatively low infection rate (Mao, 1990). On the other hand, dogs have a habit of eating human faeces. The schistosome eggs in human faeces ingested by dogs may then be excreted in the dog faeces in a viable state and still hatch. Therefore, dogs are considered to serve a dual role in the transmission of schistosomiasis (Zheng et al., 1990a,b,c).

5.2.5 Other domestic animal hosts

Other domestic animal reservoirs, including horses, donkeys and mules, are found to have a relatively low prevalence of *S. japonicum* infection and low intensities of infection, and they are mostly found in mountain areas. These animals seldom go to wet areas serving as snail habitats, and thus have a low risk of infection. It is therefore considered that these domestic animals play little role in the transmission of schistosomiasis (Ministry of Agriculture, 1998; Ministry of Health 2006).

5.2.6 Relative transmission index

It is now widely accepted that bovines, particularly water buffaloes, play a major role in the transmission of schistosomiasis in The People's Republic of China. Mathematical models estimate that up to 75% of transmission is attributable to bovines in the lake and marshland areas, as they are naturally infected with schistosomes and deposit more eggs into the environment than humans or any other animal hosts (Gray et al., 2009; Guo et al., 2006). However, the major infectious sources of schistosomiasis have been found to vary in different endemic areas. For example, a cross-sectional survey conducted in two villages along the Yangtze River valley in Anhui Province in 2003 with the aim of assessing the relative contribution of humans and domestic animals to schistosomiasis transmission showed that the prevalence and intensity of *S. japonicum* infection both varied significantly between host species and between the two villages investigated. Likewise the total daily egg excretion and RTI varied significantly between the two villages. Water buffaloes were responsible for about 90% of the transmission in one village, whereas its contribution in the other village was only 4.5%;

Table 7 Prevalence, intensity, total daily egg excretion (TDEE) and relative transmission index (RTI) of *S. japonicum*–infected hosts in Chenqiao village of Anhui Province

Species	Total no.	No. examined	No. positive	Prevalence (%)	Intensity (EPG)	TDEE	RTI (%)
Humans	2849	652	8	1.2	62	347,015	4.4
Water buffaloes	191	108	29	26.9	9.4	7,077,823	89.8
Cattle	0	0	0	0	0	0	0
Pigs	67	27	2	7.49	2	15,049	0.2
Goats	298	66	22	33.3	22.2	422,121	5.4
Dogs	310	73	2	2.7	20.5	17,239	0.2
Cats	157	34	0	0	0	0	0

Table 8 Prevalence, intensity, total daily egg excretion (TDEE) and relative transmission index (RTI) of *S. japonicum*–infected hosts in Guanghui village of Anhui Province

Species	Total no.	No. examined	No. positive	Prevalence (%)	Intensity (EPG)	TDEE	RTI (%)
Humans	2779	1216	122	10	99.6	4,435,908	80.4
Water buffaloes	78	49	4	8.2	2.7	249,246	4.5
Cattle	286	192	33	17.2	2.8	824,295	14.9
Pigs	76	49	0	0	0	0	0
Goats	76	76	0	0	0	0	0
Dogs	211	74	3	4.1	10.7	9027	0.2
Cats	150	67	1	1.5	6	261	0

the human contribution was also strikingly different in the two villages with more than 80% of the transmission determined to be resulting from humans in one village but only 4.4% in the other (Tables 7 and 8) (Wang et al., 2005). This survey revealed that schistosomiasis transmission sources may vary significantly between farming communities. Hence, it is suggested that successful schistosomiasis control in the different endemic areas in The People's Republic of China should rely on RTI determinations rather than routine prevalence and intensity determination.

6. CONTROL STRATEGIES FOR DOMESTIC ANIMAL SCHISTOSOMIASIS AND ITS EFFECTIVENESS

Since the 1950s when The People's Republic of China started the campaign to combat schistosomiasis, the control of animal schistosomiasis has been carried out almost synchronously with that of human schistosomiasis, with the strategies and approaches utilized shifting over time in order to adapt to political, socioeconomic, technological and epidemiological changes. Four relatively distinct phases may be identified in the process of schistosomiasis control in domestic animals: (1) large-scale epidemiological surveys in the 1950s; (2) case screening followed by limited drug treatment during the 1960s and 1970s; (3) mass chemotherapy with praziquantel during the 1980s and 1990s; and (4) an integrated strategy aimed at preventing environmental contamination of schistosome eggs from the early 2000s to till date (Collins et al., 2012).

Although schistosomiasis japonica is a zoonotic disease with many animals playing a role in its transmission, only bovines have been included in the national control programme besides humans, due to their vast numbers in the endemic regions, high prevalence and relatively greater contamination index (Wang et al., 2006). Accordingly, the total numbers of cattle and water buffaloes present as well as the numbers of bovines tested, found positive and treated must be reported to the schistosomiasis control authorities at the Chinese National Health and Family Planning Commission on an annual basis (Zhang et al., 2016a). The situation of bovine schistosomiasis in The People's Republic of China from 1989 to 2014 is shown in Table 9.

6.1 Chemotherapy

6.1.1 Chemotherapy drugs

Drugs used in the early stages of the control programme to treat domestic animal schistosomiasis included antimonyl potassium tartrate, furpromide, hexachloroparaxylene and metrifonate; however, they were found to have severe and even lethal side effects that had to be weighed against the benefits for the infected animals (Xiao, 2005). In 1978, a breakthrough in chemotherapy occurred when the antischistosomiasis drug praziquantel was synthesized in The People's Republic of China. Both animal experiments and clinical studies have shown that the drug possesses the characteristics of low toxicity, high efficacy, short treatment course and ease of administration. It can be widely used for treatment of both humans and domestic animals suffering from schistosomiasis. The drug has been widely used for chemotherapy since the mid-1980s after a few years of clinical trials (Dabo et al., 2013; Ojurongbe et al., 2014). The oral dose of praziquantel for cattle and water buffaloes is 30 mg/kg and 25 mg/kg, respectively. The treatment doses are lower than that used for humans (40 mg/kg for 1 day or 60 mg/kg for 2 days) because the collateral effects may be fatal, which is thought to result from portal occlusion by dead worms in heavily

Table 9 The situation of bovine schistosomiasis in The People's Republic of China from 1989 to 2014[a]

Year	No. of bovines in endemic regions	No. examined	No. of cases	Prevalence (%)	No. treated	No. of expanding chemotherapy in severe endemic regions
1989	1,306,849	602,550	27,650	4.59	25,821	–
1990	1,625,485	936,455	50,882	5.43	73,953	–
1991	1,487,233	959,172	50,954	5.31	51,302	–
1992	1,659,232	742,862	35,196	4.74	87,681	–
1993	1,558,945	618,788	22,489	3.63	123,231	–
1994	1,667,878	641,887	19,374	3.02	91,143	–
1995	1,742,907	660,486	17,731	2.68	16,590	321,611
1996	1,750,197	620,272	18,519	2.99	17,612	289,087
1997	1,824,184	626,587	15,899	2.54	15,075	340,364
1998	1,815,265	639,073	21,030	3.29	20,026	380,337
1999	1,638,433	640,559	21,457	3.35	21,626	348,901
2000	1,672,918	616,489	20,705	3.36	20,594	283,607
2001	1,404,046	575,184	31,547	5.48	31,320	234,814
2002	1,676,321	665,123	23,199	3.49	22,886	291,266
2003	1,803,808	594,522	24,461	4.11	23,848	275,554
2004	1,701,220	554,003	24,863	4.49	21,948	341,249
2005	1,764,472	916,344	33,736	3.68	32,093	426,572
2006	1,586,715	724,454	24,855	3.43	24,423	560,267
2007	1,496,477	785,855	16,624	2.10	13,909	528,506
2008	1,468,669	747,857	9988	1.34	9912	686,552
2009	1,570,300	752,779	7753	1.03	7899	748,121
2010	1,476,606	686,622	7173	1.04	7000	479,844
2011	1,410,936	753,782	5146	0.68	5220	491,983
2012	1,189,829	630,217	3297	0.52	3607	467,069
2013	962,065	221,509	633	0.29	927	434,370
2014	919,579	257,769	666	0.26	798	408,690

[a]The data come from annual reports on schistosomiasis control issued by Chinese National Health and Family Planning Commission.

infected animals (Chen, 2005). In consideration of both safety and effectiveness, the dosage mentioned is used for cattle greater than 300 kg body weight and water buffaloes greater than 400 kg of body weight with lower doses administered to smaller bovines.

Besides chemotherapy with praziquantel, artesunate and artemether were tested as early preventive drugs by killing schistosomula in cattle and water buffaloes before they develop into adult schistosomes, with positive results. However, the cost of the preventive treatment is high, which limits its large-scale application (Xiang et al., 2001).

6.1.2 Effectiveness

In the early phase of the Chinese national schistosomiasis control programme, the endemic situation was quite serious with high morbidity and mortality of domestic animals especially bovines and sheep as a result of severe schistosomiasis resulting in the closure of multiple livestock farms. Chemotherapy was lifesaving and played a great role in morbidity control between 1950s and 1970s. However, the chemotherapy drugs used in this period were comparatively toxic, usually requiring a long treatment course, such that they could not meet the requirements for large-scale use. Individual chemotherapy based on confirmed diagnosis was the main approach for schistosomiasis treatment during the 1950s until the mid-1980s when praziquantel became available. Thus chemotherapy played a comparatively limited role in the control of schistosomiasis before the mid-1980s (Xiao, 2005).

Large-scale implementation of praziquantel-based chemotherapy has revolutionized the national schistosomiasis control programme in The People's Republic of China, shifting the focus on transmission control to morbidity control. Since the mid-1980s praziquantel has become the drug of choice for treatment of both human and domestic animal schistosomiasis as the price of the drug has decreased significantly making it cost effective for widespread use. A synchronous praziquantel chemotherapy programme for both humans and bovines was initiated in the late 1980s in the lake region, firstly in Hunan Province, and then in other provinces such as Hubei, Jiangxi and Anhui. As a consequence, a significant reduction of the prevalence and intensity of *S. japonicum* infection was achieved in humans and bovines. A longitudinal study on the effectiveness of synchronous chemotherapy in 30 pilot sites of the Dongting Lake region during the period 1987 to 1994 showed that the prevalence and intensity of *S. japonicum* infection decreased from 8.2% and 5.2 in 1987 to 4.2% and 2.0 in 1994, respectively, following synchronous chemotherapy with a single dose of praziquantel of 58.9–86.3% of targeted populations (Chen et al., 1998).

From 1992 to 2001 when the World Bank Loan Project (WBLP) for Schistosomiasis Control was implemented in The People's Republic of China, a great decrease in prevalence and morbidity was achieved through the mass chemotherapy strategy. The WBLP started in eight provinces in 1992, was finalized in five of them (Anhui, Jiangsu, Jiangxi, Sichuan and Zhejiang) at the end of 1998, and continued until the end of 2001 in the three remaining provinces (Hubei, Hunan and Yunnan). The five provinces that completed the project in 1998 continued to carry out schistosomiasis control with their own funds according to the operational plan set out by the WBLP. During the 10-year implementation of the WBLP, a total of 1.7 million cattle and water buffaloes were screened and those infected were treated with praziquantel and an additional 2.2 million animals in severe endemic areas received mass chemotherapy. More than 63 million people were screened, and almost 19 million treatments were given through, both mass chemotherapy and selective treatment campaigns. In 1998, when the WBLP came to an end in five of the eight provinces, the number of infected bovines and their infection rate decreased by 55.03% and 50.31%, respectively, while the number of infected people and the infection rate of humans decreased by 49.57% and 54.69%, respectively, compared to the initial 1992 figures. The mean number of human patients diagnosed per year with acute schistosomiasis decreased from 6386 during the period from 1989 to 1991, to 1093 cases during the period between 1996 and 2000, despite severe flooding in the endemic regions in 1998 and 1999. The density of infected snails in areas with high, medium and low endemicity decreased by 75.6%, 90% and 87.5%, respectively (Table 10). In the eight provinces, the number of administrative villages with high endemicity (prevalence greater than 15%) was reduced from 4058 in 1992 to 2552 in 1998, a decrease of 37.1%, while the number of administrative villages with low endemicity (prevalence lower than 3%) rose from 26,834 in 1992 to 30,850 in 1998, an increase of 15.8% (Chen, 2005). All of these parameters mentioned above further decreased in 2001 (Chen et al., 2002). The original WBLP schistosomiasis control goals of reducing the prevalence

Table 10 The World Bank Loan Project for schistosomiasis control in The People's Republic of China: operational indicators 1992–1998

Indicator	Year		Reduction rate (%)
	1992	1998	
No. of infected people	1,733,981	874,515	49.6
% of positive results of faecal examination	6.9	3.1	54.7
No. of infected cattle and buffaloes	104,764	47,115	55
% of positive results of faecal examination	6.4	3.2	50.3
Density of infected snails(no. per **0.1 m^2) in areas of**			
High endemicity	0.0078	0.0019	75.6
Medium endemicity	0.006	0.0006	90
Low endemicity	0.0001	0.0001	87.5

in humans and bovines and reducing the density of infected snails were completely achieved.

The achievements of the WBLP for Schistosomiasis Control proved that the chemotherapy-based strategy could decrease the prevalence and morbidity of schistosomiasis rapidly, and was thus utilized widely for schistosomiasis control in The People's Republic of China, especially in the 1980s and 1990s. However, further decrease of the prevalence was difficult. Although the sources of infection were being controlled through periodic chemotherapy, the snail habitats did not change, resulting in the probability of reinfection remaining relatively high thus preventing transmission from being interrupted. In addition, concern developed that the long-term extensive praziquantel-based chemotherapy could result in the emergence of praziquantel-resistant parasites. Following the termination of the WBLP for Schistosomiasis Control in 2001, investment in schistosomiasis control programme decreased, and demographic, environmental and socioeconomic transformations led to the reemergence of schistosomiasis in certain parts of the country (Liang et al., 2006). Thus, there was growing concern that the national control programme would not reach its ultimate goal that was the elimination of the disease from The People's Republic of China.

6.2 An integrated strategy with emphasis on infectious source control

6.2.1 Underlying rationale and key technical measures

Facing the challenges posed by the reemergence of schistosomiasis, an integrated strategy for control of the disease in The People's Republic of China was proposed by The People's Republic of China's State Council in 2004 and implemented by the Chinese Ministry of Health to limit the contamination of the environment with schistosome eggs by reducing the roles of bovines and humans as sources of infection for snails. The key technical measures of this strategy include: (1) reduction of the infection source by mechanization of agriculture, facilitated by the replacement of bovines with tractors; (2) management of domestic animals by fencing of pastures or raising them confined in pens to stop the indiscriminate environmental contamination with schistosome eggs from bovine faeces; (3) improved access to clean water, facilitated by supplying tap water to homes; (4) improved sanitation, facilitated by constructing lavatories and latrines; and (5) solid waste management for certain sectors of the human population, for example, provision of on-board containers for collection of human faeces from high-risk groups such as fishermen and boatmen, and the safe disposal of collected faeces in newly constructed latrines onshore. A special feature is to reduce the number of bovines by replacing them with tractors or to fence them off or pen them if farmers show reluctance to part with their animals. Fig. 2 depicts the key technical measures of the integrated strategy for bovine source control. This strategy takes environmental and socioeconomic factors into account and is based on the understanding that the epidemiology of schistosomiasis is influenced not only by human demography and social connectivity, but also strongly affected by the presence and movement of domestic animals (McManus et al., 2009; Wang et al., 2009a,b). According to the underlying rationale, which builds on previous experience gained

(A)

(B)

(C)

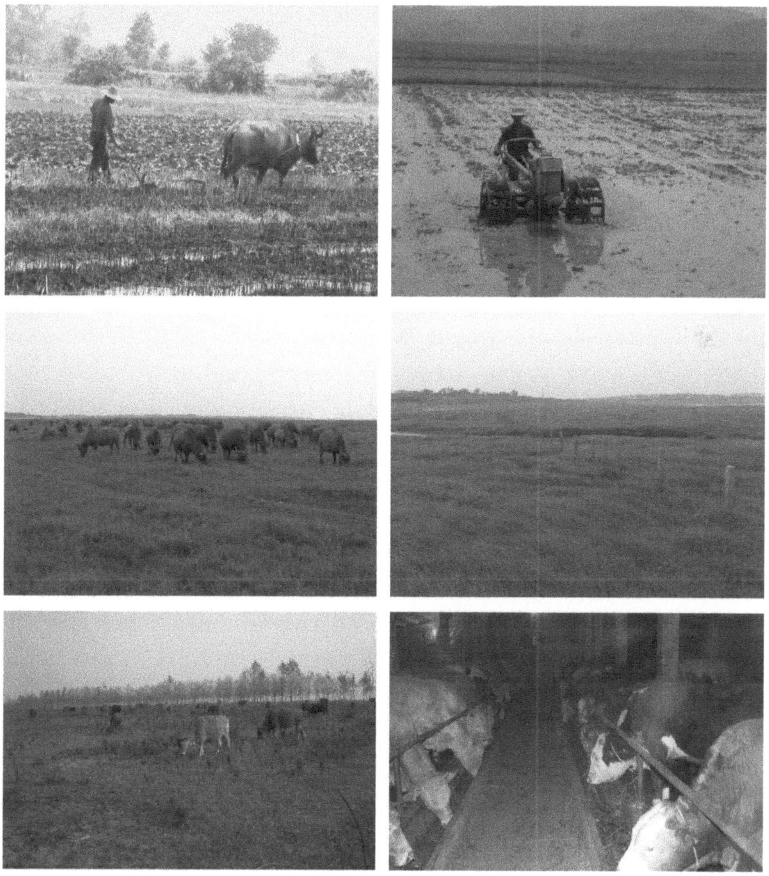

Figure 2 The key technical measures to control bovine infection source in the integrated schistosomiasis control strategy in The People's Republic of China [(A) replacing bovines with tractors for farming, (B) fencing of pastures to prevent bovines from grazing on grasslands with *O. hupensis* and (C) raising bovines in pens].

with schistosomiasis control, the main emphasis has shifted back to transmission control, while praziquantel-based morbidity control is further consolidated. This retargeting of the control approach is based on the understanding that whenever the environmental contamination with *S. japonicum* eggs from humans and domestic animals can be reduced or even eliminated, the production of cercariae in *O. hupensis* will diminish, since the lifespan of infected snails is shorter than one year (Yang et al., 2007; Zhou et al., 2005).

6.2.2 Effectiveness

The immediate goal of this integrated strategy is to effectively suppress the reemergence of schistosomiasis, while ultimately striving for its elimination. The approach has proved effective in four pilot counties in the provinces of Anhui, Hubei, Hunan and Jiangxi, where the strategy to reduce the transmission of *S. japonicum* infection from bovines and humans to snails led to a dramatic reduction in the number of infected snails in their natural habitat (Wang et al., 2009a,b). Validation of this control strategy in a pilot village in the Dongting Lake region through the construction of fences to prevent bovines from grazing on snail habitat in beach areas similarly resulted in significant reductions in the rates of *S. japonicum* infection in domestic animals, humans and *O. hupensis* (Wang et al., 2009a,b). To further evaluate the effect of the new strategy on schistosomiasis control, 40 endemic villages in Guichi District, Chizhou City, Anhui Province were selected as national pilot villages in 2006, and another 10 provincial pilot villages were respectively selected from 10 highly endemic counties in seven cities in 2007, and the key technical measure of replacing bovines with tractors for farming was carried out among the above pilot villages during the period of the pilot study. At the end of 2008, 13 national pilot villages and 6 provincial pilot villages were selected to evaluate the effect of the new integrated strategy in those villages. It was found that the prevalence of human *S. japonicum* infection decreased from 4.57% to 1.76% in national pilot villages after implementation of the new integrated strategy, with a reduction of 61.49%; and the density of infected snails decreased from 0.0067 to 0.0008 snails per 0.1 m^2, the infection rate of snails decreased from 0.28% to 0.04%, with 88.06% and 85.71% reduction rates observed, respectively (Tables 11 and 12). In the provincial pilot villages, the human *S. japonicum* infection rate decreased from 1.27% to 0.21% after 2 years of implementing the new integrated strategy, with a reduction of 83.46%, and the density of infected snails decreased from 0.0025 to 0.0003 snails per 0.1 m^2, and the

Table 11 Schistosomiasis infection status in residents of 13 national pilot villages of Anhui Province before and after the implementation of replacing bovines with tractors for farming

	Before implementation of replacing bovines with tractors					After implementation of replacing bovines with tractors					
	IHA		Kato-Katz			IHA		Kato-Katz			
Village	No. examined	No. positive	No. examined	No. positive	Infection rate of residents (%)	No. examined	No. positive	No. examined	No. positive	Infection rate of residents (%)	Reduction of infection rate in residents (%)
Nanzha	557	119	119	36	6.46	343	61	61	7	2.04	68.42
Changgang	638	142	142	44	6.90	499	110	110	5	1.00	59.71
Guifan	1587	228	228	83	5.23	1115	122	122	31	2.78	46.85
Xinhe	1450	259	259	35	2.41	814	121	121	3	0.37	84.65
Jinxing	784	137	135	36	4.66	439	57	57	3	0.68	85.41
Pufeng	1207	160	160	55	4.56	570	57	57	3	0.53	88.34
Daxing	500	88	88	37	7.40	438	59	59	11	2.51	66.08
Yongxing	783	85	85	33	4.21	696	61	61	16	2.30	45.37
Xianjin	478	85	85	28	5.86	1105	109	109	24	2.17	62.97
Jinbu	1003	105	105	39	3.89	777	74	74	15	1.93	50.36
Pailou	797	128	128	29	3.64	795	94	94	15	1.89	48.08
Waipai	330	137	137	13	3.94	300	56	56	8	2.67	32.23
Huangpen	545	99	99	19	3.49	479	95	95	6	1.25	64.18
Total	10,659	1772	1770	487	4.57	8370	1076	1076	147	1.76	61.49

Table 12 *Oncomelania* snail status in 13 national pilot villages of Anhui Province before and after the implementation of replacing bovines with tractors for farming

	Before implementation of replacing bovines with tractors				After implementation of replacing bovines with tractors				Comparison before and after the implementation of the measure		
Village	No. frames surveyed	Mean density of living snails (No./0.1 m^2)	Mean density of infected snails (No./0.1 m^2)	Infection rate of snails (%)	No. frames surveyed	Mean density of living snails (No./0.1 m^2)	Mean density of infected snails (No./0.1 m^2)	Infection rate of snails (%)	Reduction of mean density of living snails (%)	Reduction of mean density of infected snails (%)	Reduction of snail infection rate (%)
Nanzha	43	0.51	0.0000	0.00	44	0.61	0.0000	0.00	−19.61	–	–
Changgang	1651	4.03	0.0157	0.39	1665	3.08	0.0000	0.00	23.57	100.00	100.00
Guifan	3111	3.75	0.0058	0.15	3113	4.01	0.0006	0.02	−6.93	89.66	86.67
Xinhe	750	1.53	0.0067	0.44	750	1.32	0.0000	0.00	13.73	100.00	100.00
Jinxing	423	0.77	0.0000	0.00	415	0.69	0.0000	0.00	10.39	–	–
Pufeng	777	0.48	0.0000	0.00	715	0.00	0.0000	0.00	100.00	–	–
Daxing	350	3.76	0.0140	0.30	900	2.64	0.0000	0.00	29.79	100.00	100.00
Yongxing	989	1.13	0.0030	0.27	1142	0.75	0.0026	0.35	33.63	13.33	−29.63
Xianjin	0	–	–	–	0	–	–	–	–	–	–
Jinbu	0	–	–	–	0	–	–	–	–	–	–
Pailou	648	0.95	0.0015	0.16	649	0.60	0.0000	0.00	36.84	100.00	100.00
Waipai	524	0.61	0.0095	1.57	524	0.24	0.0000	0.00	60.66	100.00	100.00
Huangpen	1820	1.33	0.0055	0.41	1750	0.70	0.0023	0.33	47.37	58.18	19.51
Total	10,900	2.38	0.0067	0.28	11,667	2.05	0.0008	0. 04	13.87	88.06	85.71

snail infection decreased from 0.13% to 0.05%, with reduction rates of 88.00% and 61.54%, respectively (Tables 13 and 14). The results indicate that the integrated strategy is effective to control schistosomiasis transmission in the marshland and lake regions (Cao et al., 2012).

During 2010s, this integrated strategy was widely implemented in different types of schistosomiasis-endemic areas in The People's Republic of China, and great achievements have been obtained. The number of estimated infected people decreased from 843,000 in 2003 to 115,614 in 2014, and the number of acute cases decreased from 1114 in 2003 to only 2 in 2014. During the same period the prevalence of *S. japonicum* infection decreased from 4.1% to 0.26% in bovines. All seven remaining endemic provinces achieved infection control in 2008, and four of them further achieved transmission control between 2013 and 2014 (Hao et al., 2009; Lei et al., 2015).

7. CHALLENGES

Schistosomiasis was once a major public health concern in The People's Republic of China but is now under effective control. Since the mid-1950s, great strides have been made in the reduction of the prevalence and intensity of *S. japonicum* infection as well as in the control of schistosomiasis transmission through implementing synchronous control of the disease in domestic animals and humans (McManus et al., 2010, 2011). Currently, *S. japonicum* infection has been controlled such that the prevalence of bovine and human schistosomiasis are both under 1%, and by the end of 2015, all endemic provinces have reached the criteria of transmission control. The current major objective is to further reduce the prevalence and morbidity, and interrupt the transmission of the disease by 2020 (Zhu et al., 2016). Although the integrated strategy with emphasis on infectious source control can effectively block schistosomiasis transmission through reducing environmental contamination with schistosome eggs in *O. hupensis* habitats (Jiang and Guo, 2009; Liu et al., 2014b; Wang et al., 2009c), and its key technical measures, especially replacing bovines with mechanized tractors for farming, are being encouraged by the Chinese government in schistosomiasis endemic areas, there are still challenges being faced. The coverage of the programme is limited in some areas especially rural communities, for example, in the marshland and lake regions where cattle and water buffaloes are still the main draught power for agricultural production as well as the main source of income for many farmers, and mechanized tractors are

Table 13 Schistosomiasis infection status in residents of six provincial pilot villages of Anhui Province before and after the implementation of replacing bovines with tractors for farming

Village	Before implementation of replacing bovines with tractors					After implementation of replacing bovines with tractors					Reduction of infection rate in residents (%)
	IHA		Kato-Katz		Infection rate of residents (%)	IHA		Kato-Katz		Infection rate of residents (%)	
	No. examined	No. positive	No. examined	No. positive		No. examined	No. positive	No. examined	No. positive		
Sanli	1162	113	96	32	3.2	1016	70	70	0	0.0	100.0
Xintian	0	0	713	35	4.9	922	46	46	5	0.5	89.8
Dongcun	821	48	48	19	2.3	745	22	22	0	0.0	100.0
Nanxin	1125	173	173	53	4.7	1153	75	75	0	0.0	100.0
Xitang	1146	226	223	24	2.1	1606	526	526	9	0.6	71.4
Guanghui	0	0	1080	64	5.9	1150	105	105	0	0.0	100.0
Total	4254	560	2333	227	1.3	6592	844	844	14	0.21	83.8

Table 14 *Oncomelania* snail status in six provincial pilot villages of Anhui Province before and after the implementation of replacing bovines with tractors for farming

	Before implementation of replacing bovines with tractors				After implementation of replacing bovines with tractors				Comparison before and after the implementation of the measure		
Village	**No. frames**	**Mean density of living snails (No./0.1 m^2)**	**Mean density of infected snails (No./0.1 m^2)**	**Infection rate of snails (%)**	**No. frames**	**Mean density of living snails (No./0.1 m^2)**	**Mean density of infected snails (No./0.1 m^2)**	**Infection rate of snails (%)**	**Reduction of mean density of living snails (%)**	**Reduction of mean density of infected snails (%)**	**Reduction of snail infection rate (%)**
Sanli	813	1.70	0.0000	0.00	810	0.09	0.0000	0.00	94.71	—	—
Xintian	3453	1.36	0.0009	0.06	4417	1.04	0.0000	0.00	23.53	100.00	100.00
Dongcun	1186	17.00	0.0000	0.00	1985	0.65	0.0000	0.00	96.18	—	—
Nanxin	486	0.37	0.0514	14.04	640	0.17	0.0047	2.70	54.05	90.86	80.77
Xitang	7360	0.13	0.0005	0.40	6060	0.33	0.0000	0.00	−153.85	100.00	100.00
Guanghui	1667	0.73	0.0036	0.49	1594	0.25	0.0006	0.25	65.75	83.33	48.98
Total	14,965	1.91	0.0025	0.13	15,506	0.55	0.0003	0.05	71.20	88.00	61.54

expensive to buy and maintain and not suitable for all terrains. In addition, the dominant animal reservoir species, their numbers, susceptibility to *S. japonicum* and RTI may differ in different endemic areas (Wang et al., 2005). Hence if only bovines are involved in the national control programme, it will not likely be fully effective. In order to fulfil the objective of scientific control, the main infectious animal sources in a certain region need to be determined through epidemiological surveys. All the potential main infection sources such as cattle, water buffaloes, goats/sheep, pigs and horses, in a certain region should be assessed and then included in the local control programme accordingly, adjusting the control strategies for domestic animals as the main local reservoir hosts change over time. It is anticipated that schistosomiasis will eventually be eliminated in the near future in The People's Republic of China through sustained implementation of the integrated control strategy with emphasis on the control of both domestic animal and human infection sources.

ACKNOWLEDGEMENTS

This work was supported by grants from the The People's Republic of China–UK Global Health Support Programme (grant no. GHSP-CS-OP1) and Natural Science Foundation of Anhui Province (grant no. 1408085MH194). Many thanks to Prof. Xiao-Nong Zhou for his constructive advice during the preparation of the manuscript.

REFERENCES

Cao, Z.G., Wang, T.P., He, J.C., Zhang, S.Q., Chen, G.X., Zhang, G.H., et al., 2012. Evaluation on the effect of comprehensive control strategy of schistosomiasis with emphasis on infection source control in Anhui province. Chin. J. Prev. Med. 46, 114–118.

Chen, M.G., Feng, Z., 1999. Schistosomiasis control in China. Parasitol. Int. 48, 11–19.

Chen, Y., Xie, M.S., Wang, F.H., Wu, Z.D., 1998. Analysis on the effect of large-scale chemotherapy for the control of schistosomiasis in 30 pilot areas in Hunan Province. Chin. J. Schistosomiasis Control 10, 294–297.

Chen, X.Y., Jiang, Q.W., Wang, L.Y., Zhao, G.M., Zhao, Q., Gu, Y.A., et al., 2002. Schistosomiasis situation in the People's Republic of China in 2001. Chin. J. Schistosomiasis Control 14, 241–243.

Chen, M.G., 2005. Use of praziquantel for clinical treatment and morbidity control of schistosomiasis japonica in China: a review of 30 years' experience. Acta Trop. 96, 168–176.

Chen, M.G., 2014. Assessment of morbidity due to *Schistosoma japonicum* infection in China. Infect. Dis. Poverty 3, 6.

Collins, C., Xu, J., Tang, S.L., 2012. Schistosomiasis control and the health system in P.R. China. Infect. Dis. Poverty 1, 8.

Dabo, A., Bary, B., Kouriba, B., Sankare, O., Doumbo, O., 2013. Factors associated with coverage of praziquantel for schistosomiasis control in the community-direct intervention (CDI) approach in Mali (West Africa). Infect. Dis. Poverty 2, 11.

Faust, E.C., Meleney, H.E., 1924. Studies on schistosomiasis japonica. Am. J. Hyg. Monogr. Ser. 3, 1–339.

Fujinami, A., Nakamura, H., 1909. Experimental studies on the serological reactions in calves experimentally infected with *Schistosoma japonicum*. J. Kyoto Med. Assoc. 6, 224–252.

Gray, D.J., Williams, G.M., Li, Y., McManus, D.P., 2008. Transmission dynamics of *Schistosoma japonicum* in the lakes and marshlands of China. PLoS One 3, e4058.

Gray, D.J., Williams, G.M., Li, Y., Chen, H., Forsyth, S.J., Li, R.S., et al., 2009. A cluster-randomised intervention trial against *S. japonicum* in the Peoples' Republic of China: bovine and human transmission. PLoS One 4, e5900.

Gryseels, B., Polman, K., Clerinx, J., Kestens, L., 2006. Human schistosomiasis. Lancet 368, 1106–1118.

Guo, J.G., Ross, A.G.P., Lin, D.D., Williams, G.M., Chen, H.G., Li, Y.S., et al., 2001. A baseline study on the importance of bovines for human *Schistosoma japonicum* infection around Poyang Lake, China. Am. J. Trop. Med. Hyg. 65, 272–278.

Guo, J., Li, Y., Gray, D., Ning, A., Hu, G., Chen, H., et al., 2006. A drug-based intervention study on the importance of buffaloes for human *Schistosoma japonicum* infection around Poyang Lake, Peoples' Republic of China. Am. J. Trop. Med. Hyg. 74, 335–341.

Hao, Y., Zheng, H., Zhu, R., Guo, J.G., Wu, X.H., Wang, L.Y., et al., 2009. Schistosomiasis situation in the People's Republic of China in 2008. Chin. J. Schistosomiasis Control 21, 451–456,463.

He, Y.X., Yang, H.Z., Mao, S.P., 1960. Experimental studies on the host specificity of *Schistosoma japonicum* I. Developmental rate, distribution and survival of the worms in mammalian hosts. Chin. Med. J. 46, 470–475.

Hunan Medical College, 1979. Study on an Ancient Female Corpse Unearthed in Mawangdui, Changsha, Hunan. Beijing Publishing House for Cultural Relics (in Chinese).

Jiang, W.S., Guo, J.G., 2009. Control of livestock infection source for anti-schistosomiasis. Int. J. Med. Parasit. Dis. 36, 236–240.

Jin, Z.F., 1990. Survey on *Schistosoma japonicum* infection of domestic animals in Su Jia He Po domestic farm of Hanshou country. Chin. J. Schistosomiasis Control 2, 80–81.

Lei, Z.L., Zhang, L.J., Xu, Z.M., Dang, H., Xu, J., Lv, S., et al., 2015. Endemic status of schistosomiasis in People's Republic of China in 2014. Chin. J. Schistosomiasis Control 27, 563–569.

Li, J.Y., Lin, D.D., 2007. Epidemiology and control of schistosomiasis japonica in domestic animals in China. J. Trop. Dis. Parasitol. 5, 125–128.

Li, S.K., Zhu, Z.L., Jin, B.R., 1965. Non-susceptibility of *Microtus fortis* to *S. japonicum* infection. Trans. Parasitol. 2, 103.

Li, H., Liu, J.M., Song, J.X., Ma, S.C., Wang, Q., He, L., et al., 2014a. Domestic animal schistosomiasis in 2012 in China. Chin. J. Anim. Infect. Dis. 22, 68–71.

Li, Y.S., McManus, D.P., Lin, D.D., Williams, G.M., Harn, D.A., Ross, A.G., et al., 2014b. The *Schistosoma japonicum* self-cure phenomenon in water buffaloes: potential impact on the control and elimination of schistosomiasis in China. Int. J. Parasitol. 44, 167–171.

Li, Z.J., Ge, J., Dai, J.R., Wen, L.Y., Lin, D.D., Madsen, H., et al., 2016. Biology and control of snail intermediate host of *Schistosoma japonicum* in the People's Republic of China. Adv. Parasitol. 92.

Liang, S., Yang, C.H., Zhong, B., Qiu, D., 2006. Re-emerging schistosomiasis in hilly and mountainous areas of Sichuan, China. Bull. World Health Organ. 84, 139–144.

Liu, J.S., Rong, S.M., Chen, P.J., Liu, Z.H., Mo, G.Y., 1992. Experimental observation on several species of wild rats infected artificially with *S. japonicum*. Chin. J. Schistosomiasis Control 4, 350–351.

Liu, X.P., Wang, T.P., Wang, Q.Z., Yin, X.M., Zhou, L., Wang, F.F., et al., 2013. Infection status of sources of schistosomiasis japonica in marshland and hilly regions. J. Pathog. Biol. 8, 445–447.

Liu, L., Yang, G.J., Zhu, H.R., Yang, K., Ai, L., 2014a. Knowledge of, attitudes towards, and practice relating to schistosomiasis in two subtypes of a mountainous region of the People's Republic of China. Infect. Dis. Poverty 3, 16.

Liu, Z.C., He, H.B., Yi, P., Yu, J.H., Xu, X.J., Xia, M., et al., 2014b. Role of controlling livestock infection in management of infected *Oncomelania hupensis* in schistosomiasis endemic areas. Chin. J. Vector Biol. Control 25, 35–38.

Liu, Y.X., 1991. Influence of *Schistosma japonicum* infection on body weight of goats. Chin. J. Schistosomiasis Control 5, 311.

Logan, O.T., 1905. A case of dysentery in Hunan Province caused by the trematode *Schistosoma japonicum* 1905. China Med. Mission. J. 19, 243–245.

Mao, S.B., 1990. Biology of Schistosome and Schistosomiasis Control. The first version. Beijing Publishing House of People's Health.

McManus, D.P., Li, Y., Gray, D.J., Ross, A.G., 2009. Conquering 'snail fever': schistosomiasis and its control in China. Expert Rev. Anti Infect. Ther. 7, 473–485.

McManus, D.P., Gray, D.J., Li, Y., Feng, Z., Williams, G.M., Stewart, D., et al., 2010. Schistosomiasis in the People's Republic of China: the era of the Three Gorges Dam. Clin. Microbiol. Rev. 23, 442–466.

McManus, D.P., Gray, D.J., Ross, A.G., Williams, G.M., He, H.B., Li, Y.S., 2011. Schistosomiasis research in the Dongting lake region and its impact on local and national treatment and control in China. PLoS Negl. Trop. Dis. 5, e1053.

Ministry of Agriculture, 1998. Manual for Animal Schistosomiasis Control. Chinese Publishing House of Agricultural Science and Technology (in Chinese), Beijing.

Ministry of Health, 1993. People's Republic of China: Epidemiological Situation of Schistosomiasis in China-Results from a Nation-wide Sampling Survey in 1989. Chengdu Science and Technology University Press (in Chinese).

Ministry of Health, 1998. Epidemic Status of Schistosomiasis in China – Results from a Nation-wide Sampling Survey in 1995. Nanjing University Press (in Chinese).

Ministry of Health, 2000. People's Republic of China. Manual of Schistosomiasis Control. Shanghai Publishing House of Technique and Science.

Ministry of Health, 2006. Epidemic Status of Schistosomiasis in China-Results from a Nationwide Sampling Survey in 2004. Shanghai Publishing House for Sciences and Technology (in Chinese).

National Research Committee on Schistosomiasis, 1957. Compilation of Research Data for Schistosomiasis. Shanghai Publishing House of Health (in Chinese).

National Schistosomiasis Research Committee, 1959. Conclusion of the national symposium on the control of domestic animal schistosomiasis. In: A Corpus of Control of Schistosomiasis in Domestic Animals. Shanghai Publishing House for Sciences and Technology (in Chinese).

Ojurongbe, O., Sina-Agbaje, O.R., Busari, A., Okorie, P.N., Ojurongbe, T.A., Akindele, A.A., 2014. Efficacy of praziquantel in the treatment of *Schistosoma haematobium* infection among school-age children in rural communities of Abeokuta, Nigeria. Infect. Dis. Poverty 3, 30.

Qian, B.Z., Tan, Y., Bogh, O., Henrik, J., Maria, V., Shi, X.H., et al., 2002. Experimental studies on congenital transmission of *Schistosoma japonicum*. Chin. J. Schistosomiasis Control 14, 25–27.

Salam, R.A., Maredia, H., Das, J.K., Lassi, Z.S., Bhutta, Z.A., 2014. Community-based interventions for the prevention and control of helmintic neglected tropical diseases. Infect. Dis. Poverty 3, 23.

Shen, W., 1992. Review and suggestions for domestic animals schistosomiasis control. Chin. J. Schistosomiasis Control 4, 82–84.

Shi, Z.G., Hu, S.G., Zhou, Q.Y., Wang, Z.K., Zhang, Z.G., 1992. The role of pigs in schistosomiasis transmission in Yujiang village. Chin. J. Schistosomiasis Control 4, 293–295.

Shi, L., Li, W., Wu, F., Zhang, J.F., Yang, K., Zhou, X.N., 2016. Epidemiological features and control progress of schistosomiasis in waterway-network region in P.R. China. Adv. Parasitol. 92.

Sleigh, A., Li, X., Jackson, S., Huang, K., 1998. Eradication of schistosomiasis in Guangxi, China. Part 1: Setting, strategies, operations, and outcomes, 1953–1992. Bull. World Health Organ. 76, 361–372.

Su, Z.W., Hu, C.Q., Fu, Y., Chen, W., Huang, X.B., 1994. The role of different hosts on the transmission of schistosomiasis in the lake regions. Chin. J. Parasitol. Parasit. Dis. 12, 48–51.

Su, L.Q., Wu, X., Fan, C.Z., 1999. Analysis on the role of main reservoirs on transmission of schistosomiasis in high mountainous regions in Yunnan Province. J. Pract. Parasit. Dis. 7, 27–28.

Tambo, E., Ai, L., Zhou, X., Chen, J.H., Hu, W., Bergquist, R., 2014. Surveillance-response systems: the key to elimination of tropical diseases. Infect. Dis. Poverty 3, 17.

Tan, B., 1997. Survey on *Schistosoma japonicum* infection of goats. Chin. J. Schistosomiasis Control 9, 18.

Tang, L.H., Xu, L.Q., Chen, Y.D., 2012. Parasitic Disease Control and Research in China. Beijing Publishing House for Sciences and Technology.

Wang, T.P., Ge, J.H., Wu, W.D., Zhang, S.Q., Lu, D.B., Zhang, G.H., et al., 1998. Infection sources of schistosomiasis and their role in the transmission in lake and marshland regions in Anhui Province. Chin. J. Schistosomiasis Control 11, 196–199.

Wang, G.L., Yang, G.R., Wu, X., Fan, C.Z., Xiong, M.T., Tao, K.H., et al., 2000. The role of various hosts on transmission of schistosomiasis at Yongli village of Weishan County. Chin. J. Schistosomiasis Control 12, 122–123.

Wang, T.P., Vang Johansen, M., Zhang, S.Q., Wang, F.F., Wu, W.D., Zhang, G.H., et al., 2005. Transmission of *Schistosoma japonicum* by humans and domestic animals in the Yangtze River valley, Anhui province, China. Acta Trop. 96, 198–204.

Wang, T.P., Zhang, S.Q., Wu, W.D., Zhang, G.H., Lu, D.B., Ornbjerg, N., et al., 2006. Treatment and reinfection of water buffaloes and cattle infected with *Schistosoma japonicum* in Yangtze River Valley, Anhui province, China. J. Parasitol. 92, 1088–1091.

Wang, L.D., Utzinger, J., Zhou, X.N., 2008. Schistosomiasis control: experiences and lessons from China. Lancet 372, 1793–1795.

Wang, L.D., Chen, H.G., Guo, J.G., Zeng, X.J., Hong, X.L., Xiong, J.J., et al., 2009a. A strategy to control transmission of *Schistosoma japonicum* in China. N. Eng. J. Med. 360, 121–128.

Wang, L.D., Guo, J.G., Wu, X.H., Chen, H.G., Wang, T.P., Zhu, S.P., et al., 2009b. China's new strategy to block *Schistosoma japonicum* transmission: experiences and impact beyond schistosomiasis. Trop. Med. Int. Health 14, 1475–1483.

Wang, T.P., Cao, Z.G., Chen, H.G., Zhou, X.N., 2009c. Changes of control strategy and improvement of schistosomiasis control in China. Chin. J. Schistosomiasis Control 21, 241–242.

Wang, X.Y., 1959. Abortion in cattle. In: Ministry of Health, People's Republic of China (Ed.), Control of Domestic Animal Schistosomiasis. Shanghai Science and Technology Press.

Wei, D.X., Yang, W.Y., Huang, S.Q., Lu, Y.F., Su, T.C., Ma, J.H., et al., 1980. Parasitological studies on the ancient corpse of the Western Han Dynasty unearthed from Tomb No. 188 on Phoenix Hill at Jiangling County. Acta Wuhan Med. Coll. 3, 1–6.

Willingham, A.L., Johansen, M.V., Bøgh, H.O., Ito, A., Andreassen, J., Lindberg, R., et al., 1999. Congenital transmission of *Schistosoma japonicum* in pigs. Am. J. Trop. Med. Hyg. 60, 311–312.

Xiang, J., Yuan, Z.S., Xiang, J.Y., Xu, H., Liu, J.W., Xu, Z.M., et al., 2001. Observation on the preventive effect of artesunate against *S. japonicum* of farm cattle. Chin. J. Schistosomiasis Control 13, 360–361.

Xiao, S.H., 2005. Development of antischistosomal drugs in China, with particular consideration to praziquantel and the artemisinins. Acta Trop. 96, 153–167.

Xu, M.S., Wang, H., 1997. Survey on outbreak of acute schistosomiasis in bovines and goats imported from non-endemic areas in Shatan village. Chin. J. Schistosomiasis Control 9, 272–273.

Xu, F.S., Gu, X.G., Qiu, D.C., Li, Y.X., Yin, H.Z., Zhao, L.G., et al., 2001. A quantitative study on reservoirs of *Schistosoma japonicum* at Chuanxing of Xichang City. J. Pract. Parasit. Dis. 9, 159–160.

Yang, Z., Yang, H., 1996. Survey on infection status of *S. japonicum* in cattle in mountainous region of Leqiu, Yunnan Province. Chin. J. Schistosomiasis Control 8, 182.

Yang, G.J., Utzinger, J., Sun, L.P., Hong, Q.B., Vounatsou, P., Tanner, M., et al., 2007. Effect of temperature on the development of *Schistosoma japonicum* within *Oncomelania hupensis*, and hibernation of *O. hupensis*. Parasitol. Res. 100, 695–700.

Yin, Z.C., Qian, X.H., Wu, Z.S., 2003. An analysis of the current situation of cattle and water buffalo schistosomiasis in Sichuan Province in 2001. Parasitoses Infect. Dis. 9, 104–106.

Zhang, Q., Qing, S.T., Zhu, C.X., Hu, X.G., 1998. A survey on goats infected with *Schistosoma japonicum* outside embankment in Matang, Yueyang County. Chin. J. Schistosomiasis Control 11, 253.

Zhang, L.J., Li, S.Z., Wen, L.Y., Lin, D.D., Abe, E.M., Zhu, R., et al., 2016a. Establishment and function of schistosomiasis surveillance system towards elimination in the People's Republic of China. Adv. Parasitol. 92.

Zhang, S.Q., Sun, C.S., Wang, M., Lin, D.D., Zhou, X.N., Wang, T.P., 2016b. Epidemiological features and control effectiveness of schistosomiasis in lake and marshland region in the People's Republic of China. Adv. Parasitol. 92.

Zheng, J., Bi, S.Z., Qiu, Z.L., Gao, H.Z., Pu, H.Z., 1990a. Farther observation on status of the eggs excreted after dogs eating feces with schistosome eggs. Chin. J. Schistosomiasis Control 2, 65–67.

Zheng, J., Qian, K., Yao, B.Y., Zhu, H.Q., Chen, Z.H., Zhang, R., 1990b. Studies on distribution characteristics of infection sources of schistosomiasis in mountainous regions. Chin. J. Schistosomiasis Control 2, 24–27.

Zheng, J., Qian, K., Yao, B.Y., Zhu, H.Q., Chen, Z.H., Zhang, R., 1990c. Study on the distribution pattern of schistosomiasis infection sources in mountainous regions. Chin. J. Schistosomiasis Control 3, 24–26.

Zheng, Q., Vanderslott, S., Jiang, B., Xu, L.L., Liu, C.S., Huo, L.L., 2013. Research gaps for three main tropical diseases in the People's Republic of China. Infect. Dis. Poverty 2, 15.

Zhou, X.N., Wang, L.Y., Chen, M.G., Wu, X.H., Jiang, Q.W., Chen, X.Y., et al., 2005. The public health significance and control of schistosomiasis in China-then and now. Acta Trop. 96, 97–105.

Zhu, H., Yap, P., Utzinger, J., Jia, T.W., Li, S.Z., Huang, X.B., et al., 2016. Policy support and resources mobilization for the national schistosomiasis control programme in the People's Republic of China. Adv. Parasitol. 92.

CHAPTER ELEVEN

Health Education as an Important Component in the National Schistosomiasis Control Programme in The People's Republic of China

L. Chen*, B. Zhong*[,1], J. Xu[§,¶,||], R.-Z. Li*, C.-L. Cao[§,¶]

*Sichuan Provincial Center for Disease Control and Prevention, Chengdu, The People's Republic of China
[§]National Institute of Parasitic Diseases, Chinese Center for Disease Control and Prevention, Shanghai, The People's Republic of China
[¶]WHO Collaborating Center for Tropical Diseases, Shanghai, The People's Republic of China
[||]Key Laboratory of Parasite and Vector Biology of the Chinese Ministry of Health, Shanghai, The People's Republic of China
[1]Corresponding author: E-mail: zhongbo1968@163.com

Contents

Abstract

Schistosomiasis control programme in The People's Republic of China had promoted the mass mobilization of health education in various forms, such as films, drama, traditional opera, poems, slogans, posters, exhibits. This paper is trying to review the impacts

Advances in Parasitology, Volume 92
ISSN 0065-308X
http://dx.doi.org/10.1016/bs.apar.2016.03.004

of those forms on different endemic settings and targeted populations. In the future, health education and health promotion will still be the effective strategy and one of the interventions in the national control programme for schistosomiasis and other infectious diseases, even in the pre- or posttransmission stages. With the social and economic development and improvement of people's living standard, it is necessary to establish a sustainable mechanism, in combination of health education with health guarantee of improving the quality of life, improving the production and living conditions, changing the unhealthy production methods and lifestyle of the residents in the endemic areas, in order to reach the goal of schistosomiasis elimination in The People's Republic of China.

1. BACKGROUND

Schistosomiasis is a contagious, regional and natural foci disease, which has severely harmful human health, impaired social stability and economy in the world (Chen, 2014). It is not just an infectious disease caused by pathogens, but an unhealthy behaviour. In The People's Republic of China, human can be infected with *Schistosoma japonicum* through contacting water where infested with cercaria, one of larval stage of the parasite (Ministry of Health, 2000a,b; WHO, 2002; Xu et al., 2016). After 1984, WHO proposed a new strategy for schistosomiasis control programme, with an emphasis on human and human's behaviour, which took consideration of health education as one of the major intervention measures in the national schistosomiasis control programme (Ministry of Health, 2000a,b; Zhou et al., 2005).

Health education is to help individuals and communities change insanitary behaviour to healthy behaviour, through activities on information, education, communication (IEC). Health promotion depends on social behaviour and strategies, which can extensively organize and coordinates involved relevant parties, communities, families and individuals to hold up health (Tian, 2005). Health education is one of the important strategies for health promotion, and it also provides circumstance in policy-making to support health education.

In the global level, health education began as hygiene classes in some countries such as America and Britain in the 1880s. America is one of the earliest countries which developed health education. Since 1920s, America, Britain and Soviet Union had formally established organizations of health education, which finally developed to the professional level. The great progress of health education was presented in the 1960s and 1970s, with the increase of knowledge in chronic diseases and more needs for primary health care. WHO had emphasized that health education was the first task of primary health care in the Alma-Ata Declaration (WHO, 1978).

In The People's Republic of China, schistosomiasis due to human infection with *S. japonicum* has been seriously prevalent in the country since the 1950s (Cao et al., 2016; Chen, 2014). With great efforts paid by the government involved with communities in last six decades, great achievements in control of schistosomiasis have been gained in The People's Republic of China. As one of the components in the control strategy in the national schistosomiasis control programme, health education through mobilization of health education had been performed in many aspects, such as promotion of mass mobilization, knowledge of education including life cycle of *S. japonicum*, clinical manifestation and sequels, control principle and so on (Liu et al., 2014). There were many forms for the education approaches, such as films, drama, traditional opera, poems, slogans, posters, exhibits, although only propagation and education of health care presented in the early stage (Mao, 1990).

In 1984, WHO recommended the new strategy from transmission control to the morbidity control for the national schistosomiasis control programme. The emphasis of prevention alerted to change unhealthy behaviour (Mott,1992). In the 1990s, The People's Republic of China introduced the World Bank Loan Project (WBLP) on schistosomiasis control, the health education as one of the strategy components had expanded gradually, which promoted for increasing the awareness rate of people, changing behaviour of contacting water for residents, and raising patient's willingness to prevent from infection with *S. japonicum* (Sun, 2002; Liu et al., 2000; Li, 2000; Hu et al., 2001). Since then, The People's Republic of China accepted the concept for health education as major interventions, and carried out goal-oriented, planned, organized, and evaluated health education activity, which improved the national schistosomiasis control programme by standardization of activities.

In the 21st century, the integrated control strategy has implemented in the national schistosomiasis control programme in The People's Republic of China, with health education as one of the most important measures leading to elimination of reservoir transmission. Health education continued to target the specific population through intersectorial cooperation and community's involvement, and also kept the same steps with the development of communities, supports by governmental policy and the improvement of environment. Health promotion with the development of health education had become the primary measure in the national schistosomiasis control programme, and greatly supported the health system development in The People's Republic of China (Collins et al., 2012).

2. APPLICATION OF HEALTH EDUCATION AND HEALTH PROMOTION IN THE NATIONAL SCHISTOSOMIASIS CONTROL PROGRAMME

2.1 Behaviour identification study of the target population

Health education is a goal-oriented, planned, organized and evaluated intervention. Target population and their behaviour should be identified before interventions are carried out.

In most epidemic areas of The People's Republic of China, water contact pattern of adult males is majorly involved by agriculture activities, such as transplanting rice seedlings, cutting grassland and fishing. Females' water contact patterns include household activities such as washing clothes and vegetables. Major water contact patterns in children include swimming, playing with water and fishing (Zheng and Zheng, 2000; Liu et al., 1992, 1994; Gu, 1993). Chen Ming investigated water contact behaviours of people in beach epidemic areas and found that cutting grass, fishing and catching shrimp were the most major contact patterns, followed by swimming and bathing. Most contacting appeared in summer and autumn, followed by spring and winter. Farmers have more chances to contact water than others (Chen et al., 1990). Hu et al. (1997) investigated that the major water contact patterns in adult females were washing clothes in stream, river or lake. The investigation of hilly epidemic areas showed that the major water contact patterns included domestic contact and agriculture product such as washing clothes and vegetables, transplanting. The peak of water exposure of adults is in the agriculturally busy season. Farming and washing were the major water contact patterns of adults in epidemic areas (He et al., 1996; Zhong et al., 2006).

Students are prone to acute infection after water contacting as they lack immunity against schistosomiasis infection (Zhou et al., 1997). About 50% of acute cases in The People's Republic of China were students in 2003–05. Many investigations of Sichuan province showed that over 50% acute schistosomiasis patients were students and the major infection modes were entertaining water contact such as swimming and playing water (Xia et al., 2006; Liu et al., 2016). The period between July and June is the peak of schistosomiasis outbreaks. The percentage of acute infections in boys was much higher than that in girls (Gu et al., 1990; Wu et al., 2006). Some research showed that health education has an obvious effect on entertaining water contact behaviour rather than household and agriculture activities (Wei et al., 2000a,b). Health education to change people's behaviour is better to carrying out in students. Research on people's behaviour changes in epidemic areas showed that there was no difference in behaviours between the males and the females, although the males had more knowledge than that of the females. The reason is that males as the major labour are taken more attentions to the control activities such as medical treatment and snail surveys, but the agriculture activities are inevitable for both the males and females, it is almost impossible to change water contact patterns for the agriculture activities (Song et al., 2010; Huang and Manderson, 2003).

It is an indisputable strategy to reduce the morbidity of schistosomiasis through changing peoples' dangerous behaviours by health education. After behaviour identification in different populations, students are identified as a target population for health education (MOH, 1993). In areas of comprehensive measures implemented, it is important to improve residents' acceptance of measures and increase their engagement. Rural women have an important impact on their children and family in the dissemination of knowledge and conducting of behaviours. They can avoid water contact by household activities through reconstructing water supply project. With development of economy, population migrating become very frequently between epidemic and nonepidemic areas, the migrant population accounted almost 30% of rural labour. Especially in transmission-interrupted areas, migrant population becomes the source of transmission of schistosomiasis, which introduced the returning of schistosomiasis (Sun et al., 2002). Migrant population becomes new target population of health education in control of schistosomiasis.

Success of health education is depended on identification of the different targeted populations, because of water contact patterns differed in different people, also human behaviour caused different impact on transmission of the disease, though susceptibility is the same in different sexes and ages. According to characteristics of targeted populations, different health education interventions should be provided from reality conditions, emphasizing on interaction of different populations (Dabo et al., 2013; Salam et al., 2014a,b).

2.2 Health education for the target population

2.2.1 Application methods

2.2.1.1 Students

There were three typical methodologies targeting to the students from primary or high school, and were used in the last three decades in the national schistosomiasis control programme in The People's Republic of China.

First, after the World Bank Loan Project (WBLP) on schistosomiasis control in 2000, the purpose of health education changed to focus on reducing infested-water contact due to amusement behaviour, so that gathering intrapersonal spread-permeation mode was introduced into all endemic provinces. The national schistosomiasis control programme designed and provided IEC materials, such as foldout and sheet. In the recognition and support of the government, schools in the key epidemic areas are asked to take classes of schistosomiasis health education (Wang et al., 2002; Ojurongbe et al., 2014), and knowledge of schistosomiasis prevention presented in the health textbooks in the school. These activities were also supported by the 'National Regulations for Schistosomiasis Control' issued by the central government of The People's Republic of China in 2006. This regulation indicated that government at or above county level should call for schools that are located in schistosomiasis endemic area teaching students on knowledge of schistosomiasis prevention.

Second, during the 1990s, provinces supported by the WBLP carried out 'four-one' activity in primary schools in all endemic counties. The activity included one class, one special lecture, one extracurricular activity and one essay, which were all relative to improve the EIC of schistosomiasis (Liu et al., 1995). Particularly those activities in summer holidays were good time to intensify health education intervention to students and it can reduce exposure opportunities to schistosome infection, even acute schistosomiasis (Chang et al., 2003). The research targeting to the primary students in Poyang Lake showed that it was a good mode through audition education, skills training, supplying drug, in combination with rewards and punishment (Hu et al., 1995). It was also noticed that application of popular science cartoons and albums in combination with health education information well fit into local education settings in Poyang Lake. The major EIC teaching students with methods of no-contacting water and self-protection had got good result with the widespread in schools of seriously endemic areas (Wei et al., 2000a,b).

Third, the mode of 'children hands in parents' hands' was carried out in Sichuan (Liu et al., 2016). Students, after getting knowledge on schistosomiasis control in school, were asked to transmit the knowledge to their families and surrounding communities, which significantly extended the coverage area of health education. It was also proposed a method that permeates knowledge of schistosomiasis control through building a chain of doctor, teacher, student, family, neighbour and society (Jiang et al., 1998). The method was very easily applied in the endemic areas of the developing countries due to low investment with high effectiveness and no extra work to students.

2.2.1.2 Residents

The most important approach for the residents, including working people and housewives, in endemic areas to introduce intervention methods and prevention knowledge is through multimedia distribution, such as radio broadcasts and television programs, etc. Because of the wide distribution of those people in lake areas, the chances for contacting fishermen are relied on type of media broadcasts, such as warning signs, posters, mobile radio broadcasting, and other multimedia or person to person methods. For large scale interventions, local public health networks in connection with clinicians coordinate to provide technical skills and deliver information regarding snail eradication in order to create effective intervention measures for local residents, particularly for adult population.

Results from research have made evident that 'preventative values = education + prevention skills training' which has been used as an intervention model on housewives in endemic areas. It has been successful in overcoming ingrained tendencies that local residents easily use available infected water for washing and other daily life activities, and has prevented from the parasite reinfection following chemotherapy (Xu et al., 2002). Better results have gained in two case studies, one was that awarding a competition prize among participants of a group after arrangement of small group discussion; the other one was giving 1 min of health education prior to clinical treatment to the patients (Liu et al., 1995). A different method for adult males was also tried with 'patient compliance for schistosomiasis screening and chemotherapy = education + prevention skills training' which had made advanced health education in the field of schistosomiasis control. As a result, target population's compliance rate was greatly increased after interventions (Hu et al., 2000).

2.2.1.3 Migrant population

With the development of society and economy, the migrant population has been increasing (Zhang et al., 2016). More than 200 million surplus labours in the rural area of The People's Republic of China have migrated into cities or economically developed areas. Among these surplus labours, at least 30 million mobile population, who flowed to cities were originally from schistosomiasis endemic areas. This migrated pattern has brought new difficulties in schistosomiasis control programme in The People's Republic of China (Zheng, 2003; Zhou et al., 2007). Although migrant population, as a special group, has no causal relationship to the schistosomiasis epidemic, the combination of its flow characteristics and the spread factor of schistosomiasis are likely to lead to increasing transmission of schistosomiasis. Compared to the population of permanent residents in the endemic areas, the migrant population has a higher infection rate, higher liquidity, and lower rate of knowledge about schistosomiasis prevention, which not only seriously affected the outflow of schistosomiasis control and its consolidation, but also to bring the inflow of schistosomiasis epidemic risks (Cao and Guo, 2010; Coa et al., 2011). In recent years, because of the mobile population and environmental changes, acute infections occurred in some areas even after transmission interrupted for years (Yuan et al., 2005; Zhou et al., 2008; Ye et al., 2007; Qi et al., 2010). The control of infectious sources from mobile population is one of the main tasks in the transmission-controlled region now, and it has gradually been an important approach in control of infection sources in these areas.

For boatmen in the lake area, building public toilets in human gathering sites or centres (parked), installing and using stool collection containers on board were initialized. The fishing boat people with higher education level, as schistosomiasis volunteers, taught their own experiences to their companions about the benefits of using the stool collector and legal obligation (Gao et al., 2009). After the intervention, with their consciousness enhanced and unhealthy behaviour changed, the risk of schistosomiasis infection was reduced. In mountainous area, due to emigrant population and their habits with potential risk of schistosomiasis infection, short message service of mobile phone companies was promoted for spreading knowledge of schistosomiasis prevention and examination and treatment information to emigrant population. The degree of people's acceptation is higher, it also has better effect to improve its rates of screening and treatment compliance as well as schistosomiasis knowledge and awareness of mobile population (Chen et al., 2013). As the migrants are generally not at a high education level, the health education materials have to made as easy as possible for them to understand, including pictures, music, animation, etc. Intervention measures through radio, television and other mass media-based can significantly improve the schistosomiasis awareness rate and knowledge of the mobile population (Wei, 2014a,b; Fan and Xu, 2009a,b).

2.2.2 Application of educational materials

In the intervention activities of health education, educational materials are of certain importance and information transmission is especially need to be concerned. According to strategies and transmission data of health education, accuracy of information and engaging design are critical for materials application that are easily disseminatable and attractive to readers. Regardless of the medium, information for dissemination should be scientifically accurate, interesting, digestible, and memorable to be accepted by the target population (Cao et al., 2009).

Since 1996, The People's Republic of China has produced a large amount of materials in a variety of media, which can be classified as audio—visual, print media, and various daily articles. Audio—visual media included film, television, video, tape recording, and slides, etc. (Figs 1—4). Print media included magazines and literature, posters, pamphlets, and newspaper, etc. (Figs 5 and 6). Daily articles included fans, shirts, towels, umbrellas, chopsticks, aprons, pencil boxes, and pins, etc. (Figs 7—14). These objects and media increase residents' awareness and also encourage the adoption of better healthy behaviours. In Anhui Province, it was discovered that different populations had different levels of access to different materials. For example, local adult proportion of access to television or film was higher than mobile populations ($P < 0.01$), higher grade students had much

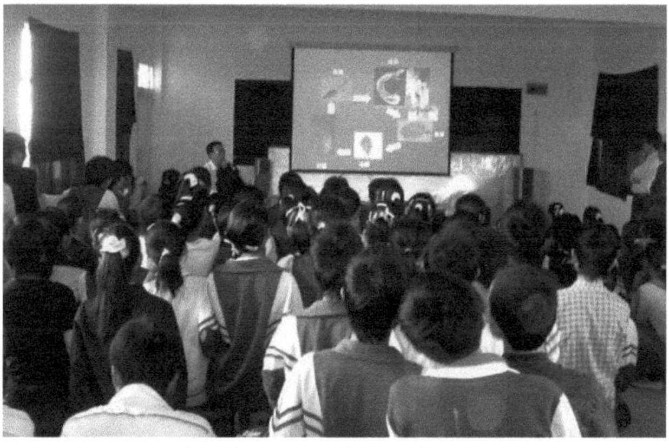

Figure 1 Playing the life history slides of *Schistosoma japonicum*.

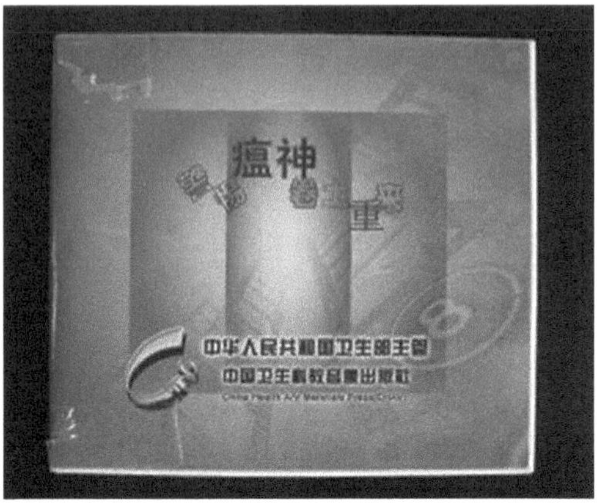

Figure 2 The video on schistosomiasis control in The People's Republic of China.

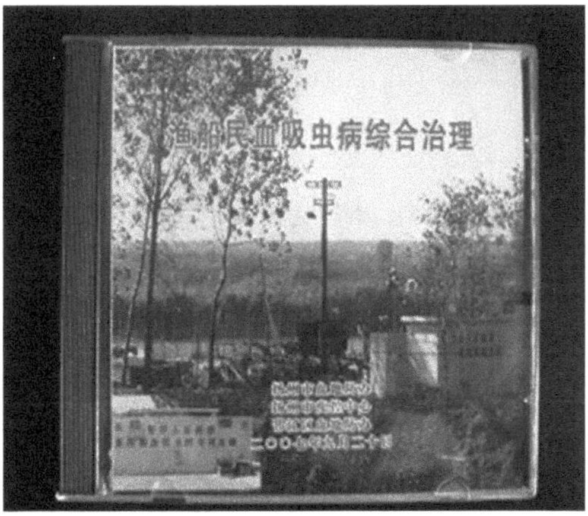

Figure 3 The video on schistosomiasis control measures in mobile boat fishermen.

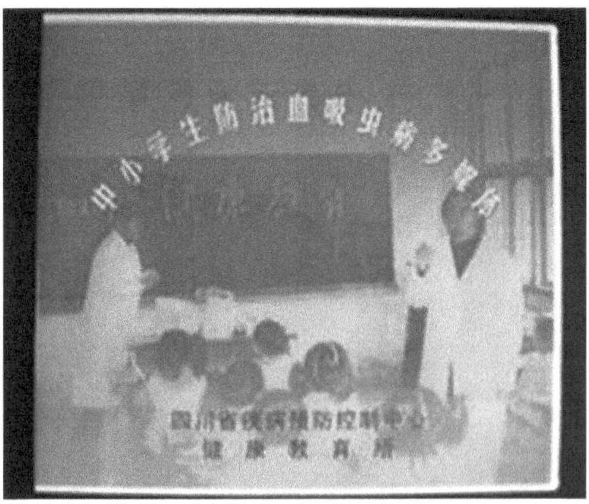

Figure 4 The video on schistosomiasis control in primary and middle school students.

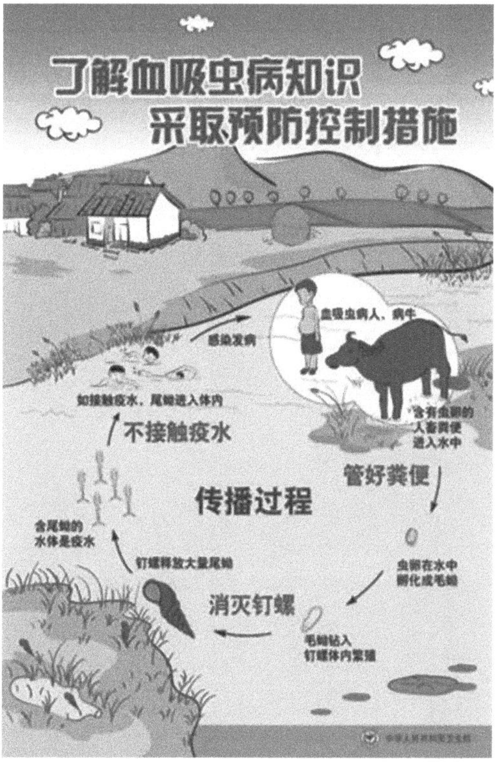
了解血吸虫病知识
采取预防控制措施
不接触疫水
传播过程
管好粪便
消灭钉螺

Figure 5 The poster on the life history of Schistosoma japonicum.

more access to audio–visual material than lower grade students ($P < 0.05$); local adults access to newspaper, pamphlets, and posters was higher than mobile populations ($P < 0.01$), higher grade students had more access to posters than lower grade students ($P < 0.05$) (Li et al., 2013). It has also revealed that educational materials in the form of television and practical information are most liked by students, adult males, and females. In particular, the dissemination of information better focus on brevity and intelligibility, with concise text and illustration, and printed on articles of daily use as the medium of choice for acceptance and approval (Chen et al., 2009a,b). It is better making educational materials to be bilingual, for example in Yi and Chinese in Puge County of Liangshan Autonomous Prefecture, where the Yi people make up the majority of the population, to raise awareness of schistosomiasis prevention and give basic knowledge to improve local residents hygiene, with the goal of schistosomiasis control (Wu et al., 2009).

During production and dissemination of materials, standards and optimization of the production process are divided into following four steps. First,

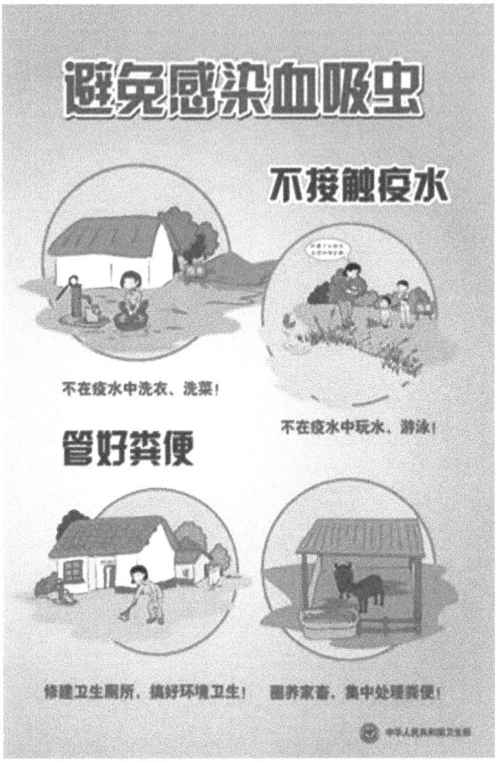
避免感染血吸虫
不接触疫水
不在疫水中洗衣、洗菜！
不在疫水中玩水、游泳！
管好粪便
修建卫生厕所，搞好环境卫生！
圈养家畜，集中处理粪便！

Figure 6 The poster on schistosomiasis prevention behavior.

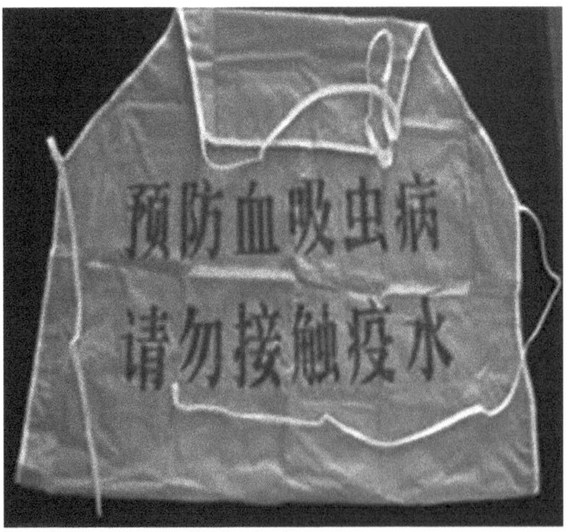

Figure 7 The apron printed information on schistosomiasis control.

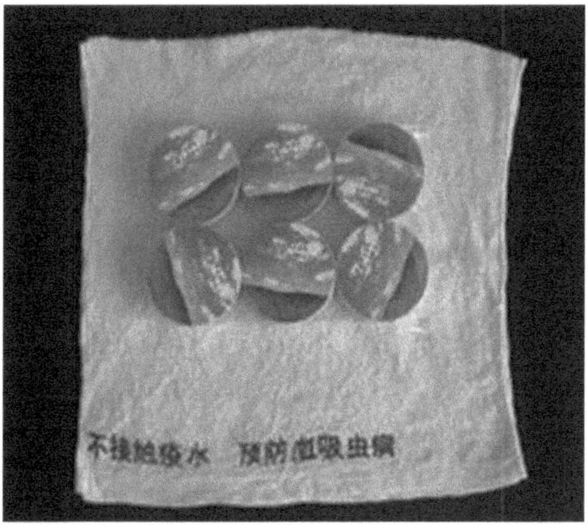

Figure 8 The compressed towel printed information on schistosomiasis control.

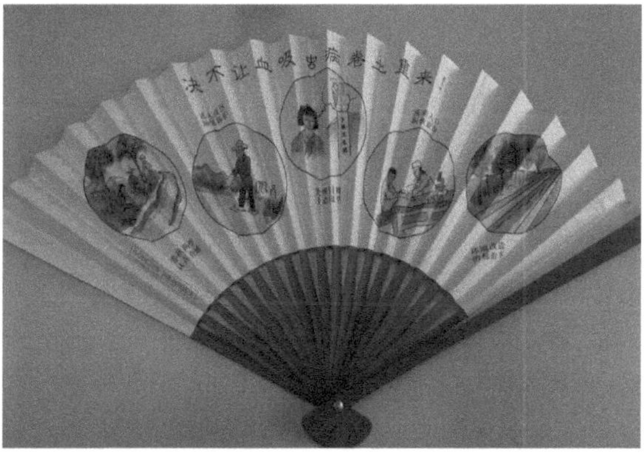
决不让血吸虫病卷土重来

Figure 9 The fan printed information on schistosomiasis control.

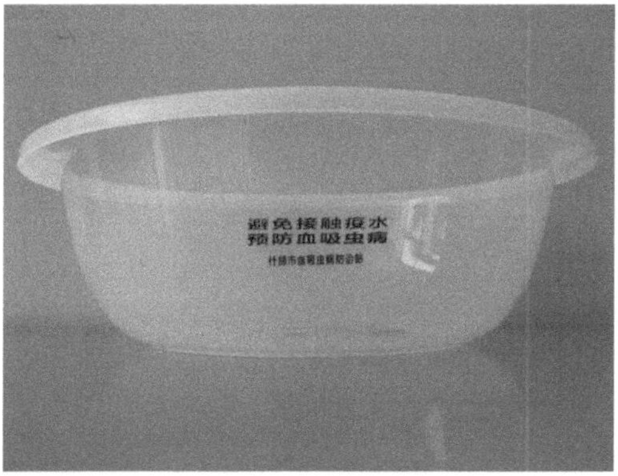
避免接触疫水
预防血吸虫病

Figure 10 The wash basin printed information on schistosomiasis control.

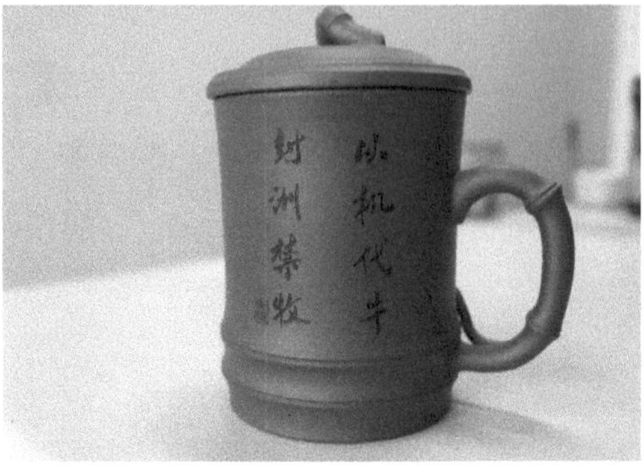

Figure 11 The cup printed information on schistosomiasis control.

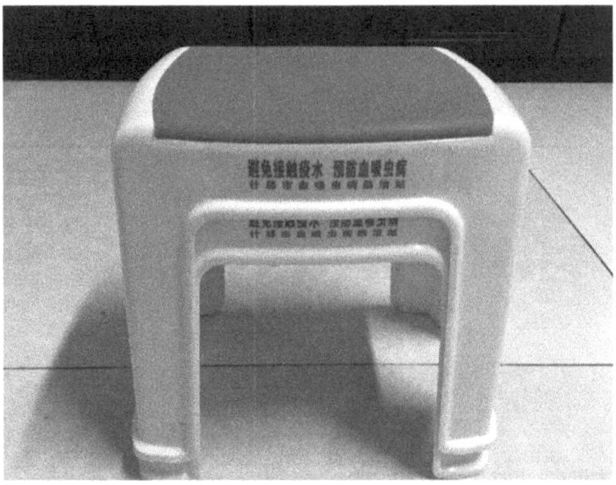

Figure 12 The stool printed information on schistosomiasis control.

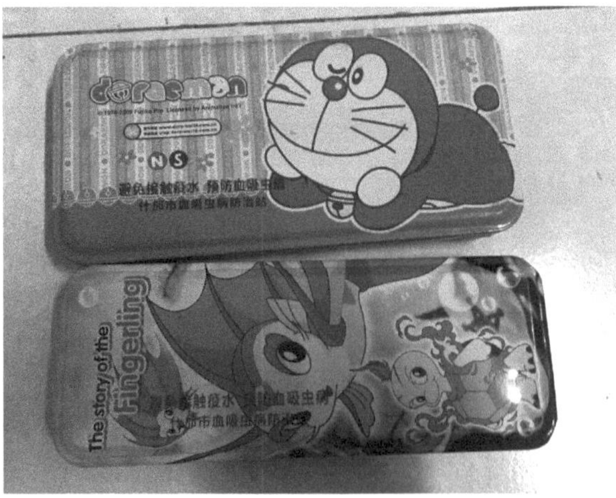

Figure 13 The pencil-boxes printed information on schistosomiasis control.

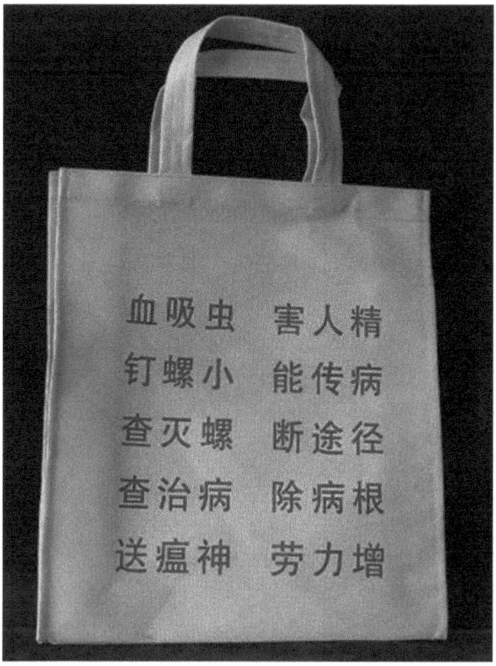

Figure 14 The nonwoven shopping bag printed information on schistosomiasis control.

analysis of needs and resources should be undertaken prior to design of materials. Second, pre-trials of the designed material need to take place to allow for timely correction prior to use. Third, the materials, such as 'The health knowledge of schistosomiasis control calendar' and 'The health education box of schistosomiasis control', used for the small group discussion and the consultation of experts need to be carefully selected in the pre-trials of the materials. Finally, postimplementation evaluation is encouraged after the link between dissemination and use was taken into account. Results showed that after three pre-trials in expert consultants and corrections, the level for understanding of the materials by target population was increased by over 90%; then it was only time to finalize the materials' designing and samples were produced (Hu et al., 2005; Zhang et al., 2004). Qualitative analysis after the distribution of educational materials, such as 'The poster of schistosomiasis control', is normally made by taking random samples of different populations, such as students, housewives, village leaders, doctors, teachers, and other important groups, to systematically evaluate effectiveness of different media and materials in educating different groups on schistosomiasis prevention. In summary, the critical information contained in the posters was able to be understood and accepted by primary students as well as other important groups. These results reemphasize the importance for focus, scientific accuracy, and human interest when designing health education materials (Sun et al., 2005).

2.3 The effectiveness of health education

2.3.1 Increase the awareness and promote behaviour change

Health education was introduced as one of the important measures of schistosomiasis control following schistosomiasis control program supported by WBLP operation in The People's Republic of China during 1992 to 1998. Therefore, the information education and communication of schistosomiasis control was explored widely, and experiences of different health education model to target populations were concluded. Meanwhile, the effectiveness was obviously. At the end of the WBLP, health education has become one of main measures of schistosomiasis control in The People's Republic of China. The health education on knowledge of schistosomiasis control and prevention behavior increased target populations' knowledge and changed their behavior. The pupil's high infection risk behaviors of infested water contact were changed as one of the most high light effect. As one of the most important supplementary measures for WHO chemotherapy-based strategy, health education can improve the chemotherapy compliance of the target population and reduce the infection rate of the population. Based on health education, in combination with mass chemotherapy strategy can effectively control schistosomiasis infection or reinfection, especially in the control of acute infection of schistosomiasis (Liu et al., 1999; Hu et al., 1999a,b; Wang et al., 1999; Hu et al., 1999a,b).

To understand what effectiveness had been gained in The People's Republic of China on health education for schistosomiasis prevention, two pair of search terms such as 'Xuexichong (schistosome)' + 'Jiankangjiaoyu (healthy family)', and 'Schistosomiasis' + 'Health Education' were used to retrieve published literatures from the Chinese biomedical literature database and the PubMed database during 2004–14. Statistical analysis of literatures was done in the inclusion criteria to complete the evaluation of project design. It retrieved up-to-standard related 25 references, including 9 articles on adult articles (which specifically for adult male 2, adult female 1), 8 on students, 8 on mobile population (Table 1; Wei, 2014a,b; Chu and Cheng, 2014; Li et al., 2008, 2014; Chen et al., 2009a,b; Zhou et al., 2013; Wu et al., 2013; Wang et al., 2008, 2010, 2012; Xie and Fu, 2012; Yang et al., 2012; Song et al., 2010; Chen et al., 2008, 2009a,b; Liu et al., 2009a,b; Fan and Xu, 2009a,b; Zhang et al., 2006a,b, 2008a,b; Qu et al., 2008; Ji et al., 2006; Qiu et al., 2006; Ma and Mao, 2014).

It was found that health education in The People's Republic of China pays special attention to the various targeted population in the endemic area, such as adult residents, students and migrant population over the past decade (Table 1), which is consistent with the priorities of the current health education programme on schistosomiasis elimination in The People's Republic of China. Results from various groups of intervention showed that the highest increased rate was on the range of knowledge about schistosomiasis prevention awareness, which was one of the most obvious indicators for change of health education intervention. On the part of behavior changing, there is huge difference among reference, which associated with behaviour evaluation. For example, it has been shown that health behaviour change in target population required a long process and associated with the economic status and living environment among many factors, so that those rely solely on health education maybe difficult to achieve the expected outcomes. The infection rates did not reported in many reference due to short-term health education probably. It is necessary that evaluation to the outcome of long-term health education.

2.3.2 The role of health promoting role

The role of health promoting in the national schistosomiasis control programme along with other measures is important to achieve the goal of schistosomiasis elimination, and it has been showed the nature of the health education should be low cost, quick and have long-term effects and high social benefits. For instance, health education by spreading schistosomiasis prevention knowledge widely has not only enhanced the consciousness of target population, change the behaviour of local people in contact with the contaminated water, but also can effectively promote the implementation of the periodic chemotherapy, improve the snail control in local environment, and ensure the integrated strategy on schistosomiasis control is well performed, such as safe water supply and waste management. Research in the lake region showed that health education along with chemotherapy strategy targeting both people and animals can control the epidemics efficiently with lower costs (Cao et al., 2006). Exploration in view of performing the health education intervention to three target populations including students, adult men, and adult women has been carried out by comparing cost-effectiveness. Results showed that after

Table 1 The intervention effect of all kinds of target population

Area	Target population	The intervention effect							
		Awareness rate (%)		Attitude accuracy (%)		Correct behaviour rate (%)		Infection rate (%)	
		Before the intervention	After the intervention	Before the intervention	After the intervention	Before the intervention	After the intervention	Before the intervention	After the intervention
Anhui	Floating population	10.00	93.80	9.10	91.90	38.80	93.20	/	/
Yunnan	Student	75.98	97.73	73.18	96.59	68.72	95.45	/	/
Yunnan	Adult	72.03	98.03	69.23	96.71	65.73	94.74	/	/
Hubei	Student	89.45	96.75	91.04	98.01	88.47	100	/	/
Jiangsu	Floating population	62.00	94.20	83.80	97.70	50.50	91.90	/	/
Jiangxi	Student	26.47	99.51	17.04	100	16.67	73.04	2.94	0.00
Jiangxi	Floating population	7.96	96.39	/	/	0.00	98.23	/	/
Sichuan	Floating population	56.19	71.38	/	/	60.68	67.30	/	/
Jiangsu	Student	63.73	10.00	/	/	64.46	100	/	/
Jiangsu	Adult	60.71	99.67	80.17	99.89	36.93	90.13	10.29[a]	0.60
Hunan	Adult	73.27	98.36	87.80	99.67	75.49	92.84	9.30	2.67
Jiangxi	Adult male	67.35	91.92	56.44	97.98	46.46	92.08	/	/
Zhejiang	Floating population	33.50	90.10	/	/	34.50	93.20	/	/

Jiangsu	Floating population	23.85	95.70	/	/	6.59	53.42	27.95[a]	8.15
Sichuan	Adult	79.55	91.57	39.96	81.13	74.86	91.65	28[b]	0.00
Sichuan	Student	73.77	91.47	32.52	83.10	72.87	90.61	18[b]	0.00
Jiangxi	Student	8.99	94.38	55.06	98.88	85.45	98.13	13.94	2.25
Hubei	Floating population	36.88	98.45	53.46	97.95	47.37	98.01	12.45	2.41
Jiangsu	Floating population	23.38	69.41			47.80	85.49	/	/
Jiangxi	Adult female	55.34	84.85	67.96	95.96	90.53	94.93	19.42	7.14
Hunan	Adult	23.68	85.21	/	/	70.97	99.42	20.02	7.17
Anhui	Adult	77.50	95.98	/	/	/	/	4.11	3.06
Jiangsu	Student	51.30	90.40	/	/	47.20	92.40	/	/
Jiangxi	Student	26.47	99.02	35.29	95.10	84.84	97.23	9.80	0.98
Jiangxi	Adult male	73.79	93.29	53.05	92.07	41.46	90.24	11.59	10.37

"/" = not reported.
[a]The positive rate of blood detect.
[b]The case of acute schistosomiasis infection.

implementation of targeted health education intervention, the infection rates of *S. japonicum* in the three groups of students, adult female, adult male fell down by 1% per 100 people with cost of 4.69, 5.32 and 17.53 yuan, respectively, while the cost of reducing the infection rates by 1% per 100 people through chemotherapy measure was 15.52 yuan. From a short-term pilot result, the cost-effectiveness in adult male is not better than that of chemotherapy, but the chemotherapy compliance was improved in adult male, can significantly reduce the infection rate (Liu et al., 2005). A cost–benefit analysis based on video intervention for housewives and children were performed in the experimental and control areas, to improve the self-protection consciousness, establishing beliefs to treat as early as possible. Results showed that the cost–benefit ratio was 1:10.11, and it also affected other family members in terms of reducing schistosomiasis infection rate (Lv et al., 1998). Another research was done to improve the participation in the mass detection of snails through implementation of health education intervention; it was found that the unit cost for snail detection in the transmission interrupted area was 1054 yuan and 14,703 yuan before and after health education, respectively (Fang et al., 2005). It is visible that there is a big gap in estimate costs to examine snails through health education. Therefore, it made clear enough on the responsibility and obligation through health education to strengthen public consciousness in endemic area, so that the whole society is significantly promoted to involve in the national schistosomiasis control programme.

2.4 Effectiveness of health promotion

To strengthen knowledge through education and dissemination in the targeted population, it is necessary to promote the community development and the environmental transformation, which is an effective way for health promotion at home and abroad. Health promotion is the development and expansion of health education. While the promotion of providing education and dissemination of health information to the targeted population also depend on the development of community, the leading role of government policies, multisectoral cooperation and participation as well as improvement of human environment and transformation of natural environment. Many studies have concluded that health education alone can only bring changes in the behaviours of residents who contact infested water in the recreational activities in the endemic areas, but will not bring significant changes in their behaviours on contacting infested water in the productive activities. Currently, in most of schistosomiasis epidemic areas in The People's

Republic of China, it is very difficult to completely eliminate the chance for human contact with infested water. To make better life, a lot of farmers have to contact water while catching fishes, shrimps or farming in the fields, but due to limited economic resources they cannot afford protective equipments and will inevitably come into having chances in contact with infected water. Because of no safe drinking-water projects, it is inevitable that residents in the snail-infested areas will come into contact with infected water in nonproductive activities (such as laundry, washing vegetables, washing hands, etc.). Faced with this situation, if there is no substitute method, health education alone cannot change this situation. Only health education, along with the economic development at community level, can gradually eliminate these risk behaviours, control and eventually eliminate schistosomiasis at local contexts. Moreover, the effect produced by this approach is fundamental and long term.

With health assurance of quality of life as a starting point, health promotion will incorporate health planning with health education as the centre into the policies and leading role of community government. In particular, implementation, not only reduction of the risky behaviours of residents in the endemic areas, will be regarded as a behavioural target, but also government policy support, multisectoral cooperation and participation and environmental reform will be regarded as a behavioural target. Target population also includes community leaders, decision-makers and key personnel of relevant departments. Based on preparation, distribution and training of health education materials, it is necessary to carry out social mobilization, coordinate multisectoral cooperation, be the adviser of government health planning, coordinate multisectoral interests and conflicts, timely investigate and analyse the effectiveness of community development and environmental reform, and timely and effectively disseminate it to the target population. In information exchange, it is necessary to transform from changing unhealthy behaviours of individuals to changing behaviours through changing community group behaviours and improve from simply changing knowledge education and personal behaviours to improving and emphasizing community development, environmental reform and risky behaviours.

The Law of The People's Republic of China on the Prevention and Treatment of Schistosomiasis, promulgated by the Chinese government in 2006, clearly requires more activities on agricultural mechanization, rural latrine improvement, biogas tank construction, construction or improvement of drinking water facilities both for human and livestock. The relevant government departments of the State Council have given priority to the relevant projects in the higher transmission regions, and raise requirements for all levels of governments to increase the input for the schistosomiasis control in the endemic areas. *The Long-term Plan of Prevention and Control of Schistosomiasis (2004–15)* proposed the integrated control strategy with an emphasis on controlling the infection sources for block transmission. These political documents provided the basis and guarantee for implementation of the health promotion activities in a long term. Therefore, health promotion based on health education is a fundamental step in control of schistosomiasis. For instance, research report in the lake areas with high endemicity showed that the schistosomiasis infection rate in the pilot villages fell down by 53.3%, and no cases of acute schistosomiasis occurred, after implementation of integrated control strategy for 5 years, while the infection rate in the control villages was increased and cases of acute schistosomiasis occurred frequently (Chen et al., 2006). To coordinate with the implementation of these measures, the promotional materials in Yi language and Chinese were prepared to publicize and improve the basic knowledge on schistosomiasis control, enhance the health awareness of the villagers, and gradually change the poor health habits. After implementation for 4 years, the awareness rate of knowledge on schistosomiasis prevention increased from 28% to 85%, the toilet usage gradually reached 90%; the infection rate of human decreased from 14.45% to 0.88% with a decline rate of 93.91%; the infection rate of livestock decreased from 12.89% to 0.54% with a decrease rate of 95.81%; no infected snails appeared for two consecutive years (Wu et al., 2009).

In mountainous region, the integrated strategy with focus on drinking water projects for both human and livestock, such as mountain pond rectification, irrigation cannel reconstruction, and miniature hydraulic engineering projects, has been promoted in wider areas. All those projects coupled with farmland renovation and ecological agriculture alteration have achieved transmission control or elimination for schistosomiasis (Zhong et al., 2002; Liang et al., 2007). On the other hand, these integrated control measures have improved the local agricultural production and economic development. Due to active involvement by local communities, high acceptance of those integrated measures was observed (Zhang et al., 2008a,b).

It is worth noting that, it is necessary to closely integrate schistosomiasis health education with various engineering projects which can produce more impacts to the communities, such as improving the awareness of disease control, acceptance to relevant control activities. Particularly, in the planning and implementation of health promotion programmes, health education intervention need to fit into targeted households with an assistance of broadcast and posters for mobilization and advocacy, thereby ensuring the success of the project implementation.

2.5 Case studies

2.5.1 Health education of schistosomiasis control knowledge shared by volunteers from the boatmen to fishery community: a new health education model in marshland and lake regions

Schistosomiasis japonica is a water-related parasitic disease caused by contact with infested water (Lv et al., 2013). The boat fishermen living along the Yangtze River basin frequently contact water due to production and living, and significantly higher prevalence and intensity of *S. japonicum* infection has been reported which was higher than that of general populations (Li et al., 2003, 2006; Ross et al., 1997; Li and Yu, 1991). The boat fishermen are migrating throughout the years, and they frequently pour schistosome eggs—contaminated faeces into water. It has been shown that boat fishermen have virtually become the predominant source of infection in the lake region (Hong et al., 2011). In addition, the management of these populations is of great difficulty since they migrate across the Yangtze River, which severely threatens the progress towards the elimination of schistosomiasis. A new model of schistosomiasis control health education was therefore developed with the aim to improve the awareness of schistosomiasis control and alter incorrect behaviours, thereby reducing the likelihood of infection and transmission of *S. japonicum* among boat fishermen.

First, a group of active, respected boat fishermen with high education levels are selected as health education volunteers (one volunteer for 10 boats). Second, the volunteers receive training pertaining to schistosomiasis prevention and control by professional staff from local disease control and prevention to ensure that the volunteers seize the techniques of health education regarding schistosomiasis prevention and control knowledge. Third, the volunteers transmit the schistosomiasis prevention knowledge to the massive boat fishermen (one volunteer is responsible for fishermen living in 10 boats), and participates in health education interventions targeting the boat fishermen. Finally, the volunteers help professional staff to alter the incorrect behaviours, remind the implementation of self-protective measures and prohibit the pouring of the contaminated faeces into water. They also help to record the use of faeces container in boats and the use of harmless public toilets at fixed anchor points. A questionnaire survey was conducted to evaluate the effectiveness of such a health education model on schistosomiasis control among the boat fishermen, and results showed that the 3-year (2005–07) implementation of this health education model increased the awareness of schistosomiasis control knowledge and percentage of correct schistosomiasis control behaviour from 23.85% and 6.59% to 95.7% and 53.42%, the use of harmless public toilets and on-boat faecal container from 0% to 80.21% and 54.52%, respectively, while the seroprevalence of *S. japonicum* decreased from 27.95% in 2004 to 19.24%, 12.27% and 8.15% from 2005 to 2007, respectively (Liu et al., 2009a,b). The results demonstrate that the model of health education of schistosomiasis prevention and control knowledge transmitted by volunteers in the same boat improve the awareness of schistosomiasis prevention and control knowledge and correct the undesirable health habits, which play an active role in the prevention and control of schistosomiasis among the boat fishermen. Further expanded studies are required to assess the effectiveness of this health education model in the major schistosomiasis endemic foci of marshland and lake regions in The People's Republic of China.

3. PROSPECTS AND CHALLENGES

In 1984, with the advent of chemotherapy drugs praziquantel, the Expert Committee of the World Health Organization adjusted the strategies of schistosomiasis control and proposed that the target of schistosomiasis control in underdeveloped countries should be morbidity control based on chemotherapy. In these underdeveloped countries, it is difficult to rely on multiple and comprehensive control measures to eradicate schistosomiasis or interrupt its transmission in terms of human and financial resources (WHO, 1984; Mtethiwa et al., 2015). It also pointed out that because the schistosomiasis infection was closely related to people's agriculture activities and lifestyles, health education should be one of the important components in the disease control strategies. Since then, The People's Republic of China carried out a pilot project with disease control as the strategy in the heavy endemic areas, and gradually introduced this strategy concept. After implementation of the WBLP on schistosomiasis control in 1992, the endemic areas in The People's Republic of China implemented with the disease control strategy, carried out the schistosomiasis control measures based on chemotherapy and with snail elimination as the focus, and gradually regarded health education as an important measure for disease control. Therefore health education gradually enters the scientific and standardized track with the WBLP in The People's Republic of China. After 2004, The People's Republic of China enhanced the national schistosomiasis control programme with the integrated strategy based on controlling the infectious sources, continued to regard health education as an important measure for schistosomiasis control programme. Through multisectorial collaboration, the integrated strategy was performed successfully, such as reconstructing water supply and lavatory, replacing cattle with machine, returning farmland to forest, social and economic development and new rural construction with schistosomiasis control health education, so that health promotion started to play an important role in improving the schistosomiasis control knowledge and awareness among the masses in the endemic areas and changing their behaviours and lifestyle (Paudel et al., 2013).

During several decades of schistosomiasis health education work, The People's Republic of China has accumulated a great deal of experience in schistosomiasis control. But up to now, most reports and literatures focus on research of health education intervention mode or method, and there is no systematic research on the health communication strategy of schistosomiasis control, including communicators, information, communication mode, audiences, feedback, effect evaluation and a series of key processes throughout the entire communication process. Most research studies are quantitative, and there are few literatures on qualitative research, which cannot fully reflect the implementation and effectiveness of schistosomiasis health education in The People's Republic of China. In addition, the floating population is still the important and weak link in the current prevention and control work. Exploration and effectiveness evaluation of some health education intervention mode in few inflow and outflow areas cannot achieve large-scale promotion and application in terms of control and prevention. In the next stage, in accordance with the law on schistosomiasis prevention and control, schistosomiasis management methods on floating population shall be developed according to the local situation, the responsibilities of health, public security, agriculture, foreign population management. Other relevant departments shall be regulated, and schistosomiasis health education on floating population shall be established and improved. With social progress, economic development and environmental changes, the target groups of health education may also change, and it will be an eternal topic to explore suitable health education intervention models and measures for new target groups.

In 1985, WHO proposed that health education in endemic areas was a continuous process which should be continued with the deepening of the prevention and control work. However, after the implementation of countermeasures achieved a certain effect and the epidemic situation is reduced to a low level, many areas will immediately stop or relax the prevention and control work. And what is the first to be ignored is health education as an auxiliary control measure, then the awareness of schistosomiasis control of local residents will be weakening, and it is hard to correct bad habits. Once infection source is imported, it is prone to repeated outbreaks, and then more investment and effort will be required to control the epidemic situation. WHO experts believe that a successful schistosomiasis prevention and control program should include three aspects: (1) recognize the importance of schistosomiasis as public health; (2) local leaders are willing to use resources for prevention and control; (3) be prepared to use public health infrastructures for the distribution and maintenance of prevention and intervention (WHO, 1984, 1985). Therefore, on the premise that the Chinese government attaches great importance to schistosomiasis and increase investment in this respect, we should enhance the publicity of the importance of schistosomiasis prevention and control, enable the leaders at all levels in the schistosomiasis endemic areas to have a sufficient understanding of the longevity, arduousness and usualness of schistosomiasis prevention and control, expand and consolidate schistosomiasis prevention and control achievements in combination of the socioeconomic development in the endemic areas, respect disease control and the coordination of social and economic development and environmental protection, and establish a sustainable work mechanism (WHO, 1985; Tambo et al., 2014).

4. CONCLUSION

In the national schistosomiasis control programme, health education and health promotion plays a positive role in mobilizing the masses, mobilizing the community and promoting the prevention and control measures, and has become one of the main measures to control schistosomiasis. For a long time in the future, health education and health promotion will still be the effective strategy and means in schistosomiasis and other diseases control (Zhen et al., 2013; Bieri et al., 2013; Das et al., 2014; Salam et al., 2014a,b; Koroma and Lv, 2015). With the social and economic development and improvement of people's living standard, it is necessary to establish a sustainable mechanism, combine health education with health guarantee of improving the quality of life, improve the production and living conditions, change the unhealthy production methods and lifestyle of the residents in the endemic areas, and ultimately control and eliminate the schistosomiasis (Collins et al., 2012).

ACKNOWLEDGEMENT

This paper was supported by China–UK Global Health Support Programme (GHSP OP203).

REFERENCES

Bieri, F.A., Yuan, L.P., Li, Y.S., He, Y.K., Bedford, A., Li, R.S., et al., 2013. Development of an educational cartoon to prevent worm infections in Chinese schoolchildren. Infect. Dis. Poverty 2, 29.

Cao, C.L., Guo, J.G., 2010. Schistosome infection and control of migration population. Chin. J. Schistosomiasis Control 4, 388–390 (in Chinese).

Cao, Q., Tan, X.D., Kong, Q.L., Xu, X.J., 2006. Reforming latrine for schistosomiasis control in Hubei. J. Public Health Prev. Med. 6, 28–29+32 (in Chinese).

Cao, C.L., Liang, Y.S., Guo, J.G., Wang, L.P., Sun, L.P., Wu, X.H., Hu, G.H., Wang, W., Ru, W.W., Ma, J.H., Xu, X.J., Gao, Y., Zhou, X.N., 2009. Establishment and applying for the national appraisal system of materials of health education for schistosomiasis control. Chin. J. Schistosomiasis Control 1, 43–46+83 (in Chinese).

Cao, C.L., Chen, L., Wan, X.X., Liu, Q., Cai, X.P., Bao, Z.P., Zhong, B., Guo, J.G., 2011. Investigation on migration regularity and schistosome infection of migrant population in mountainous regions. Chin. J. Schistosomiasis Control 2, 145–147 (in Chinese).

Cao, Z.G., Zhao, Y.E., Willingham, A.L., Wang, T.P., 2016. Towards the elimination of schistosomiasis japonica through control of the disease in domestic animals in the People's Republic of China: a tale of over 60 years. Adv. Parasitol. 92.

Chang, Y.G., Zheng, S.F., Liao, Y.S., 2003. Effects of health education in school before summer vacation. Chin. J. Schistosomiasis Control 15, 188 (in Chinese).

Chen, M.G., 2014. Assessment of morbidity due to *Schistosoma japonicum* infection in China. Infect. Dis. Poverty 3, 6.

Chen, M., Yuan, H.C., Jiang, Q.W., 1990. The quantitative study in endemic area of schistosomiasis japonica of water contact. Chin. J. Schistosomiasis Control 1, 28–33 (in Chinese).

Chen, G.X., Han, S.M., Wang, M.S., He, Z.G., Ni, Y., 2006. Analysis of the effect on the comprehensive measures of replacing cattle by machine and reconstructing water supply and lavatory to control the schistosomiasis for five years. J. Trop. Dis. Parasitol. 3, 160–163 (in Chinese).

Chen, H.Y., Hu, J., Song, K.Y., Xiong, Z.W., Hu, G.H., Hu, W.C., Peng, G.H., Ge, J., Fan, Y.B., 2008. Longitudinal observation of health education in the control of schistosomiasis for 16 years in students of heavy epidemic areas in Poyang Lake region. Chin. J. Zoonoses 12, 1149–1152 (in Chinese).

Chen, H.Y., Hu, G.H., Song, K.Y., Xiong, Z.W., Hu, J., Yang, P.Y., Hu, G.H., Hu, W.C., Yu, S.S., Fu, G.L., Liu, G.H., Qi, J.C., Ge, J., Wan, B.P., 2009a. Establishment and application of school-based health promotion and intervention model of schistosomiasis in lake-type endemic area. Chin. J. Parasitol. Parasit. Dis. 2, 125–129+134 (in Chinese).

Chen, L., Zhong, B., Qiu, D.C., Luan, R.S., 2009b. Analysis on knowledge, attitude, practice of schistosomiasis control of population in endemic areas of Sichuan. J. Prev. Med. Inf. 5, 416–419 (in Chinese).

Chen, L., Cao, C.L., Bao, Z.P., Wan, X.X., Liu, Q., Zhong, B., Qiu, D.C., Guo, J.G., 2013. Study on schistosomiasis control to migrant population by new pattern. Mod. Prev. Med. 9, 1754–1756 (in Chinese).

Chu, L.P., Cheng, B., 2014. In the evaluation of patients with schistosomiasis demonstration school health education effect of developing areas. J. Public Health Prev. Med. 1, 126–128 (in Chinese).
Collins, C., Xu, J., Tang, S., 2012. Schistosomiasis control and the health system in P.R. China. Infect. Dis. Poverty 1, 8.
Dabo, A., Bary, B., Kouriba, B., Sankare, O., Doumbo, O., 2013. Factors associated with coverage of praziquantel for schistosomiasis control in the community-direct intervention (CDI) approach in Mali (West Africa). Infect. Dis. Poverty 2, 11.
Das, J.K., Salam, R.A., Arshad, A., Maredia, H., Bhutta, Z.A., 2014. Community based interventions for the prevention and control of non-helmintic NTD. Infect. Dis. Poverty 3, 24.
Fan, F.N., Xu, J.Y., 2009a. Effect of health education for schistosomiasis control on floating population in Cixi City. Chin. J. Schistosomiasis Control 6, 499–514 (in Chinese).
Fan, F.N., Xu, J.Y., 2009b. Health education of migrant population in Cixi City. Chin. J. Schistosomiasis Control 6, 499–514 (in Chinese).
Fang, R.L., Fang, W.X., Hu, Y., Xiao, H.M., 2005. Effect of health education on comprehensive prevention and control of schistosomiasis transmission blocking area. J. Trop. Dis. Parasitol. 2, 105–106 (in Chinese).
Gao, Y., Sun, L.P., Wu, H.H., Yang, J., Hong, Q.B., Tian, Z.X., Ma, Y.C., Tang, M.L., Huang, Y.X., Liang, Y.S., Hu, X.S., 2009. Study on schistosomiasis control measures in mobile boat fishermen II Effect of comprehensive measures with emphasis on management of boat fishermen feces for schistosomiasis control. Chin. J. Schistosomiasis Control 4, 262–266 (in Chinese).
Gu, X.G., Wang, W.N., Zhao, W.X., 1990. Investigation report of acute schistosomiasis in hilly areas of Sichuan. Chin. J. Schistosomiasis Control 2, 62–66 (in Chinese).
Gu, X.G., 1993. Study on the epidemic law and control strategy of schistosomiasis in Sichuan Province. J. Prev. Med. Inf. S1, 21–22 (in Chinese).
He, N., Yuan, H.C., Jiang, Q.W., Zhang, S.J., 1996. Quantitative study on the hilly endemic area of water contact. Chin. J. Schistosomiasis Control 1, 1–5 (in Chinese).
Hong, Q.B., Yang, K., Huang, Y.X., Sun, L.P., Yang, G.J., Gao, Y., Gao, Y., Zhang, L.H., Zhou, M., Steinmann, P., Liang, Y.S., 2011. Effectiveness of a comprehensive schistosomiasis japonica control program in Jiangsu Province, China, from 2005 to 2008. Acta Trop. 120, S151–S157.
Hu, G.H., Lin, D.D., Zeng, X.J., 1995. Health education for primary school students in Poyang Lake District. Chin. J. Health Educ. 11, 34–36 (in Chinese).
Hu, G.H., Liu, J.X., Lin, D.D., Kang, Z.H., Xiong, Y.L., Chen, T.H., 1997. The role of health education in adult women in the marshland endemic area of schistosomiasis control. Chin. J. Parasit. Dis. Parasit. Dis. 5, 47–50 (in Chinese).
Hu, G.H., Lin, D.D., Zhang, S.J., Zeng, X.J., Kang, Z.H., Chen, G.J., 1999a. Evaluation on effectiveness of health education for schistosomiasis control in highly endemic area of Poyang Lake region. Chin. J. Public Health 10, 83–84 (in Chinese).
Hu, G.H., Zhang, J., Wang, L.Z., Su, J.C., Tong, Y., Wu, L.S., Du, H.G., Lv, S.B., 1999b. Effectiveness of health education in Schistosomiasis controlled areas. Chin. J. Parasit. Dis. Control Prev. 4, 55–56 (in Chinese).
Hu, G.H., Lin, D.D., Zhang, S.J., 2000. Study on the intervention model of health education for schistosomiasis. Chin. J. Schistosomiasis Control 14, 283 (in Chinese).
Hu, G.H., Lin, H., Li, D., Wang, L.Z., Zhao, S.S., Ye, B.X., Wan, B.P., Pu, Z.L., 2001. Final evaluation of health education for schistosomiasis control of World Bank Loan Projection in Jiangxi Province. Chin. J. Parasit. Dis. Control 3, 45–48 (in Chinese).
Hu, G.H., Li, H.Z., Zhou, X.N., Wu, X.H., Tang, B.L., Gu, X.N., Li, S.Z., Bai, G.H., Ge, J., 2005. Development and pretest of the calendar of health education for schistosomiasis control. Chin. J. Schistosomiasis Control 4, 287–289 (in Chinese).

Huang, Y.X., Manderson, L., 2003. Chinese rural people's perceptions of schistosomiasis and other diseases. Chin. J. Schistosomiasis Control 2, 108–115.

Ji, H., He, J.C., Zhuang, X.D., Zhang, S.Q., Zhang, G.H., Gao, F.H., 2006. Implementation and evaluation of health education for schistosomiasis control in Anhui Province from 2003 to 2005. Parasitoses Infect. Dis. 3, 119–121 (in Chinese).

Jiang, Z., Li, D.Q., Du, S.R., 1998. Research on knowledge in primary school students in advanced schistosomiasis infiltration education. Chin. Prim. Health Care 12, 44–46.

Koroma, M., Lv, S., 2015. Ebola wreaks havoc in Sierra Leone. Infect. Dis. Poverty 4, 10.

Li, Y.S., Yu, D.B., 1991. *Schistosoma japonicum* infection among migrant fishermen in the Dongting Lake region of China. Trans. R. Soc. Trop. Med. Hyg. 85, 623–625.

Li, Y.S., He, Y.K., Zeng, Q.R., McManus, D.P., 2003. Epidemiological and morbidity assessment of *Schistosoma japonicum* infection in a migrant fisherman community, the Dongting Lake region, China. Trans. R. Soc. Trop. Med. Hyg. 97, 177–181.

Li, Y., Zeng, Q., Ellis, M.K., Xiong, T., Balen, J., McManus, D.P., 2006. $CD4^+$ T-cell counts, $CD4^+/CD8^+$ T-cell count ratios, and antibody levels in migrant fishermen infected with *Schistosoma japonicum* in the Dongting Lake, China. Am. J. Trop. Med. Hyg. 75, 910–913.

Li, D., Hu, W.C., Hu, G.H., Zhang, J., Lin, D.D., Zhang, J., Huang, M.J., Jiang, W.S., Kang, Z.H., Qiu, L., 2008. Longitudinal investigation on effectiveness of health schistosomiasis control among adult women in heavy endemic areas for 13 years. Chin. J. Schistosomiasis Control 2, 144–146 (in Chinese).

Li, T.T., He, J.C., Wang, H., Zhang, G.H., Gao, F.H., 2013. Investigation on current situation of health education materials for schistosomiasis control in Anhui Province. J. Trop. Dis. Parasitol. 3, 149–152 (in Chinese).

Li, B.G., Chen, S.R., Li, W.B., Luo, J.J., 2014. Effect of health education combined with source control on schistosomiasis control in Mountainous areas. J. Prev. Med. Inf. 7, 519–523 (in Chinese).

Li, K.L., 2000. Evaluation report on the implementation of health education for the World Bank loan schistosomiasis control project in Yunnan Province. J. Pract. Parasit. Dis. 4, 178–179 (in Chinese).

Liang, L., Gong, Q., Zhang, H., Tao, W., Zhao, P., Chen, P.L., 2007. Effect evaluation of comprehensive control of schistosomiasis in Pujiang County 2001–2005. Parasitoses Infect. Dis. 1, 26–27 (in Chinese).

Liu, B.Z., Liu, C.Y., Zhang, G.S., 1992. Endemic characteristics of schistosomiasis in hilly areas. Chin. J. Schistosomiasis Control 4, 305–307 (in Chinese).

Liu, Q.H., Liu, B.Z., Chen, Y.W., 1994. Investigation of schistosomiasis epidemic area of Sichuan village in cognition and related behavior. J. Pract. Parasit. Dis. 2, 8–11 (in Chinese).

Liu, Q.H., Liu, B.Z., Chen, Y.W., Chen, Z., Liu, G.D., Wang, Q., He, G.Z., Xiong, S.R., Chen, Y., 1995. Health education for mid-term evaluation of World Bank Loan Project for schistosomiasis control in Sichuan Province. J. Pract. Parasit. Dis. 3, 114–116 (in Chinese).

Liu, Q.H., Chen, Y.W., Liu, B.Z., Wang, Q., Shan, J.Z., Luo, Y., Liu, Z.X., 1999. Study on enhancement of schistosomiasis chemotherapy compliance by health education. Chin. J. Schistosomiasis Control 1, 11–14 (in Chinese).

Liu, Q.H., Chen, Y.W., Liu, B.Z., Chen, Z., Wang, M.P., Zhang, W., Xiong, M.E., Kang, J.X., Dong, Y.C., Chen, Y., 2000. Final report on evaluation of health education in the World Bank loan for Schistosomiasis control program in Sichuan. J. Pract. Parasit. Dis. 2, 61–65 (in Chinese).

Liu, Z.Y., Dai, Y.H., Xu, X.J., Li, C.M., Zhang, D.P., 2005. Study on intervention modes and cost effect of health education for schistosomiasis. J. Trop. Med. 1, 34–37+77 (in Chinese).

Liu, X.L., Ma, Y.C., Wang, F.B., 2009a. Effect of health education on schistosomiasis control in fishermen and boatmen. Chin. J. Schistosomiasis Control 21, 424–425.
Liu, X.L., Ma, Y.C., Wang, F.B., 2009b. Effect of health education on schistosomiasis control in fishermen and boatmen. Chin. J. Schistosomiasis Control 5, 424–425 (in Chinese).
Liu, L., Yang, G.J., Zhu, H.R., Yang, K., Ai, L., 2014. Knowledge of, attitudes towards, and practice relating to schistosomiasis in two subtypes of a mountainous region of the People's Republic of China. Infect. Dis. Poverty 3, 16.
Liu, Y., Zhou, Y.B., Li, R.Z., Wan, J.J., Yang, Y., Qiu, D.C., et al., 2016. Epidemiological features and control effectiveness of schistosomiasis in mountainous and hilly region of the People's Republic of China. Adv. Parasitol. 92.
Lv, G.Y., Yang, X.X., Xu, X.J., Su, Z.M., Wan, G.G., Yuan, T.X., Xiao, Y.L., Zeng, R.X., Huang, Y.J., Wu, J.A., 1998. Analysis of schistosomiasis housewife care seeking of children benefit and to promote health education. Chin. J. Health Educ. 1, 35–36 (in Chinese).
Lv, S., Tian, L.G., Liu, Q., Qian, M.B., Fu, Q., Steinmann, P., Chen, J.X., Yang, G.J., Yang, K., Zhou, X.N., 2013. Water-related parasitic diseases in China. Int. J. Environ. Res. Public Health 10, 1977–2016.
Ma, S.C., Mao, Y.S., 2014. Evaluation on schistosomiasis health education in workers of shipyards along the Yangtze River in Hexian County. J. Trop. Dis. Parasitol. 4, 233–234+244 (in Chinese).
Mao, S.B., 1990. Schistosomiasis Biology and Schistosomiasis Control. People's Health Publishing House (in Chinese).
Ministry of Health of the People's Republic of China, 2000a. Schistosomiasis Control Manual. Shanghai Science and Technology Press (in Chinese).
Ministry of Health of the People's Republic of China, 2000b. Guide for Health Education of Schistosomiasis. Beijing Medical University Press (in Chinese).
MOH, 1993. Guidelines for the Implementation of the World Bank Loan for Schistosomiasis Control Projects in China. Science and Technology Press (in Chinese).
Mott, K.E., 1992. Schistosomiasis control: everybody's business. In: Beijing: International Symposium on Schistosomiasis.
Mtethiwa, A.H., Nkwengulila, G., Bakuza, J., Sikawa, D., Kazembe, A., 2015. Extent of morbidity associated with schistosomiasis infection in Malawi: a review paper. Infect. Dis. Poverty 4, 25.
Ojurongbe, O., Sina-Agbaje, O.R., Busari, A., Okorie, P.N., Ojurongbe, T.A., Akindele, A.A., 2014. Efficacy of praziquantel in the treatment of *Schistosoma haematobium* infection among school-age children in rural communities of Abeokuta, Nigeria. Infect. Dis. Poverty 3, 30.
Paudel, M., Acharya, B., Adhikari, M., 2013. Social determinants that lead to poor knowledge about, and inappropriate precautionary practices towards, avian influenza among butchers in Kathmandu, Nepal. Infect. Dis. Poverty 2, 10.
Qi, J.C., Hu, G.H., Peng, G.H., Wan, B.P., Hu, W.C., Zhang, Z.Z., 2010. Investigation of schistosome infection among fishermen in the Poyang Lake area. J. Pathog. Biol. 1, 71+25 (in Chinese).
Qiu, C.G., Hu, G.H., Hu, W.C., Gu, X.N., Ge, J., Zhang, J., Huang, M.J., Qiu, L., Liu, Z.H., Xiong, G.L., 2006. Expanded application of health education for schistosomiasis control in adult men. Parasitoses Infect. Dis. 4, 173–176 (in Chinese).
Qu, G.S., Hu, D.Z., Zhou, Y.C., Xu, W.Z., 2008. Embankment schistosomiasis in heavy endemic areas based on health education and control effect of infection rate of residents. Pract. Prev. Med. 1, 138–139 (in Chinese).
Ross, A.G., Yuesheng, L., Sleigh, A.S., Yi, L., Williams, G.M., Wu, W.Z., Xinsong, L., Yongkang, H., McManus, D.P., 1997. Epidemiologic features of *Schistosoma japonicum*

among fishermen and other occupational groups in the Dongting Lake region (Hunan Province) of China. Am. J. Trop. Med. Hyg. 57, 302–308.
Salam, R.A., Haroon, S., Ahmed, H.H., Das, J.K., Bhutta, Z.A., 2014a. Impact of community-based interventions on HIV knowledge, attitudes, and transmission. Infect. Dis. Poverty 3, 26.
Salam, R.A., Maredia, H., Das, J.K., Lassi, Z.S., Bhutta, Z.A., 2014b. Community-based interventions for the prevention and control of helmintic neglected tropical diseases. Infect. Dis. Poverty 3, 23.
Song, K.Y., Yin, H., Hu, G.H., Chen, H.Y., Ge, J., Peng, G.H., Zhang, J., Zhang, J., Hu, Z.H., Hu, W.C., 2010. Longitudinal observation on effect of health education for adult male residents for 18 years in heavy epidemic areas of schistosomiasis around Poyang Lake region. Chin. J. Schistosomiasis Control 22, 242–246 (in Chinese).
Sun, J.G., Wang, L.Y., Li, J.H., Hao, Y., Li, Y.B., Li, F.B., 2002. Final evaluation of health education in the World Bank loan national schistosomiasis control program. Chin. J. Health Educ. 18, 210–216 (in Chinese).
Sun, J.G., Dai, Y.H., Yin, L.R., Zhong, G.T., Zhang, Z.R., Liu, Z.Y., Zhang, G., 2005. Effectiveness of posters of prevention and control of schistosomiasis. Chin. J. Health Educ. 2, 77–78 (in Chinese).
Sun, D.K., 2002. Effect evaluation of health education for floating population in Jinhu County. Chin. J. Health Educ. 18, 797–798 (in Chinese).
Tambo, E., Ai, L., Zhou, X., Chen, J.H., Hu, W., Bergquist, R., et al., 2014. Surveillance-response systems: the key to elimination of tropical diseases. Infect. Dis. Poverty 3, 17.
Tian, B.C., 2005. Practical Methods of Health Education and Health Promotion. Peking University Medical Press (in Chinese).
Wang, Q.Z., Zhang, S.Q., Wang, T.P., Xiao, X., Zhang, G.H., Lv, D.B., Zhu, C.G., Fang, G.R., Su, G.B., Yao, Z.Q., 1999. Longitudinal study on schistosomiasis control effect of extended chemotherapy combined with health education in islet endemic area. J. Trop. Dis. Parasitol. 4, 209–212 (in Chinese).
Wang, L.P., Li, B., Shen, Y.P., Wu, W., Zhu, Y.C., Zhao, Y.J., 2002. Evaluation on the effect of the health education of schistosomiasis in Jiangsu Province. Chin. J. Health Educ. 4, 25–27 (in Chinese).
Wang, A.P., Gu, C.Y., Wu, M.Y., Zhou, Z.L., Chen, H., Zhu, S.Y., 2008. Effect of health education intervention for schistosomiasis control among nonnative personnel in Changzhou City. Chin. J. Schistosomiasis Control 4, 300–301 (in Chinese).
Wang, Y.L., Zhou, H., Liang, J.X., Guo, X.H., Ouyang, S.W., He, W.L., 2010. Effect of health education on schistosomiasis control in high endemic areas of marshland and lake regions. Chin. J. Schistosomiasis Control 4, 397–398 (in Chinese).
Wang, Z., Lin, C.P., Wang, H., Tang, W.G., Wang, Y., 2012. Impact assessment of health education on schistosomiasis among high school students in Wanzhou area of Three Gorges Reservoir. Chin. J. Evidence Based Med. 3, 274–277 (in Chinese).
Wei, W.Y., Yuan, L.P., Jiang, Q.X., 2000a. Study on health education to reduce the primary water contact behavior. Chin. J. Schistosomiasis Control 12, 143–145 (in Chinese).
Wei, W.Y., Yuan, L.P., Jiang, Q.X., Peng, A.G., Zhou, D.R., 2000b. Study on health education to reduce the primary water contact behavior. Chin. J. Schistosomiasis Control 3, 143–145 (in Chinese).
Wei, D.H., 2014a. To evaluate the effect of health education in Nanjing area fishermen. Mod. Prev. Med. 2, 277–278 (in Chinese).
Wei, D.H., 2014b. Evalution on the effectiveness of health education on schistosomiasis for fishermen and boatmen in the Nanjing area. Mod. Prev. Med. 2, 277–278 (in Chinese).
WHO, 1978. Declaration of Alma-Ata. WHO Chron. 32 (11), 428–430.
WHO, 1984. World Health Organization new strategy on schistosomiasis control. Southeast Asia J. Trop. Med. Public Health 15, 469–470.

WHO, 1985. Report of a World Health Organization expert committee. The control of schistosomiasis. WHO Tech. Rep. Ser. 728, 81–86.
WHO, 2002. In: WHO. Geneva (Ed.), Prevention and Control of Schistosomiasis and Soil-transmitted Helminthiasis, pp. 1–57.
Wu, Z.S., Zhang, X.S., Zhong, B., 2006. Analysis of acute schistosomiasis in Sichuan Province from 2003 to 2005. Chin. J. Schistosomiasis Control 18, 386–387 (in Chinese).
Wu, Z.S., Yi, H.W.L., Zhang, X.S., Wang, S.A., Xu, L., Liu, G.M., Liu, H.B., Zhou, Y.B., Xiao, Y.M., Wang, T.G., Qiu, D.C., 2009. Schistosomiasis epidemic characteristic and effectiveness for comprehensive measure with emphasis on infectious resource control in high mountainous area in Sichuan Province. Parasitoses Infect. Dis. 3, 126–130 (in Chinese).
Wu, G.S., Hong, X.L., Hu, Z.H., Xu, S.W., Fu, G.L., Hu, S.Z., Hu, M.W., Fan, Y.L., Li, X.G., 2013. Effect of health education on prevention from schistosome infection in engineering construction workers in Poyang Lake area. Chin. J. Schistosomiasis Control 6, 677–678 (in Chinese).
Xia, G., Zhang, J., Zhao, S., Wang, L.Y., 2006. Study on control strategies of acute infection of *Schistosoma japonicum* in school children. Chin. J. Schistosomiasis Control 1, 71–73 (in Chinese).
Xie, C.Y., Fu, H.S., 2012. Effect of health education on schistosomiasis control in high endemic areas of marshland and lake regions. Chin. J. Schistosomiasis Control 3, 362–363 (in Chinese).
Xu, L.W., Hu, G.H., Zhang, J., 2002. Effectiveness of the spread application of intervention modes on health education for schistosomiasis control among adult women. Chin. J. Schistosomiasis Control 14, 283 (in Chinese).
Xu, J., Steinman, P., Maybe, D., Zhou, X.N., Lv, S., Li, S.Z., et al., 2016. Evolution of the national schistosomiasis control programmes in the People's Republic of China. Adv. Parasitol. 92.
Yang, P.Y., Li, L.W., Li, Z.J., Wan, G.B., Xiong, G.Q., Zeng, H., Chen, Z.G., 2012. Effect of comprehensive intervention of schistosomiasis control in construction workers in Poyang Lake region. Chin. J. Schistosomiasis Control 6, 718–719 (in Chinese).
Ye, L.P., Xu, G.Z., Lu, F., 2007. Management and monitoring of floating population in Ningbo in 2003 -2005. Dis. Surveill. 22, 101–103 (in Chinese).
Yuan, G.P., Guo, Z.P., Gu, M.M., 2005. Surveillance report on the consolidation of schistosomiasis in Baoshan District, Shanghai. Shanghai J. Prev. Med. 17, 320–321 (in Chinese).
Zhang, J., Hu, G.H., Yang, X.Y., Ge, J., Chen, N.G., Huang, M.J., Li, D., Kang, Z.H., 2004. Report on development and pretest of the box of health education for schistosomiasis control. Chin. J. Schistosomiasis Control 4, 443–445 (in Chinese).
Zhang, J., Hu, W.C., Hu, G.H., Kang, Z.H., Chen, N.G., Huang, M.J., Ge, J., Chen, Y.P., 2006a. Effect of schistosomiasis health education combined with behavior interventi0n on Schistosoma infection control in students of heavy endemic areas. Chin. J. Schistosomiasis Control 6, 410 (in Chinese).
Zhang, K., Ye, J.M., Wang, S., 2006b. Effect of health education of schistosomiasis control among students in Qixia District, Nanjing City. Chin. J. Schistosomiasis Control 6, 410 (in Chinese).
Zhang, Y., Wang, T., Zhong, B., Chen, L., Liao, B., 2008a. Impact of rural community construction and industrial structure adjustment on the transmission control of schistosomiasis. Parasitoses Infect. Dis. 1, 41–42 (in Chinese).
Zhang, Y.Q., Zhang, W., Xiong, Y.Q., Wang, Z.C., Sun, W.S., Tian, J.P., Yang, H., Wang, W.L., Xu, Q.C., Yang, R., Zhang, J., Zhang, R., Yang, F.L., Hu, H.J., 2008b.

Effect of health education on transient population from schistosomiasis free area. Parasitoses Infect. Dis. 4, 182–184 (in Chinese).

Zhang, L.J., Li, S.Z., Wen, L.Y., Lin, D.D., Abe, E.M., Zhu, R., et al., 2016. Establishment and function of schistosomiasis surveillance system towards elimination in the People's Republic of China. Adv. Parasitol. 92.

Zheng, Q.S., Zheng, J., 2000. Social Medicine and Schistosomiasis. Tianjin Science and Technology Press (in Chinese).

Zheng, Q., Vanderslott, S., Jiang, B., Xu, L.L., Liu, C.S., Huo, L.L., et al., 2013. Research gaps for three main tropical diseases in the People's Republic of China. Infect. Dis. Poverty 2, 15.

Zheng, J., 2003. Present situation and Prospect of schistosomiasis control in China. Chin. J. Schistosomiasis Control 15, 1–2 (in Chinese).

Zhong, B., Qiu, D.C., Wen, S., Wei, J.B., Shan, J.Z., Gong, Q., Li, S.Q., Gu, X.G., 2002. Comparison on schistosomiasis control strategies in Changqiu mountain area, Sichuan Province. J. Pract. Parasit. Dis. 1, 1–4 (in Chinese).

Zhong, B., Liang, S., Zhang, Y., Lai, Y.H., Chen, L., Yin, H.Z., Zhao, Y.M., Lv, J.Q., Qiu, D.C., 2006. Water exposure modes and times of different population in mountainous schistosomiasis endemic areas near Qionghai lake. Chin. J. Prev. Med. 4, 239–243 (in Chinese).

Zhou, H., He, Y.K., Luo, X.S., Yu, X.L., 1997. Study of children behavior with schistosomiasis in Dongting Lake. Chin. J. Sch. Health 4, 275 (in Chinese).

Zhou, X.N., Wang, L.Y., Chen, M.G., Wu, X.H., Jiang, Q.W., Chen, X.Y., et al., 2005. The public health significance and control of schistosomiasis in China-then and now. Acta Trop. 96, 97–105.

Zhou, X.N., Cai, L., Zhang, X.P., 2007. Potential risks for transmission of schistosomiasis caused by Mobile population in Shanghai. Chin. J. Parasitol. Parasit. Dis. 25, 180–184 (in Chinese).

Zhou, L.S., Shen, P., Ping, J.M., 2008. Infection status of migration population and its influencing factors. Chin. J. Zoonoses 24, 397–398 (in Chinese).

Zhou, X., Chen, R.S., Zheng, D.R., Li, J.R., Cheng, X.B., Ao, J.Q., Liu, H.X., 2013. Effect of health education intervention in schools of Yanrui town, Yushan county. Chin. J. Schistosomiasis Control 6, 675–676 (in Chinese).

CHAPTER TWELVE

Policy Support and Resources Mobilization for the National Schistosomiasis Control Programme in The People's Republic of China

H. Zhu*, P. Yap[§,¶], J. Utzinger[§,¶], T.-W. Jia[||,], S.-Z. Li[||,**,§§], X.-B. Huang*, S.-X. Cai*[,1]**

*Hubei Provincial Center for Disease Control and Prevention, Wuhan, The People's Republic of China
[§]Swiss Tropical and Public Health Institute, Basel, Switzerland
[¶]University of Basel, Basel, Switzerland
[||]National Institute of Parasitic Diseases, Chinese Center for Disease Control and Prevention, Shanghai, The People's Republic of China
**WHO Collaborating Centre for Tropical Diseases, Shanghai, The People's Republic of China
[§§]Key Laboratory of Parasite and Vector Biology, MOH, Shanghai, The People's Republic of China
[1]Corresponding author: E-mail: 441711219@qq.com

Contents

Advances in Parasitology, Volume 92
ISSN 0065-308X
http://dx.doi.org/10.1016/bs.apar.2016.03.002

Abstract

Schistosomiasis remains a public health problem in many developing countries around the world. After the founding of The People's Republic of China, from 1949 till date, all levels of government, from central to local, have been attaching great importance to schistosomiasis control in The People's Republic of China. With considerable policy support and resources mobilization, the national schistosomiasis control programmes have been implemented during the past 65 years. Here, we summarize the successful experience of schistosomiasis control during the process. Recommendations for the future management of the Chinese national schistosomiasis elimination programme are put forward after considering the remaining challenges, shortcomings and lessons learnt from 65 years of schistosomiasis control drives in The People's Republic of China. They will help to sustain past achievements, foster the attainment of the ultimate goal of schistosomiasis elimination for the country and provide reference for schistosomiasis control programme in other countries.

1. INTRODUCTION

Schistosomiasis remains a public health problem in many developing countries around the world (Mazigo et al., 2013), and is a major limiting factor in the development of local economies (Zhou et al., 2002). After the founding of The People's Republic of China, all levels of government, from central to local, have been attaching great importance to schistosomiasis control. Such efforts have also been integrated into sustainable social and economic development planning. After more than 60 years of constant efforts in the control of schistosomiasis, the Chinese government has made remarkable achievements, which can be a learning basis for many developing countries (Xu et al., 2016a,b). At present, schistosomiasis elimination has been identified as the new target in The People's Republic of China (Lei and Zhou, 2015).

This chapter reviews the process and successful experiences of schistosomiasis control in The People's Republic of China for the past 65 years, from 1949 to 2014. The control programme can be divided into four stages, namely in the early years after the founding of The People's Republic of China from 1949 to 1959, in the later 20th century from 1960s to 1980s, from the late 1980s to the end of the 20th century and the 21st century (Xu et al., 2016a,b). At each stage, the successful experiences have been summarized into three aspects, namely national policy support and measures, resource mobilization and effect of schistosomiasis control. Such a summary provides the basis for designing an elimination programme against schistosomiasis in The People's Republic of China and be potentially used as a reference for developing schistosomiasis control programmes in other developing countries.

2. IN THE EARLY YEARS AFTER THE FOUNDING OF THE PEOPLE'S REPUBLIC OF CHINA FROM 1949 TO 1959

2.1 Background

Before the founding of The People's Republic of China, schistosomiasis was a pandemic disease in southern China (Chen, 2014), causing great harm to people's life and health. After the founding of The People's Republic of China, the Central Committee of the Communist Party of China (CPC), headed by Chairman Mao Zedong, considered schistosomiasis a major public health problem and attached great importance to its control (Shi, 2011). Eliminating schistosomiasis was considered a serious political task at that time. Although the whole country was mobilized to make unremitting efforts to eliminate the disease, the work of schistosomiasis control was exceptionally arduous due to limited economic and technological conditions at that time.

2.2 Policy support and measures

2.2.1 To determine the organizational leadership of schistosomiasis control

Due to the urgency and difficulty in schistosomiasis control in the early days, the Central Committee of CPC set up the organizational leadership for the control programme promptly in November 1955. The leading group was also called the 'nine people group'. Subsequently, leading groups were found at different levels of party committee, including in the provincial party committee, municipal party committee, county party committee and town party committee, which lead the local work of schistosomiasis control (Fig. 1). In addition, specific responsibilities and actions at five levels of leadership were clearly stated. Firstly, a regular meeting system was established. Secondly, a regular reporting system, which reflected the true progress and problems of schistosomiasis control was set up (Zhang et al., 2016). Thirdly,

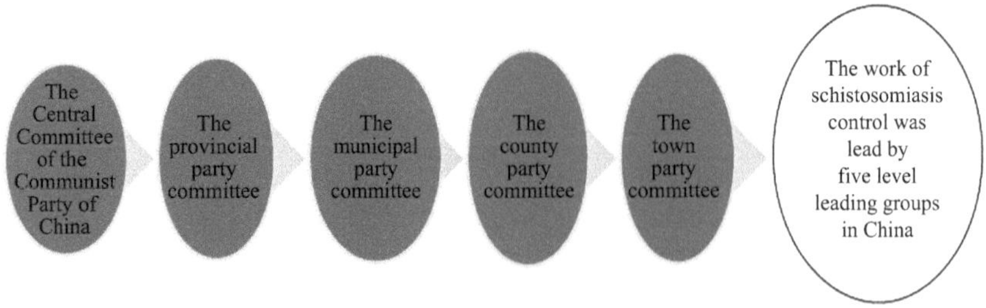

Figure 1 The leadership hierarchy for the work of schistosomiasis control in the 1950s in The People's Republic of China.

the local schistosomiasis control planning was sought to be assessed and reformulated each year. The leading group of the Central Committee of CPC performed its duties fully and consecutive national work conferences on schistosomiasis control were held thrice in Shanghai in a span of 2 years (Shi, 2011). Directives of the state council for schistosomiasis elimination were issued by Premier Zhou Enlai on 20 April 1957, and the council issued the highest level of government documents on schistosomiasis control (Wang, 2011). A notice on implementing the directives of schistosomiasis elimination was published by the Central Committee of CPC on 23 April 1957, which expressed the terms that all provincial party committees, municipal party committees of schistosomiasis endemic areas and the party groups of the relevant departments under the state council should ensure the execution of the state council's instructions. From then on, the relevant provincial communist party had to submit a report on schistosomiasis control every 6 months to the Central Committee of CPC.

2.2.2 To strengthening the legal system management

At this stage, setting up a legal system governing the control of infectious disease, including schistosomiasis, was required. The infectious disease management law of The People's Republic of China passed in 1955 was the first health law for the management of infectious diseases issued by the highest authority of the state after the founding of The People's Republic of China. With this law, the prevention and treatment of infectious diseases were brought into the ambit of legal system management for the first time (Zhou, 2004). Initially, only scientific management system of schistosomiasis control was set up at that time in The People's Republic of China, where schistosomiasis was listed as a 'c' class infectious disease in the law. By setting up a proper legal management system, a comprehensive set of regulations and principles as well as prevention and treatment measures for schistosomiasis were clarified. This included the responsibilities of the citizens, social organizations and relevant government departments (Cao et al., 2016). In addition, the law reflected science and humanity as more attention was directed at protecting the individual privacy of patients with infectious diseases (Li and Shen, 2006; Yao and Xu, 2005). Furthermore, the reporting and releasing system of epidemic became more effective as witnessed in the legal infectious disease reporting system carried out in the 1950s in The People's Republic of China. Therefore, the transparency of infectious disease control was strengthened and the citizens' right to know was respected according to the above approach.

2.2.3 To strengthen the top scientific planning

In order to strengthen the scientific aspect of the control programme, technology support measures were also put forward by the professional institutions in The People's Republic of China. For example, the national expert advisory committee of schistosomiasis control of CPC was established in December 1955, only one month after establishment of the leading group of the Central Committee of CPC. Subsequently, the comprehensive measures for schistosomiasis control were put forward by the national expert advisory committee of schistosomiasis control of CPC (Shi, 2011). The prevention and control of schistosomiasis and other infectious diseases were included in the national agricultural development outline (draft), which was passed by the Political Bureau of the Central Committee of CPC, in January 1956. From 1956 to 1967, infectious diseases research projects, including work on schistosomiasis, were considered important goals and formed the basis for the planning of science and technology development in The People's Republic of China. The drugs for the control of *Oncomelania hupensis*, oral therapy for infected patients and traditional Chinese medicine (TCM) therapy also received much attention during the planning (Li et al., 2016).

2.3 Resources mobilization

2.3.1 Integrating organizations at all levels from central to local for schistosomiasis control

The work of schistosomiasis control was lead uniformly by the office of the leading group of the Central Committee of CPC. Resources from different departments (including health, agriculture, water conservancy, education and civil affairs) and various organizations (including army, trade unions, communist youth league and women workers committee) were integrated for the control of all endemic areas. Besides, resources of organizations from different endemic provinces including Jiangsu, Zhejiang, Fujian, Anhui and Shanghai were integrated for the national control of schistosomiasis. In addition, the schistosomiasis control bureau, under the Ministry of Health, was established in Shanghai in July 1957 to strength the leadership of schistosomiasis control. All these activities had led to improved coordination and cooperation between the central schistosomiasis control institutions (Wang, 2011).

2.3.2 Integrating professional institutions for schistosomiasis control

Schistosomiasis control was regarded as the most important work under disease control during this time period. Therefore, different levels of leading groups of CPC for schistosomiasis control were established after the central leadership group was established. They included the provincial, the municipality, the county and the township committees of CPC. Various levels of expert advisory committee for schistosomiasis control have also been successively set up during the same period. At a local level, there were people in charge of the schistosomiasis control work in villages. In 1953, stations of disease control and prevention had already been established in provinces, cities (municipalities) and counties (districts) across the whole country. These stations became the professional network for disease control unit of the CPC and the state to implement the strategy and measures of public health (Li, 2013). By August 1957, a total of 19 professional institutions, 236 stations and 1346 groups were established specifically for schistosomiasis control in The People's Republic of China.

2.3.3 Integrating scientific research institution

To strengthen the scientific research work on schistosomiasis, the human and financial resources from medical colleges and institutions working on schistosomiasis control in different areas, including Jiangsu province, Zhejiang province, Anhui province and Shanghai, were systematically integrated by the national expert advisory committee of schistosomiasis control of CPC. In addition, under the leadership of the national expert advisory committee of schistosomiasis control of CPC, different levels of scientific research institution were established in provinces, cities and counties (districts) (Wang, 2011). Besides the scientific research organization mentioned above, national and local institutions and laboratories of TCM, were also integrated. All of them played an important role of schistosomiasis control.

2.3.4 Integrating the strength of the people in endemic area

After the directives of schistosomiasis elimination were published by the state council and the basic policies of 'health work should be combined with the mass movement' were implemented in 1957, all masses and organizations were mobilized to carry out the work of schistosomiasis control with vigour and vitality. These organizations could be divided mainly into two kinds, namely mass organizations of treatment and mass organizations of prevention, which included the snail control team, investigation team of infection rate and emergency response team, who played important roles in snail control, faeces of human and livestock management, and daily sanitation and hygiene management. For example, in order to play its role properly, Jiangsu Province integrated their treatment and prevention units with their social medical organization by establishing a joint clinic. During this period, similar mass organizations of prevention and treatment were also established in endemic provinces, so as to implement the principle of mass prevention and treatment into practice.

2.4 Effect of prevention and control

Through the implementation of measures mentioned in Section 2.3, the following achievements have been achieved in the 1950s in The People's Republic of China.

Firstly, through a national large-scale epidemiological investigation on schistosomiasis, the distribution of schistosomiasis epidemic areas in 1959 were verified, and they were found to be located along the south of the Yangtze River of The People's Republic of China, including 12 provinces (autonomous regions and municipalities directly under the central government), namely Jiangsu, Zhejiang, Anhui, Hunan, Hubei, Jiangxi, Fujian, Guangdong, Guangxi, Sichuan, Yunnan and Shangha. There were 449 epidemic counties (cities, areas), 3563 epidemic towns, resulting in more than 11.6 million patients, 1.20 million cattle infected by schistosome, and an area coverage of 14.3 billion m^2 of snail. The high epidemic areas of schistosomiasis were also located along the Yangtze River and its connected lakes, such as Dongting Lake, Poyang Lake and Tai Lake. The epidemic in other provinces, such as Yunnan, Fujian, Guangxi and Guangdong provinces, were relatively light (Chen and Feng, 1999; Tang, 2012). According to the epidemiological characteristics and snail-ridden environments, the areas endemic with schistosomiasis were divided into three types in The People's Republic of China, namely marshland, hilly and water network areas (Liu et al., 2016; Shi et al., 2016; Zhang et al., 2016).

Secondly, successful experience of schistosomiasis control was documented in a systematic and comprehensive way including the scientific achievements and the invention of the masses during the work of schistosomiasis control. The national compilation of schistosomiasis research data has been published every year since 1955, and a guiding 'schistosomiasis control manual' was published for the first time in 1956. The ordinance of schistosomiasis control (draft) was also made available, and consisted of 7 chapters and 33 articles. Promulgation and implementation of the ordinance play an important role in promoting the work of schistosomiasis control.

Finally, Yujiang County in Jiangxi Province was the first county to achieve schistosomiasis elimination in June 1958. Chairman Mao wrote a brilliant poem entitled 'Send away the god of plague' when he heard the good news. This poem greatly inspired the passion of scientific researchers for schistosomiasis control and the people who resided in endemic areas. The will and determination to send away the god of plague was formed since then (Wang et al., 2009a,b,c). By the end of 1958, the number of schistosomiasis-infected patients who have received treatment was more than 4.3 million, and many areas have completely eliminated the harm with schistosome infection (Zhang, 2014). The Health Minister, Li De Quan, said 'schistosomiasis has basically been eliminated in 65% of the epidemic areas' during a meeting, which summarized achievements for 10 years worth of health work since the founding of The People's Republic of China in 1959 (Wang, 2011). Through masses mobilization in 1950s, great achievements had been obtained including achieving the goal of basic elimination of schistosomiasis and protecting people's health, thus resulting in the promotion of national productivity and economy.

3. IN THE 20TH CENTURY FROM 1960S TO 1980S

3.1 Background

During 1960s to 1980s, the main task of schistosomiasis control was large-scale snail control, combined with irrigation and water conservancy construction by people who resided in endemic areas. It was inspired by the successful experiences of Yujiang County. It was also based on the global strategy of schistosomiasis control, which emphasized snail elimination and the condition of rural social economy at that time in The People's Republic of China (Mao, 1990). Due to the occurrence of natural disasters and famines in 1960s, a huge negative impact was inflicted on health prevention between 1966 and 1976, causing the work of schistosomiasis control to be severely disrupted. The process of schistosomiasis control was halted, leading to a serious reemergence of schistosomiasis. The leading groups and professional organizations for schistosomiasis control were dissolved at different levels, namely the national, provincial, municipal (city) and county (district) levels (Wang et al., 1989). After 1970s, the process of schistosomiasis control began to develop steadily, with a national overhaul and recovery. Some epidemic prevention institutions were rebuilt. During this period, the effective policies and measures for schistosomiasis control were made once again under the leadership of the CPC and government, which played an important guidance for schistosomiasis control (Cai, 2013).

3.2 Policy support and measures

3.2.1 Continue to give policy guarantee and promoting

The management model of schistosomiasis control consisted of leadership of local party committees at different levels, which were led uniformly by the leading group of the Central Committee of CPC. The coordination work of party committees, at different levels, and the relevant government departments were all completed by the leading group of the Central Committee of CPC. They were also responsible for the formulation and implementation of schistosomiasis control planning. In addition, a network of the specialized institutions of epidemic areas were formed at three levels, namely provincial, municipal (city) and county (district). By the end of 1960s, the epidemic reporting network has been set up throughout the urban and rural areas of the whole country (Zhou, 2004). The expert advisory committee of schistosomiasis control has set up at a later stage, and its responsibilities included: technical guidance and supervision for the implementation and application of the technical scheme and new technologies, setting standards, evaluation of control efforts and summarizing work experiences.

3.2.2 Following the principles of combining schistosomiasis control with agricultural production, combining mass movement with science and technology and combining temporary work with regular work

The movement of mass prevention and control involved mobilizing all party members and citizens. During this period, the financial costs of schistosomiasis control were shouldered by the state, collectives and individuals. The early and advanced stage of schistosomiasis were both given priority and treated. And according to the patient's socioeconomic status, different charging strategies, namely full, discounted and at no cost, were applied. Meanwhile, snail control was given priority than water conservancy.

3.2.3 Following the comprehensive strategy on emphasis of snail elimination

Schistosomiasis elimination was the main goal at that time. Schistosomiasis control workers strictly observed the following principles: active control, comprehensive measures of prevention and control, and performing work as circumstances permit. The comprehensive control strategy which emphasizes on snails elimination was implemented, and combined with the basic construction of irrigation and water conservancy depending on local economic conditions (Dai, 2001). In addition, other measures, including the treatment of patients and infected livestock, transforming the ecological habitat of snails, personal protection, waste management and safe water provision, were also implemented. A 5-year plan of schistosomiasis scientific research from 1963 to 1967 was formulated in 1963 (Zhang and Cai, 2013), in which great importance was attached to the research on the snail as a vector, snail control methods and the treatment for advanced schistosomiasis.

3.3 Resources mobilization

3.3.1 Continue to integrate the professional schistosomiasis control institution

The national professional institutions and organizations of schistosomiasis control were improved and expanded (Fig. 2). By the mid-1980s, there was a total of more than 260 professional institutions in the province, municipal (city) and county (district), more than 1620 professional institutions in towns and subdistrict, more than 16,000 professionals, and about 10 part-time staff in each village (Zheng, 1988).

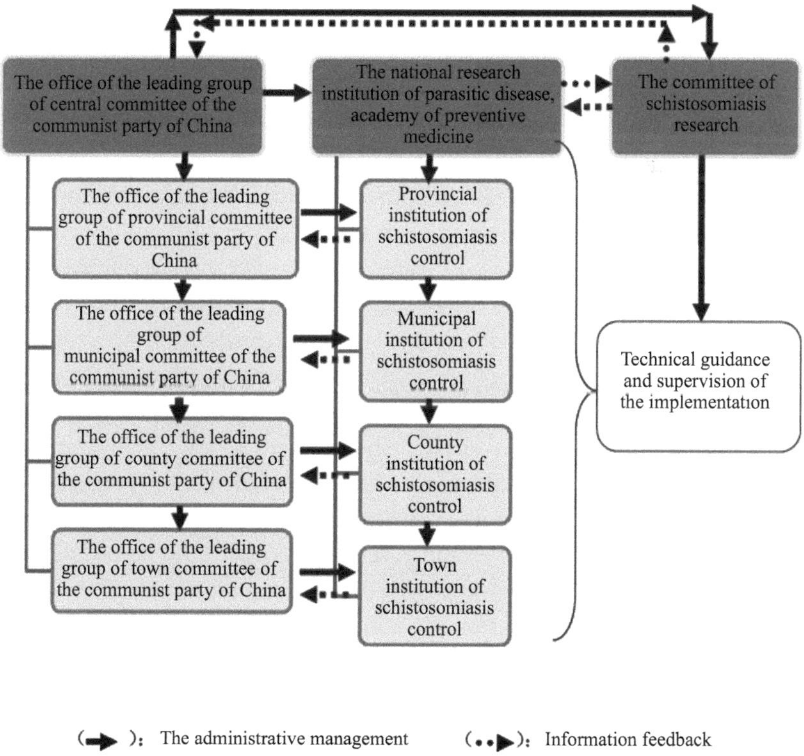

Figure 2 The work model of leadership and professional institution of schistosomiasis control at five levels in the early 1980s of The People's Republic of China.

3.3.2 Integration and development of zone defence force

Due to its regional distribution, a document numbering as No. 12 was issued by the Central Committee of CPC in 1970 indicated that 'adjacent area of the provincial, municipal (city), district (county) should carry forward the spirit of collaboration of communism through close cooperation, work together and strive to complete the task', as well as the same hydrographic net of adjacent areas (eg, around Dongting Lake), in 1970. Accordingly, after the collaboration plan of schistosomiasis elimination between Hunan and Hubei provinces was made by the two provinces and their adjacent areas with 11 county and 2 farms, a huge range of activities for disease control were carried out. From then on, it has a growing influence on schistosomiasis control in the whole country. Because of the concern, support and good organization from the party and government in The People's Republic of China, more collaborations between provinces and individuals were included in the work, resulting in the achievement of the goals for schistosomiasis control.

3.4 Effect of prevention and control

Through implementation of the strategy, which emphasized on snail control according to the target of schistosomiasis control, the progress of schistosomiasis control was hastened in The People's Republic of China. The measures included survey of snail population and mass snail control, survey of infection rate and provision of chemotherapy to infected patients and livestock, and transforming the ecological environment of snail combined with the infrastructure of irrigation and water conservancy in endemic areas.

By the end of 1984, 11 million patients with schistosomiasis were treated and 11 billion m^2 of snail-ridden areas were eliminated. The number of counties that has eliminated schistosomiasis increased. Within 370 endemic counties nationwide, 76 counties reached the standard of schistosomiasis elimination and 193 counties reached the standard of basic schistosomiasis elimination (during 1956–95, the goals for schistosomiasis prevention and control were divided into two level, namely, elimination and basic elimination. 'Elimination' and 'basic elimination' were equal to the later technical term of 'interruption' and 'transmission control', respectively). For example, hilly areas or water network areas of Guangdong Province, Shanghai, Fujian Province and Guangxi Province reached the standard of schistosomiasis elimination (Zhou et al., 2010). Finally, the national standard for elimination of schistosomiasis and basic elimination of schistosomiasis were promulgated and implemented, guiding future work of schistosomiasis control (Chen, 2005).

4. FROM THE LATE 1980S TO THE END OF THE 20TH CENTURY

4.1 Background

Due to reforms in the national and the increasing needs of the development of health work, the leading group of the Central Committee of CPC and organizations and institutions were cancelled by the Central Committee of CPC in 1986. Subsequently, the work of schistosomiasis control was handed over to the Ministry of Health, where the Bureau for Disease Control was established. The Bureau for Disease Control was renamed to be the Department of Endemic Disease Control in 1989, and the latter was further renamed to be the National Endemic Disease Control office in 1994. After being restructured in 1998, the disease control department guided the work of schistosomiasis control countrywide. Under the leadership of the Ministry of Health, the Schistosomiasis Expert Advisory Committee was established and consisted of experts from the national institutions of schistosomiasis control, medical colleges and different provinces. These experts provided consultation and assisted in decision making. Since the 1980s, the collective ownership economy gradually transformed to the household contract responsibility system in rural The People's Republic of China. Due to changes in the economy system and opening up of markets in The People's Republic of China, the epidemic prevention system was also subjected to modification. It was difficult to organize the mass movement of large-scale snail control, and to assemble the resources of disease control. The idea of 'send away the god of plague' became history (Chen, 2005) and schistosomiasis infections began to rise again in areas where measures of schistosomiasis control failed to be carried out. Meanwhile, it was discovered that the target of schistosomiasis elimination in the marshland and some hilly areas was difficult to achieve with only emphasis on snail control as there were other natural environment and economic factors influencing the progress. The government paid high attention to the schistosomiasis resurgence in The People's Republic of China. Comrade Deng Xiaoping commented: 'It is beneficial for the people to control endemic diseases.' in 1984. Comrade Jiang Zemin said in the letter to the Five Province's Schistosomiasis Control Conference in 1989, 'It is the duty of the governments at all levels of schistosomiasis endemic areas to carry out schistosomiasis control and elimination', which contributed to a new wave of efforts in sending away the god of plague through mobilization of the available resources in the early 1990s.

At the same time, schistosomiasis control strategy and target have been adjusted by the WHO Expert Committee in 1984. They pointed out that health education should be an important part in the disease control strategy as transmission of schistosomiasis was closely related to people's work and living style. The emphasis on preventive chemotherapy was also gradually introduced in The People's Republic of China, and pilot work on control was carried out in heavy endemic areas.

4.2 Policy support and measures

In the mid-1980s, WHO put forward and carried out the strategy of 'disease control' through the administration of praziquantel, which was a high efficient, cheap and safe drug (Dabo et al., 2013; Ojurongbe et al., 2014). The People's Republic of China also started to adjust the strategy of schistosomiasis control by adopting integrated control involving both chemotherapy administration to humans and livestock and snail control in susceptible areas (Zhou et a1., 2005; Utzinger et al., 2005; Guo and Zheng, 2000; Zheng and Guo, 2000).

4.2.1 Strengthening the leadership and adjusting strategy

In view of the severe epidemic situation at that time, the five provinces of marshland areas meeting was held in Nanchang City in December 1989, which called for 'sending away the god of plague by mobilization once more'. After 1989, the State Council strengthened the leadership of schistosomiasis control and various measures of schistosomiasis control were adopted. They included planning for prevention and control, increasing the investment, coordinating the power of different departments, adjusting the strategy, advocating the control strategy consisting of three steps (namely infection control, transmission control and interruption) and improving the management mechanism. The State Council issued the file on 'decision on strengthening schistosomiasis prevention and control' in 1990. Five provinces of marshland areas were defined as focus throughout the country in the file. Regular meeting were set up to solve the important problems during the progress of implementation. During the period of Chinese eighth five-year planning (1991—95), the Central Committee of CPC and the government of endemic areas at different levels invested funds of 1 billion yuan for schistosomiasis control (source: National Conference of Schistosomiasis Control in 1997).

4.2.2 Expert consultation, suggestions and decisions

The Expert Advisory Committee of Schistosomiasis of the Ministry of Health was founded in 1987. For decades, the expert consulting organization has provided lots of scientific suggestion and advice of schistosomiasis control for the government, including guidelines, policies, planning, control strategy and technical guidance.

4.2.3 Making planning, scientific revention and control

Since the 1980s, the health policy focus on science and technology was put forward in The People's Republic of China. Attention was given to schistosomiasis control during the national planning. The national schistosomiasis control planning from 1987 to 1990 emphasized the importance of scientific research. The Schistosomiasis Expert Advisory Committee of Ministry of Health played an important role in schistosomiasis control, by working on inventing new drugs for snail control with high efficiency, low toxicity and low price through scientific research (Cai and Zhang, 2012). The State Council issued "the national eighth five-year plan of comprehensive control of schistosomiasis" in 1991, in which schistosomiasis control was accepted into the overall planning of economic and social development at different levels of government. The national eighth five-year plan of scientific research of schistosomiasis control has strengthened the scientific research of schistosomiasis control. The national health education implementation planning was made since 1992, where health education was accepted into the overall plan of schistosomiasis control. The purpose of health education was to mobilize the whole society to support schistosomiasis control, and to change the behaviour of target groups who are in close contact with infected water. The State Council issued 'The national ninth five-year plan of comprehensive control of schistosomiasis' in 1997, where the important position and role of science and technology in schistosomiasis control was provided with more attention by the government after 1980s. The government no longer relied on mass movement and participation for schistosomiasis control, but developed the science and technology for it instead.

4.3 Resources Mobilization

4.3.1 The resources of World Bank Loan Project

In face of the severe endemic situation due to a rebound of schistosomiasis, and insufficient investment for schistosomiasis control, Chinese government decided to actively strive for the World Bank Loan Project (WBLP). Foreign capital and advanced technology and management were introduced to make up for the inadequacy of government investment and the lack of technical and management skills. The project was implemented from 1992 to 2001 (Collins et al., 2012). The endemic disease control department of the

Ministry of Health and foreign loan office were responsible for the implementation of the project. Within the 10-year period, the total investment for the project amounted to 1.088 billion yuan, including the World Bank loan of RMB 491 million yuan and the Chinese government of different levels matching fund of RMB 597 million yuan (Tables 1–4). The projects covered 219 counties of 8 provinces (Hubei, Hunan, Jiangxi, Anhui, Jiangsu, Zhejiang, Yunnan and Sichuan). The total goals of the project were to control the epidemic of schistosomiasis and to interrupt transmission of schistosomiasis in some areas in The People's Republic of China. All project activities were planned till the end of 1998, while three provinces Hunan, Hubei and Yunnan continued till 2001 due to further demands. The project had support from the State Development Planning

Table 1 Planned and actual input of WBLP for schistosomiasis control in The People's Republic of China (in 10,000 RMB)

	Loan	Matching fund	Loan/ matching	Total input	Present value of input in 2001
Planned input	41,590	47,390	1.14	88,980	125,462
Actual input	49,092	59,702	1.22	108,794	108,794
Difference between planned and actual input	−7502	−12,312	1.64	−19,814	16,668

The exchange rate of US$ to RMB was 1:5.8 in 1992 and 1:8.2 in 2001.

Table 2 Use of the WBLP for schistosomiasis control according to different components in The People's Republic of China (in 10,000 RMB)

	Loan		Matching fund		Total	
Item	**Fund**	**%**	**Fund**	**%**	**Fund**	**%**
Case screening	4113.86	3.78	8750.09	8.04	12,863.94	11.82
Chemotherapy	10,589.02	9.73	10,267.01	9.44	20,852.03	19.17
Snail survey and elimination	27,925.19	25.67	20,004.53	18.39	47,929.63	44.06
Health education	539.18	0.5	2923.03	2.69	3462.21	3.18
Training	541.62	0.5	1857.66	1.71	2399.29	2.21
Project management	2055.19	1.89	11,507.08	10.58	13,562.27	12.47
Disease surveillance	217.33	0.2	1251.49	1.15	1468.82	1.35
Operational research	1252.46	1.15	868.01	0.8	2120.47	1.95
Others	1858.2	1.71	2273.49	2.09	4135.78	3.8
Total	49,092.06	45.12	59,702.37	54.88	108,794.43	100

Table 3 Input of chemotherapy drugs and molluscicide from the WBLP for schistosomiasis control in The People's Republic of China

	Praziquantel for humans (tablet)		Praziquantel for animals (kg)		Niclosamide (kg)	
Year	**No. purchased**	**No. actually used**	**No. purchased**	**No. actually used**	**No. purchased**	**No. actually used**
1992	46,641,517	40,867,249	4195.44	3145.07	174,027.00	162,855.98
1993	65,491,334	39,449,465	5968.59	3209.96	506,421.20	349,094.87
1994	37,928,859	31,854,397	1998.67	3245.96	283,698.10	326,904.80
1995	23,802,962	22,137,618	3728.73	2128.72	310,666.10	326,029.80
1996	34,675,780	21,265,729	3001.02	2226.93	659,520.30	394,261.14
1997	39,986,723	20,522,793	2916.81	2104.52	537,744.20	487,691.30
1998	25,535,193	21,626,767	1805.09	2425.10	254,404.60	309,463.33
1999	11,300,888	14,750,499	988.37	1557.69	141,743.80	222,526.81
2000	10,010,955	14,282,098	926.57	1522.83	164,973.30	209,650.70
2001	8,817,210	11,045,398	880.97	1201.88	165,028.40	117,526.60
Total	304,191,421	237,802,013	26,410.26	22,768.65	3,198,227.00	2,906,005.34

Note: Only included in the Table of the data from 1999 to 2000 all those from Hunan, Hubei, Yunnan and Jiangxi provinces; 2001 all those from Hubei, Yunnan and Jiangxi provinces

Table 4 The input and payment for schistosomiasis control between 1997 and 2001 in The People's Republic of China (in 10,000 RMB)

	Government input			Payment for							
Year	Province	Prefecture and county	Total	Salary	Case finding and chemotherapy	Snail survey and elimination	Health education and training	Project management	Surveillance	Equipment	Others
1997	6052.77	13,415.60	19,468.37	10,599.09	1772.17	2747.44	742.92	1093.24	355.57	717.62	1353.11
1998	6385.90	15,462.46	21,848.36	11,799.19	2009.88	3421.88	840.02	1284.32	349.57	1055.80	1357.78
1999	6629.74	16,007.47	22,637.21	12,835.99	1719.25	2988.96	627.49	834.35	726.30	1168.93	1778.95
2000	6712.05	15,788.76	22,500.81	14,105.25	2435.25	3165.98	869.91	888.94	724.88	1000.61	1444.53
2001	8385.40	18,748.44	27,133.84	15,671.53	2304.55	4072.54	984.39	953.43	3779.07	1073.33	1595.39
Total	34,165.86	79,422.73	113,588.59	65,011.05	10,241.10	16,396.80	4064.73	5054.28	5935.39	5016.29	7529.76

World Bank Loan Program completion report on infectious and endemic disease control project schistosomiasis control component of The People's Republic of China (1992–2001). Department of Disease Control, Ministry of Health, The People's Republic of China. Foreign Loan Office, Ministry of Health, The People's Republic of China.

Commission and the Ministry of Finance, with multisectoral participation including health, agriculture, water conservancy and the state drug administration departments. During the project, there were 63,375,009 person-time with case screening, 18,925,688 person-time with chemotherapy, 1,688,428 cattle with case screening and 2,234,634 cattle with treatment. In addition, 9.64 billion m^2 of area was surveyed for snails, snail elimination with molluscicide was performed on 2.85 billion m^2, and snail elimination via environmental modification was conducted on 1.05 billion m^2. An estimated 7.47 million people benefited from the project (Chen, 2005).

4.3.2 Continuing to integrate the resources of regional defence

The regional defence agreement of five provinces of schistosomiasis control was made in 1985 including Jiangsu, Anhui, Jiangxi, Hunan and Hubei. It was decided that classified guidance of schistosomiasis control should be carried out in the five provinces of marshland, paying special attention to the integrated control strategy. It was also demanded that acute schistosomiasis control should be a main component in the control work for the five provinces. Control included snail survey and elimination, case screening, chemotherapy of human and animal at the same time, and strengthening control of migrant population, so as to promote the progress of schistosomiasis control.

4.3.3 The integration of regional resources of comprehensive control

The State Council issued 'a decision on strengthening schistosomiasis control' in 1990, where the schistosomiasis leading group of five provinces, namely Hunan, Hubei, Jiangxi, Anhui and Jiangsu, comprised of the vice-governor or the local leader of schistosomiasis leadership team. This group unified commands and coordination and played an important role in schistosomiasis control.

4.3.4 Strengthening personnel training and scientific research

A series of technical training activities were carried out during the WBLP, and a national network of health education was also preliminarily established. The management and professional technical personnel having both ability and political integrity were selected to go abroad to study, and related experts were organized to go abroad to inspect and conduct academic exchanges at the same time. This resulted in a large number of elite people being trained and the quality of technical personnel improved together with the strengthening the international communication and cooperation ability.

A series of applied scientific research work was also carried out during the project, including a total number of 245 research projects approved and funded by joint research management committee (JRMC). Finally, a total number of 278 papers were published, 25 research projects won awards at or above the provincial level, and 7 research projects won the national patent through 6 years JRMC activity. These fruitful research results obtained have played a positive role in promoting the progress of schistosomiasis control in The People's Republic of China. To accommodate the need for applied research and training at that time in The People's Republic of China, the junior college classes and professional courses on schistosomiasis control were held in Nanjing Medical College, Hubei Medical College and Shanghai University of Medicine.

4.4 Effect of prevention and control

The WBLP, which lasted for 10 years was an important part of the national 'eighth five-year plan and ninth five-year plan' in The People's Republic of China, which funded for schistosomiasis control and accumulated valuable

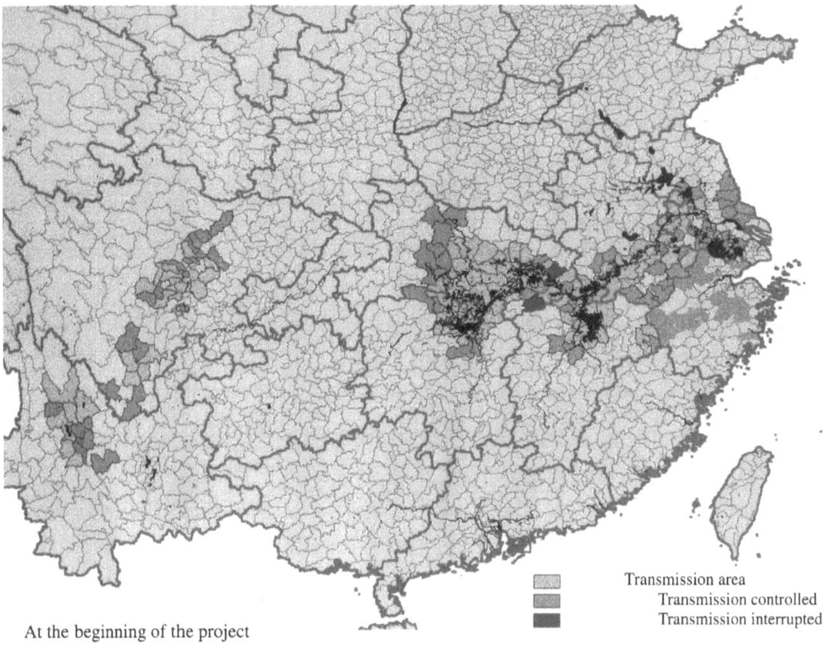

Figure 3 The distribution of the project counties and endemic situation of WBLP of schistosomiasis control in The People's Republic of China (at the beginning of the project).

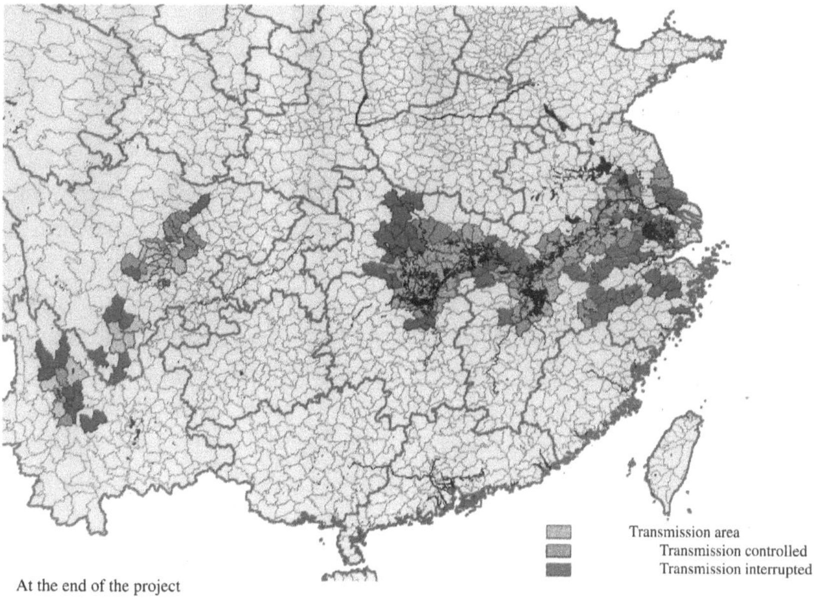

Figure 4 The distribution of the project counties and endemic situation of WBLP of schistosomiasis control in The People's Republic of China (at the end of the project). *WBLP completion report on infectious and endemic disease control project schistosomiasis control component of The People's Republic of China (1992–2001). Department of Disease Control, Ministry of Health, The People's Republic of China; Foreign Loan Office, Ministry of Health, The People's Republic of China.*

experience. The number of endemic areas of schistosomiasis decreased yearly (Figs 3 and 4) through the implementation of the project. From 1992 to 2001, 47 counties achieved transmission control and 82 counties achieved transmission interruption. The number of highly endemic areas of administrative villages fell by 37.1% and the moderately endemic areas fell by 29.0%, but the low endemic areas increased by 15.0%. The epidemic of schistosomiasis was effectively controlled through the implementation of the project. By the end of 2002, the national infection rate of human and livestock fell 55.0% and 50.0%, respectively, from before the project was implemented in 1992. The national density of infected snails in endemic areas decreased by 75%. In Zhejiang province, schistosomiasis transmission was interrupted in 1995 (Chen et a1., 2005) and thus, achieving one of the goals of the project.

Compared with the early years of The People's Republic of China, the infection rates in the province, county and town decreased by 59.0%, 74.2% and 72.0% respectively; total number of schistosomiasis patients decreased by 93.0% and patients with advanced schistosomiasis decreased by 95.7% in 2002. There were 913 cases of acute schistosomiasis in 2002. In contrast, there were about 10,000 cases of acute infection, and 1000 people dying from acute infection each year in the early foundation of The People's Republic of China. In addition, national cattle infection rate decreased by 85.5%, areas containing snail reduced by 75.4% in 2002. During this period, the National Regulations of Schistosomiasis Control passed the administrative approval by Ministry of Health after repeated modifications. The 'Criteria for control and elimination of schistosomiasis (GB15976-1995) in The People's Republic of China' was issued for the first time. The 'Chinese Journal of Schistosomiasis Control' was established and the 'Handbook of Schistosomiasis Control'' was modified. A lot of news on schistosomiasis control and the epidemic were reported by the central and local newspapers and radio stations, bringing them to the attention of the national and local leaders (Wang et a1., 1989).

5. SINCE THE 21ST CENTURY

5.1 Background

In the early 21st century, there was a significant rebound of schistosoma epidemics in the Yangtze River basin and some hilly areas due to biological, natural and social economic factors (Zhou et al., 2004; Wang et al., 2004).

1. The ecological environment of endemic regions had changed because of the implementation of measures for flood diversion after the flood in 1998. Measures included building of embankments and returning farmland to lake. However, this change of environment has led to the proliferation of *oncomelania* snail—infested areas (Yang et a1., 2005).
2. New epidemic characteristics and regularity of schistosomiasis thus emerged due to the changes of environment. For example, after the completion of the Three Gorges Dam, the extension of the flooding period caused the infectious season to be longer in areas with snails, such as Dongting Lake and Poyang Lake. Global climate change also increased schistosomiasis transmission intensity in some areas (Zhou et al., 2002, 2008; Wu et al., 2007).
3. The development of animal husbandry led to a more important role of the animal host in schistosomiasis transmission.
4. Chemical molluscicide (especially for aquatic animals) caused serious pollution in the environment, limiting the scope of application of molluscicide.

5. Compliance with long-term and repeated chemotherapy in humans and livestock dropped yearly. Infectious source increased since synchronous chemotherapy of human and livestock could not be carried out. Furthermore the only effective drug, praziquantel, had a potential risk of resistance (Wang and Liang, 2007) because of its wide-range use for a long time in the endemic areas.
6. The increase in social and economic developments brought along a rise in population mobility and livestock trading. Therefore, the frequency of contact with infected water, and reinfection of human and animal increased (Zuo et al., 2003).
7. Since 2000s, the society and the mass people have paid more attention to the market economy system; however, due to the change of people's ideology and behaviour, schistosomiasis control was ignored to some extent and some measures were hard to carried out at one time (Li et al., 2002; Cai et al., 2003; Yin et al., 2002).
8. After the WBLP on schistosomiasis control ended in 2001, there was a serious shortage of funding, causing schistosomiasis control in the country to be more passive.
9. The current technology and measures cannot satisfy the needs of the current schistosomiasis control programme, hence it was difficult to effectively control the disease.

Thus, at the beginning of the 21st century, there was a significant rebound of schistosomiasis epidemics in The People's Republic of China. As a result, the total number of patients countrywide remains at around 800,000 from 1998 to 2005, and 700,000 of them are from the five marshland provinces. Cattle infection rate was around 4–5%, with an increased spread of snails. The risk of infection with schistosome was rising, with new areas of infected snails estimated to be about 9 million m^2 each year in the marshland areas (Chen et al., 2011). The endemic status of schistosomiasis in The People's Republic of China showed that the task of schistosomiasis control was still urgent. The continuous rise in endemic status lasted for 3 years, increasing the risk of human and animal infected by schistosome (Chen et al., 2002, 2003; Xiao et al., 2004). In addition, it was difficult to reach the goal of transmission interruption through snail elimination in the marshland areas, such as Hunan, Hubei, Jiangxi, Anhui and Jiangsu Provinces, as well as the hilly areas, including Sichuan and Yunnan provinces, where the snails were widely distributed, and the ecological environment were complex. Therefore, during 2000s the emphasis on schistosomiasis control is in marshland and hilly endemic areas (Cao et al., 2003).

5.2 Policy support and measures

To curb the rebound trend of schistosomiasis endemic status, the Central Committee of the CPC paid important attention to effectively control schistosomiasis by quickly adopting a series of measures. The administrative institutions, including the State Council and the Ministry of Health, announced 141 files to guide the national schistosomiasis control from 2003 to 2007 (Fig. 5). The State Council leading group of schistosomiasis control was established in February 2004. And the notice of strengthening the control of schistosomiasis further was issued by the State Council in May 2004. The national conference of schistosomiasis control was held in Yueyang City one week after the notice was issued, in order to accelerate the process of schistosomiasis control. Since then, there were important adjustment and propulsion from the national planning and policies, legal management, financial investment and technical standards.

5.2.1 Establishing a new period national planning

The 'National Program of Schistosomiasis Control in Mid- and Long Term (2004–15)' was organized in July 2004. The goal and objectives of schistosomiasis control were clearly clarified in these national programs. The timeline for reaching goals and the national standards in the endemic areas in The

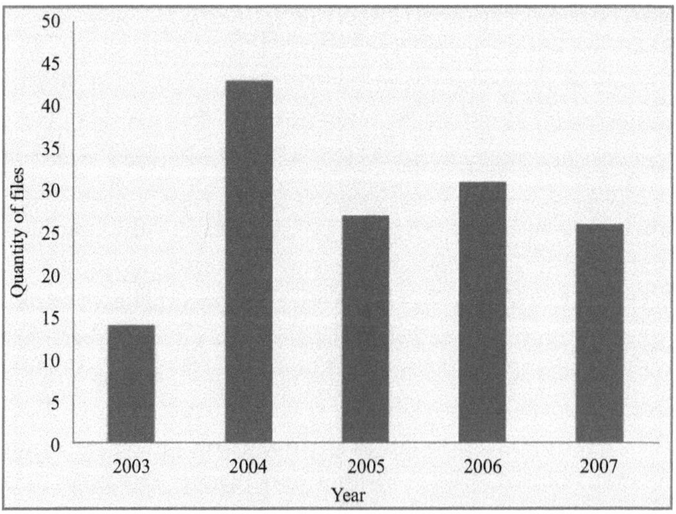

Figure 5 Documents issued by Chinese government (the State Council and the Ministry of Health) from 2003 to 2007. *The department of disease control of the Ministry of Health. 'Documents compilation of schistosomiasis and parasitic disease control (2003–07)'.*

People's Republic of China, including infection control, transmission control and interruption, was clearly stated. With the support of all departments, the central fiscal transfer payments programme was quickly implemented, thus achieving the expected results. At the same time, the management model of this project also became the best example for disease prevention and control in The People's Republic of China (Zhou et al., 2011) because of its specific goals, scientific strategies and specific measures, which took into account the vital interests of the people in endemic areas. The 'National Program of Schistosomiasis Comprehensive Control (2004–08)' was organized by multiministries and commissions in October 2004. The central government allocated special funds to carry out comprehensive control of schistosomiasis in heavy endemic areas, focussing on 163 key counties (city, district). The 'National Program of Schistosomiasis Comprehensive Control (2009–15)' was organized in 2010 and reaffirmed the overall goal of schistosomiasis control in The People's Republic of China. The 'National Program of Animal Disease Control for the Mid- and Long Term (2012–20)' was organized in 2012. In addition, suggestions for the twelfth five-year plan of the national economy and social development made by the Central Committee of the CPC were passed during the fifth plenary session of the 17th of the communist party. It was an important task to 'improve the system of public health and medical service' during the "twelfth five-year' period. According to the policy, a basic public health system, including schistosomiasis control, was to be provided in the future.

5.2.2 The application of comprehensive control strategy 'on the emphasis of infection source control'

With the rapid development of economy in the 21st century, the epidemic reduced gradually in endemic area. Based on results from epidemiological studies and a further understanding of the characteristics and regularity of schistosomiasis in The People's Republic of China, Chinese scholars paid more attention to the two transmission stages of schistosomiasis, namely the miracidium and snail. It was considered that the waste management of human and livestock was an effective way to control infection and reinfection of schistosome (Lin et al., 2009). The comprehensive control strategy 'on the emphasis of infection source control' was officially announced and implemented in 2006 (Chen et al., 2009; Wang, 2005; Wang et al., 2009a,b,c). The central government arranged special funds for water conservancy, agriculture, health and forestry for schistosomiasis control. The comprehensive control strategy 'on the emphasis of infection source control' was implemented in endemic areas, through the project resources and the increased investment from the local government. The notice of 'further strengthening the infectious source control of schistosomiasis' was issued to the relevant provinces and the ministries by the State Council general office via an urgent telegram in October 2007. Prohibition of countermeasures to control grazing in the areas of snail habitats was extended since 2008. It was indicated that the Central Committee and the State Council were equally concerned with fighting the 'god of plague', flood prevention and disaster relief and people in the endemic areas were inspired to fight schistosomiasis. In addition, the research institute of parasitic disease of Chinese academy of preventive medicine was renamed to the National Institute of Parasitic Disease, Chinese Center for Disease Control and Prevention, in 2002. The national and provincial institutes of parasitic disease made up a scientific research base, which provided guidance for the scientific research of disease control. Three levels of institute (station) of schistosomiasis control, namely municipal (city), county (district) and countryside (town) were still playing a role to organize the implementation of measures. This led to an effective implementation of the measures of the comprehensive control strategy.

5.2.3 Further improving the legal management of schistosomiasis control

The law on the prevention and control of infectious diseases was formally implemented on 1 December 2004, in which schistosomiasis was promoted from 'c' to 'b' class of infectious diseases (Zhou, 2004). The regulations on schistosomiasis control were issued by the State Council in 2006. It was demanded that the comprehensive control measures must be implemented. From then on, the legalization of schistosomiasis control allowed the programme to have organization and management, forming a new work mechanism where the government-led ministries and departments cooperated, experts and technical personnel supported and the masses participated (Zhou et al., 2010).

5.2.4 Increasing National Finance investment

After the outbreak of severe acute respiratory syndrome (SARS) in 2003 (Wang, 2004), the Chinese government paid great importance to the public health and disease prevention and control. The National Finance increased finance investment on schistosomiasis control, making it part of the central financial transfer payment project. The total number of special funds allocated for endemic areas was over 11.2 billion yuan from the central government since 2004 (data source: Deputy Prime Minister Liu Yandong, speech on the National Conference of Schistosomiasis Control in 2014).

5.2.5 Making standards and technical specification

The 'Technical guidance for water conservancy combined with schistosomiasis prevention' was issued by the Ministry of Water Conservancy in 2005. And the 'Criteria for control and elimination of schistosomiasis (GB15976-2006) in The People's Republic of China' was issued in 2006, which replaced the 'Criteria for control and elimination of schistosomiasis (GB15976-1995) in The People's Republic of China'. In the same year, 'National specifications on schistosomiasis prevention and control' was issued, which made the implementation of schistosomiasis control more scientific and standardized.

5.3 Resources mobilization

5.3.1 Comprehensive control

With the present economic and social developments, the construction of new socialist rural areas has become an important work. The local governments invested lots of money for it, including agricultural mechanization, safe drinking water, the use of biogas and construction of nonhazardous sanitary latrines. These funds were made up of health project funds from the central transfer payments, construction funds such as agriculture, water conservancy, forestry and land (Yang et al., 2016), as well as matching funds from central project supporting funds from the local governments and routine funds of the schistosomiasis control project. This did not only guarantee a smooth development in all the endemic provinces, municipalities (cities), counties (districts), but also improved the efficiency of schistosomiasis control under the construction of a new socialist countryside. In endemic areas of schistosomiasis, the safe drinking water problem of 6 million people were solved, 1.62 million nonhazardous sanitary latrines were built, 490,000 biogas were built, 430,000 cattle were killed, 760 thousands sets of new agricultural machinery were introduced to replaced cattle, 1183 km of the river channel revetment were constructed, 0.17 billion m^2 of paddy fields were changed to dry land, 1272 km of river and lake beach were forbidden from grazing by fence, 20 billion m^2 of prevention forest were built since 2011. The government of Hubei Province invested 240 million yuan to implement cattle elimination, 200,000 head of cattle were killed for 4 consecutive years from 2011 to 2014. Thus, the infectious source of livestock was controlled efficiently by lots of measures, such as promoting the whole county with comprehensive control, establishing agricultural cooperatives and carrying out the 'no oxen county' campaign (data source: Deputy Prime Minister Liu Yandong, speech on the National Conference of Schistosomiasis Control in 2014). Local governments at all levels worked according to the demands of 'building a harmonious society, constructing new countryside' and implemented comprehensive control measures, with emphasis on infectious source – timely suggested by the Ministry of Health. The process of schistosomiasis control were effectively promoted in The People's Republic of China due to the priority of the resources and strategies, methods and technology, and efforts to ensure achievement of anticipated goal (Lin et al., 2007; Yi et al., 2009a,b; Wang et al., 2009a,b,c). For example, the State Council approved the implementation of the national rural drinking water safety project and solved the drinking water safety problem for 353 million rural residents and more than 24 million students and teachers from 2005 to 2012. In addition, The People's Republic of China has also allocated 18.5 billion yuan to the construction of prevention and control system for animal disease and a comprehensive schistosomiasis control (Li, 2013). The pilot counties for schistosomiasis-integrated control were set up by the State Council leading group in different endemic areas for the first time, including Jinxian County in Jiangxi Province, AnXiang County in Hunan Province, Hanchuan County in Hubei Province, Guichi County in Anhui Province and Puge County in Sichuan Province. They were the representatives of schistosomiasis-integrated control through implementation of all proposed measures (Yu et al., 2006). Subsequently, provinces also carried out the pilot work in heavy endemic counties with effective results (Zhang et al., 2009; Zhu et al., 2009; Yang et al., 2009; Yi et al., 2009a,b).

5.3.2 Multisectoral cooperation

The planning has been implemented after 2005. The comprehensive and scientific prevention and control were strengthened under the unified leadership of the central government, and the close cooperation of ministries of agriculture, forestry, water conservancy, health and others, as well as the guarantee of organization, funding, laws and regulations, technology, institutions and personnel. According to different ecological environment and epidemic characteristics in endemic areas, distinct goals for prevention and control were made and thus a varied package of control measures was carried out to control schistosomiasis. Measures included eliminating and replacing cattle with machine, adjusting agricultural industry structure, eliminating snails by aquaculture, forestry, improving irrigation system, river regulation, eliminating the source of infection by improvement of water supplier and construction of sanitary latrines, building the biogas, synchronous chemotherapy for human and livestock, case screening and treatment, health education (Liu et al., 2014; Cao et al., 2016; Yang et al., 2016) and others.

5.3.3 Provinces and ministries union

The work mechanism among the Ministry of Health, the Ministry of Agriculture, and provinces in heavy endemic areas was established in order to promote the process of schistosomiasis control in The People's Republic of China. The government of Hubei Province launched the new work mechanism of schistosomiasis control with the Ministry of Health and the Ministry of Agriculture in 2008. The strategy of prevention and control with emphasis on infectious source were strongly performed in 33 key counties. This strategy integrated the resources from the department of agriculture, water conservancy, land, health, forestry, transportation, including the leading group of government, departments union, action of the central and local, and thus allowed power and resources to be concentrated. Due to 'the implementation of comprehensive control in the whole county' in heavy endemic areas, the infection rate was reduced further and the achievements were consolidated in Hubei Province. The unified actions for schistosomiasis control between the government of Hunan Province and the Ministry of Health were carried out in 2010. According to the principle of 'overall planning, comprehensive control, showing emphasis', the control measures, focussing on management of infection sources, were carried out in 14 counties (districts) in heavy endemic areas of the Dongting Lake and along the Yangtze River. It was also combined with new rural construction in order to eliminate the cause of schistosomiasis.

5.3.4 Clearing responsibility

To strengthen the leadership of schistosomiasis control, lots of governments at different levels included the programme into their overall planning for local economy and social development and the management target of government, such as signing the 'target responsibility' and 'responsibility contract'. Various forms of responsibility system, including clearing responsibility, task and objectives and the regular evaluation system were set up. It was also important to evaluate the performance of the cadres. Related research work of schistosomiasis control has been carried out in-depth by the relevant ministries and commissions of the State Council and the governments at all levels in The People's Republic of China.

5.4 Effect of prevention and control

The above-mentioned strategy and measures further controlled the schistosoma epidemics in The People's Republic of China, and infection rate hit a record low in history (Figs 6–10). By the end of 2008, five provinces, namely, Jiangsu, Anhui, Jiangxi, Hubei and Hunan in marshland endemic areas and Yunnan Province in hilly endemic areas achieved the standard of infection control. Sichuan and Yunnan provinces achieved the standard of transmission control in 2008 and 2009, respectively. This meant the medium-term objectives of the national long-term planning of schistosomiasis

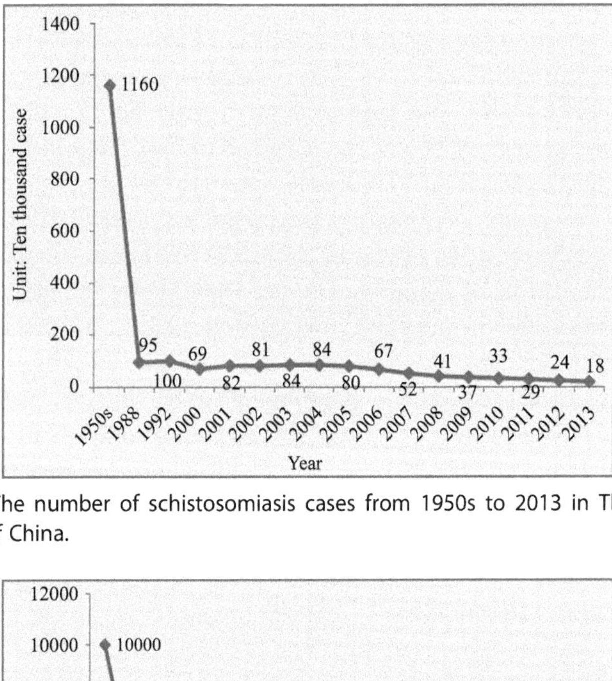

Figure 6 The number of schistosomiasis cases from 1950s to 2013 in The People's Republic of China.

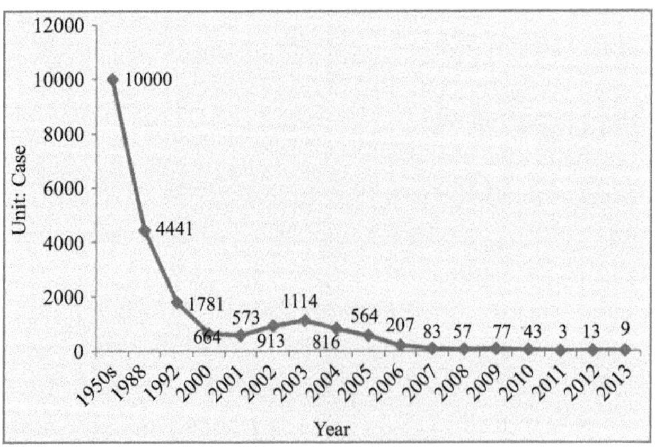

Figure 7 The number of acute schistosomiasis cases from 1950s to 2013 in The People's Republic of China.

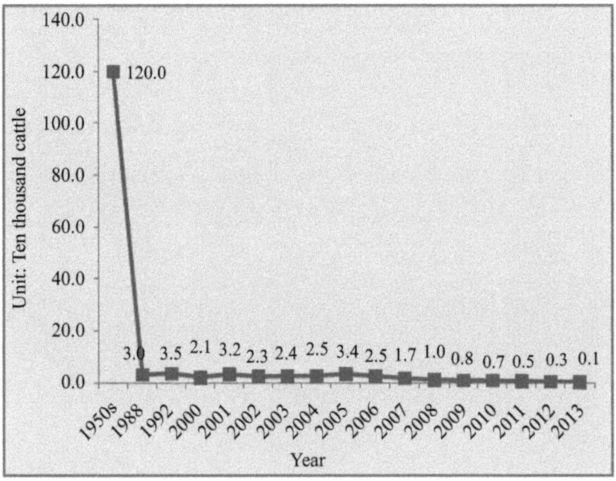

Figure 8 The number of infectious cattle with *Schistosoma japonicum* from 1950s to 2013 in The People's Republic of China.

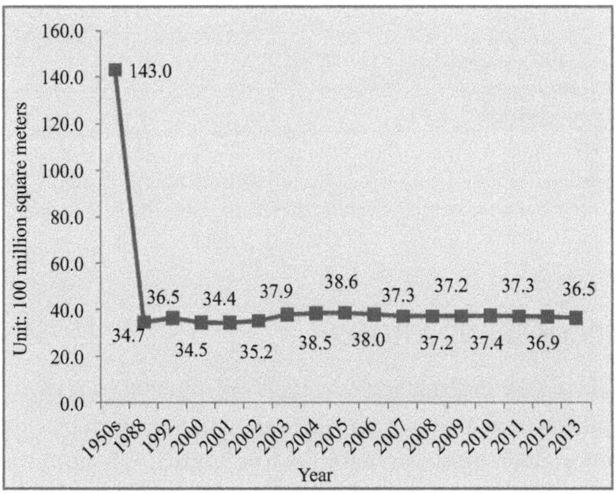

Figure 9 The snail areas from 1950s to 2013 in The People's Republic of China.

control were achieved (Hao et al., 2009; The Ministry of Health et al., 2008; Hao et al., 2010; Li et al., 2009). Jiangsu and Hubei provinces achieved the standard of transmission control in 2010 and 2013, respectively, causing the final objectives of national long-term planning of schistosomiasis control to be achieved. Besides, the infection rate in three provinces Anhui, Jiangxi and Hunan reduced yearly. All of them will achieve the final objectives of national long-term planning of schistosomiasis control as scheduled by the end of 2015.

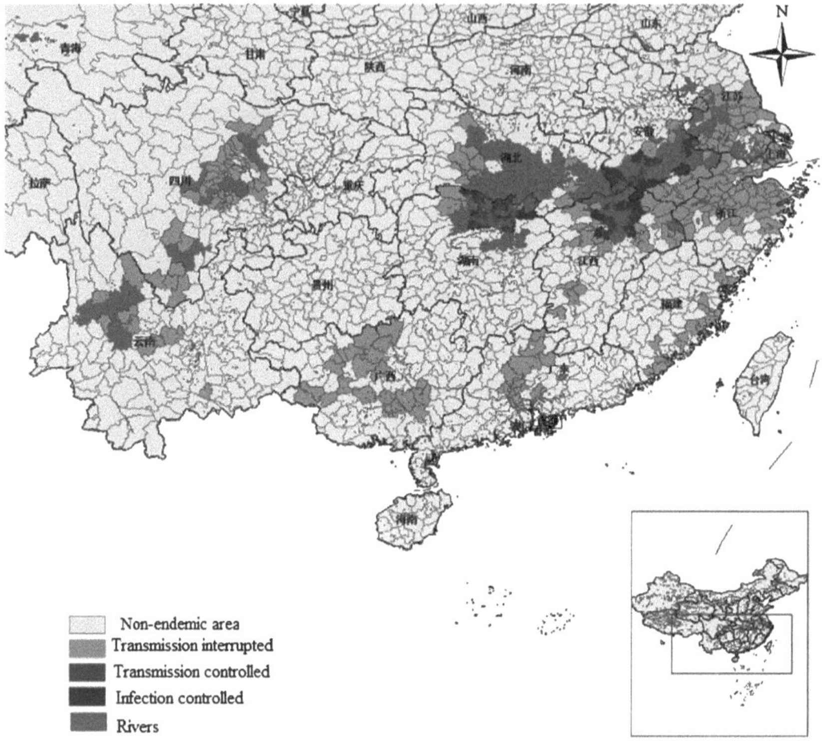

Figure 10 The distribution of endemic status of schistosomiasis in 2013 in The People's Republic of China. *Endemic status of schistosomiasis in The People's Republic of China in 2013.*

6. RECOMMENDATIONS

Reviewing the brilliant achievements of schistosomiasis control in since mid-1950s, the experiences, which were suited to the development of society and economy at different stages, have been accumulated from the prevention work in The People's Republic of China (Fig. 11). In The People's Republic of China, the major experience of policy evolution of schistosomiasis control was that, we had depended mainly on the mass movement from the 1950s, on the progress of scientific and technological in the 1980s, and then attached great importance to the ecological comprehensive control since the 21st century. Therefore, it gives us the inspirations as follows.

6.1 Government leading

Schistosomiasis control was always an important topic in the field of public health in The People's Republic of China. Moreover, it is valid only due to

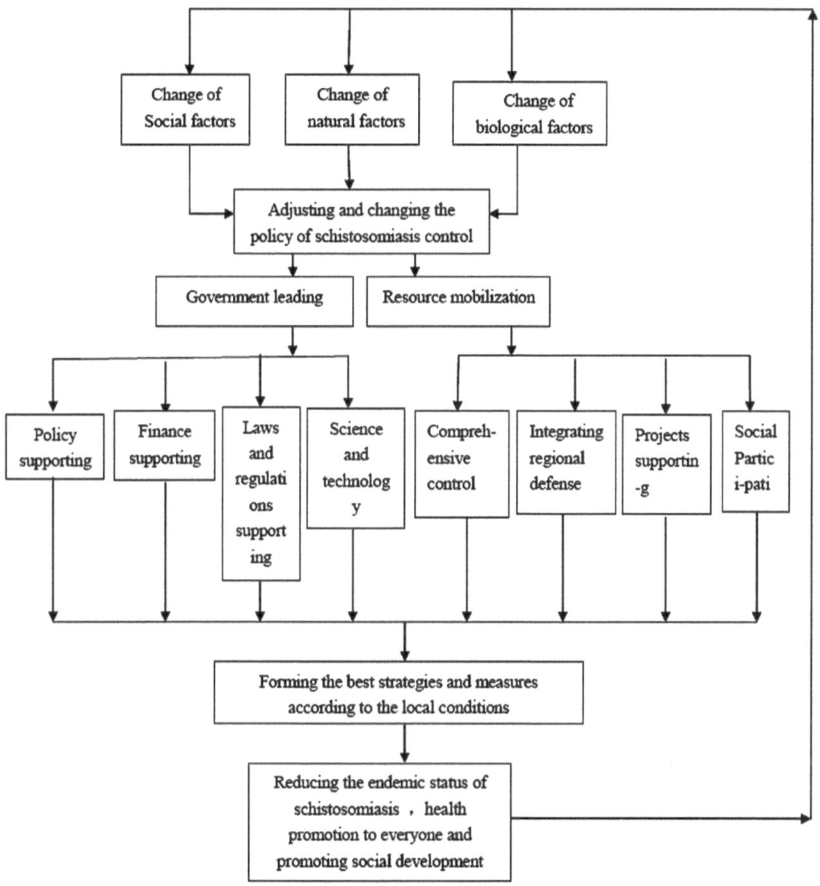

Figure 11 Model pattern of policy support and resources mobilization for the National Schistosomiasis Control Programme in The People's Republic of China.

the unified leadership and policy support from the government, whether it is in the early years where the country has a relatively backward social economy, or in 2010s with the rapid development of social economy (Table 5). There were three rebound epidemics of schistosomiasis in The People's Republic of China: the first one was influenced by the cultural revolution during the 1960s, the second was influenced by the reform of market economy system during the 1980s and the third was affected by the multiple factors of the natural environment and social economy around the 20th century. The CPC and the government paid great importance to schistosomiasis control. The policy system of schistosomiasis control was formed by strengthening the leadership according to the measures of issuing a series of policy

Table 5 The schedule of National Conference of Schistosomiasis Control organized by the Central Committee of the CPC and the government in The People's Republic of China, from 1950s to 2014

Time	Name of conference	Place (Provinces/ Municipalities)	Organizer
November 1955	The First National Conference on Schistosomiasis Control	Shanghai	The Central Committee of the CPC
March 1956	The Second National Conference on Schistosomiasis Control	Shanghai	The Central Committee of the CPC
December 1956	The Third National Conference on Schistosomiasis Control	Shanghai	The Central Committee of the CPC
December 1989	The Conference on Schistosomiasis Control from Five Provinces in Marshland Areas	Jiangxi Province	The State Council
November 1990	The National Conference on Schistosomiasis Control	Hubei Province	The State Council
1991	The National Conference on Schistosomiasis Control	Hunan Province	The State Council
December 1992	The National Conference on Schistosomiasis Control	Anhui Province	The State Council
November 1993	The National Conference on Schistosomiasis Control	Jiangsu Province	The State Council
November 1994	The National Conference on Schistosomiasis Control	Beijing	The State Council
December 1995	The Conference on Schistosomiasis Controlfrom the Ministry of Agriculture	Yunnan Province	The Ministry of Agriculture
November 1997	The National Conference on Schistosomiasis Control	Beijing	The State Council
March 1999	The National Conference on Schistosomiasis Control	Beijing	The State Council

June 2000	The Conference on Schistosomiasis Control from the Ministry of Agriculture	Guangxi Province	The Ministry of Agriculture
May 2002	The Conference on Schistosomiasis Control from the Ministry of Agriculture	Jiangxi Province	The Ministry of Agriculture
August 2003	The Conference on Zone Defence of Schistosomiasis Control from Five Provinces in Marshland Areas	Jiangsu Province	The Ministry of Health
May 2004	The National Conference on Schistosomiasis Control	Hunan Province	The State Council
May 2006	The National Conference on Schistosomiasis Control	Jiangxi Province	The State Council
December 2009	The Conference on Schistosomiasis Control from the Ministry of Agriculture	Anhui Province	The Ministry of Agriculture
September 2010	The National Conference on Schistosomiasis Control	Hubei Province	The State Council
November 2011	The Conference on Schistosomiasis Control from the Ministry of Agriculture	Yunnan Province	The Ministry of Agriculture
December 2012	The Conference on Schistosomiasis Control from the Ministry of Agriculture	Hunan Province	The Ministry of Agriculture
May 2013	The Conference on Schistosomiasis Control from the State Forestry Bureau	Anhui Province	The State Forestry Bureau
November 2014	The National Conference on Schistosomiasis Control	Hunan Province	The State Council

document on schistosomiasis control from central to local government, and making central planning and local specific measures. Therefore, the mode of schistosomiasis control depended on the leadership of the government, who indicated the direction of the development and laid the foundation in future. In addition, disease control and prevention was upgraded to the national polity level, where promoting disease control and prevention by political authority formed the solid foundation of schistosomiasis elimination.

6.2 National planning

A series of planning has been made from the central government to the local governments in The People's Republic of China, effectively promoted by the implementation process of schistosomiasis control, by setting phased objectives and the final target in the long term. Measures were adjusted according to local conditions and epidemic situation, and from strategies to specific measures all were integrated to allow a comprehensive control programme to be rolled out. Experiences from The People's Republic of China showed that the prevalence of schistosomiasis could be controlled effectively with well-planned and executed national control programmes and a certain amount of investment (Zhou et al., 2009).

6.3 Comprehensive control

Schistosomiasis is a public health concern and its control involves the departments of agriculture, forestry, water conservancy, forestry and environment. Thus the control programme depends on the cooperation of different departments, and is difficult to be implemented by the department of health alone. Remarkable achievements of schistosomiasis control were achieved in The People's Republic of China, because it has always paid important attention to combine coordination with development between different departments, integrate resources from the whole society, conform to the trend of social development, closely combine with the economic construction and implement comprehensive control measures according to the local condition.

6.4 Science and technology leading

Strategies for schistosomiasis control has been continually improved in The People's Republic of China with the development of society and economy, the progress of science and technology, and the adjustment of strategies from WHO. All the corrections were made using scientific research as the guide. Practice shows that the promotion of science and technology was the key in speeding up the progress of schistosomiasis control. Difficulties and bottlenecks from schistosomiasis control were defeated relying on the progress of science and technology (Chen et al., 2016). The level of disease prevention and control are improved relying on the guidance of science and technology. Concurrently, it is important to assemble a professional high-quality team who can carry out the scientific prevention and control measures.

6.5 Social participation

In the early years of The People's Republic of China, the whole society was mobilized to join in the infectious diseases control, including the fundamental interests of the masses, social politics and economic development. The basis of schistosomiasis control relied closely on the masses during the 1950s. Remarkable results were achieved by organizing the masses movement at that time even though the science and technology were underdeveloped. Hence, people were the main force of the elimination of schistosomiasis then. Nowadays, schistosomiasis control still need the organizations and institutions of disease prevention and control with the leadership of the party committees at all levels. We still need the understanding and support of the whole society to carry out extensive social mobilization and participation (Salam et al., 2014). And we hope to create a healthy environment by sending 'the god of plague' away together.

7. CHALLENGES

Across the 65 years of history in schistosomiasis control in The People's Republic of China, precious and rich experiences in terms of policy support and resource mobilization were accumulated, providing a powerful guarantee to promote the process of national prevention and control. But two main problems need to be emphasized on the macrocontrol of policy in future, as follows: Firstly, it was not given enough attention to the schistosomiasis control, which is complex in nature, its economic benefits were always ignored. Therefore, there was a lack in assessment on strategy, especially on comparative assessment on economic benefit analysis of strategy and the rational allocation of resources. Secondly, the investment of schistosomiasis control was under a budgeting system responsible by the state. When the proposed measures did not work, nobody but the state had to bear the economic losses. It also means that there is no competition for investment of schistosomiasis control, so there is no push for an effective use of national resources (Zhou et al., 2010).

8. THE WAY FORWARD

The national conference on schistosomiasis control was held by the State Council in November 2014. Premier Li Keqiang, the Standing Committee of the Political Bureau of the CPC Central Committee made important instructions for the meeting: '... sweeping "the god of plague" into history, and bringing the clean, peace and health to all people.' Vice Premier Liu Yandong, the Committee of the Political Bureau of the CPC Central Committee stressed that the control planning of the next 10 years must be made as soon as possible at the meeting. We must strive to improve the professional technology in order to win the battle of schistosomiasis control in the next 10 years, and strive to realize schistosomiasis elimination. With the social and economic developments, the level of people's life and culture has gradually improved. The government invests more financial and material resources to schistosomiasis control, therefore people will be able to choose a healthy life, far away from schistosomiasis (Jiang et al., 2010). We believe that we will achieve the goal of schistosomiasis elimination as early as possible, and the long-cherished wish of sending 'the god of plague' will be finally realized through the leadership of the party and government, and the joint efforts from the whole society in the near future (Zheng et al., 2013).

The time of cooperation for the development of improved global public health is approaching (Xu et al., 2016a,b). The global elimination of schistosomiasis in 2025 was passed on the World Health Assembly in 2012. The United Nations summit put forward 'sustainable development goals after 2015' on 'Rio + 20' in 2014, including the global elimination of schistosomiasis. Currently, one-third of global population is threatened by schistosomiasis in The People's Republic of China. In order to achieve global sustainable development, it is important to control schistosomiasis well in The People's Republic of China. As a responsible and big country, we should response positively to the international initiative, by speeding up the pace of schistosomiasis elimination (Tambo et al., 2014). This will in turn benefit both the people of The People's Republic of China and the international community.

REFERENCES

Cai, J., 2013. Science and Technology Planning and Effectiveness of Schistosomiasis Since the Reform and Opening of Our Country. Master's thesis,7,52 (in Chinese).
Cai, J., Zhang, X.L., 2012. The role of theory of modern science and technology in schistosomiasis control. In: The Joint Conference Papers of National Science Theory and Subject Construction, and Science and Technology in 2012 (in Chinese).

Cai, K.P., Chen, Y., Hu, Y.H., Huang, S.Y., 2003. The epidemics changes of schistosomiasis in resettlement areas against hills in Dongting Lake region. Pract. Prev. Med. 10, 457–459 (in Chinese).
Cao, Z.G., Zhao, Y.E., Willingham, A.L., Wang, T.P., 2016. Towards the elimination of schistosomiasis japonica through control of the disease in domestic animals in the People's Republic of China: a tale of over 60 years. Adv. Parasitol. 92.
Cao, L., Hu, G.H., Guo, J.G., 2003. The influence of new drugs and new technology development to the strategy of schistosomiasis control in China. Chin. J. Parasit. Dis. Con. 16, 380–382 (in Chinese).
Chen, M.G., 2014. Assessment of morbidity due to *Schistosoma japonicum* infection in China. Infect. Dis. Poverty 3, 6.
Chen, M.G., Feng, Z., 1999. Schistosomiasis control in China. Parasitol. Int. 48, 11–19.
Chen, S.B., Ai, L., Hu, W., Xu, J., Bergquist, R., Qin, Z.Q., et al., 2016. New anti-schistosome approaches in the People's Republic of China: development of diagnostics, vaccines and other new techniques belonging to the 'omics' group. Adv. Parasitol. 92.
Chen, H.G., Xie, S.Y., Zeng, X.J., Huang, X.B., Wang, T.P., Li, Y.S., Liang, Y.S., Zhou, X.N., 2011. Current endemic situation and control strategy of schistosomiasis in lake and marshland regions in China. Chin. J. Schisto. Control 23, 5–9 (in Chinese).
Chen, H.G., Zeng, X.J., Xiong, J.J., Jiang, W.S., Hong, X.L., Hu, S.Z., Guo, J.G., 2009. Study on comprehensive schistosomiasis control strategy with emphasis on infectious source control in Poyang Lake areas. Chin. J. Schisto. Control 21, 243–249 (in Chinese).
Chen, X.Y., 2005. Changing control strategies and management system for schistosomiasis in China. Dr. Theses 1, 115 (in Chinese).
Chen, X.Y., Jiang, Q.W., Wang, L.Y., Zhao, G.M., Zhao, Q., Gu, G.A., Wei, J.G., Hao, Y., 2002. Schistosomiasis situation in the People's Republic of China in 2001. Chin. J. Schisto. Control 14, 241–243 (in Chinese).
Chen, X.Y., Wang, L.Y., Cai, J.M., Zhou, X.N., Zhen, J., Guo, J.G., Wu, X.H., Engels, D., Chen, M.G., 2005. Schistosomiasis control in China: the impact of a 10-year world bank loan Project (1992–2001). Bull. World Health Organization 83, 43–48.
Chen, X.Y., Wu, X., Wang, L.Y., Dang, H., Wang, Q., Zhen, J., Guo, J.G., Jiang, Q.W., Zhao, G.M., Zhou, X.N., 2003. Schistosomiasis situation in the People's Republic of China in 2002. Chin. J. Schisto. Control 15, 241–244 (in Chinese).
Collins, C., Xu, J., Tang, S., 2012. Schistosomiasis control and the health system in P. R. China. Infect. Dis. Poverty 1, 8.
Dabo, A., Bary, B., Kouriba, B., Sankare, O., Doumbo, O., 2013. Factors associated with coverage of praziquantel for schistosomiasis control in the community-direct intervention (CDI) approach in Mali (West Africa). Infect. Dis. Poverty 2, 11.
Dai, G.Q., 2001. Analysis of the control strategy of schistosomiasis. Chin. J. Dis. Control Prev. 5, 97–98 (in Chinese).
Guo, J.G., Zheng, J., 2000. Schistosomiasis endemic and control in China. Chin. J. Dis. Control Prev. 4, 289–293 (in Chinese).
Hao, Y., Zhen, H., Zhu, R., Guo, J.G., Wang, L.Y., Chen, Z., Zhou, X.N., 2010. Schistosomiasis situation in the People's Republic of China in 2009. Chin. J. Schisto. Control 22, 521–527 (in Chinese).
Hao, Y., Zhen, H., Zhu, R., Guo, J.G., Wu, X.H., Wang, L.Y., Chen, Z., Zhou, X.N., 2009. Schistosomiasis situation in the People's Republic of China in 2008. Chin. J. Schisto. Control 21, 451–456 (in Chinese).
Jiang, M.S., Zhen, R., Zhao, Q.P., Dong, H.F., Guo, Y., 2010. Social epidemiological thinking about schistosomiasis. Chin. J. Schisto. Control 22, 201–205 (in Chinese).
Lei, Z.L., Zhou, X.L., 2015. Eradication of schistosomiasis: a new target and a new task for the National schistosomiasis control porgramme in the People's Republic of China. Chin. J. Schisto. Control 27, 1–4 (in Chinese).

Li, Z.J., Ge, J., Dai, J.R., Wen, L.Y., Lin, D.D., Madsen, H., et al., 2016. Biology and control of snail intermediate host of *Schistosoma japonicum* in the People's Republic of China. Adv. Parasitol. 92.

Li, B., 2013. Report on the implementation of the infectious diseases control and the law of the prevention and control of infectious diseases of the State Council. Cap. J. Public Health 7, 193–195 (in Chinese).

Li, K.L., Yang, G.H., Duan, S.S., Xia, G.H., 2002. Re-emergence of schistosomiasis in Dali city after the criteria of transmission control were met. Chin. J. Parasitol. Parasit. Dis. 20, 235–237 (in Chinese).

Li, S.Z., Luz, A., Wang, X.H., Xu, L.L., Wang, Q., Qian, Y.J., Wu, X.H., Guo, J.G., Xia, G., Wang, L.Y., Zhou, X.N., 2009. Schistosomiasis in China: acute infections during 2005–2008. Chin. Med. J. (Engl.) 122, 1009–1014.

Li, Z.Q., Shen, M.Y., 2006. The importance and practical significance of the law on the prevention and control of infectious diseases. J. China Inst. Ind. Relat. 20, 88–90 (in Chinese).

Lin, D.D., Wu, X.H., Jiang, Q.W., Lin, J.J., Zhou, X.N., 2009. Strategic emphasis for research development of schistosomiasis control in China. Chin. J. Schisto. Control 21, 1–5 (in Chinese).

Lin, D.D., Wu, H.W., Wu, G.L., Zhou, X.N., 2007. Review and evaluation on optimal combined strategies for schistosomiasis control in China. Chin. J. Schisto. Control 19, 234–236 (in Chinese).

Liu, L., Yang, G.J., Zhu, H.R., Yang, K., Ai, L., 2014. Knowledge of, attitudes towards, and practice relating to schistosomiasis in two subtypes of a mountainous region of the People's Republic of China. Infect. Dis. Poverty 3, 16.

Liu, Y., Zhou, Y.B., Li, R.Z., Wan, J.J., Yang, Y., Qiu, D.C., et al., 2016. Epidemiological features and control effectiveness of schistosomiasis in mountainous and hilly region of the People's Republic of China. Adv. Parasitol. 92.

Mao, S.B., 1990. Schistosoma Biology and Schistosomiasis Control. People's Medical Publishing House, pp. 699–700 (in Chinese).

Mazigo, H.D., Nuwaha, F., Wilson, S., Kinung'hi, S.M., Morona, D., Waihenya, R., et al., 2013. Epidemiology and interactions of human immunodeficiency virus – 1 and *Schistosoma mansoni* in sub-Saharan Africa. Infect. Dis. Poverty 2, 2.

Ministry of Health, National Development and Reform Commission, Ministry of Finance, The Ministry of Agriculture, Ministry of Water Resources, Forestry Bureau, 2008. The national mid-long term planning for schistosomiasis control (2004–2015). The department of disease control of Health Ministry. Lit. Compil. Schisto. Parasit. Dis. Control 48, 53.

Ojurongbe, O., Sina-Agbaje, O.R., Busari, A., Okorie, P.N., Ojurongbe, T.A., Akindele, A.A., 2014. Efficacy of praziquantel in the treatment of *Schistosoma haematobium* infection among school-age children in rural communities of Abeokuta, Nigeria. Infect. Dis. Poverty 3, 30.

Salam, R.A., Maredia, H., Das, J.K., Lassi, Z.S., Bhutta, Z.A., 2014. Community-based interventions for the prevention and control of helmintic neglected tropical diseases. Infect. Dis. Poverty 3, 23.

Shi, L., Li, W., Wu, F., Zhang, J.F., Yang, K., Zhou, X.N., 2016. Epidemiological features and control progress of schistosomiasis in waterway-network region in P. R. China. Adv. Parasitol. 92.

Shi, L.Y., 2011. The leadership and the importance of schistosomiasis control attached by the Central Committee of the Communist Party of China in the early of New China. Lit. Party Hist. Acad. Ed. 4, 4–24 (in Chinese).

Tambo, E., Ai, L., Zhou, X., Chen, J.H., Hu, W., Bergquist, R., et al., 2014. Surveillance-response systems: the key to elimination of tropical diseases. Infect. Dis. Poverty 3, 17.

Tang, L.H., 2012. Parasitic Disease Control and Research in China (I). Beijing Science and Technology Press, pp. 3–26 (in Chinese).
Utzinger, J., Zhou, X.N., Chen, M.G., Bergquist, R., 2005. Conquering schistosomiasis in China: the long march. Acta Trop. 96, 69–96.
Wang, L.D., Chen, H.G., Guo, J.G., Zeng, X.J., Hong, X.L., Xiong, J.J., Wu, X.H., Wang, X.H., Wang, L.Y., Xia, G., Hao, Y., Chin, D.P., Zhou, X.N., 2009a. A strategy to control transmission of *Schistosoma japonicum* in China. N. Engl. J. Med. 360, 121–128.
Wang, X.Y., Zou, H., Yang, Y.B., Wang, X.H., Huang, X.P., Wang, J.C., 2009b. Retrospect and prospect of schistosomiasis control strategy in China – celebrating the achievement of schistosomiasis control on the 60th anniversary since the founding of new China. Jiangxi Sci. 27, 871–876 (in Chinese).
Wang, G.Z., 2011. Enlightenment on the integration of organization resources of schistosomiasis control by the Central Committee of the Communist Party of China in the 1950 s. Res. Teach. Party Hist. 3, 89–96 (in Chinese).
Wang, H.Z., Jia, Y.D., Guo, J.P., Xia, C., 1989. Retrospect of schistosomiasis control for 40th years in China. Chin. J. Health Serv. Manage. 6, 344–346 (in Chinese).
Wang, L.D., 2004. Problems and countermeasures of major infectious disease control in China. Natl. Med. J. China 84, 1944–1947 (in Chinese).
Wang, L.D., 2005. The management of feces for human and animal is the key to schistosomiasis control in china. Chin. J. Epidemiol. 26, 929–930 (in Chinese).
Wang, L.D., Zhou, X.N., Chen, H.G., Guo, J.G., Zeng, X.J., Hong, X.L., Xiong, J.J., Wu, X.H., Wang, L.Y., Xia, G., Hao, Y., 2009c. A new strategy to control transmission of *Schistosoma japonicum*. Eng. Sci. 11, 37–43 (in Chinese).
Wang, R.B., Wang, T.P., Wang, L.Y., Guo, J.G., Yu, Q., Xu, J., Gao, F.H., Yin, Z.C., Zhou, X.N., 2004. Study on the re-emerging of schistosomiasis epidemics in areas already under control and interruption. Chin. J. Epidemiol. 25, 564–567 (in Chinese).
Wang, W., Liang, Y.S., 2007. Progress on research of resistance of schistosome to praziquantel. Int. J. Med. Parasit. Dis. 34, 291–296 (in Chinese).
Wu, X.H., Xu, X.J., Xiao, B.Z., Wang, R.B., Dai, Y.H., Xu, J., Wu, C.G., Wei, F.H., Zhou, X.N., Zheng, J., 2007. Study on the risk factors of schistosomiasis transmission in the Three Gorges Reservoir AreasIIInfluence of the socioeconomic development on schistosomiasis transmission. Chin. J. Schisto. Control 19, 183–187 (in Chinese).
Xiao, D.L., Yu, Q., Dang, H., Guo, J.G., Zhou, X.N., Wang, L.Y., 2004. Schistosomiasis situation in the People's Republic of China in 2003. Chin. J. Schisto. Control 16, 401–404 (in Chinese).
Xu, J., Bergquist, R., Qian, Y.J., Wang, Q., Yu, Q., Peeling, R., et al., 2016a. China-Africa and China-Asia collaboration on schistosomiasis control: a SWOT analysis. Adv. Parasitol. 92.
Xu, J., Steinman, P., Maybe, D., Zhou, X.N., Lv, S., Li, S.Z., et al., 2016b. Evolution of the national schistosomiasis control programmes in the People's Republic of China. Adv. Parasitol. 92.
Yang, Y., Zhou, Y.B., Song, X.X., Li, S.Z., Zhong, B., Wang, T.P., et al., 2016. Integrated control strategy of schistosomiasis in the People's Republic of China: projects involving agriculture, water-conservancy, forestry, sanitation and environmental modification. Adv. Parasitol. 92.
Yang, G.J., Vounatsou, P., Zhou, X.N., Utzinger, J., Tanner, M., 2005. A review of geographic information system and remote sensing with applications to the epidemiology and control of schistosomiasis in China. Acta Trop. 96, 117–129.
Yang, K., Li, H.J., Yang, W.C., Shi, X.W., Qi, Y.L., 2009. Effect of comprehensive schistosomiasis control measures with emphasis on infectious source control in dam areas of mountainous region, Yunnan Province. Chin. J. Schisto. Control 21, 272–275 (in Chinese).

Yao, Y.H., Xu, G.J., 2005. The promulgation and implementation of the Law of the prevention and control of infectious diseases and the development trend of preventive medicine. Mod. Prev. Med. 32, 756–757 (in Chinese).
Yi, D.H., Yi, P., Liu, Y.C., Li, Y.S., Quan, M.Z., Xiao, S.Y., 2009a. Practice and thought of schistosomiasis control with an emphasis on control sources of infection in Dongting Lake area. Chin. J. Schisto. Control 21, 161–164 (in Chinese).
Yi, H.W.L., Zhou, Y.B., Liu, G.M., Wu, Z.S., Wang, S.A., Xu, L., Liu, H.B., Jiang, Q.W., 2009b. Effect of four-year comprehensive schistosomiasis control in Puge county, Sichuan province. Chin. J. Schisto. Control 21, 276–279 (in Chinese).
Yin, Z.C., Gu, X.G., Qiu, D.C., Qian, X.H., Wu, Z.S., 2002. Schistosomiasis situation in Sichuan province – report of sampling survey in 2001. J. Pract. Parasit. Dis. 10, 97–103 (in Chinese).
Yu, Q., Zhao, G.M., Guo, J.G., 2006. Evolvement of comprehensive strategy on schistosomiasis control in various control phases in China. J. Pathog. Biol. 1, 470–473 (in Chinese).
Zhang, S.Q., Sun, C.S., Wang, M., Lin, D.D., Zhou, X.N., Wang, T.P., 2016. Epidemiological features and control effectiveness of schistosomiasis in lake and marshland region in the People's Republic of China. Adv. Parasitol. 92.
Zhang, S.Q., Pan, X.P., Wang, T.P., Li, Y.Q., Tian, X.G., Ke, Z.M., He, J.C., 2009. Preliminary effect of comprehensive measures with emphasis on infections source control for schistosomiasis control in islet endemic regions. Chin. J. Schisto. Control 21, 259–261 (in Chinese).
Zhang, X.L., 2014. Theory of the development for Mao zedong and schistosomiasis control in new China. Lit. Party Hist. Acad. Ed. 4, 33–36 (in Chinese).
Zhang, X.L., Cai, J., 2013. The evolution and action of science policy for schistosomiasis control and in China. Soft Sci. Health 27, 765–767 (in Chinese).
Zheng, Q., Vanderslott, S., Jiang, B., Xu, L.L., Liu, C.S., Huo, L.L., et al., 2013. Research gaps for three main tropical diseases in the People's Republic of China. Infect. Dis. Poverty 2, 15.
Zheng, G., 1988. History of preventive medicine in new China (Volume 3 Disease control and prevention). People's Med. Publ. House 239, 284 (in Chinese).
Zheng, J., Guo, J.G., 2000. The status of animal hosts in schistosomiasis transmission of China. Chin. J. Zoonoses 16, 87–88 (in Chinese).
Zhou, X.N., Yang, G.J., Sun, L.P., Hong, Q.B., Yang, K., Wang, R.B., Hua, Z.H., 2002. Potential impact on the spread of schistosomiasis from global warming. Chin. J. Epidemiol. 23 (83), 86 (in Chinese).
Zhou, X.N., Guo, J.G., Yang, K., Wang, X.H., Hong, Q.B., Sun, L.P., Malone, J., Kristensen, T., Bergquist, N., Utzinger, J., 2008. Potential impact of climate change on schistosomiasis transmission in China. Am. J. Trop. Med. Hyg. 78, 188–194.
Zhou, X.N., Jia, T.W., Guo, J.G., Wang, L.Y., Jiang, Q.W., 2010. Project management model and its evolution in schistosomiasis control programme of China. Chin. J. Schisto. Control 22, 1–4 (in Chinese).
Zhou, X.N., Lin, D.D., Wang, T.P., Chen, H.G., Guo, J.G., Liang, Y.S., Qiu, D.C., Dong, X.Q., Li, S.Z., 2011. Control strategy of schistosomiasis and key points in the 12th five-year plan in China. Chin. J. Schisto. Control 23, 1–4 (in Chinese).
Zhou, X.N., Wang, L.Y., Chen, M.G., Wu, X.H., Jiang, Q.W., Chen, X.Y., Zhen, J., Utzinger, J., 2005. The public health significance and control of schistosomiasis in China-then and now. Acta Trop. 96, 97–105.
Zhou, X.N., Wang, T.P., Lin, D.D., Wu, X.H., 2009. Current strategy and its effect on control of schistosomiasis transmission in China. Int. J. Med. Parasit. Dis. 36, 266–273 (in Chinese).

Zhou, X.N., Wang, T.P., Wang, L.Y., Guo, J.G., Yu, Q., Xu, J., Wang, R.B., Chen, Z., Jia, T.W., 2004. The current status of schistosomiasis epidemics in China. Chin. J. Epidemiol. 25, 555–558 (in Chinese).
Zhou, X.Z., 2004. Studying and implementing the Law on the prevention and control of infectious diseases and in accordance with the law to carry out infectious diseases control. Chin. J. Nurs. 39, 949–951 (in Chinese).
Zhu, H., Cai, S.X., Huang, X.B., Tu, Z.W., Cao, M.M., Dai, L.F., Gao, H., Chen, Y.Y., Li, G., Xiao, Y., Zhou, X.R., 2009. Preliminary effect of comprehensive measures with emphasis on infectious source control for schistosomiasis control in Hubei Province. Chin. J. Schisto. Control 21, 267–271 (in Chinese).
Zuo, X., Wei, X.Y., Ding, F.X., Li, C.D., Yuan, Q.M., Kong, D.H., Shen, W.R., Zhou, J.W., 2003. Epidemiology investigation on livestock epidemic of schistosomiasis. Chin J. Vet. Med. 39, 21–22 (in Chinese).

CHAPTER THIRTEEN

New Anti-*Schistosoma* Approaches in The People's Republic of China: Development of Diagnostics, Vaccines and Other New Techniques Belonging to the 'Omics' Group

S.-B. Chen[*,§,¶], **L. Ai**[*,§,¶], **W. Hu**[*,§,¶,||], **J. Xu**[*,§,¶], **R. Bergquist**[#], **Z.-Q. Qin**[*,§,¶,1], **J.-H. Chen**[*,§,¶,1]

*National Institute of Parasitic Diseases, Chinese Center for Disease Control and Prevention, Shanghai, The People's Republic of China

§Key Laboratory of Parasite and Vector Biology of the Chinese Ministry of Health, Shanghai, The People's Republic of China

¶WHO Collaborating Center for Tropical Diseases, Shanghai, The People's Republic of China

||Fudan University, Shanghai, The People's Republic of China

#Geospatial Health, University of Naples Federico II, Naples, Italy

1Corresponding authors: E-mail: junhuchen@hotmail.com; qinzq1008@hotmail.com

Contents

Advances in Parasitology, Volume 92
ISSN 0065-308X
http://dx.doi.org/10.1016/bs.apar.2016.02.007

Abstract

A new national schistosomiasis elimination programme will be implemented for the period 2016–20. To support this approach, we have performed a systematic review to assess anti-schistosome approaches in The People's Republic of China and defined research priorities for the coming years. A systematic search was conducted for articles published from January 2000 to March 2015 in international journals. Totally 410 references were published in English between 2000 and 2015 related to schistosomiasis after unrelated references and reviews or comments were further excluded. A set of research priorities has been identified for the near future that would improve the progress toward schistosomiasis elimination in The People's Republic of China. In particular, there is a lack of sensitive and specific tests for the detection of schistosomiasis cases with low parasite burdens, as well as an effective vaccine against schistosomiasis, and there is a need for surveillance tools that can evaluate the epidemic status for guiding the elimination strategy. Hence, we think that schistosomiasis control and elimination will be improved in The People's Republic of China through development of new tools.

1. INTRODUCTION

The recent publication of the genome of *Schistosoma haematobium* represents a useful addition to the previously released genomes and transcriptomes of *Schistosoma mansoni* and *Schistosoma japonicum* (Berriman et al., 2009; Hu et al., 2003; Neafsey et al., 2012; Protasio et al., 2012; Consortium, S.j.G.S.a.F.A., 2009; Verjovski-Almeida et al., 2003). The unravelling of the genomes of the three schistosome species that case the great majority of human infection has provided research opportunities on many aspects of schistosome biology. This genomic information is an extremely valuable resource for global postgenomic research activities, such as DNA microarray profiling, proteomics, immunomics, metabolomics and glycomics that make up the core of the 'omics' group of disciplines (Hokke et al., 2007; Lier et al., 2009). Although this approach to the study of schistosome biology is still in its initial stage, there are important technological advances, not only for new diagnostics, and vaccines, but also for our understanding of disease mechanisms, host–parasite interactions and transmission biology based on the genomic resources of the different schistosome species (Brindley et al., 2009; Lustigman et al., 2012).

Screening of potential vaccine and diagnostic antigens and development of new anti-schistosome tools by high-throughput proteogenomic approaches remain a research priority (Chen et al., 2014; Gaze et al., 2014). Firstly, in spite of the existence of the safe and highly effective drug praziquantel (PZQ) for schistosomiasis treatment, disease transmission cannot be control by chemotherapy alone, eg, mass treatment does not prevent reinfection, and the potential risk of parasite resistance is a potential threat when mass drug administration is repeated for the long term (Tambo et al., 2015). Therefore, vaccination strategies represent an important supplementary component alongside chemotherapy for sustainable control of schistosomiasis (Hotez et al., 2010; McManus and Loukas, 2008). Secondly, most of the currently available diagnostic antibody-detection techniques, based on whole-schistosome crude extracts, as have low specificity and poor reproducibility (Zhang et al., 2015). Thus, improved direct, diagnostic tests with high specificity and sensitivity, are required to determine transmission interruption and elimination of schistosomiasis following control efforts (You and McManus, 2015; Zheng et al., 2013). Thirdly, the availability of functional genomic tools for investigating the schistosome biology, eg, RNA interference (RNAi) (Lustigman et al., 2012) is still limited. Control of schistosomiasis in The People's Republic of China requires more than chemotherapy alone and preferably new approaches based on omics, such as new vaccines and other new techniques in the future (Chen et al., 2012). The aim of this the review is to identify new tools under development and inform about which anti-schistosome tools are already now available.

2. MATERIAL AND METHODS

2.1 Search strategies and selection criteria

A systematic search was conducted for articles published from January 2000 to March 2015 in international journals in the Medline database through PubMed, the database of the National Library of Medicine in the United States. We used the following search criteria, ie, (schistosomiasis japonica or *S. japonicum* [Title/Abstract]) AND The People's Republic of China AND English [Language] AND ('2000/01/01' [Date − Create]: '2015/03/31' [Date − Create]) (Fig. 1). The references were exported from PubMed into Endnote X1 (Thompson Reuters, San Francisco, USA), duplicates were removed and the file was transferred to Excel 2007 (Microsoft Corp, Seattle, USA).

Each article was assigned to at least one of the following subjects based on the keywords included in the reference: omics (genomics, RNAomics, proteomics, transcriptomics, metabolomics, immunomics, glycomics), vaccines, new techniques (molecular diagnosis, immunodiagnosis, genotyping, crystal structure, RNAi). We excluded the following articles: review, education, software, comment, book, health promotion and commercial-related topics.

2.2 Statistical analysis

Data were processed using Excel (Microsoft, WA, USA) filters. Excel was also used to compute index analysis for references published in PubMed.

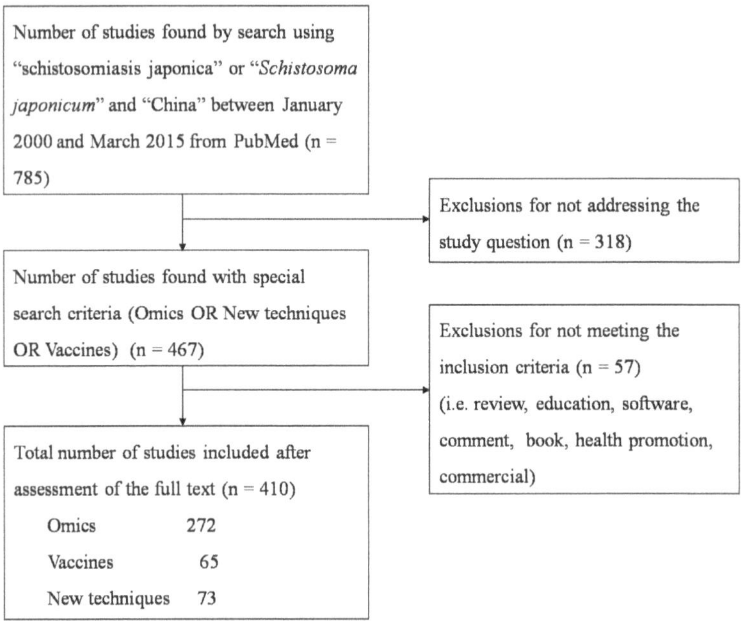

Figure 1 ***Flowchart visualizing the procedure for identifying relevant articles.*** Articles about 'schistosomiasis japonica' or *Schistosoma japonicum* from January 2000 to March 2015 in international journals from PubMed (n = 785). Articles did not address the study question were excluded from the search results (n = 318); review, education, software, comment, book, health promotion, commercial were also excluded (n = 57). Remaining articles were categorized according to subject, including omics (n = 272), vaccines (n = 65), new techniques (n = 73).

3. CURRENT RESEARCH STATE

3.1 General information

An exponential increase of references published in PubMed ($R^2 = 0.730$) was observed for the period January 2000 to March 2015 (Fig. 2).

Fourteen journals published 10 or more articles each on *S. japonicum* research in The People's Republic of China during January 2000 and March 2015 (Table 1). *Parasitology Research* and *Acta Tropica* are the top two journals for publication of *S. japonicum* research in The People's Republic of China. In addition, relevant works from Chinese researchers were also published in *New England Journal of Medicine* (Wang et al., 2009), *Lancet* (Wang et al., 2008), *Lancet Infectious Diseases* (Wang et al., 2008), *Nature* (Consortium, S.j.G.S.a.F.A., 2009), *Nature Genetics* (Hu et al., 2003).

Fifteen academic and research organizations in The People's Republic of China published 10 or more articles on *S. japonicum* research searched from PubMed from January 2000 to March 2015 (Table 2). National Institute of Parasitic Diseases, Chinese Center for Disease Control and Prevention (The People's Republic of China CDC) is the topest research institution for publication of *S. japonicum* research in The People's Republic of China.

3.2 Omics

In total, 272 references were found for —omics of *S. japonicum* in The People's Republic of China from PubMed with English language after unrelated references and reviews or comments were excluded from the search results.

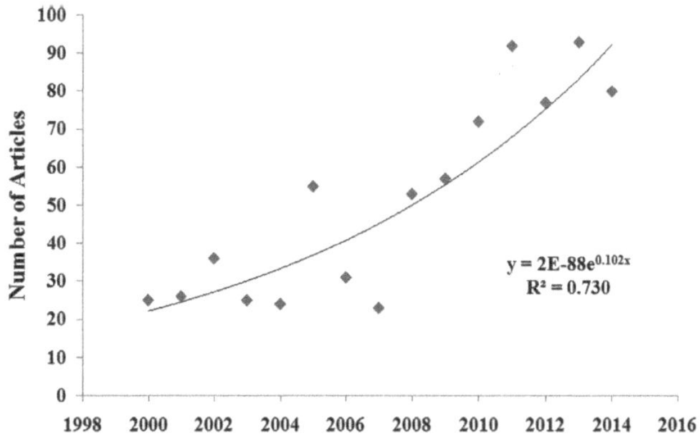

Figure 2 Distribution of references for *Schistosoma japonicum* research in The People's Republic of China in PubMed.

Table 1 Journals having published 10 or more articles on *Schistosoma japonicum* research in The People's Republic of China (PubMed search)

Journal	Articles
Parasitology Research	106
Acta Tropica	70
Parasites and Vectors	39
PLoS One	39
PLoS Neglected Tropical Diseases	36
Parasitology International	26
Experimental Parasitology	25
American Journal of Tropical Medicine and Hygiene	23
International Journal of Parasitology	23
Parasitology	23
Southeast Asian Journal of Tropical Medicine and Public Health	21
Annals of Tropical Medicine and Parasitology	14
Vaccine	14
Transactions of the Royal Society of Tropical Medicine and Hygiene	10

Table 2 Fifteen institutes in The People's Republic of China published 10 or more articles on *Schistosoma japonicum* research

Institution	Articles
National Institute of Parasitic Disease, China CDC	80
Jiangsu Institute of Parasitic Disease	53
Huazhong University of Science and Technology	48
Nanjing Medical University	47
Shanghai Veterinary Research Institute, CAAS	47
Fudan University	29
Central South University	28
Wuhan University	23
Sun Yat-sen University	22
Anhui Medical University	19
Hunan Institute of Parasitic Diseases	14
Tongji University	14
Soochow University	13
Chinese Academy of Medical Sciences & Peking Union Medical College	13
Guangzhou Medical University	10

CAAS, Chinese Academy of Agricultural Sciences.

The remaining references were categorized according to subject, including genomics (18.38%), RNAomics (4.78%), transcriptomics (8.09%), proteomics (39.34%), immunomics (26.47%), metabolomics (2.57%) and glycomics (0.37%) (Fig. 3). Systems biology and functional genomics aim to integrate 'omic' information for a better understanding of cellular biology.

3.2.1 Genomics

The genome of *S. japonicum* was deciphered and published in 2009 under the efforts from Chinese researchers (Consortium, S.j.G.S.a.F.A., 2009). The genome of *S. japonicum* (397 Mb) has eight chromosomes, including seven pairs of autosomal chromosomes and one pair of ZW type sexual chromosomes and encompass 13,469 protein-coding genes.

3.2.2 RNAomics

Unlike messenger RNAs (mRNAs), small noncoding RNAs (sncRNAs) represent a group of nontranslatable transcripts which are approximately 18–30 nucleotides in length and serve as critical regulators to silence or activate specific target genes in fungi, plants and metazoans (Bartel, 2009; Brennecke et al., 2007; Molnar et al., 2010). Three main components of sncRNAs, small interfering RNAs (siRNAs), microRNAs (miRNAs) and Piwi-interacting RNAs (piRNAs) have been well established and extensively studied (Kim, 2005). Using protocols similar to conventional transcriptomic research, which can be outlined as RNA isolation, library construction and sequencing (Cheng and Jin, 2012), vast numbers of schistosomal siRNAs and miRNAs have been successfully detected in

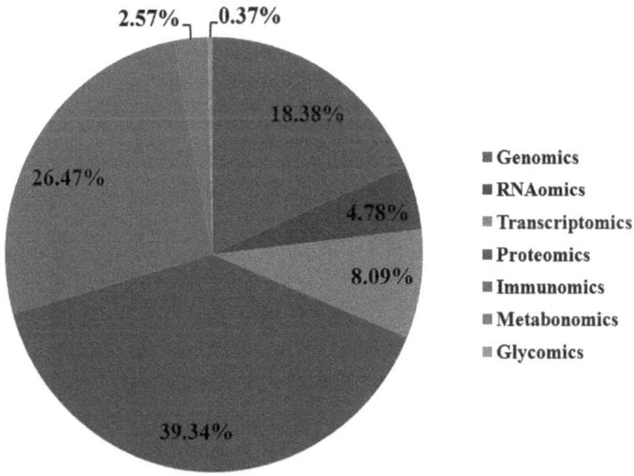

Figure 3 Percentage distribution of references for omics on *Schistosoma japonicum* in The People's Republic of China.

S. japonicum by Chinese researchers (Dai et al., 2014; Hao et al., 2010; Wu et al., 2014; Xue et al., 2008).

3.2.3 Proteomics

Gene expression is the creation of a product (most often a protein) based on the transfer of information from a gene. This process involves several steps and relationship between the transcriptional and the translational level is not always straightforward. Proteomic analysis plays an important role as it aiming at the characterization and comparison of functions, abundance and subcellular localization of numerous gene products derived from single or multiple samples (Chuan et al., 2010). Taking a schistosomal specimen as example, it would first be separated by one-dimensional gel electrophoresis (1DGE) or 2DGE, subsequently subjecting isolated bands or spots to digestion followed by matrix-assisted laser desorption/ionization time-of-flight mass spectrometry (MALDI-TOF MS) (Wang et al., 2013) or liquid chromatography—tandem mass spectrometry (LC-MS/MS) (Cao et al., 2015) depending on the method of separation chosen. This process would eventually provide information on the specimen's protein identities through by database searches (van Hellemond et al., 2007). Heretofore, schistosomal proteomics has been applied to the investigation and comparison of protein compositions in various developmental stages and between the two genders (Cheng et al., 2005; Liu et al., 2009, 2014)

3.2.4 Transcripomics

The continuing release of updated and new helminth, genome sequences has catalysed the emergence of transcriptomic analyses, which are providing unprecedented approach to understanding biological function that should eventually result in novel control interventions. *Schistosoma japonicum* transcripomics research commenced from the establishment of complementary DNA (cDNA) expression libraries, which has generated expressed sequence tags (ESTs) from nearly all stages of *S. japonicum* (Peng et al., 2003). After the numerous ESTs data have been obtained, microarray and serial analysis of gene expression technology have been applied to profile schistosome transcripts of from different stages and/or under distinct conditions. These applications can be classified into four main categories: (1) characterization of individual cell/tissue types; (2) profilation of intact organisms and life cycles (Chai et al., 2006); (3) study of parasite—host interactions and effect of chemotherapy (You et al., 2009) and (4) study of gene expression differences between geographical isolates or species.

3.2.5 Metabolomics

Metabolomics is the study of metabolites that appear in response to outside influences, eg, infections. Thus, each infection produces specific, cellular processes that reveal themselves as unique chemical fingerprints that can be used for profiling. For example, such a strategy was used to investigate the metabolic responses of Syrian hamsters (SLAC) experimentally infected with *S. japonicum* using various spectroscopic methods, eg, high resolution ^1H nuclear magnetic resonance spectroscopy, MS and capillary electrophoresis, coupled with various data-mining technologies. Several metabolites related to schistosome infection have been profiled, eg, in urine samples from hamsters infected with *S. japonicum* (Wang et al., 2006), as well as in blood and multiple tissue samples from rodents coinfected with *S. japonicum* and *Necator americanus*) (Wu et al., 2010).

3.2.6 Immunomics

Immunomics is a study that combines proteomics with serology and aims at ascertaining the interaction between host immune system and exotic antigens after pathogen invasion. Early schistosomal immunomics utilized combined 2D Western blotting and MS to identify and compare proteins recognized in serum samples from patients exposed for *S. japonicum* cercariae before and after PZQ treatment or testing the situation at different ages and infection intensities. Utilizing immunomics together with a protein microarray has also been applied in an attempt to seek prospective vaccine targets (Driguez et al., 2010). This advanced technology consists of several steps including gene selection, cell-free expression, chip printing and serological probing (Chen et al., 2010, 2014, 2015; Fan et al., 2013). An immunomics approach to schistosome antigen discovery was used in seeking antibody signatures in naturally resistant and chronically infected individuals from endemic areas (Gaze et al., 2014). Screening diagnostic candidates for schistosomiasis from tegument proteins of adult *S. japonicum* using an immunoproteomic approach has also been attempted (Zhang et al., 2015).

3.2.7 Glycomics

The name glycomics, formed to follow the convention established by genomics, proteomics, etc., refers to systematic study of glycan structures, including genetic, physiologic and pathologic aspects. It has been well accepted that glycans play critical role in the induction of innate immune responses during schistosome—host interplay, the profiling of schistosomal protein- and/or lipid-conjugated glycan or free glycan elements was addressed even before the screening of schistosomal transcriptomics and proteomics. However, it is not clear what kind of worm glycans can affect the infected host to mount IgG responses and whether mounted anti-glycan IgG responses are protective. The research group from The People's Republic of China discovered that both periodate-resistant periodate-sensitive glycans are antigenic, and dominant anti-glycan IgG responses can play important roles in protective immunity in schistosome-infected host (Gong et al., 2015).

3.3 Schistosomiasis vaccine development in The People's Republic of China

Although PZQ is current cornerstone of schistosomiasis control strategy, there is a need to find a complementary approach that can provide a more long-term prevention. The solution would be immunization with an anti-schistosome vaccine combined with PZQ treatment (Bergquist et al., 2005).

Some of the leading *S. japonicum* vaccine candidates, the protective efficacies of which in different host animals are summarized in Table 3, are discussed later.

Table 3 The current *Schistosoma japonicum* vaccine candidates

Schistosome antigen (protein or cDNA)	Experimental animal (worm reduction): Mouse	Experimental animal (worm reduction): Domestic animals (pig, water buffalo)	References
Attenuated carcarie	33–77%	80–90%	Lin et al. (2011)
Attenuated carcarie		89%	Shi et al. (1993)
Adult worm SjGST 26–28	26–32%	25–69%	Wei et al. (2008)
Adult worm Sj31–32	28%		Wang et al. (2008)
Adult worm SjTPI[a]	21–25%		Dai et al. (2014)
Adult worm SjTPI[a] (i.m.)[b]	50%		Dai et al. (2014)
Adult worm Sj23	27–35%	32–59%	Wang et al. (2014)
Mimotope peptide[c]	26–32%		Wang et al. (2005), Wu et al. (2006)

Some of the leading *S. japonicum* vaccine candidates are discussed, the protective efficacies of these and other molecules in different host animals are summarized.
[a]Triosephosphate isomerase.
[b]Intramuscular injection.
[c]Recombinant Sj338 protein.

3.3.1 Live attenuated vaccines

The initial approach to the development of a schistosome vaccine in The People's Republic of China relied predominantly on live attenuated cercarial vaccines. Cercariae and schistosomula, attenuated in various ways (gamma rays, X-rays, ultraviolet irradiation), have been reported to elicit high levels of protective immunity against schistosomiasis. Irradiated schistosome cercariae confer protection against infection in experimental animal challenge models. For example, water buffaloes vaccinated with irradiation-attenuated *S. japonicum* cercariae, developed 89% resistance to reinfection (Shi et al., 1993). In addition, Chinese researchers have reported that high levels of protective efficacy (77.62%, 88.8% and 99.78% reduction in worm burden, liver eggs and faecal eggs, respectively) against *S. japonicum* challenge were obtained with an ultraviolet-attenuated cercarial vaccine in pigs (Lin et al., 2011). The killing mechanism might be mediated through effective IFN-γ response and strong antibody-mediated response (Lin et al., 2011). Live vaccines are suitable for inducing protection in the laboratory but are not considered for vaccinating humans or domestic animals in the field. The reasons for this include: (1) production costs and labour-intensive efforts required to obtain large numbers of cercariae from infected *Oncomelania* snails; (2) the difficulties in standardizing the dose of ionizing radiation to induce cercarial attenuation and (3) the potential toxicity of administering a live vaccine. To circumvent these problems, Chinese scientists have attempted to improve the protection expressed by the attenuated cercarial vaccines by substituting chemically defined schistosomal antigens genetically engineered in bacteria or yeasts or virus. To date, promising results have been obtained with three major classes of recombinant vaccines, ie, plasmid DNA vaccines, mimotope-based peptide vaccines and vaccines based on viral vectors.

3.3.2 Plasmid DNA vaccines

DNA vaccines use a plasmid containing the gene(s) that code for an immunogenic protein(s) of interest (Zhang et al., 2015). Until recently, no licensed DNA vaccine is commercially available; however, this technology has gained considerable attention, and several products are at various developmental or experimental trial stages, eg, a recombinant plasmid DNA vaccine, pVAX1/SjTGR that is currently being tested in BALB/c mice. The recombinant plasmid, administrated by a 'gene gun', has achieved an average protective efficacy assessed as 27.8–38.8% worm reduction and 40.4–44.5% of liver egg count reduction. All animals vaccinated with pVAX1/SjTGR developed significant specific anti-SjTGR antibodies. Moreover, animals immunized by the gene gun exhibited a splenocyte proliferative response, with an increase in IFN-γ and IL-4 cytokines (Cao et al., 2013). Purified vaccine antigens are often poorly immunogenic, even when produced as recombinant subunit vaccines, and require additional components, such as adjuvants, to stimulate protective immunity based on antibodies and effector-T cells. Adjuvants are currently widely used in animal models, but they are rarely used in human. Immune stimulation by cytokines has been successful in the control of *S. japonicum* infection of poultry as experimental animal (Wei et al., 2008). For example, enhancement of a vaccine-induced immune response was achieved by co-administration of a DNA vaccine encoding for *S. japonicum* 14 kDa fatty acid binding protein (SjFABP) or *S. japonicum* 26 kDa GST with IL-18 (Wei et al., 2009). In both cases, significant increase in the humoral immune responses has been reported. In another study, cimetidine (CIM), a histamine-2-receptor antagonist, as an adjuvant, with pEGFP-Sj26GST (the recombinant plasmid containing enhanced green fluorescent protein gene and the gene encoding 26 kDa glutathione S-transferase of *S. japonicum*) DNA vaccine to immunize mice. The results showed a reduction of both worm and egg burdens in the pEGFP-Sj26GST + CIM group (79.0% and 68.4%, respectively), significantly higher than that in pEGFP-Sj26GST alone group (27.0% and 22.5%, respectively). Compared with the pEGFP-Sj26GST alone group, mice immunized with pEGFP-Sj26GST plus CIM showed an elevated level of IFN-γ and IL-12 and a low level of IL-10 in splenocytes, while the levels of IL-4 and IL-5 showed no difference between the two groups (Li et al., 2011). Wang X reported that by using levamisole (LMS) as an adjuvant enhances cell-mediated immunity in DNA vaccination; VR1012-SjGST-32, in an LMS formulation in the murine challenge model. Compared to controls, the VR1012-SjGST-32 plus LMS reduced worm and egg burdens, as well as, the associated immunopathological complications significantly in liver, apparently associated with a Th1-type response. Together, these results suggest that the LMS as a potential schistosome DNA vaccine adjuvant can be useful for prevention, possibly mediated through the induction of a strong Th1-response (Chen et al., 2012). DNA vaccines have some limitations, since most DNA vaccines are administered by injection, which makes their application difficult in large commercial application. APAMAM dendrimers as a novel vaccine delivery vector will assist in protecting the vaccine against enzymatic degradation and may enhance the immunoreactivity of DNA vaccine and increase the protective effect of the SjC23DNA vaccine against *S. japonicum* infection (Wang et al., 2014).

3.3.3 Mimotope-based peptide vaccines

One interesting approach toward the discovery of new antigens with biotechnological applications is based on phage display technology (Clark and March, 2004). Phage display has been used to identify mimotopes (peptides that mimic linear, discontinuous, and even nonpeptide epitopes) to be employed as vaccine candidates (Arnon et al., 2000). The mimotope peptide vaccines are derived from pathogen protein or a portion of the genome coding for immunogenic epitope. A study has demonstrated that in an effort to identify protective epitopes in Sj338 and increase the level of protection in murine vaccination all four of these phages demonstrated 34.2% worm reduction compared to controls vaccinated with the M13 clone (Xu et al., 2007). Although at experimental stages of development, mimotope peptide vaccines have been shown to be promising for schistosomiasis control, some researchers have focused on developing multiepitope peptide vaccines, eg, clones from a phage library were selected by innate resistance antibodies present in sera samples of rats and *Microtus fortis*, respectively. Expression analyses and immunization study using the screened and enriched mimotope peptides yielded significant humoral and cell-mediated immune responses that resulted in >30% protection after challenge with *S. japonicum* cercariae (Ouyang et al., 2003; Wang et al., 2005). These data suggest that mimotope peptides are potential vaccine candidates.

3.3.4 Viral vector-based vaccines

The use of viral vectors to deliver gene(s) of interest has been studied extensively. Remarkably, the ability of adenovirus vector to persist in cells without causing pathology as well as their tropism to various dividing and nondividing cells allows sustained antigen release. It is also possible to package and express different immunogenic protein subunits in vector-based vaccines without the necessary use of a whole virulent organism. Experimental recombinant vector vaccines have been developed against *S. japonicum*. For example, intramuscular rAdV-SjTPI.opt (triosephosphate isomerase from *S. japonicum* (SjTPI)) provided a consistent and repeatable higher protective effect in mice (more than 50%). These findings may be due to the associated higher levels of specific Th1, antibody responses and partially lower level of IL-17A (Dai et al., 2014). Similarly, Hu have constructed a modified adenoviral vector system that may serve as an alternative delivery vehicle for schistosome vaccine development (Hu et al., 2014).

3.4 New techniques

In total, 73 references were found for new techniques of *S. japonicum* in The People's Republic of China from PubMed with English language after unrelated references and reviews or comments were excluded from the search results. The remaining references were categorized according to subject, including immunodiagnosis (63.01%), molecular diagnosis (16.43%), RNAi (10.96%), genotyping (5.48%) and crystal structure (4.11%) (Fig. 4).

3.4.1 Immunodiagnosis

Immunodiagnostic techniques have a high sensitivity, are easy to perform and are an excellent epidemiological tool for the screening of target populations in schistosome-endemic areas (Zhang et al., 2016). Many variations of indirect immunodiagnostic assays in schistosomiasis diagnosis include the circumoval precipitin test and indirect haemagglutination assay (IHA) which have been widely used historically, and dipstick dye immunoassay and enzyme-linked immonosorbent assay (ELISA), using soluble egg antigen (SEA) as the source of target antigen, is the most widely used technique currently (You and McManus, 2015; Zhu, 2005). Diagnosis based on the detection of antibodies is very sensitive and relatively repeatable, tractable and time-saving compared with traditional direct parasitological methods. Early indirect immunodiagnosis relied on the crude extracts of worm components, like microsomal extract, gut-associated polysaccharide, nonfractionated extracts of eggs, etc. However, early

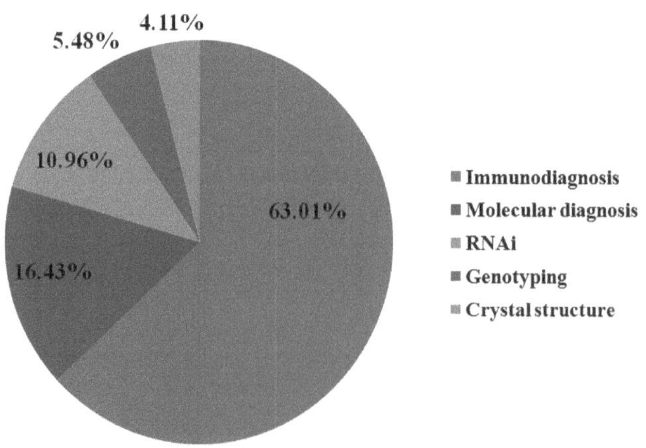

Figure 4 Percentage distribution of references for new techniques of *Schistosoma japonicum* in The People's Republic of China.

indirect immunodiagnosis relied on the crude extracts of worm components including microsomal extract, gut-associated polysaccharide and nonfractionated extracts of eggs, which faces a cross-reaction problem (Jin et al., 2010). Furthermore, antibody-based serological assays are not quantitative and usually fail to discriminate between previous exposure and current infection. Although it is difficult to avoid innate drawbacks like these, these diagnostic techniques could be improved to some extent by the use of selected recombinant antigens. Owing to the enormous amount of gene sequence information procured by the genomics and transcriptomics research, together with screening methods including proteomics, immunomics as well as some bioinformatics tools, many promising diagnostic antigens have been identified and their immunogenicity have been successfully tested (Zhang et al., 2009, 2015), vastly enriching the diagnostic antigen tool box.

Transcriptomic resources have provided cDNA expression libraries. Combined serological screening and immunological verification, schistosomal antigens with high immunogenicity could be identified in cDNA expression libraries and finally be applied for antibody-based immunodiagnosis of schistosomiasis (Zhou et al., 2010) used rabbit sera collected on day 21 postinfection in an antigenic screening of a previously constructed cercariae cDNA expression library of *S. japonicum* (Fung et al., 2002). Likewise, another group of Chinese researchers (Zhou et al., 2009) used human saliva instead of rabbit sera to screen a cDNA expression library of *S. japonicum* eggs, which resulted in the detection of the Sj13 antigen. The following ELISA assay exhibited 92.5% sensitivity and 92.1% specificity of salivary IgG detection with recombinant Sj13. Given the easy-accessibility and noninvasiveness of the saliva samples, saliva/Sj13 was asserted as a promising alternative to serological test for schistosomiasis. In addition, numerous antigens sorted from the cDNA expression library established in 2003 (Hu et al., 2003), which including 43,707 ESTs derived from adult *S. japonicum* and their eggs. Furthermore, bioinformatics techniques also served as screening tools to seek antigen candidates for indirect immunological diagnosis in the *S. japonicum* genome. In another study, immunomics was also employed to uncover prospective diagnosis antigens for schistosomiasis (Zhong et al., 2010).

Early immunoassays have shown that schistosome-derived antigens, such as adult worm antigen (AWA), SEA and various circulating antigens (Zhao et al., 2012) are released into the host circulatory system/excreta in infected humans and other hosts, which facilitates the research on direct immunological diagnosis of schistosomiasis. Circulating anodic antigen

(CAA) and circulating cathodic antigen are by far the most extensively used antigens for the antigen-based immunodiagnosis of schistosomiasis and methods for the detection of circulating antigens encompass sandwich ELISA, IHA, time-resolved immunofluorometric assay, magnetic bead immunoassay, reagent strips and liquid-phase piezoelectric immunosensor. Compared with the two foregoing diagnostic methods, the detection of circulating antigens is more suitable for drug efficacy trials owing to its high specificity and the ability to discriminate between previous exposure and current infection. The significantly higher prevalence of active schistosome infections by the urine and serum upconverting phosphor lateral-flow CAA assays has implications for the national control and elimination programme, particularly in respect to case-finding and intervention strategies while the downward trend in prevalence and intensity of *S. japonicum* infection in The People's Republic of China has reached a level (van Dam et al., 2015). It is important to mention this here as this technique is in fact more sensitive than the molecular techniques since they target antigens emitted from the worm in the blood, while the latter approach generally targets egg antigens leaving the body with the faeces.

3.4.2 Molecular diagnosis

Given the existence of *S. japonicum* DNA in host serum derived from dead schistosomula, tegument shedding of worm or inactive eggs (Xu et al., 2013), molecular diagnosis based on the polymerase chain reaction (PCR) has become a promising alternative to overcome the innate shortcomings of etiological diagnosis and immunodiagnosis for schistosomiasis. Since the publication of the usefulness of the PCR for detecting *S. mansoni* DNA in human faecal and serum sample (Pontes et al., 2002), PCR-based molecular diagnosis has been applied to the detection of schistosomes in multiple diagnostic field works and several novel technologies, such as real-time PCR (RT-PCR), PCR-ELISA and loop-mediated isothermal amplification (Tambo et al., 2014; Xu et al., 2010), etc. have been added to the tool box in addition to conventional PCR for boosting the detection sensitivity. Empirical evidence shows that molecular diagnosis of schistosomiasis has both high sensitivity and high specificity, enabling detection during the larval stage or at least before eggs are released in the host, and can use various materials, eg, faeces, serum, plasma and urine as samples. These reasons suffice to convince users that they are superior to conventional diagnostic approaches. Factors that impact the result of molecular diagnosis are various and the choice of amplified products is definitely among them. However,

confined by the inaccessibility to the schistosomal genome sequence, in the pregenomic era, researchers could only select PCR targets with limited candidates.

A large-scale selection had been conducted to seek suitable target sequences among 25 retrotransposons identified along with the publication of the genome of *S. japonicum* to achieve a specific and sensitive diagnosis (Consortium, S.j.G.S.a.F.A., 2009; Guo et al., 2012). To begin with, primer pairs were designed for the 25 candidates with *Sj*R2, a previously described molecular diagnostic target, serving as positive control. A series of diluted genomic *S. japonicum* DNA were used as templates in a PCR assay to amplify the target fragments and judge the sensitivity of those 25 candidates. The result showed that in addition to *Sj*R2, a new non-LTR retrotransposon named *Sj*CHGCS19, with the PCR product of 303-bp in length, had high sensitivity for detecting *S. japonicum* DNA. Coincidentally, bioinformatics research showed that both *Sj*CHGCS19 and *Sj*R2 have higher genome proportions, repetitive complete copies and partial copies and more active ESTs compared with other candidates in the *S. japonicum* genome, which may also outline the general features of ideal targets for PCR diagnosis of schistosomiasis.

Parasite-derived miRNA strands, similar to genomic DNA, are also present in host biofluids, eg, plasma, serum, urine and saliva, which support their potential as biomarkers for the molecular diagnosis of schistosomiasis. Besides, in response to the invasion of pathogens, some characteristic changes of the host's miRNA profile might appear, which can also serve as a hint of an infection event. Nowadays, the available sequences of schistosomal miRNAs, in association with those approaches established for the profiling of miRNAs, eg, stem-loop RT-PCR, miRNA array and high-throughput sequencing have paved the way for the use of miRNA-based molecular diagnosis of schistosomiasis in the future.

3.4.3 RNA interference

RNAi is a potent gene silencing process triggered by exogenous double-stranded (ds) RNA. Knockdown of genes using RNAi has proven to be a powerful technique for investigating a variety of gene functions in schistosomes (Britton et al., 2012; Krautz-Peterson et al., 2010). Schistosomes undergo many morphological and physiological transformations during development as a result of profound changes in gene expression when moving from one stage of the life cycle to the next. Proteins containing zinc finger (ZF) motifs usually play an important role in DNA recognition, RNA packaging and transcriptional activation. In a study, Liu et al. (2015) cloned the open reading frame of *S. japonicum* SjZFP1, which encodes a ZF protein, analysed the cDNA sequence of SjZFP1 and examined the expression of SjZFP1 mRNA from various developmental stages. This research group also tested the effects of RNAi with respect to worm burden, spawning and egg hatching. The results suggest that the SjZFP1 gene might be important for parasite development and egg production in the vertebrate host, as well as egg hatching in the water.

The worms survive in the capillary networks in the abdomen of the final host, where thioredoxin glutathione reductase (TGR) activity helps them to survive in the aerobic environment (Wang et al., 2014) synthesized four small interfering RNAs (siRNA S1, S2, S3 and S4) using them to target and knock out the SjTGR gene. The knockout effect of the siRNAs resulting in closing down the thioredoxin reductase activity of SjTGR were evaluated in vitro. The results of this study indicate that SjTGR may play an important role in the clearance of oxygen free radicals and protection of *S. japonicum* parasites against oxidative damage.

3.4.4 Genotyping

In the present study, intersimple sequence repeats (ISSRs) markers were used to examine the genetic variability of *S. japonicum* isolates from different provinces in The People's Republic of China, using *S. japonicum* from Japan and *S. mansoni* from Puerto Rico for comparison. Of the 30 primers screened, 4 produced highly reproducible ISSR fragments. Using these primers, 107 discernible DNA fragments were generated with 105 (98.13%) being polymorphic, indicating considerable genetic variation among the examined *S. japonicum* isolates. The percentage of polymorphic bands among *S. japonicum* isolates from The People's Republic of China and Japan was 82.2%, 43.9% among mountainous type isolates and 64.5% among lake/marshland type isolates from The People's Republic of China. Unweighted pair group method analysis revealed that all of the *S. japonicum* samples were grouped into two clades, the first containing Chinese isolates and the other Japanese ones. Within the cluster of *S. japonicum* isolates from The People's Republic of China, isolates from mountainous Sichuan and Yunnan provinces grouped together, whereas isolates from lake/marshland regions (Anhui, Jiangsu and Hubei provinces) clustered together. The results demonstrated that the ISSR markers are useful for studying genetic diversity and population structure of *S. japonicum* isolates from The People's Republic of China (Wang and Li, 1990; Zhao et al., 2009).

3.4.5 Crystal structure

Thioredoxin-glutathione system of *S. japonicum* plays a critical role in maintaining the redox balance in parasite, which is a potential target for development of novel anti-schistosomal agents. Researchers cloned the gene of *S. japonicum* thioredoxin (SjTrx) from cDNA, expressed and purified the recombinant SjTrx in *Escherichia coli*. Functional assay shows that SjTrx catalyses the dithiothreitol reduction of insulin disulphide bonds. The coupling assay of SjTrx with its endogenous reductase, TGR from *S. japonicum* (SjTGR), supports its biological function to maintain the redox homoeostasis in the cell. Furthermore, the crystal structure of SjTrx in the oxidized state was determined at 2.0 Å resolution, revealing a typical architecture of thioredoxin fold. The structural information of SjTrx provides us important clues for understanding the maintenance function of redox homoeostasis in *S. japonicum* and pathogenesis of this chronic disease (Alicino et al., 2015).

4. CONCLUSIONS AND RECOMMENDATIONS

An exponentially increasing number of references published in both of English and Chinese from PubMed was observed by our systematic search for published articles on *S. japonicum* research covering the 2000–15 timeframe. In total 410 references were published in English. Articles on omics were the largest proportion of articles published in English during the latest 15 years.

Although we think that schistosomiasis control and elimination will be improved in The People's Republic of China through development of new tools facilitating the march toward schistosomiasis control and elimination in The People's Republic of China, a series of research gaps were identified that could hinder progress (Zheng et al., 2013). For example, there is a lack of sensitive and specific tests for the detection of schistosomiasis cases with low intensity of infection, and there is a need for a vaccine that can reduce symptoms and slow transmission. Hence, They need to be regarded as one component, albeit a very important one, of integrated schistosomiasis control programs that complement existing strategies.

ACKNOWLEDGEMENTS

This work was supported in part by the Foundation of National Science and Technology Major Program (Grant No. 2012ZX10004-220), the National Natural Science Foundation of The People's Republic of China (Grant No. 30400256) and the International S&T Cooperation Programme of The People's Republic of China (Grant No. 2014DFA31130).

REFERENCES

Alicino, C., Bragazzi, N.L., Faccio, V., Amicizia, D., Panatto, D., Gasparini, R., et al., 2015. Assessing Ebola-related web search behaviour: insights and implications from an analytical study of Google Trends-based query volumes. Infect. Dis. Poverty 4, 54.

Arnon, R., Tarrab-Hazdai, R., Steward, M., 2000. A mimotope peptide-based vaccine against *Schistosoma mansoni*: synthesis and characterization. Immunology 101 (4), 555–562.

Bartel, D.P., 2009. MicroRNAs: target recognition and regulatory functions. Cell 136 (2), 215–233.

Bergquist, N.R., Leonardo, L.R., Mitchell, G.F., 2005. Vaccine-linked chemotherapy: can schistosomiasis control benefit from an integrated approach? Trends Parasitol. 21 (3), 112–117.

Berriman, M., Haas, B.J., LoVerde, P.T., Wilson, R.A., Dillon, G.P., Cerqueira, G.C., et al., 2009. The genome of the blood fluke *Schistosoma mansoni*. Nature 460, 352–358.

Brennecke, J., Aravin, A.A., Stark, A., Dus, M., Kellis, M., Sachidanandam, R., Hannon, G.J., et al., 2007. Discrete small RNA-generating loci as master regulators of transposon activity in *Drosophila*. Cell 128 (6), 1089–1103.

Brindley, P.J., Mitreva, M., Ghedin, E., Lustigman, S., 2009. Helminth genomics: the implications for human health. PLoS Neglected Trop. Dis. 3, e538.

Britton, C., Samarasinghe, B., Knox, D.P., 2012. Ups and downs of RNA interference in parasitic nematodes. Exp. Parasitol. 132 (1), 56–61.

Cao, X., Fu, Z., Zhang, M., Han, Y., Han, Q., Lu, K., et al., 2015. Excretory/secretory proteome of 14-day schistosomula, *Schistosoma japonicum*. J. Proteomics. http://dx.doi.org/10.1016/j.jprot.2015.10.001 pii:S1874–3919(15)30145-7.

Cao, Y., Zhao, B., Han, Y., Zhang, J., Li, X., Qiu, C., Wu, X., et al., 2013. Gene gun bombardment with DNA-coated golden particles enhanced the protective effect of a DNA vaccine based on thioredoxin glutathione reductase of *Schistosoma japonicum*. Biomed. Res. Int. 2013, 952416.

Chai, M., McManus, D.P., McInnes, R., Moertel, L., Tran, M., Loukas, A., Jonesa, M.K., et al., 2006. Transcriptome profiling of lung schistosomula, in vitro cultured schistosomula and adult *Schistosoma japonicum*. Cell Mol. Life Sci. 63 (7–8), 919–929.

Chen, J.H., Jung, J.W., Wang, Y., Ha, K.S., Lu, F., Lim, C.S., Takeo, S., et al., 2010. Immunoproteomics profiling of blood stage *Plasmodium vivax* infection by high-throughput screening assays. J. Proteome Res. 9 (12), 6479–6489.

Chen, J.H., Wang, H., Chen, J.X., Bergquist, R., Tanner, M., Utzinger, J., et al., 2012. Frontiers of parasitology research in the People's Republic of China: infection, diagnosis, protection and surveillance. Parasit. Vectors 5, 221.

Chen, J.H., Zhang, T., Ju, C., Xu, B., Lu, Y., Mo, X.J., et al., 2014. An integrated immunoproteomics and bioinformatics approach for the analysis of *Schistosoma japonicum* tegument proteins. J. Proteomics 98, 289–299.

Chen, J.H., Chen, S.B., Wang, Y., Ju, C., Zhang, T., Xu, B., Shen, H.M., et al., 2015. An immunomics approach for the analysis of natural antibody responses to *Plasmodium vivax* infection. Mol. Biosyst. 11 (8), 2354–2363.

Cheng, G., Jin, Y., 2012. MicroRNAs: potentially important regulators for schistosome development and therapeutic targets against schistosomiasis. Parasitology 139 (5), 669–679.

Cheng, G.F., Lin, J.J., Feng, X.G., Fu, Z.Q., Jin, Y.M., Yuan, C.X., Zhou, Y.C., et al., 2005. Proteomic analysis of differentially expressed proteins between the male and female worm of *Schistosoma japonicum* after pairing. Proteomics 5 (2), 511–521.

Chuan, J., Feng, Z., Brindley, P.J., McManus, D.P., Han, Z., Jianxin, P., Hu, W., et al., 2010. Our wormy world genomics, proteomics and transcriptomics in east and southeast Asia. Adv. Parasitol. 73, 327–371.

Clark, J.R., March, J.B., 2004. Bacteriophage-mediated nucleic acid immunisation. FEMS Immunol. Med. Microbiol. 40 (1), 21–26.

Consortium, S.j.G.S.a.F.A, 2009. The *Schistosoma japonicum* genome reveals features of host-parasite interplay. Nature 460 (7253), 345–351.

Dai, Y., Wang, X., Zhao, S., Tang, J., Zhang, L., Dai, J., et al., 2014. Construction and evaluation of replication-defective recombinant optimized triosephosphate isomerase adenoviral vaccination in *Schistosoma japonicum* challenged mice. Vaccine 32 (7), 771–778.

Driguez, P., Doolan, D.L., Loukas, A., Felgner, P.L., McManus, D.P., 2010. Schistosomiasis vaccine discovery using immunomics. Parasit. Vectors 3, 4.

Fan, Y.T., Wang, Y., Ju, C., Zhang, T., Xu, B., Hu, W., Chen, J.H., et al., 2013. Systematic analysis of natural antibody responses to *P. falciparum* merozoite antigens by protein arrays. J. Proteomics 78, 148–158.

Fung, M.C., Lau, M.T., Chen, X.G., 2002. Expressed sequence tag (EST) analysis of a *Schistosoma japonicum* cercariae cDNA library. Acta Trop. 82 (2), 215–224.

Gaze, S., Driguez, P., Pearson, M.S., Mendes, T., Doolan, D.L., Trieu, A., et al., 2014. An immunomics approach to schistosome antigen discovery: antibody signatures of naturally resistant and chronically infected individuals from endemic areas. PLoS Pathog. 10 (3), e1004033.

Gong, W., Huang, F., Ma, Y., Bai, H., Yin, L., Li, J., et al., 2015. Protective immunity against *Schistosoma japonicum* infection can be provided by IgG antibodies towards periodate-sensitive or periodate-resistant glycans. Parasit. Vectors 8, 234.

Guo, J.J., Zheng, H.J., Xu, J., Zhu, X.Q., Wang, S.Y., Xia, C.M., 2012. Sensitive and specific target sequences selected from retrotransposons of *Schistosoma japonicum* for the diagnosis of schistosomiasis. PLoS Neglected Trop. Dis. 6 (3), e1579.

Hao, L., Cai, P., Jiang, N., Wang, H., Chen, Q., 2010. Identification and characterization of microRNAs and endogenous siRNAs in *Schistosoma japonicum*. BMC Genomics 11, 55.

Hokke, C.H., Fitzpatrick, J.M., Hoffmann, K.F., 2007. Integrating transcriptome, proteome and glycome analyses of *Schistosoma* biology. Trends Parasitol. 23, 165–174.

Hotez, P.J., Bethony, J.M., Diemert, D.J., Pearson, M., Loukas, A., 2010. Developing vaccines to combat hookworm infection and intestinal schistosomiasis. Nat. Rev. Microbiol. 8, 814–826.

Hu, C., Zhu, L., Luo, R., Dao, J., Zhao, J., Shi, Y., Li, H., et al., 2014. Evaluation of protective immune response in mice by vaccination the recombinant adenovirus for expressing Schistosomajaponicum inhibitor apoptosis protein. Parasitol. Res. 113 (11), 4261–4269.

Hu, W., Yan, Q., Shen, D.K., Liu, F., Zhu, Z.D., Song, H.D., Xu, X.R., et al., 2003. Evolutionary and biomedical implications of a *Schistosoma japonicum* complementary DNA resource. Nat. Genet. 35 (2), 139–147.

Jin, Y.M., Lu, K., Zhou, W.F., Fu, Z.Q., Liu, J.M., Shi, Y.J., Li, H., et al., 2010. Comparison of recombinant proteins from *Schistosoma japonicum* for schistosomiasis diagnosis. Clin. Vaccine Immunol. 17 (3), 476–480.

Kim, V.N., 2005. Small RNAs: classification, biogenesis, and function. Mol. Cells 19 (1), 1–15.

Krautz-Peterson, G., Bhardwaj, R., Faghiri, Z., Tararam, C.A., Skelly, P.J., 2010. RNA interference in schistosomes: machinery and methodology. Parasitology 137 (3), 485–495.

Li, M.J., Lei, J.H., Wang, T., Lu, S.J., Guan, F., Liu, W.Q., Li, Y.L., et al., 2011. Cimetidine enhances the protective effect of GST DNA vaccine against *Schistosoma japonicum*. Exp. Parasitol. 128 (4), 427–432.

Lier, T., Simonsen, G.S., Wang, T., Lu, D., Haukland, H.H., Vennervald, B.J., et al., 2009. Real-time polymerase chain reaction for detection of low-intensity *Schistosoma japonicum* infections in China. Am. J. Trop. Med. Hyg. 81, 428–432.
Lin, D., Tian, F., Wu, H., Gao, Y., Wu, J., Zhang, D., Ji, M., et al., 2011. Multiple vaccinations with UV-attenuated cercariae in pig enhance protective immunity against *Schistosoma japonicum* infection as compared to single vaccination. Parasit. Vectors 4, 103.
Liu, F., Cui, S.J., Hu, W., Feng, Z., Wang, Z.Q., Han, Z.G., 2009. Excretory/secretory proteome of the adult developmental stage of human blood fluke, *Schistosoma japonicum*. Mol. Cell Proteomics 8 (6), 1236–1251.
Liu, L., Yang, G.J., Zhu, H.R., Yang, K., Ai, L., 2014. Knowledge of, attitudes towards, and practice relating to schistosomiasis in two subtypes of a mountainous region of the People's Republic of China. Infect. Dis. Poverty 3, 16.
Liu, X., Liu, J.M., Song, Z.Y., Xing, R.H., Jin, Y.M., Guo, Y.H., Li, H., et al., 2015. The molecular characterization and RNAi silencing of SjZFP1 in *Schistosoma japonicum*. Parasitol. Res. 114 (3), 903–911.
Lustigman, S., Geldhof, P., Grant, W.N., Osei-Atweneboana, M.Y., Sripa, B., Basanez, M.G., 2012. A research agenda for helminth diseases of humans: basic research and enabling technologies to support control and elimination of helminthiases. PLoS Neglected Trop. Dis. 6, e1445.
McManus, D.P., Loukas, A., 2008. Current status of vaccines for schistosomiasis. Clin. Microbiol. Rev. 21, 225–242.
Molnar, A., Melnyk, C.W., Bassett, A., Hardcastle, T.J., Dunn, R., Baulcombe, D.C., 2010. Small silencing RNAs in plants are mobile and direct epigenetic modification in recipient cells. Science 328 (5980), 872–875.
Neafsey, D.E., Galinsky, K., Jiang, R.H., Young, L., Sykes, S.M., Saif, S., et al., 2012. The malaria parasite *Plasmodium vivax* exhibits greater genetic diversity than *Plasmodium falciparum*. Nat. Genet. 44, 1046–1050.
Ouyang, L., Yi, X., Zeng, X., Zhou, J., Wang, Q., McReynolds, L., 2003. Partial protection induced by phage library-selected peptides mimicking epitopes of *Schistosoma japonicum*. Chin. Med. J. Engl. 116 (1), 138–141.
Peng, H.J., Chen, X.G., Wang, X.Z., Lun, Z.R., 2003. Analysis of the gene expression profile of *Schistosoma japonicum* cercariae by a strategy based on expressed sequence tags. Parasitol. Res. 90 (4), 287–293.
Pontes, L.A., Dias-Neto, E., Rabello, A., 2002. Detection by polymerase chain reaction of *Schistosoma mansoni* DNA in human serum and feces. Am. J. Trop. Med. Hyg. 66 (2), 157–162.
Protasio, A.V., Tsai, I.J., Babbage, A., Nichol, S., Hunt, M., Aslett, M.A., et al., 2012. A systematically improved high quality genome and transcriptome of the human blood fluke *Schistosoma mansoni*. PLoS Neglected Trop. Dis. 6, e1455.
Shi, Y.E., Jiang, C.F., Han, J.J., Li, Y.L., Ruppel, A., 1993. Immunization of pigs against infection with *Schistosoma japonicum* using ultraviolet-attenuated cercariae. Parasitology 106 (Pt 5), 459–462.
Tambo, E., Ai, L., Zhou, X., Chen, J.H., Hu, W., Bergquist, R., et al., 2014. Surveillance-response systems: the key to elimination of tropical diseases. Infect. Dis. Poverty 3, 17.
Tambo, E., Khater, E.I., Chen, J.H., Bergquist, R., Zhou, X.N., 2015. Nobel prize for the artemisinin and ivermectin discoveries: a great boost towards elimination of the global infectious diseases of poverty. Infect. Dis. Poverty 4, 58.
van Dam, G.J., Xu, J., Bergquist, R., de Dood, C.J., Utzinger, J., Qin, Z.Q., et al., 2015. An ultra-sensitive assay targeting the circulating anodic antigen for the diagnosis of *Schistosoma japonicum* in a low-endemic area, People's Republic of China. Acta Trop. 141 (Pt B), 190–197.

van Hellemond, J.J., van Balkom, B.W., Tielens, A.G.M., 2007. Schistosome biology and proteomics: progress and challenges. Exp. Parasitol. 117 (3), 267–274.

Verjovski-Almeida, S., DeMarco, R., Martins, E.A., Guimaraes, P.E., Ojopi, E.P., Paquola, A.C., et al., 2003. Transcriptome analysis of the acoelomate human parasite *Schistosoma mansoni*. Nat. Genet. 35, 148–157.

Wang, J., Zhao, F., Yu, C.X., Xiao, D., Song, L.J., Yin, X.R., Shen, S., et al., 2013. Identification of proteins inducing short-lived antibody responses from excreted/secretory products of *Schistosoma japonicum* adult worms by immunoproteomic analysis. J. Proteomics 87, 53–67.

Wang, L., Utzinger, J., Zhou, X.N., 2008. Schistosomiasis control: experiences and lessons from China. Lancet 372 (9652), 1793–1795.

Wang, L.D., Chen, H.G., Guo, J.G., Zeng, X.J., Hong, X.L., Xiong, J.J., Wu, X.H., et al., 2009. A strategy to control transmission of *Schistosoma japonicum* in China. N. Engl. J. Med. 360 (2), 121–128.

Wang, M., Yi, X.Y., Li, X.P., Zhou, D.M., Larry, M., Zeng, X.F., 2005. Phage displaying peptides mimic schistosoma antigenic epitopes selected by rat natural antibodies and protective immunity induced by their immunization in mice. World J. Gastroenterol. 11 (19), 2960–2966.

Wang, X., Li, S., 1990. Study on rapid ELISA using PVC for immunodiagnosis of schistosomiasis and its application. Chin. J. Schisto. Control 2, 31–35 (in Chinese).

Wang, X., Dai, Y., Zhao, S., Tang, J., Li, H., Xing, Y., et al., 2014. PAMAM-Lys, a novel vaccine delivery vector, enhances the protective effects of the SjC23 DNA vaccine against *Schistosoma japonicum* infection. PLoS One 9 (1), e86578.

Wang, Y., Utzinger, J., Xiao, S.-H., Xue, J., Nicholson, J.K., Tanner, M., Singer, B.H., et al., 2006. System level metabolic effects of a *Schistosoma japonicum* infection in the Syrian hamster. Mol. Biochem. Parasitol. 146 (1), 1–9.

Wei, F., Liu, Q., Gao, S., Shang, L., Zhai, Y., Men, J., Jiang, L., et al., 2008. Enhancement by IL-18 of the protective effect of a *Schistosoma japonicum* 26 kDa GST plasmid DNA vaccine in mice. Vaccine 26 (33), 4145–4149.

Wei, F., Liu, Q., Zhai, Y., Fu, Z., Liu, W., Shang, L., Men, J., et al., 2009. IL-18 enhances protective effect in mice immunized with a *Schistosoma japonicum* FABP DNA vaccine. Acta Trop. 111 (3), 284–288.

Wu, H.W., Hu, X.M., Wang, Y., Kurtis, J.D., Zeng, F.J., McGarvey, S.T., Wu, G.L., et al., 2006. Protective immunity induced by phage displayed mitochondrial related peptides of *Schistosoma japonicum*. Acta. Trop. 99 (2-3), 200–207.

Wu, J.F., Holmes, E., Xue, J., Xiao, S.H., Singer, B.H., Tang, H.R., Utzinger, J., et al., 2010. Metabolic alterations in the hamster co-infected with *Schistosoma japonicum* and *Necator americanus*. Int. J. Parasitol. 40 (6), 695–703.

Wu, J.Y., Zhou, Y.B., Li, L.H., Zheng, S.B., Liang, S., Coatsworth, A., et al., 2014. Identification of optimum scopes of environmental factors for snails using spatial analysis techniques in Dongting Lake Region, China. Parasit. Vectors 7, 216.

Xu, J., Chen, N.G., Feng, T., Wang, E.M., Wu, X.H., Chen, H.G., et al., 2007. Effectiveness of routinely used assays for the diagnosis of schistosomiasis japonica in the field. Chin. J. Parasitol. Parasit. Dis. 25, 175–179 (in Chinese).

Xu, J., Rong, R., Zhang, H.Q., Shi, C.J., Zhu, X.Q., Xia, C.M., 2010. Sensitive and rapid detection of *Schistosoma japonicum* DNA by loop-mediated isothermal amplification (LAMP). Int. J. Parasitol. 40 (3), 327–331.

Xu, J., Liu, A., Guo, J.J., Wang, B., Qiu, S.J., Sun, H., Guan, W., et al., 2013. The sources and metabolic dynamics of *Schistosoma japonicum* DNA in serum of the host. Parasitol. Res. 112 (1), 129–133.

Xue, X., Sun J., Zhang, Q., Wang, Z., Huang, Y., Pan, W., 2008. Identification and characterization of novel microRNAs from *Schistosoma japonicum*.

You, H., Zhang, W., Moertel, L., McManus, D.P., Gobert, G.N., 2009. Transcriptional profiles of adult male and female *Schistosoma japonicum* in response to insulin reveal increased expression of genes involved in growth and development. Int. J. Parasitol. 39 (14), 1551–1559.

You, H., McManus, D.P., 2015. Vaccines and diagnostics for zoonotic schistosomiasis japonica. Parasitology 142 (2), 271–289.

Zhang, J.F., Xu, J., Bergquist, R., Yu, L.L., Yan, X.L., Zhu, H.Q., et al., 2016. Development and application of diagnostics in the national schistosomiasis control programme in the People's Republic of China. Adv. Parasitol. 92.

Zhang, M., Fu, Z., Li, C., Han, Y., Cao, X., Han, H., et al., 2015. Screening diagnostic candidates for schistosomiasis from tegument proteins of adult *Schistosoma japonicum* using an immunoproteomic approach. PLoS Neglected Trop. Dis. 9 (2), e0003454.

Zhang, Y.Y., Luo, J.P., Liu, Y.M., Wang, Q.Z., Chen, J.H., Xu, M.X., et al., 2009. Evaluation of Kato-Katz examination method in three areas with low-level endemicity of schistosomiasis japonica in China: a Bayesian modeling approach. Acta Trop. 112, 16–22.

Zhao, G.H., Li, J., Zou, F.C., Mo, X.H., Yuan, Z.G., Lin, R.Q., Weng, Y.B., et al., 2009. ISSR, an effective molecular approach for studying genetic variability among *Schistosoma japonicum* isolates from different provinces in mainland China. Infect. Genet. Evol. 9 (5), 903–907.

Zhao, G.H., Li, J., Blair, D., Li, X.Y., Elsheikha, H.M., Lin, R.Q., Zou, F.C., et al., 2012. Biotechnological advances in the diagnosis, species differentiation and phylogenetic analysis of *Schistosoma* spp. Biotechnol. Adv. 30 (6), 1381–1389.

Zheng, Q., Vanderslott, S., Jiang, B., Xu, L.L., Liu, C.S., Huo, L.L., et al., 2013. Research gaps for three main tropical diseases in the People's Republic of China. Infect. Dis. Poverty 2, 15.

Zhong, Z.R., Zhou, H.B., Li, X.Y., Luo, Q.L., Song, X.R., Wang, W., Wen, H.Q., et al., 2010. Serological proteome-oriented screening and application of antigens for the diagnosis of *Schistosomiasis japonica*. Acta Trop. 116 (1), 1–8.

Zhou, X.H., Wu, J.Y., Huang, X.Q., Kunnon, S.P., Zhu, X.Q., Chen, X.G., 2010. Identification and characterization of *Schistosoma japonicum* Sjp40, a potential antigen candidate for the early diagnosis of schistosomiasis. Diagn. Microbiol. Infect. Dis. 67 (4), 337–345.

Zhou, Y.P., Wu, Z.D., Yang, L.L., Sun, X., You, X., Yu, X.B., Hu, W., et al., 2009. Cloning, molecular characterization of a 13-kDa antigen from *Schistosoma japonicum*, Sj13, a putative salivary diagnosis candidate for Schistosomiasis japonica. Parasitol. Res. 105 (5), 1435–1444.

Zhu, Y.C., 2005. Immunodiagnosis and its role in schistosomiasis control in China: a review. Acta Trop. 96 (2–3), 130–136.

CHAPTER FOURTEEN

Development and Application of Diagnostics in the National Schistosomiasis Control Programme in The People's Republic of China

J.-F. Zhang[*,**,§§], J. Xu[§,¶,||], R. Bergquist[#], L.-L. Yu[*], X.-L. Yan[*], H.-Q. Zhu[§,¶,||], L.-Y. Wen[*,¶¶,1]

[*]Zhejiang Academy of Medical Sciences, Hangzhou, Zhejiang, The People's Republic of China
[§]National Institute of Parasitic Diseases, Chinese Centre for Disease Control and Prevention, Shanghai, The People's Republic of China
[¶]WHO Collaborating Center for Tropical Diseases, Shanghai, The People's Republic of China
[||]Key Laboratory of Parasite and Vector Biology, Ministry of Health, Shanghai, The People's Republic of China
[#]Geospatial Health, University of Naples Federico II, Naples, Italy
[**]Jiangsu Institute of Parasitic Diseases, Key Laboratory of Parasitic Disease Control and Prevention (Ministry of Health), Jiangsu Provincial Key Laboratory of Parasite Molecular Biology, Wuxi, The People's Republic of China
[§§]Public Health Research Center, Jiangnan University, Wuxi, The People's Republic of China
[¶¶]Institute of Parasitic Diseases, Zhejiang Academy of Medical Sciences, Hangzhou, The People's Republic of China
[1]Corresponding authors: E-mail: xfmjing@163.com; wenliyong@126.com

Contents

Advances in Parasitology, Volume 92
ISSN 0065-308X
http://dx.doi.org/10.1016/bs.apar.2016.02.008

Abstract

Schistosomiasis, caused by *Schistosoma japonicum* infection to human, has a documented history of more than 2100 years in The People's Republic of China. In spite of great progress in controlling the disease, it is still one of the most serious parasitic diseases in the country. The study and use of diagnostic techniques play an important role in the targeting of chemotherapy that has been continuously applied in the national schistosomiasis control programme for several decades. This paper reviews the development and application of parasitological, immunodiagnostic and molecular diagnostic technology for *S. japonicum* in The People's Republic of China with a brief mention of diagnostic imagery, such as ultrasound and radiology. When analysing the efficacy and performance characteristics of the main diagnostic techniques in current use, it becomes apparent that approaches that worked well in the past are less suitable now as successful control has shifted the endemic situation towards control and interruption of transmission. The conclusion is that a mutable approach must be adopted choosing the most appropriate diagnostic technique for each control stage (and area), thus modifying the methodology according to the prevailing diagnostic needs in terms of sensitivity and specificity.

1. INTRODUCTION

Schistosomiasis in The People's Republic of China is confined to infection by *Schistosoma japonicum*. The first report of a human case where the clinical symptoms were directly connected with this parasite was made by an American physician working in The People's Republic of China (Chen, 2014; Logan, 1905). After that, only sporadic reports are available in English, but in the mid-1950s, there were more than 11 million known infected cases (Chen and Feng, 1999; Mao and Shao, 1982; Xu et al., 2016). Thanks to sustained, strong control efforts started then, both prevalence rates and the intensity of infection in the endemic areas have dramatically declined since then resulting in a drop to an estimated 185,000 people in 2013 (Lei et al., 2014; Wang, 2006). According to the criteria for schistosomiasis control and elimination issued by the Chinese Ministry of Health, the stages for the national schistosomiasis control programme are classified according to the prevailing prevalence level, ie, morbidity control stage when prevalence is over than 5%, infection control stage when prevalence at 1–5%, and transmission control stage when prevalence less than 1%, while absence of local cases for 5 years signifies transmission interruption and the continued absence of cases for another 5 years means that elimination has been achieved (Zhou et al., 2011; Zhu et al., 2016). Case finding and treatment, assessment of morbidity as well as evaluation of control strategies all build on the results of diagnostic tests, so it can emphatically be said that diagnosis is the essential basis of treatment and central to the control of schistosomiasis (Collins et al., 2012; Feldmeier and Poggensee, 1993).

The current, widely used diagnostic methodology can be divided into parasitological techniques (detection of parasite eggs or miracidia in the faeces) and immunologic approaches (detection of specific antibodies or circulating schistosome antigens). Parasitological techniques such as the Kato-Katz thick-smear method and the miracidium hatching technique are used to determine if there is infection and usually serve as reference to evaluate other diagnostic tools (Bergquist et al., 2009; Wu, 2002). Indirect approaches including immunodiagnostic techniques have superior sensitivity and are rapid as well as affordable. Antibody-based immunoassays are useful for large-scale screening but positive titres abate only slowly making it impossible to differentiate between current and cured infections. On the other hand, antibody techniques are highly effective for surveying areas from where infection has been eliminated (Hillyer et al., 1999). The detection of circulating antigens (CAg) is not only the most reliable technique (if the latest, high-sensitivity techniques are used – see the later discussion), but also the most direct one as the amount of released antigens from the adult worms in the host changes in direct relation to a change in the worm burden, while the excretion of eggs from the infected host is somewhat uneven (Engels et al., 1996), a variable that would be even more pronounced in the case of *S. japonicum* as this species tends to release its eggs in aggregates. In addition, the development of molecular biotechnology, including the polymerase chain reaction (PCR) and the loop-mediated isothermal amplification (LAMP), both based on the gene cloning amplification, has been developed and successfully transferred from the laboratory to the field (Lier et al., 2009; Xia et al., 2009; Xu et al., 2010, 2015).

Integration of diagnostic tools into national control programmes requires collaboration between research laboratories, epidemiologists and control programme managers, defining assays in terms of sensitivity, specificity and predictive values (Dabo et al., 2015). Big differences exist between different endemic areas and stages of control in terms of prevalence and infection intensity. Diagnostic tools and strategies should therefore vary according to the perceived prevalence level and attention should be paid to the prevailing socioeconomic situation. This article reviews the development and application of parasitological, immunodiagnostic and molecular diagnostic technology for *S. japonicum* infection in The People's Republic of China with a brief mention of imaging techniques such as ultrasound and radiology. The currently most important diagnostic approaches useful for epidemiological survey against the backdrop of the historical record are also discussed.

2. HISTORICAL REVIEW OF DIAGNOSTIC TOOLS

2.1 Parasitological methods

The diagnosis of active *S. japonicum* infection consists of the detection of viable schistosome eggs in faeces or tissue biopsies. Direct smear, sedimentation, formol-ether concentration (Allen and Ridley, 1970), Kato-Katz thick smear (Katz et al., 1972), the hatching test (Qiu and Xue, 1990) and rectal biopsy can be used to diagnose schistosome infection. All these techniques require microscope and well-trained laboratory technicians. Although of little importance in the endemic areas, it should be pointed out that acute schistosomiasis, particularly in the very early stages and in 'immunologically naive' patients, could sometimes remain undiagnosed by the exclusive use of stool examination.

2.1.1 Stool examination

The detection of eggs or miracidia in stool samples is the traditional way to confirm an infection with *S. japonicum*. For quantification of faecal egg counts, the Kato-Katz method, originally developed in the mid-1950s by the Japanese researchers Kato and Miura (1954) and later standardized by the introduction of a 41.7 mg templates by Katz et al. (1972) in Brazil, is the most broadly used technique in epidemiological surveys pertaining to intestinal schistosomiasis. The number of eggs per gram (EPG) faeces is used as an index of the intensity of infection dividing cases into three categories: light infection (EPG <100), medium infection ($100 \leq$ EPG < 400) and heavy infection (EPG ≥ 400) as recommended by the World Health Organization (WHO, 2002). In spite of reduced utility with regard to light infections, the Kato-Katz thick stool smear remains the most commonly used technique for general prevalence mapping and field-based control of schistosomiasis.

Among other traditional tests, the hatching test, based on the positive phototrophic behaviour of schistosome miracidia, relies on the observation of released miracidia from parasite eggs hatched in faeces diluted in water and allowed to sediment (Qiu and Xue, 1990). The sensitivity of hatching technique is supposedly higher than the Kato-Katz thick-smear method due to the large volume of faeces investigated (Zhu et al., 2014). Sometimes, the hatching technique, followed by microscopic examination of faecal sediment, can be implemented to improve sensitivity (Xu et al., 2007). However, the result is influenced by temperature, quality of the water added and examiner experience. The slight improvement of sensitivity achieved may not justify wider use due to the added time and cost required.

2.1.2 Tissue biopsy

When a schistosome infection is suspected but no eggs are found in faeces after multiple examinations, proctoscopy combined with rectal biopsy could be attempted to find eggs deposited in the intestinal mucosa. However, this is a clinical, hospital-based approach that does not play a role in large-scale, control schemes. In addition, the use of this approach in practice is limited as it has a low level of acceptance by patients and physicians alike due to associated complications, such as bleeding and the high possibility of sampling error (Yu et al., 1989).

2.2 Imaging techniques

Radiology, now generally replaced by computer tomography (CT) and magnetic resonance imaging (MRI) when searching for schistosome-induced hepatic or hepatosplenic enlargement, must be carried out in a hospital environment. Ultrasonography (US), on the other hand, represents a more versatile approach with several advantages. Not only can the technology be adopted for field use, but it is also less costly while still capable of demonstrating the classical features of periportal fibrosis (appearing as a netlike echogenic pattern in *S. japonicum* infection), hepatic granuloma and gallbladder thickening. The US approach is especially helpful for documenting advanced schistosomiasis. However, the technique is not only useful in the diagnosis and differential diagnosis of advanced schistosomiasis, but also for the guidance of treatment and evaluation of therapeutic effects and, furthermore, for risk prediction of portal hypertension and upper gastrointestinal haemorrhage (Wu et al., 2015). The introduction of portable US equipment broadened the applicability of diagnostic, imagery investigations in endemic community settings.

Although the US technology originated in 1940s and was not used for schistosomiasis investigations until the 1980s (Zhou et al., 2009), it has now overtaken the other imaging techniques in importance. However, the diagnostic characteristics of all three methodologies are similar in that they are noninvasive and record the damage of intra-abdominal organs in a straightforward way. Imaging approaches are therefore particularly suitable for the diagnosis of ectopic schistosomiasis, eg, neuroschistosomiasis (Ross et al., 2012). Together with CT and MRI, US facilitates the detection of lesions, such as pathological enlargements and tissue oedema, which is suitable for location before clinical, invasive procedures (Fang and Xu, 2014; Li, 2015; Lv and Pei, 2007; Shen et al., 2012; Wang et al., 2014; Yang, 2015). While CT and MRI are not routinely used for schistosomiasis diagnosis in resource-poor areas for economic reasons and US is particularly useful in the field, all three techniques require highly qualified users with medical education and special training.

2.3 Immunological tests

Immunological tests for schistosomiasis diagnosis have a long history in The People's Republic of China. These tests were developed to detect the antibody or circulating schistosome antigens based on various labelling techniques emphasizing advantages such as high sensitivity, easy use and rapidity.

2.3.1 The intradermal test

The earliest test based on immune reactions in The People's Republic of China is the intradermal test (ID) introduced by Gan (1936), who adopted this approach from work described for other schistosome species. Antigens aimed at the detection of specific IgE antibodies were extracted from fresh or frozen adult worms, eggs, miracidia or cercaria and their diagnostic efficacy was evaluated in a trial. The advantages of ID, such as ease of use, low cost and high sensitivity (estimated at 90%) facilitated its implementation in the early 1950s in the national schistosomiasis control programme to investigate the distribution and prevalence of schistosomiasis japonica (Maegraith, 1958; Mao and Shao, 1982). However, the specificity was low, so it was soon replaced by other tests.

2.3.2 The circumoval precipitin test

This assay was originally described by Liu et al. (1958) and widely used in The People's Republic of China in the remaining part of last century. Circumoval precipitin test (COPT) substitutes intact fresh parasite eggs for the antigen preparation, which normally consists of schistosome eggs that have been lyophilized or subjected to heat and/or ultrasound. It has a high sensitivity (94–99%) and adequate specificity with low, false positive rates in healthy people from nonendemic areas (2–4%) (Li, 1991). After effective treatment for 4 years, alternatively 3–8 years, the negative reversion rates were 82.5% and 80–83%, respectively (Li, 1991). However, with repeated treatments in the controlled areas leading to very low rates of prevalence and intensity of infection, the sensitivity of the test declined to 70–80% (Song et al., 2003). The technique is, however, comparatively complicated and time-consuming (48 h for recording the results in the laboratory) and requires microscopy, issues that limit its wider application in endemic areas these days.

2.3.3 The indirect haemagglutination assay

Soluble antigen preparations are necessary for tests relying on agglutination of microscopic particles, eg, sheep erythrocytes as used in the indirect haemagglutination assay (IHA), a test first employed for the diagnosis of *S. japonicum* in The People's Republic of China by Tao (Shi et al., 1980). Erythrocytes sensitized with schistosomes antigens in a first step will agglutinate when antibodies against such antigens in patients' serum samples combine with the antigens on the cell surfaces. After multiple modifications by Chinese scientists, the diagnostic efficacy and stability of IHA have been improved significantly. The sensitivity of IHA has thus reached 93–100%, while the false positive rate in healthy people from nonendemic areas have come down to 2–3%, and which have the diagnostic value in early infection (Chen et al., 2011a; Wang et al., 2010; Yang et al., 2009). After effective, periodical treatment for 3 years or more, most former schistosomiasis patients turn negative in the test. IHA remains a widely used general immunoassay in The People's Republic of China, secondary only to COPT in having been used for more than 50 years (Zhu et al., 2009).

2.3.4 The enzyme-linked immunosorbent assay

Enzyme-linked immunosorbent assay (ELISA) detects the presence of specific antibodies (or antigens) in samples based on the specific combination of antibody and antigen made visible by the addition of secondary antibodies labelled with an enzyme-substrate (Engvall and Perlmann, 1971). Yan and Lv (1978) were the first to develop and use ELISA for the diagnosis of schistosomiasis in The People's Republic of China. The sensitivity of routine applications of ELISA based on SEA reaches 95–99% in *S. japonicum* egg-positive individuals with a conversion rate of 59–60% 1–2 years after effective treatment, while the false positive rates in a nonendemic area remain low at 1–4% (Li, 1991). Special treatment of the antigens or modification of the assay components can improve the diagnostic efficacy of ELISA and extend its application. Various ELISA modifications, including the

Falcon assay screening test (FAST-ELISA), the avidin-biotin-peroxidase complex assay (ABC-ELISA) and the fractioned-antigen (FA-ELISA), have been explored and developed for antibody detection (Wang and Li, 1990; Zhang et al., 1986; Zhu et al., 1996). In the past 20 years, many assays based on recombinant peptide antigens have reported excellent sensitivity and specificity, eg, rSj26GST (Xie et al., 1995), rSj23HD (Ren et al., 2001), rSj32 (Shu et al., 1998). The rSP13-ELISA tool developed by Dr Xu et al. (2014b) have shown substantial advantages over simple egg-detection and SEA-ELISA, including adequate sensitivity and specificity needed in areas characterized by low levels of transmission. Application of such tools may allow identification of cases with low-intensity infections for targeted treatment (Zhou, 2014).

With the advent of the hybridoma technique by Kohler and Milstein (1975), a number of monoclonal antibodies reactive with specific schistosome antigens were developed in The People's Republic of China and used for the detection of CAg (Zhu, 2005). Using nitrocellulose and other paper membranes as carrier, Yan et al. developed a dot-ELISA kit with a monoclonal antibody against the *S. japonicum* circulating cathodic antigen (CCA) linked with peroxidase, which detected 90.6% and 83.2% of acute and chronic schistosomiasis patients, respectively (Yan et al., 1990). Although various ELISA-based monoclonal antibody assays on for antigen detection were explored by Chinese scientists, they are not widely used due to unsatisfactory sensitivity in patients, especially with light infections (Guan and Shi, 1996; Yi et al., 1995). As an ELISA reader is required for most kits and the delay before it is possible to inspect the results is usually 2–3 h, ELISA is mainly a laboratory-based tool that cannot be easily adapted for large-scale use in field settings.

2.3.5 Rapid diagnostic kits

As diagnosis in the field needs to be settled at the point of care, which means minutes rather than waiting a few hours as the case is with ELISA-type assays. To that end, rapid diagnostic kits based on immunofiltration or immunochromatography principles with dyes or colloid metals as markers have been developed. For example, Ding et al. (1998) developed the dot immunogold filtration assay (DIGFA) for schistosomiasis japonica diagnosis based on SEA as antigen and rabbit–antihuman IgG labelled with colloidal gold as probe, while Tang et al. (2008) developed the assay further by using a sheep antihuman IgM immunogold conjugate as probe to detect specific IgM anti-*S. japonicum* antibody that produced positive rates for acute and chronic schistosomiasis at 100% and 96% sensitivity, respectively. The specificity was also good, with only 3% of patients infected with *Paragonimus westermani* reacting positively in the test (Tang et al., 2008). The dipstick dye immunoassay (DDIA) is another rapid diagnostic approach, which is basically a chromatography technique with SEA labelled with a dye as indicator. It was first produced by He et al. (2000) and further developed by Zhu et al. and Song et al. (Song, et al. 2003; Zhu, et al. 2002; Zhu, 2005). This test has a high sensitivity for both acute and chronic cases of schistosomiasis (97% and 94–97%, respectively) and specificity of 97% when tested with healthy people from nonendemic communities. This assay was also adopted for *Schistosomiasis mekongi* diagnosis (Zhu et al., 2005b), while Ding and Yu modified the technique and made it capable of the detection of specific antibodies also in whole-blood samples, ie, the dipstick latex immunochromatography assay (DLIA). It has high sensitivity (95% for serum and 94% for whole-blood) and specificity (95% for serum and 97% for whole-blood) with no cross-reaction with *Clonorchis* or intestinal nematodes including *Angiostrongylus cantonensis* (Ding et al., 2010; Yu et al., 2011). All the rapid diagnostic assays mentioned previously are suitable for general field screenings since they can be read within 5–10 min without need of a microscope or other special equipment.

It should finally be mentioned that recent advances in the detection of CAg have solved the problem of low sensitivity that has plagued this approach for decades. The upconverting phosphate lateral flow (UCP-LF) (Corstjens et al., 2014; van Dam et al., 2013) presents previously unimaginable sensitivity (a few worm pairs) and specificity (Corstjens et al., 2014). A small-scale field trial conducted in a low-endemic areas in The People's Republic of China has shown that UCP-LF can be used for the diagnosis of *S. japonicum* infection based on the excretion of CCA in urine samples (van Dam et al., 2015), a fact that will aid complacency. The assay exhibited a much higher sensitivity than that of the Kato-Katz technique and detected a significant number of egg-negative cases.

2.4 Techniques based on molecular biotechnology

Better diagnostic tests for schistosomiasis are needed both in the field and in the clinic. Future research for the diagnosis of aetiology may depend on molecular tools such as PCR- or LAMP-based approaches. Improved results have been achieved with multiplex PCR (amplification of several different DNA sequences simultaneously) and real-time PCR (monitoring the amplification of a targeted DNA molecule continuously rather than only at its end) (ten Hove et al., 2008).

PCR has shown great sensitivity and specificity for the detection of *Schistosoma* DNA in a variety of samples (Gomes et al., 2010; Pontes et al., 2003;

ten Hove et al., 2008). After Lier et al. proved the feasibility of molecular methods for detecting *S. japonicum* DNA (Lier et al., 2006, 2008, 2009), Xia et al. developed a specific PCR assay for the highly repetitive retrotransposon SjR2 of *S. japonicum* DNA based on an animal model infected with *S. japonicum* detecting *S. japonicum* DNA down at 0.8 pg (10^{-12} g), which approaches the level of one EPG of stool. *Schistosoma japonicum* DNA could be detected in sera at the first week postinfection and became negative 10 weeks posttreatment (Xia et al., 2009). Fung et al. (2012) developed a faecal PCR assay using the same primer to detect *S. japonicum* infection in humans and bovines in The People's Republic of China. The test was highly sensitive, detecting *S. japonicum* DNA at 0.5 EPG of stool.

Based on the sequence of SjR2, a LAMP assay, without requirement of a thermocycling machine or electrophoresis equipment, was designed and the results showed that this method was able to detect 0.08 fg (10^{-15} g) S. *japonicum* DNA, which was 10^4 times more sensitive than conventional PCR (Xu et al., 2010, 2015). The test has a high sensitivity of 95–97% for the diagnosis of *S. japonicum* infected patients with the lowest intensity (EPG <10) (Xu et al., 2015). After treatment with praziquantel, the negative conversion rate increased from 23.4% to 83.0% at 3 months and 9 months posttreatment according to LAMP, where the seroconversion rate remained at a low level (25.5% by ELISA and 31.9% by IHA) even 9 months after treatment (Xu et al., 2010, 2015).

These studies presented previously demonstrate that PCR and LAMP are effective diagnostic tools for early diagnosis and evaluation of therapy effectiveness for *S. japonicum* infection in schistosomiasis-endemic areas with low-intensity infection. However, the dependence on expensive apparatus and the need for specialized, trained technicians, restrict the widespread applications of PCR for testing under field conditions (Guo et al., 2012; Kato-Hayashi et al., 2015; Sandoval et al., 2006). As LAMP has the potential value for field use, further studies based on real field settings need to be conducted to evaluate their diagnostic efficacy and operational characteristics. However, it should be borne in mind that stool examination may fail depending on the timing of release of parasite eggs in the stool.

3. DIAGNOSTIC APPLICATIONS IN THE NATIONAL SCHISTOSOMIASIS CONTROL PROGRAMME

Since the 1950s when the national campaign against schistosomiasis began in The People's Republic of China, the application and development of diagnostic techniques have undergone shifts. However, an approach that is useful in practice is almost always a compromise between quality and quantity because the techniques needed for large-scale application must be based on cost-effectiveness, precision, simplicity and stability (Bergquist et al., 2009). The key of the matter is the required continuous adaption of the diagnostic focus to the stage of control. Fig. 1 shows the various stages of a schistosomiasis control programme juxtaposed with the type of diagnostic tools that should be employed to reach the set goals.

3.1 The morbidity control stage

At the early stage after the founding of The People's Republic of China, there were a large number of people affected by schistosomiasis, and hence high infection prevalence and infection intensity were very common, especially during the 1950–1980 period. Treatment of patients with severe illness to save their life and rescue the workforce was the primary task. The etiologic diagnostic techniques, including direct stool smear examination, sedimentation, concentration and hatching, combined with a questionnaire approach, were almost compulsory in the identification of individuals for mass chemotherapy because of high infection intensity and toxicity of available effective drugs, eg, antimonials, for treatment. The parasitological techniques had a better diagnostic efficacy, while the immunodiagnostic approach commonly produced false positive results that increased the number of individuals receiving unnecessary chemotherapy. Eventually, immunodiagnostics were only adapted for screening prior to further parasitological examination. In the national general survey initiated in 1956, the strategy of first screening populations by ID followed by stool examination for those who reacted positively when subjected to ID testing made it possible to rapidly understand the distribution and endemic characteristics of schistosomiasis.

The development and release of praziquantel for clinical use in the 1970s was a milestone for schistosomiasis control (Tambo et al., 2015). High efficacy against all species of human schistosomiasis, use in single oral dose and with none or only mild side effects made praziquantel highly attractive, and when the cost fell dramatically in the 1990s, it could be used for mass drug administration (MDA). Along with the reduced intensity of infection that resulted, the limited sensitivity of the parasitological, diagnostic techniques in use became apparent and control programme managers looked for replacements, such as immunological techniques based on both antigen and antibody detection (Bergquist et al., 2009, 2015; Doenhoff

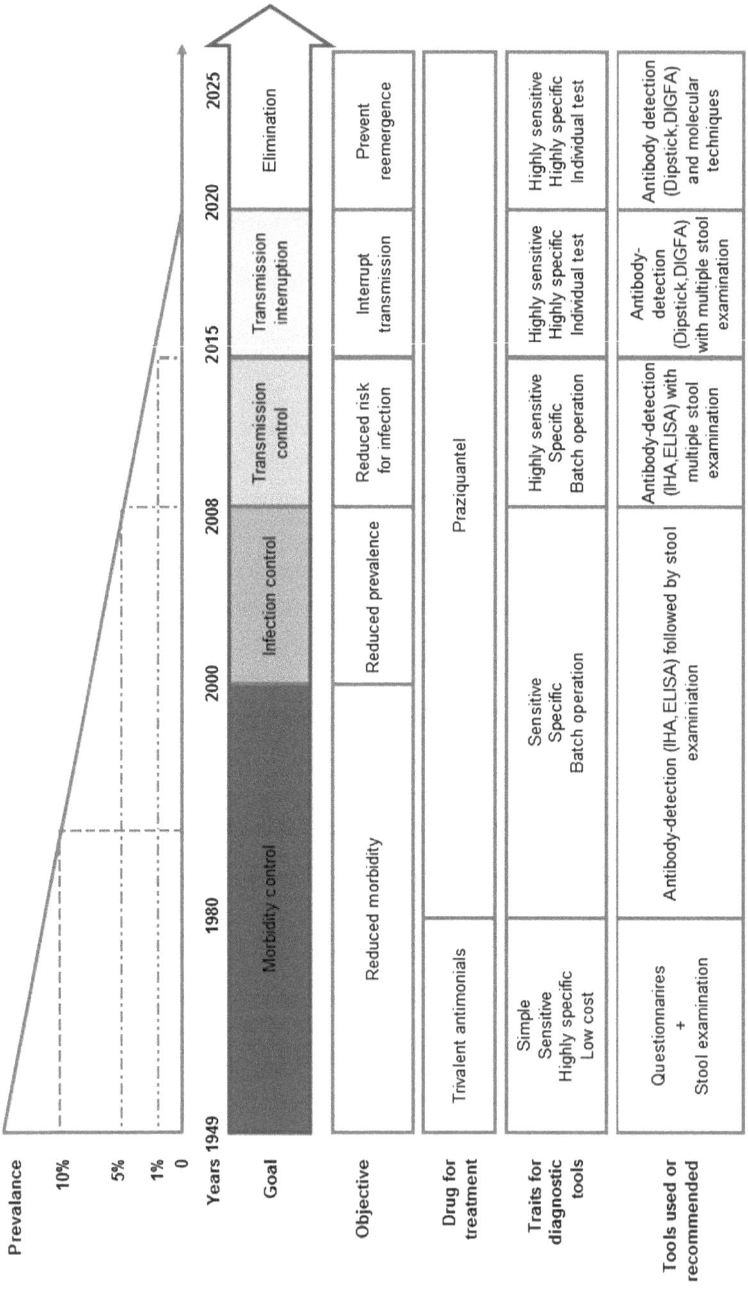

Figure 1 Diagnostic tools shift with the control stage and drug used for schistosomiasis control in The People's Republic of China.

et al., 2004; van Lieshout et al., 2000; Wu, 2002). In the implementation of 10-year World Bank Loan Project (WBLP) for schistosomiasis control initiated in 1992 (Chen et al., 2005) in The People's Republic of China aiming for morbidity control, diagnostic strategies varied according to prevalence strata and chemotherapy strategies. For instance, in areas of high endemicity (prevalence ≥15%), all individuals between 6 and 60 years old without examination were given yearly treatment. In areas of medium endemicity (15% > prevalence > 3%) and low endemicity (prevalence <3%), residents or special populations were screened by Kato-Katz method or a serological test (ELISA, COPT or IHA). The final evaluation in 2002 showed that infection rates in humans had decreased by 55% (Chen et al., 2005).

The way used for the epidemiological surveys was performed in differed methodologies according to perceived infection status and diagnostic techniques available. Direct stool examination was the only method to evaluate the prevalence of schistosomiasis in the first national sampling survey in 1989. With the development of immunological techniques and the decrease of infection intensity and prevalence in some endemic areas, direct stool examination was only used in highly endemic areas, while serological survey followed by stool examination were used where morbidity control had been reached. In the national survey conducted in 2004 after the WBLP terminated, prevalence was estimated using ELISA screening prior to stool examination as the endemicity of schistosomiasis had then decreased significantly in most endemic counties (Chen, 2014).

3.2 The infection control stage

Once morbidity is under control, infection control through decreasing prevalence and prevention of reinfection is the next target. This situation, characterized by less MDA and predominantly low-intensity infections, requires more sensitive diagnostic techniques to support the distribution of chemotherapy. In 2004, a medium- and long-term national strategic plan for schistosomiasis control was initiated in The People's Republic of China to face the challenges after the termination of the WBLP. To reach the medium goal for infection control by 2008, diagnostic and chemotherapy strategies were determined according to the prevalence of schistosomiasis based on the situation at the administrative village level. Apart from inquiry examinations conducted in villages with prevalence higher than 10%, serological methods were implemented annually, every 2 years or every 3 years for residents aged 6–65 years in villages with an estimated prevalence of 5–10%, 1–5%, 0–1%, respectively. Once infected snails were detected, serological survey would be conducted no matter the estimated prevalence of schistosomiasis in the same year (Ministry of Health, 2005; Zhou et al., 2007).

In areas having reached the stage of infection control, the survey tools shifted from direct Kato-Katz for all to initial immunological screening to increase the diagnostic efficiency and compliance rate of residents being examined (Zhu et al., 2009). A system with primary immunodiagnostic screen followed by Kato-Katz tests for the antibody-positive individuals (Balen et al., 2007; Utzinger et al., 2005) was advised. This approach is currently widely used in the Chinese national control programme as well as for community surveys and field studies. In addition, to evaluate the effect of interventions conducted and understand the changes in the endemic areas, the number of national sentinel sites was enlarged from 14 in 6 endemic provinces in 1990 to 80 in 9 endemic provinces and potential prevalent areas in Chongqing city with potential risk of endemics in 2005 in the national surveillance system due to the decrease of prevalence and general improvement of the situation (Cao et al., 2016; Zhu et al., 2011).

3.3 The transmission control stage

With the implementation of integrated control strategy based on interventions to reduce the rate of transmission of *S. japonicum* infection from cattle and humans to snails in the national control programme, the prevalence of schistosomiasis decreased to the lowest level in history and infection control was reached nationwide in 2008 (Hao et al., 2009; Wang et al., 2009). The whole country is now moving forward to transmission control, ie, nationwide prevalence <1% based at the village level (Utzinger et al., 2005; Zhou et al., 2005). At this phase, selective chemotherapy with praziquantel becomes the main strategy due to the significant decrease of infection rate in humans. However, this stage requires considerably more sensitive diagnostic tools to accurately identify infected individuals. At this stage, the Kato-Katz 'missing rate' increases significantly and can reach as high as 80% when the level of prevalence, accompanied by much lower infection intensities, falls to the <1% level (Lin et al., 2008; Zhu et al., 2005a). At egg excretion levels from the host below 100 EPG of stool, it becomes increasingly difficult to unequivocally determine whether or not there is an infection (Feldmeier and Poggensee, 1993). Although multiple Kato-Katz thick smears per sample, or increasing the frequency of stool sample collection, would boost diagnostic sensitivity (Huang et al., 2007; Xu et al., 2011a; Zhu et al., 2005a), this approach could not be used at a large scale due to the workload and increased costs as well as the risk of waning compliancy.

The Chinese criteria of schistosomiasis control and elimination recommend evaluating whether a place has reached the stage of transmission by an immunological assay followed by the hatching test as it is regarded as more sensitive than the Kato-Katz technique. Conducting multiple methods for the same stool sample at the same time would also increase the sensitivity of the diagnostic strategy. This approach has been integrated into the revised national surveillance system since 2011 (Zhang et al., 2012). An analysis shows that the parasitological final positive rates for individuals testing positively serologically have increased from 4.6% by the Kato-Katz method and 5.9% by the hatching technique to 7.1% when these two methods are used in combination (Zhu et al., 2013b).

3.4 The stage of transmission interruption and elimination

The People's Republic of China has now reached the stage when the priority is shifting from traditional monitoring to surveillance and response with the focus on reinfection in areas targeted for elimination (Cao et al., 2016; Xu et al., 2014a; Zhou et al., 2013). The most urgent need at this time is reliable assessment of control efficacy and the determination of target populations for chemotherapy in different areas as well as certification of elimination using sensitive and specific assays. The immunological techniques needed now must be fast, highly sensitive and specific. Various approaches fulfil these requirements, eg, molecular methods such as PCR, real-time PCR and LAMP could be conducted in well-equipment hospitals and laboratories; the latter can even be used in the field (Zhang et al., 2016).

The UCP-LF test (Corstjens et al., 2014; van Dam et al., 2013), on the other hand, detects CAg at a previously unimaginable sensitivity and specificity making it possible to detect infections due to only a few worm pairs (Corstjens et al., 2014). The other great advantage with this approach is that it can detect CAg both in serum and urine, the latter being more acceptable to the general public should allow the large number of test that will be needed in the elimination phase. However, further technical improvements may be needed to make the test more convenient, simple and applicable for large-scale field operations.

4. QUALITY CONTROL

Diagnosis would supply information for planning the control activities as well as assessing the strategy or effects of control measures. As many factors, such as laboratory conditions, diagnostic methods/assays chosen, technician capacity, etc. impact the quality of the final diagnosis (Tokmalaev and Bezborodov, 1982). The People's Republic of China has strengthened monitoring and management with respect to diagnostic activities. For example, criteria for schistosomiasis diagnosis have been issued to provide guidance for the technical staff and standardize the diagnostic approach. Guidelines are regularly updated by the Ministry of Health with consideration to available technology and supplies as well as the stage of control and clinical symptoms, including history of water contact, previous laboratory examinations (Minstry of Health, 2006). These criteria define the principles and basis for diagnosis and differentiation between acute, chronic and advanced cases.

Assessment of the efficacy, reliability and operational characteristics of assays in use are important for the assurance of the diagnostic accuracy. With the development and implementation of CAg assays in The People's Republic of China, three collaborative studies were conducted (in 1993, 1995 and 1996) to evaluate all existing CAg kits. In 1993, eight assays using monoclonal or polyclonal probes were evaluated and the results showed that most of the tests had low sensitivities ranging from 15% to 73% in chronic and light infection, respectively (Yi et al., 1995). The evaluation conducted in 1995 showed that 10 of 14 kits investigated had a specificity above 90% but only four assays showed a sensitivity higher than 60% (Guan and Shi, 1996). In 1996, 12 CAg kits displayed a similar diagnostic efficacy as in 1995 (Feng et al., 1998). These evaluations demonstrate that the CAg kits evaluated were inappropriate for use by the schistosomiasis control programme at that time, especially in endemic areas characterized by low-level infections. At the same time, nine assays for antibody detection were evaluated and the results showed that most kits had a specificity over 90% and sensitivity higher than 80% in chronic infection (Feng et al., 1998). Comprehensive evaluations conducted in 2004 and 2008, respectively, also showed that the sensitivity and specificity both were above 90% for most reagents (Xu et al., 2005, 2011b). A field evaluation conducted later proved that these antibody-based assays were acceptable as tools for community survey and for targeting chemotherapy.

The results of the assessments mentioned previously demonstrate that many diagnostic methods in use need to be controlled for quality, and when they are investigated the standards are often not good enough. Before 2008, many assays for schistosomiasis diagnosis were used without having passed certification by the State Food and Drug Administration (SFDA) in The People's Republic of China. However, the evaluations carried out provided data for that the manufacturer could use to apply for licence from SFDA. Until now, nine kits have been accredited by SFDA, which indicates that the situation is improving and already some assays are quality controlled with good results (Table 1).

To strengthening the capacity for schistosomiasis diagnostics, the Chinese Centres for Disease Control (China CDC) organizes since 2009 a diagnostic platform run through a set of reference or sentinel laboratories for external quality control activities, and also holds training courses. So far, one national diagnostic centre has been established in the National Institute of Parasitic Disease, Shanghai, The People's Republic of China. It is responsible for assay assessments; external control and improvement of the diagnostic quality control scheme; planning and organizing training activities; and providing technical support for subordinate laboratories. Further, 12 reference laboratories at the provincial institutes and 16 sentinel laboratories at the county level were set up in charge of the activities related with diagnostic activities (Qin et al., 2013; Zhang et al., 2016). Subsequently, several provinces established their own diagnostic platforms to enhance management of diagnostics. Chen et al. (2011b) organized three external control activities focused on the hatching technique in 2006, 2008 and 2009, respectively. The average accuracy rates of the hatching technique in 18, 28 and 33 laboratories in Zhejiang

Table 1 Immunodiagnostic assay kits for schistosomiasis diagnosis registered and accredited by The People's Republic of China Food and Drug Administration

Type of assay	Probe/target	Company
IHA[a]	SEA/IgG	Yueyang Xunchao Biotechnology Co., Ltd.
IHA[a]	SEA/IgG	Anhui Anji Medical Technology Co., Ltd.
DIGFA[b]	SEA/IgG	Yueyang Xunchao Biotechnology Co., Ltd.
DIGFA[b]	SEA/IgG	Sichuan Maike Biotechnology Co., Ltd.
DIGFA[b]	SEA/IgG	Shanghai Jikong Biotechnology Co., Ltd.
DDIA[c]	SEA/IgG	Wuxi Saide Technology Development Co., Ltd.
MPAIA[d]	SEA/IgG	Beijing Beiaikang Biological technology Co., Ltd.
ELISA[e]	SEA/IgG	Shenzhen Huakang Biomedical Engineering Co., Ltd.
ELISA[e]	Not clear/ Circulating antigen	Sichuan Maike Biotechnology Co., Ltd.

[a]Indirect haemagglutination assay.
[b]Dot immunogold filtration assay.
[c]Dipstick dye immunoassay kit.
[d]Magnetic particle antibody immunoassay.
[e]Enzyme-linked immunosorbent assay.

Province (where transmission was interrupted in 1995) were 88.9%, 100% and 93.9%, respectively. The diagnostic capacity was strengthened through repeated training and control activities.

5. CURRENT CHALLENGES

In the process of schistosomiasis control, rapid and reliable diagnostic techniques are necessary and important to identify targets accurately for treatment. Current diagnostic technology for schistosomiasis is useful in The People's Republic of China but big challenges exist when moving towards elimination.

Firstly, the stability and quality of the diagnostic assays are overestimated. Although most diagnostic kits/assays performed excellent diagnostic efficacy based on laboratory evaluation, or in a small-scale field assessment, their sensitivity and/or specificity normally decreased when evaluated in the field (Xu et al., 2007; Zhou et al., 2011) Although there are several immunological kits accredited by SFDA, the quality of immunological diagnosis kits available in the market is uneven (Xin et al., 2006). Novel approaches, such as PCR and LAMP, demonstrating excellent sensitivity and specificity as reported, mainly focused on laboratory evaluation, still need multicentre assessment both in laboratories and field settings as there are more factors, such as storage, transportation and operation, etc., influences the diagnostic efficacy and stability of the results. Because of the high sensitivity of PCR and LAMP, attention must be paid to the possibility of false positive by potential pollution in the laboratory.

Secondly, the endemic status is underestimated due to the current diagnostic strategy. The currently available antibody-based serological assays cannot distinguish active infection from previous infection or reinfection, which makes it difficult to determine prevalence directly. Theoretically, if the sensitivity of a screening tool is less than 100%, the sensitivity of current diagnostic strategy using serological screening followed by stool examination will be lower than that of direct stool examination, which hinders the process of schistosomiasis elimination due to missed infected cases although they may be very few. Although detection of schistosome CAg is regarded as an effective approach in theory, only the UCP-LF approach has shown the sensitivity required; other assays that have been tested demonstrated an unsatisfactory specificity and insufficient sensitivity, especially in patients with light infections, eg, chronic cases. Further studies should be considered to explore assay systems based on defined antigens or particular antigenic epitopes and corresponding isotype-restricted antibody responses in combination with the advantages of antibody or antigen detection, which are duration and titre dependent.

Thirdly, the diagnostic capacity in control stations is weak and needs to be strengthened. Feng et al. (2011) conducted a survey showing the poor quality of diagnostic laboratories in charge of national surveillance for schistosomiasis. The results showed that the average age of laboratory staff was 40.93 ± 9.56 years old and 69% of the personnel were older than 35 years, 86% of whom had an education background below the BA degree. Also the equipment in most laboratories needs to be improved and updated. In addition, the diagnostic capacity varied significantly among different places (Wang et al., 2015; Zang et al., 2013). Zhu et al. (2013a) prepared specimen panels with eight common helminth eggs, which was examined by 48 personnel from Hubei and Hunan Provinces. Schistosome eggs were misdiagnosed by 6% of the technicians and negative smears were misdiagnosed by half of them. This results clearly show that the diagnostic capacity must be strengthened, which should include training and modernizing outdated equipment.

6. CONCLUSIONS

Above all, the use of appropriate, sensitive diagnostic tools to identify infected individuals is imperative to control and prevent the morbidity caused by schistosomiasis. Control that appropriate diagnostic tools are applied would be extremely helpful in implementing strategies for the control and elimination of schistosomiasis. The persistence of the disease in some regions where schistosomiasis remains endemic despite massive and integrated control programmes conducted continuously may be partially due to lack of accurate diagnostic tools for case detection and community screening. The most widely used diagnostic approaches in The People's Republic of China are stool examination by Kato-Katz method, the hatching technique, while immunological assays, especially antibody detection, are used for screening. Usually, parasitological tests are performed after a positive screening test to establish a definitive diagnosis.

A variety of diagnostic techniques, ranging from basic microscopic detection to sophisticated molecular approaches, have been developed for detection of schistosome infections. The ideal diagnostic test (or set of tests) should provide an accurate diagnosis preferably performed once, be cost-effective in terms of labour, sample processing, equipment and reagents.

Implementation of appropriate diagnostic tools for all endemic areas and targeted populations remains a determining factor in the acceleration of the progress of the national schistosomiasis control programme in The People's Republic of China. As the next goal is to interrupt the transmission and then finally eliminate schistosomiasis, the test to be used for case detection at this stage needs to have very high sensitivity and specificity as most endemic areas are characterized by low transmission and low prevalence. As the test systems in current use do not meet the stringent criteria that will dominate at the elimination stage, it is imperative to develop more effective approaches for case finding and surveillance.

To ensure the accuracy and reliability of data obtained through diagnostic work, diagnostic capacity building should be strengthened through external quality control and professional training. The quality of the diagnostic tools in use should be monitored based on laboratory or field assessments using the national schistosomiasis laboratory network platforms. As schistosomiasis japonica is a zoonotic disease, this would apply also for the veterinary sciences with respect to the diagnosis of schistosomiasis in livestock (Cao et al., 2016; Yang et al., 2016). These activities will be very important for monitoring the elimination of schistosomiasis.

ACKNOWLEDGEMENTS

This manuscript was supported by the National Natural Science Foundation of The People's Republic of China (grant no. 81301454) and China–UK Global Health Support Programme (grant no.: GHSP-CS-OP1-01).

REFERENCES

Allen, A.V., Ridley, D.S., 1970. Further observations on the formol-ether concentration technique for faecal parasites. J. Clin. Pathol. 23, 545–546.

Balen, J., Zhao, Z.Y., Williams, G.M., McManus, D.P., Raso, G., Utzinger, J., et al., 2007. Prevalence, intensity and associated morbidity of *Schistosoma japonicum* infection in the Dongting Lake region, China. Bull. World Health Organ. 85, 519–526.

Bergquist, R., Johansen, M.V., Utzinger, J., 2009. Diagnostic dilemmas in helminthology: what tools to use and when? Trends Parasitol. 25, 151–156.

Bergquist, R., Yang, G.J., Knopp, S., Utzinger, J., Tanner, M., 2015. Surveillance and response: tools and approaches for the elimination stage of neglected tropical diseases. Acta Trop. 141, 229–234.

Cao, Z.G., Zhao, Y.E., Willingham, A.L., Wang, T.P., 2016. Towards the elimination of schistosomiasis japonica through control of the disease in domestic animals in the People's Republic of China: a tale of over 60 years. Adv. Parasitol. 92.

Chen, M.G., Feng, Z., 1999. Schistosomiasis control in China. Parasitol. Int. 48, 11–19.

Chen, X.Y., Wang, L.Y., Jiming, C., Zhou, X.N., Zheng, J., Guo, J.G., et al., 2005. Schistosomiasis control in China: the impact of a 10-year World Bank Loan Project (1992–2001). Bull. World Health Organ. 83, 43–48.

Chen, N.G., Lin, D.D., Xie, S.Y., Wang, Q.Z., Tang, L., liu, Y.M., et al., 2011a. Diagnostic efficiency of indirect hemagglutination assay kit for antibody detection of schistosomiasis japonica. Chin. J. Schistosomiasis Control 23, 377–380 (in Chinese).

Chen, W., Zhu, M.D., Yan, X.L., Lin, L.J., Zhang, J.F., Li, L., et al., 2011b. Quality control assessments of feces examination for schistosomiasis in province-level laboratories of Zhejiang Province. Chin. J. Schistosomiasis Control 23, 318–320 (in Chinese).

Chen, M.G., 2014. Assessment of morbidity due to *Schistosoma japonicum* infection in China. Infect. Dis. Poverty 3, 6.

Collins, C., Xu, J., Tang, S., 2012. Schistosomiasis control and the health system in P.R. China. Infect. Dis. Poverty 1, 8.

Corstjens, P.L., De Dood, C.J., Kornelis, D., Fat, E.M., Wilson, R.A., Kariuki, T.M., et al., 2014. Tools for diagnosis, monitoring and screening of *Schistosoma* infections utilizing lateral-flow based assays and upconverting phosphor labels. Parasitology 141, 1841–1855.

Dabo, A., Diarra, A.Z., Machault, V., Toure, O., Niambele, D.S., Kante, A., et al., 2015. Urban schistosomiasis and associated determinant factors among school children in Bamako, Mali, West Africa. Infect. Dis. Poverty 4, 4.

Ding, J.Z., Gan, X.X., Shen, H.Y., Shen, L.Y., Yu, J., 1998. Establishment and application of dot immunogold filtration assay for detection of anti-schistosome antibodies. Chin. J. Parasit. Dis. Control 11, 308–310 (in Chinese).

Ding, J.Z., Yu, L.L., Lou, D., Yan, X.L., Lu, S.H., Zhu, M.M., et al., 2010. Development and evaluation of a rapid immunochromatography assay for detection of the antibody against schistosoma japonica in whole-blood sample. Acta Parasit. Med. Entomol. Sin. 4, 198–202 (in Chinese).

Doenhoff, M.J., Chiodini, P.L., Hamilton, J.V., 2004. Specific and sensitive diagnosis of schistosome infection: can it be done with antibodies? Trends Parasitol. 20, 35–39.

Engels, D., Sinzinkayo, E., Gryseels, B., 1996. Day-to-day egg count fluctuation in Schistosoma mansoni infection and its operational implications. Am. J. Trop. Med. Hyg. 54, 319–324.

Engvall, E., Perlmann, P., 1971. Enzyme-linked immunosorbent assay (ELISA). Quantitative assay of immunoglobulin G. Immunochemistry 8, 871–874.

Fang, Y., Xu, L.H., 2014. Value of ultrasound in diagnosis of liver disease for chronic schistosomiasis. Chin. J. Schistosomiasis Control 29, 234 (in Chinese).

Feldmeier, H., Poggensee, G., 1993. Diagnostic techniques in schistosomiasis control. A review. Acta Trop. 52, 205–220.

Feng, Z., Qiu, L.Z., Chen, M.G., Qian, Z.L., Lu, P., Zhang, Y.H., et al., 1998. Current status analysis of schistosomiasis diagnostic reagents from results of parallel testing and monitoring in China. Chin. J. Parasitol. Parasit. Dis. 16, 321–325 (in Chinese).

Feng, T., Xu, J., Hang, D.R., Wu, Z.S., Tang, L., Wang, Q.Z., et al., 2011. Conditions of schistosomiasis laboratories at county level. Chin. J. Schistosomiasis Control 23, 370–376 (in Chinese).

Fung, M.S., Xiao, N., Wang, S., Carlton, E.J., 2012. Field evaluation of a PCR test for *Schistosoma japonicum* egg detection in low-prevalence regions of China. Am. J. Trop. Med. Hyg. 87, 1053–1058.

Gan, H.R., 1936. The intradermal test for antigen of *Schistosoma japonicum*. Chin. Med. J. 1, 387 (in Chinese).

Gomes, L.I., Dos Santos Marques, L.H., Enk, M.J., de Oliveira, M.C., Coelho, P.M., Rabello, A., 2010. Development and evaluation of a sensitive PCR-ELISA system for detection of schistosoma infection in feces. PLoS Negl. Trop. Dis. 4, e664.

Guan, X.H., Shi, Y.E., 1996. Collaborative study on evaluation of immunodiagnostic assays in schistosomiasis japonica by treatment efficacy assessment. Chin. Med. J. 109, 659–664 (in Chinese).

Guo, J.J., Zheng, H.J., Xu, J., Zhu, X.Q., Wang, S.Y., Xia, C.M., 2012. Sensitive and specific target sequences selected from retrotransposons of *Schistosoma japonicum* for the diagnosis of schistosomiasis. PLoS Negl. Trop. Dis. 6, e1579.

Hao, Y., Yi, D.H., Zhang, X.F., Xiong, J.J., Yuan, W.Z., Hu, S.J., et al., 2009. Assessment report on infection control of schistosomiasis in China, 2008. Chin. J. Schistosomiasis Control 21, 457–463 (in Chinese).

He, W., Zhu, Y.C., Hua, W., Liu, Y., 2000. Development of a rapid immunodiagnosis assay for schistosomiasis-colloidal dye strip immunoassay. Chin. J. Schistosomiasis Control 12, 18–20 (in Chinese).

Hillyer, G.V., Tsang, V.C., Vivas-Gonzalez, B.E., Noh, J., Ahn, L.H., Vorndam, V., 1999. Age-specific decrease in seroprevalence of schistosomiasis in Puerto Rico. Am. J. Trop. Med. Hyg. 60, 313–318.

Huang, M.J., Chen, N.G., Wu, Z.Q., Zhou, F., 2007. Comparison of effect of stool hatching method and Kato-Katz in the field examination of schistosomiasis. Chin. J. Schistosomiasis Control 19, 458–459 (in Chinese).

Kato, T., Miura, M., 1954. On the comparison of some stool examination methods. Jpn. J. Parasitol. 3, 35.

Kato-Hayashi, N., Leonardo, L.R., Arevalo, N.L., Tagum, M.N., Apin, J., Agsolid, L.M., et al., 2015. Detection of active schistosome infection by cell-free circulating DNA of *Schistosoma japonicum* in highly endemic areas in Sorsogon Province, the Philippines. Acta Trop. 141, 178–183.

Katz, N., Chaves, A., Pellegrino, J., 1972. A simple device for quantitative stool thick-smear technique in schistosomiasis mansoni. Rev. Inst. Med. Trop. Sao Paulo 14, 397–400.

Kohler, G., Milstein, C., 1975. Continuous cultures of fused cells secreting antibody of predefined specificity. Nature 256, 495–497.

Lei, Z.L., Zheng, H., Zhang, L.J., Zhu, R., Xu, Z.M., Xu, J., et al., 2014. Endemic status of schistosomiasis in People's Republic of China in 2013. Chin. J. Schistosomiasis Control 26, 591–597 (in Chinese).

Li, Y.H., 1991. Advance of the Study on Immunodiagnosis of Schistosomiasis. Jiangsu Science Technology Publishing House, (in Chinese), Nanjing.

Li, L., 2015. Value of ultrasound in diagnosis of liver disease for schistosomiasis in different stages. Proc. Clin. Med. 24, 308–310 (in Chinese).

Lier, T., Simonsen, G.S., Haaheim, H., Hjelmevoll, S.O., Vennervald, B.J., Johansen, M.V., 2006. Novel real-time PCr for detection of *Schistosoma japonicum* in stool. Southeast Asian J. Trop. Med. Public Health 37, 257–264.

Lier, T., Johansen, M.V., Hjelmevoll, S.O., Vennervald, B.J., Simonsen, G.S., 2008. Real-time PCR for detection of low intensity *Schistosoma japonicum* infections in a pig model. Acta Trop. 105, 74–80.

Lier, T., Simonsen, G.S., Wang, T., Lu, D., Haukland, H.H., Vennervald, B.J., et al., 2009. Real-time polymerase chain reaction for detection of low-intensity *Schistosoma japonicum* infections in China. Am. J. Trop. Med. Hyg. 81, 428–432.

Lin, D.D., Liu, J.X., Liu, Y.M., Hu, F., Zhang, Y.Y., Xu, J.M., et al., 2008. Routine Kato-Katz technique underestimates the prevalence of *Schistosoma japonicum*: a case study in an endemic area of the People's Republic of China. Parasitol. Int. 57, 281–286.

Liu, S., Wu, Y., Lu, S., 1958. Diagnosis value of COPT for schistosomiasis: observation of 1626 clinical cases and animal experiment. Chin. Med. J. 44, 640–642 (in Chinese).

Logan, O.T., 1905. A case of dysentery in Hunan province, cause by the trematoda, *schistosoma japonicum*. China Med. Missionary J. 19, 243–245.

Lv, Q.R., Pei, Y., 2007. Value of ultrasound in diagnosis of chronic schistosomiasis in transmission interrupted areas. J. Pract. Med. Tech. 14, 706 (in Chinese).

Maegraith, B., 1958. Schistosomiasis in China. Lancet 1, 208–214.

Mao, S.P., Shao, B.R., 1982. Schistosomiasis control in the people's Republic of China. Am. J. Trop. Med. Hyg. 31, 92–99.
Ministry of Health, 2005. Technical protocols of snails detecting and control, monitoring and chemotherapy in schistosomiasis control programme. In: Commnique for the Ministry of Health of the People's Republic of China, 2, pp. 57–59 (in Chinese).
Ministry of Health, 2006. Diagnostic Criteria for Schistosomiasis (WS261-2006). In: Beijing (in Chinese).
Pontes, L.A., Oliveira, M.C., Katz, N., Dias-Neto, E., Rabello, A., 2003. Comparison of a polymerase chain reaction and the Kato-Katz technique for diagnosing infection with *Schistosoma mansoni*. Am. J. Trop. Med. Hyg. 68, 652–656.
Qin, Z.Q., Xu, J., Feng, T., Zhu, H.Q., Li, S.Z., Xiao, N., et al., 2013. Strategic thinking of the construction of national schistosomiasis laboratory network in China. Chin. J. Schistosomiasis Control 25, 329–332 (in Chinese).
Qiu, L.Z., Xue, H.C., 1990. Experimental diagnosis. In: Mao, S.P. (Ed.), Schistosome Biology and Control of Schistosomiasis. Publishing House for People's Health, Beijing, pp. 448–527.
Ren, J.G., Zhu, Y.C., Harn, D.A., Yu, C.X., Si, J., Yin, X.R., et al., 2001. Protective immunity induced with SJC23 DNA vaccine and the enhancing effect of IL-12 as an adjuvant. Chin. J. Schistosomiasis Control 13, 328–332 (in Chinese).
Ross, A.G., McManus, D.P., Farrar, J., Hunstman, R.J., Gray, D.J., Li, Y.S., 2012. Neuroschistosomiasis. J. Neurol. 259, 22–32.
Sandoval, N., Siles-Lucas, M., Perez-Arellano, J.L., Carranza, C., Puente, S., Lopez-Aban, J., et al., 2006. A new PCR-based approach for the specific amplification of DNA from different *Schistosoma* species applicable to human urine samples. Parasitology 133, 581–587.
Shen, X., Zhang, W., Wang, P.J., 2012. CT manifestation of abdomen and its pathology of patients with chronic schistosomiasis. Chin. J. Schistosomiasis Control 24, 200–202 (in Chinese).
Shi, Y.E., Han, J.J., Zhou, Z.L., Ning, C.X., 1980. Studies on the indirect hemagglutination test for the diagnosis of schistosomiasis japonica. Acta Med. Wuhan. 1, 26–31 (in Chinese).
Shu, X.H., Zhou, J.C., Cai, C., Zeng, X.F., Zeng, Q.R., Yi, X.Y., 1998. *Schistosoma japonicum*: purification and diagnostic application of recombinant 32 kDa antigen. Bull. Hunan Med. Univ. 4, 331–333 (in Chinese).
Song, H., Liang, Y., Dai, J., Ji, C., Shen, X., Li, L., et al., 2003. Evaluation on dipstick dye immunoassay for screening chemotherapy targets of schistosomiasis in a lower endemic area. Chin. J. Schistosomiasis Control 15, 102–103 (in Chinese).
Tambo, E., Khater, E.I., Chen, J.H., Bergquist, R., Zhou, X.N., 2015. Nobel prize for the artemisinin and ivermectin discoveries: a great boost towards elimination of the global infectious diseases of poverty. Infect. Dis. Poverty 4, 58.
Tang, Y., Wang, Y., Shi, X.H., Xu, W.M., Gan, X.X., 2008. Rapid detection of specific IgM against *Schistosoma japonicum* by dot immune-gold filtration assay. Int. J. Epide Infect. Dis. 35, 316–318 (in Chinese).
ten Hove, R.J., Verweij, J.J., Vereecken, K., Polman, K., Dieye, L., van Lieshout, L., 2008. Multiplex real-time PCR for the detection and quantification of *Schistosoma mansoni* and *S. haematobium* infection in stool samples collected in northern Senegal. Trans. R. Soc. Trop. Med. Hyg. 102, 179–185.
Tokmalaev, A.K., Bezborodov, N.G., 1982. Importance of endoscopic studies in an asymptomatic course of schistosomiasis. Meditsinskaia Parazitol. Parazit. Bolezn. 51, 6–10.
Utzinger, J., Zhou, X.N., Chen, M.G., Bergquist, R., 2005. Conquering schistosomiasis in China: the long march. Acta Trop. 96, 69–96.

van Dam, G.J., de Dood, C.J., Lewis, M., Deelder, A.M., van Lieshout, L., Tanke, H.J., et al., 2013. A robust dry reagent lateral flow assay for diagnosis of active schistosomiasis by detection of *Schistosoma* circulating anodic antigen. Exp. Parasitol. 135, 274–282.

van Dam, G.J., Xu, J., Bergquist, R., de Dood, C.J., Utzinger, J., Qin, Z.Q., et al., 2015. An ultra-sensitive assay targeting the circulating anodic antigen for the diagnosis of *Schistosoma japonicum* in a low-endemic area, People's Republic of China. Acta Trop. 141, 190–197.

van Lieshout, L., Polderman, A.M., Deelder, A.M., 2000. Immunodiagnosis of schistosomiasis by determination of the circulating antigens CAA and CCA, in particular in individuals with recent or light infections. Acta Trop. 77, 69–80.

Wang, X., Li, S., 1990. Study on rapid ELISA using PVC for immunodiagnosis of schistosomiasis and its application. Chin. J. Schistosomiasis Control 2, 31–35 (in Chinese).

Wang, J., Zhu, J.J., Yu, X.L., Zhao, Y.Q., 2010. The quality control of antibody detection kit (indirect hemagglutination assay) for the diagnosis of schistosomiasis. Pract. Prev. Med. 17, 376–377 (in Chinese).

Wang, Q., Huang, Y., Huang, L., Yu, W., He, W., Zhong, B., et al., 2014. Review of risk factors for human echinococcosis prevalence on the Qinghai-Tibet Plateau, China: a prospective for control options. Infect. Dis. Poverty 3, 3.

Wang, L.Y., Wang, Q., Fu, Q., Li, S.Z., Zhang, L., Xu, J., et al., 2015. Analysis on the results of theoretical testing on common parasitic diseases diagnosis: national technique competition of parasitic disease diagnosis in 2013. Int. J. Med. Parasit. Dis. 42, 176–179 (in Chinese).

Wang, L.D., 2006. Schistosomiasis Control and Its Prospect in China. People's Medical Publishing House (in Chinese), Beijing.

Wang, L.D., Chen, H.G., Guo, J.G., Zeng, X.J., Hong, X.L., Xiong, J.J., et al., 2009. A strategy to control transmission of Schistosoma japonicum in China. N. Engl. J. Med. 360, 121–128.

WHO, 2002. In: WHO (Ed.), Prevention and Control of Schistosomiasis and Soil-transmitted Helminthiasis, pp. 1–57. Geneva.

Wu, W., Feng, A., Huang, Y., 2015. Research and control of advanced schistosomiasis japonica in China. Parasitol. Res. 114, 17–27.

Wu, G.L., 2002. A historical perspective on the immunodiagnosis of schistosomiasis in China. Acta Trop. 82, 193–198.

Xia, C.M., Rong, R., Lu, Z.X., Shi, C.J., Xu, J., Zhang, H.Q., et al., 2009. *Schistosoma japonicum*: a PCR assay for the early detection and evaluation of treatment in a rabbit model. Exp. Parasitol. 121, 175–179.

Xie, K., Chen, J., Liu, S., Gong, W., Shong, G., Wu, Y., et al., 1995. Serodiagnosis of schistosomiasis japonica by a new method of immunoenzymatic assay with recombinant Sj26(rSj26) antigen. Chin. J. Schistosomiasis Control 7, 219–222 (in Chinese).

Xin, X.F., Zhang, J., Bo, S.Y., Wang, G.Z., Wang, G.Z., 2006. Quality evaluation for immunological diagnosis kits of schistosomiasis. Chin. J. Schistosomiasis Control 18, 119–121 (in Chinese).

Xu, J., Feng, T., Guo, J.G., Zheng, H., Wang, Q., Wu, X.H., et al., 2005. Comprehensive evaluation of several diagnosis agents of schistosomiasis japonica in China. Chin. J. Schistosomiasis Control 17, 116–119 (in Chinese).

Xu, J., Chen, N.G., Feng, T., Wang, E.M., Wu, X.H., Chen, H.G., et al., 2007. Effectiveness of routinely used assays for the diagnosis of schistosomiasis japonica in the field. Chin. J. Parasitol. Parasit. Dis. 25, 175–179 (in Chinese).

Xu, J., Rong, R., Zhang, H.Q., Shi, C.J., Zhu, X.Q., Xia, C.M., 2010. Sensitive and rapid detection of *Schistosoma japonicum* DNA by loop-mediated isothermal amplification (LAMP). Int. J. Parasitol. 40, 327–331.

Xu, B., Feng, Z., Xu, X.J., Hu, W., 2011a. Evaluation of Kato-Katz technique combined with stool hatching test in diagnosis of schistosomiasis japonica. Chin. J. Schistosomiasis Control 23, 321–323 (in Chinese).
Xu, J., Peeling, R.W., Chen, J.X., Wu, X.H., Wu, Z.D., Wang, S.P., et al., 2011b. Evaluation of immunoassays for the diagnosis of *Schistosoma japonicum* infection using archived sera. PLoS Negl. Trop. Dis. 5, e949.
Xu, J., Yang, K., Li, S.Z., Zhou, X.N., 2014a. Surveillance system after transmission control of schistosomiasis in P.R. China. Chin. J. Schistosomiasis Control 26, 1–5 (in Chinese).
Xu, X., Zhang, Y., Lin, D., Zhang, J., Xu, J., Liu, Y.M., et al., 2014b. Serodiagnosis of *Schistosoma japonicum* infection: genome-wide identification of a protein marker, and assessment of its diagnostic validity in a field study in China. Lancet Infect. Dis. 14, 489–497.
Xu, J., Guan, Z.X., Zhao, B., Wang, Y.Y., Cao, Y., Zhang, H.Q., et al., 2015. DNA detection of *Schistosoma japonicum*: diagnostic validity of a LAMP assay for low-intensity infection and effects of chemotherapy in humans. PLoS Negl. Trop. Dis. 9, e0003668.
Xu, J., Steinman, P., Maybe, D., Zhou, X.N., Lv, S., Li, S.Z., et al., 2016. Evolution of the national schistosomiasis control programmes in the People's Republic of China. Adv. Parasitol. 92.
Yan, Z.Z., Lv, Z.Y., 1978. The preliminary research and application on the immune enzyme marker technology. Chin. Med. J. 88, 470–473 (in Chinese).
Yan, Z.Z., Wan, W., Lu, Z., Wu, Y., 1990. Detection of circulating antigen in schistosomiasis by dot-ELISA with monoclonal antibody. Chin. J. Parasitol. Parasit. Dis. 8, 161–164 (in Chinese).
Yang, K., Zhou, X.N., Wu, X.H., Steinmann, P., Wang, X.H., Yang, G.J., et al., 2009. Landscape pattern analysis and Bayesian modeling for predicting *Oncomelania hupensis* distribution in Eryuan County, People's Republic of China. Am. J. Trop. Med. Hyg. 81, 416–423.
Yang, Y., Zhou, Y.B., Song, X.X., Li, S.Z., Zhong, B., Wang, T.P., et al., 2016. Integrated control strategy of schistosomiasis in the People's Republic of China: projects involving agriculture, water-conservancy, forestry, sanitation and environmental modification. Adv. Parasitol. 92.
Yang, M., 2015. Value of ultrasound in diagnosis of liver disease for advanced schistosomiasis. Pract. Clin. Med. 16 (81), 91 (in Chinese).
Yi, X.Y., He, Y.K., Li, Y.S., 1995. Collaborative study on detection of circulating antigen in *Schistosoma japonicum*. Chin. J. Parasitol. Parasit. Dis. 13, 277–283 (in Chinese).
Yu, Z.R., Wang, J.Z., Zheng, D.J., Xu, S.F., Ying, C.E., 1989. Diagnostic value of proctoscopy and sigmoidoscopy for schistosomiasis. Chin. Rural. Med. 7, 16–17 (in Chinese).
Yu, L.L., Ding, J.Z., Wen, L.Y., Lou, D., Yan, X.L., Lin, L.J., et al., 2011. Development of a rapid dipstick with latex immunochromatographic assay (DLIA) for diagnosis of schistosomiasis japonica. Parasit. Vectors 4, 157.
Zang, W., Li, S.Z., Zhang, L., Wang, Q., Fu, Q., Liu, W., et al., 2013. A cross analysis of proficiency at detecting helminths: the 2012 national competition parasitic disease control. J. Pathog. Biol. 8, 727–730 (in Chinese).
Zhang, W.C., Zeng, Q.R., Zhou, J.C., Wu, C., 1986. The application of biotin-avidin system in the diagnosis of schistosomiasis japonica. Chin. J. Parasitol. Parasit. Dis. 4, 8–11 (in Chinese).
Zhang, L.J., Zhu, R., Dang, H., Xu, J., Li, S.Z., Guo, J.G., 2012. Analysis of surveillance of schistosomiasis in China in 2011. Chin. J. Schistosomiasis Control 24, 627–631 (in Chinese).
Zhang, L.J., Li, S.Z., Wen, L.Y., Lin, D.D., Abe, E.M., Zhu, R., et al., 2016. Establishment and function of schistosomiasis surveillance system towards elimination in the People's Republic of China. Adv. Parasitol. 92.

Zhou, X.N., Wang, L.Y., Chen, M.G., Wu, X.H., Jiang, Q.W., Chen, X.Y., et al., 2005. The public health significance and control of schistosomiasis in China—then and now. Acta Trop. 96, 97—105.

Zhou, X.N., Guo, J.G., Wu, X.H., Jiang, Q.W., Zheng, J., Dang, H., et al., 2007. Epidemiology of schistosomiasis in the People's Republic of China, 2004. Emerg. Infect. Dis. 13, 1470—1476.

Zhou, S.F., Yu, L.X., Wang, S.P., 2009. Research progress on the detection and diagnosis of schistosomiasis. J. Trop. Med. 9, 335—340 (in Chinese).

Zhou, X.N., Xu, J., Chen, H.G., Wang, T.P., Huang, X.B., Lin, D.D., et al., 2011. Tools to support policy decisions related to treatment strategies and surveillance of Schistosomiasis japonica towards elimination. PLoS Negl. Trop. Dis. 5, e1408.

Zhou, X.N., Bergquist, R., Tanner, M., 2013. Elimination of tropical disease through surveillance and response. Infect. Dis. Poverty 2, 1.

Zhou, X.N., 2014. Value of a novel diagnostics of rSP13-ELISA toward schistosomiasis elimination in China. Sci. China Life Sci. 57, 647—648.

Zhu, Y.C., Hua, W.Q., Liu, Y.J., He, W., Xu, Y.L., Jiang, Y.D., 1996. A study on evaluation of efficacy of chemotherapy for schistosomiasis with fraction antigen of soluble egg antigen of *Schistosoma japonicum*. Chin. J. Schistosomiasis Control 8, 321—324 (in Chinese).

Zhu, Y.C., He, W., Liang, Y.S., Xu, M., Yu, C.X., Hua, W.Q., et al., 2002. Development of a rapid, simple dipstick dye immunoassay for schistosomiasis diagnosis. J. Immunol. Methods 266, 1—5 (in Chinese).

Zhu, H.Q., Cao, C.L., Gao, F.H., Guo, J.G., Bao, Z.P., Wang, X.H., et al., 2005a. Evaluation of effectiveness of modified Kato-Katz technique for diagnosis of schistosomiasis japonica. Chin. J. Schistosomiasis Control 17, 273—277 (in Chinese).

Zhu, Y.C., Socheat, D., Bounlu, K., Liang, Y.S., Sinuon, M., Insisiengmay, S., et al., 2005b. Application of dipstick dye immunoassay (DDIA) kit for the diagnosis of schistosomiasis mekongi. Acta Trop. 96, 137—141.

Zhu, R., Dang, H., Zhang, L.J., Li, H.Z., Zheng, C.J., Wu, X.H., et al., 2009. National surveillance of schistosomiasis in China, 2005—2008. Chin. J. Schistosomiasis Control 21, 358—362 (in Chinese).

Zhu, R., Zhao, G.M., Li, H.Z., Guo, J.G., 2011. Development and prospect of surveillance network of schistosomiasis in China. Chin. J. Schistosomiasis Control 23, 14—17 (in Chinese).

Zhu, H.Q., Xu, J., Zhu, R., Zhang, L.J., Tian, L.G., Xu, X.L., et al., 2013a. The establishment and use of criteria to gauge proficiency at detecting common helminth eggs. J. Pathog. Biol. 8, 141—143,154 (in Chinese).

Zhu, R., Qin, Z.Q., Feng, T., Dang, H., Zhang, L.J., Xu, J., 2013b. Assessment of effect and quality control for parasitological tests in national schistosomiasis surveillance sites. Chin. J. Schistosomiasis Control 25, 11—15 (in Chinese).

Zhu, H.Q., Xu, J., Zhu, R., Cao, C.L., Bao, Z.P., Yu, Q., et al., 2014. Comparison of the miracidium hatching test and modified Kato-Katz method for detecting *Schistosoma japonicum* in low prevalence areas of China. Southeast Asian J. Trop. Med. Public Health 45, 20—25.

Zhu, H., Yap, P., Utzinger, J., Jia, T.W., Li, S.Z., Huang, X.B., et al., 2016. Policy support and resources mobilization for the national schistosomiasis control programme in the People's Republic of China. Adv. Parasitol. 92.

Zhu, Y.C., 2005. Immunodiagnosis and its role in schistosomiasis control in China: a review. Acta Trop. 96, 130—136.

CHAPTER FIFTEEN

China—Africa and China—Asia Collaboration on Schistosomiasis Control: A SWOT Analysis

J. Xu*[§,¶], R. Bergquist[||], Y.-J. Qian*[§,¶], Q. Wang*[§,¶], Q. Yu*[§,¶], R. Peeling[#], S. Croft[#], J.-G. Guo** and X.-N. Zhou*[§,¶,1]

*National Institute of Parasitic Diseases, Chinese Center for Disease Control and Prevention, Shanghai, The People's Republic of China
[§]Key Laboratory of Parasite & Vector Biology, Ministry of Public Health, Shanghai, The People's Republic of China
[¶]WHO Collaborating Center for Tropical Diseases, Shanghai, The People's Republic of China
[||]Geospatial Health, University of Naples Federico II, Naples, Italy
[#]London School of Hygiene and Tropical Medicine, London, United Kingdom
**World Health Organization, Geneva, Switzerland
[1]Corresponding author: E-mail: zhouxn1@chinacdc.cn

Contents

Advances in Parasitology, Volume 92
ISSN 0065-308X
http://dx.doi.org/10.1016/bs.apar.2016.02.005

Abstract

Schistosomiasis, a disease caused by a trematode, parasitic worm, is a worldwide public health problem. In spite of great progress with regard to morbidity control, even elimination of this infection in recent decades, there are still challenges to overcome in sub-Saharan Africa and endemic areas in Southeast Asia. Regarded as one of the most successful countries with respect to schistosomiasis control, The People's Republic of China has accumulated considerable experience and learnt important lessons in various local settings that could benefit schistosomiasis control in other endemic countries. Based on an analysis of conceived strengths, weaknesses, opportunities and threats (SWOT) of potential collaborative activities with regard to schistosomiasis in Africa and Asia, this article addresses the importance of collaborative efforts and explores the priorities that would be expected to facilitate the transfer of Chinese experience to low- and middle-income countries in Africa and Asia.

1. INTRODUCTION

The trematode worm infection schistosomiasis has been known since antiquity and remains a major public health problem draining the economic development worldwide. According to the World Health Organization (WHO), the number of countries in tropical and subtropical areas that are endemic for this disease stands currently at 78, 50 of them in Africa and 17 in Asia (WHO, 2013). *Schistosoma mansoni* and *S. haematobium* are widespread in Africa that also harbours limited foci of *S. intercalatum* in the centre and western parts of the continent (Ross et al., 2013; WHO, 2013). In Asia, *S. japonicum* are reported in The People's Republic of China and the Philippines, while small pockets exist on the island of Sulawesi in Indonesia (Ross et al., 2013). Similarly, small pockets of *S. mekongi* exist along a short stretch of the Mekong River at the border between Cambodia and Laos

(Muth et al., 2010). In addition, *S. malayensis* which is closely related to *S. japonicum* has been reported in few sites of Malaysia (Greer et al., 1988).

S. mansoni, *S. haematobium* and *S. japonicum* are mainly responsible for the human disease burden. Recent estimates suggest that over 250 million people have schistosomiasis in the world, which translates into a global burden of 3.3 million disability-adjusted life years (DALYs) (Hotez et al., 2014), a figure even higher than the 200 million infected believed to have existed by the end of last century (Chitsulo et al., 2000). However, the true DALY figure may be almost 10 times higher as argued by King (2010). With the discovery and release for large-scale use of the safe and high-efficient anthelmintic drug praziquantel (PZQ) (Davis and Wegner, 1979) and its subsequent dramatic fall in price, chemotherapy became the backbone of schistosomiasis control programmes. Significant reduction of morbidity and prevalence of schistosomiasis was achieved, including local elimination in several countries (Barkia et al., 2011; Chen et al., 2005; Ebisawa, 1998; French et al., 2010). In recent decades, interests in schistosomiasis control and discussion of suitable strategies for elimination have been raised at international meetings (Fenwick and Savioli, 2011; Rollinson et al., 2013). Although morbidity control is still the main target, particularly in sub-Saharan Africa (SSA), the resolution passed by World Health Assembly (WHA 65.21) in 2012 calls for the increased investment in schistosomiasis control to initiate elimination programmes where appropriate (WHA, 2012).

More than 90% of populations in need of chemotherapy with PZQ live in Africa and the Middle East, where people often have scarce sanitation and lack safe water (WHO, 2013). Control and/or elimination of schistosomiasis are facing great challenges in these countries (Fenwick et al., 2006; Leonardo et al., 2002; Utzinger et al., 2009). Meanwhile, great achievements have been gained in The People's Republic of China for schistosomiasis control through more than six decades of uninterrupted national control activities (Chitsulo et al., 2000; Rollinson et al., 2013). This has led to the accumulation of a significant amount of experience of various endemic stages and surroundings and at varied degrees of economic development that should benefit schistosomiasis control in other endemic countries (Wang et al., 2008; Xu et al., 2015). As there are substantial differences between The People's Republic of China and African/Asian countries, both with respect to health system and economic situation as well control strategies and intervention approaches, the transfer of knowledge will not be straightforward. The experience gained in The People's Republic of China can be more easily duplicated in Asia than in Africa due to the difference between schistosome species and, in particular the snail intermediate hosts in the latter continent.

This article aims to review and explore the priorities of facilitating the cooperation with regard to schistosomiasis control between The People's Republic of China and African/Asian countries.

2. COOPERATION BETWEEN THE PEOPLE'S REPUBLIC OF CHINA AND ENDEMIC COUNTRIES IN AFRICA AND ASIA

Since the internal and external factors, which are either favourable or unfavourable with regard to collaboration on schistosomiasis control in geographical areas as different as The People's Republic of China and Africa (Xu et al., 2016), a thorough analysis should precede active collaboration. The differences with respect to other Asian endemic areas are less pronounced, but still need to be included in the analysis.

We chose a well-known, structured approach to identify and evaluate the strengths, weaknesses, opportunities and threats (SWOT) of the planned collaborative involvement, as it deals with internal and external factors impinging on our objective. The SWOT approach was first used for management and business analysis in the 1960s, but is nowadays widely used to find out the degree to which the internal environment of an activity matches with the external environment, ie, the 'strategic fit' (Fig. 1).

2.1 Strengths

2.1.1 Similar transmission patterns

The schistosome species in The People's Republic of China, Indonesia and the Philippines are transmitted by intermediate snail hosts different from those in Africa and in the two Southeast Asian countries Cambodia and Laos. *S. japonicum* and *S. mekongi* produce serious morbidity more often and more rapidly than other species due to higher output of eggs, which are also often released in aggregates (Chen and Mott, 1988). Although the different species have unique life cycles, people get infections through contact with water contaminated by cercaria (the infective stage of the parasite), either because of their professional (agriculture, fishing, washing) or pleasure activities such bathing (Clerinx and Van Gompel, 2011; Day et al., 1996). For this reason, school-aged children and fishermen are at a particularly high risk for infection (Alebie et al., 2014; Chipeta et al., 2013; Li et al., 2009). The distribution of schistosomiasis is strictly consistent with the snail breeding areas.

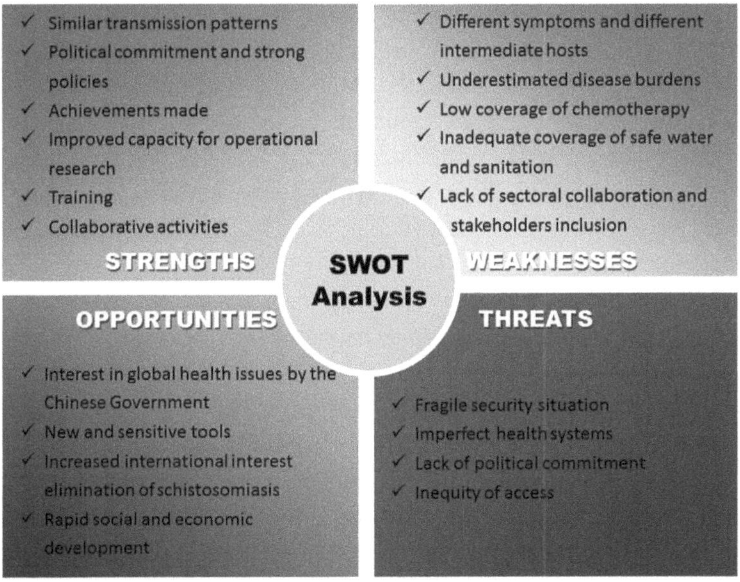

Figure 1 Strengths, weaknesses, opportunities and threats analysis on China–Africa and China–Asia collaboration on schistosomiasis control.

2.1.2 Political commitment and strong policies

Compared with other acute infectious diseases, schistosomiasis was neglected in African and most Asian countries in the past half century. Some countries, such as Brazil, Egypt, Morocco and The People's Republic of China have, however, made strong progress on its control. Recognizing the public health importance of schistosomiasis, Resolution WHA 54.19 was endorsed by Member States of the WHO in 2001 aiming to reach the target of 75% treatment coverage of school-aged children with PZQ by 2010. As the results of the decrease in prevalence and mortality led by deworming campaigns, some endemic countries have made it a goal to interrupt transmission or even elimination of the infection. For example, the Philippine government has stated that it aims to eliminate schistosomiasis as a public health problem by embarking on a vigorous, multisector approach in the endemic areas (Leonardo et al., 2008). The Zanzibar Elimination of Schistosomiasis Transmission, implemented in this part of Tanzania, shows a strong political will to eliminate schistosomiasis, which has already resulted in a significant decrease of the prevalence of this and other helminths (Knopp et al., 2012). The People's Republic of China is drafting a new national strategic plan aiming at the elimination of schistosomiasis as a public health threat from the whole country by the 2016–2025 period (Lei and Zhou, 2015).

2.1.3 Achievements made

Supported by Schistosomiasis Control Initiative (Fenwick et al., 2009) and the global network for the neglected tropical diseases (NTDs) (Liese et al., 2010), many African countries conduct chemotherapy, either for the control of schistosomiasis alone or in combined therapy schemes including also other NTDs (Mazigo et al., 2012; Savioli et al., 2009; Stothard et al., 2009). The number of people receiving treatment in WHO's African region has almost doubled, increasing from 12.37 million in 2006 to 35.56 million in 2012 (WHO, 2014). The prevalence of schistosomiasis in Cambodia, Laos, Indonesia and the Philippines has decreased to near or below 1% with the implementation of mass drug administration (MDA) (Garjito et al., 2008; Laymanivong et al., 2014; Leonardo et al., 2012; Sudomo and Pretty, 2007; Urbani et al., 2002). Many countries in Africa and Asia conduct or have already completed national surveys of human schistosomiasis prevalence as well as mapping of snail habitats (Brooker et al., 2009; Clements et al., 2008; Kabatereine et al., 2006; Leonardo et al., 2012). This information should be useful for the development of control strategies and allocation of the limited financial resources available.

2.1.4 Improved capacity for operational research

To accelerate research for schistosomiasis control and/or elimination in various parts of the world, international cooperation projects such as the Schistosomiasis Consortium for Operational Research and Evaluation (http://score.uga.edu/), CONTRAST, a multidisciplinary alliance in Africa (Bergquist, 2013), have optimized schistosomiasis control and transmission surveillance in SSA. The project on sustainable control of Asian schistosomiasis, a six-country collaboration within the Regional Network on Asian Schistosomiasis and other Helminth Zoonoses (RNAS+) supported by the Canadian International Development Agency through International Development Research Center (IDRC) was implemented to explore innovative control strategies (Zhou et al., 2015). This has led to research results being transferred or integrated into current control activities. For example, new diagnostic tools and modelling techniques were explored and implemented into national schistosomiasis control programmes (Hisakane et al., 2008; Ishikawa and Ohmae, 2009; Kato-Hayashi et al., 2013; Kirinoki et al., 2011; Obeng et al., 2008); A PZQ 'dose pole' that substitutes height for weight, validated in the Philippines and several African countries, facilitated the field administration of PZQ in situations when accurate weighing scales are unavailable (Erfe et al., 2013; Nordin et al., 2014; Palha De Sousa et al., 2014). Variations in the schistosome-intermediate host interplay have been analysed (Attwood et al., 2008a,b; Bayne, 2009; Berriman et al., 2009; Liu et al., 2006). And cost-effectiveness of control programmes and strategies for schistosomiasis elimination have been analysed (Croce et al., 2010; Tallo et al., 2008).

2.1.5 Training

To support and sustain the schistosomiasis control programmes, capacity building for governmental officials and technical staff has been strengthened to improve their technical and management skills in endemic countries. Training courses were conducted to teach the health staff how to detect and manage the schistosomiasis cases, conduct snail surveys, organize drug distribution, calculate drug requirements, and manage and analyse surveillance data (Fenwick et al., 2009; Garba et al., 2006). Through training courses and networks, government officials have been trained in communicating how to design control programs, manage chemotherapy campaign and mobilize social resources, etc. (Omedo et al., 2014; Zhou et al., 2015). To increase public knowledge how to prevent and control schistosomiasis, accurate and high-quality training materials including television sketches, radio, publicity leaflets, posters, comic strips, etc. have been designed to educate the population at large in endemic areas (Hu et al., 2005; Muth et al., 2010; Omedo et al., 2014).

2.1.6 Collaborative activities

The medical aid team sent to Algeria in 1963 was one of the first international health-related activities undertaken by the Chinese government (Liu et al., 2014). Since then, the China–Africa and China–Asia collaboration in the health field has increased through construction of hospitals, donation of medicine and equipment, sending medical teams, training health staff and malaria control. More than 23,000 Chinese medical workers have been sent to about 66 countries benefiting an estimated 270 million people. Among 49 countries supported by Chinese medical teams in 2013, 42 are in Africa and 4 in Asia (Zhu, 2013). One of the most visible cooperative research and control projects, the RNAS+ that was established in 2002 has assembled scientists and policymakers from 10 Asian countries (Leonardo and Bergquist, 2002). Activities include cooperative research projects, sharing experience and distribution of lessons for helminthiases control in Asian member countries. RNAS+ has also organized training courses and workshops related to disease control encouraging the establishment of reference laboratories and exploration of regional research priorities. To share experience on research and control of schistosomiasis and discuss the possibility of collaboration between African countries and The People's Republic of China, communication has been established between RNAS+ and its African counterpart, the research network on schistosomiasis in Africa. During 2013 and 2014, cooperation of Chinese and African institutions were further strengthened by memoranda of understanding concerning Sino-Africa collaboration. These memoranda refer to strengthening of the cooperation on schistosomiasis control and research and were signed between the Public Health Laboratory in Pemba Island, which is part of Zanzibar, a semiautonomous part of Tanzania, and Jiangsu Institute of Parasitic Diseases, The People's Republic of China, the Blue Nile Institute in Sudan and the National Institute of Parasitic Diseases, The People's Republic of China CDC, respectively. More recently, an Institution-based Network on China-Africa Cooperation for Schistosomiasis Elimination (INCAS) was established after a China-Africa cooperation workshop on schistosomiasis held in Malawi in April 2015, and further strengthened by formal technical agreement signed in October 2015 between the National Institution of Parasitic Diseases in Chinese Center for Disease Control and Prevention and 5 institutions, including University of Yaoundé I, Cameroon; Institut National De Recherche En Santé Publique, Mali; Blue Nile National Institute for Communicable Diseases University Of Gezira-Wad Medani, Sudan; National Institute for Medical Research, Mwanza Centre, Tanzania; and University of Zimbabwe, Zimbabwe.

2.2 Weaknesses

2.2.1 Different symptoms and different intermediate hosts

Although all schistosome species causing human infections have similar transmission patterns, differences exist concerning the intermediate hosts, clinical manifestations and transmission seasons. *S. japonicum* and its amphibious, dioecious *Oncomelania hupensis* snail is the sole schistosome life cycle operating in The People's Republic of China. In contrast to the African schistosome species, *S. japonicum* is zoonotic and capable of infecting more than 40 mammalian animals (Chen and Feng, 1999). *S. mekongi* in Cambodia and Laos, transmitted by the aquatic snail *Neotricula aperta*, is also zoonotic with pigs, dogs and rodents serving as reservoir hosts (Attwood, 2001; Ohmae et al., 2004). *S. mansoni*, *S. haematobium* and *S. intercalatum* in Africa depend on various aquatic and hermaphrodite host snails; for *S. mansoni Biomphalaria* spp. and *Bulinus* spp. for the latter two schistosome species (Prter et al., 1993; Rozendaal, 1997). *S. haematobium* is decidedly different as it causes urinary schistosomiasis leading to damage in the bladder, ureters and kidneys with haematuria as the most common, early symptom. All other schistosomes cause intestinal schistosomiasis of various severity stating with abdominal pain and blood in the stools, sometimes diarrhoea and increased temperature, while advanced, long-term, untreated cases have enlarged livers and spleens due to large numbers of parasite eggs, often accompanied by intestinal damage and portal hypertension. Due to the climate, there can be transmission all year around in some countries, mainly SSA, while in more temperate countries there is a marked seasonality (Adewunmi et al., 1991; Blas et al., 2004; Chandiwana et al., 1987; Sturrock et al., 2001). In addition, local temperature variations, rainfall, humidity and ecological features play an important role for presence of the intermediate hosts and thus for the transmission of schistosomiasis.

2.2.2 Underestimated disease burdens

Regardless if the true DALY figure for schistosomiasis in the world is 3.3 million (Hotez et al., 2014) or 24–29 million (King, 2010), it has been estimated that there may be about 200 million cases of schistosomiasis in Africa, 192 million of which in SSA (accounting for 25% of SSA's population) (Steinmann et al., 2006; Utzinger et al., 2009). In Asia, recent reports show the average prevalence of schistosomiasis has decreased with near 1% in Laos, Cambodia, Indonesia and the Philippines (Garjito et al., 2008; Leonardo et al., 2012; Laymanivong et al., 2014). However, we know that currently used diagnostic tools lack the sensitivity required for areas characterized by low-level infections (Bergquist, 2013) and the data may underestimate the prevalence for other reasons as well, eg, unreasonable statistic methods or low coverage of enrolment (Leonardo et al., 2012; Rollinson et al., 2013; Tallo et al., 2008). New endemic foci and resurgence of schistosomiasis in urban or rural areas have been reported recently (Blanton et al., 2015; Leonardo et al., 2015; Mwakitalu et al., 2014). On the other hand, although the mortality rate of schistosomiasis is relatively low, severe, debilitating chronic illness is caused in millions of people. It has been estimated that SSA accounts for 93% of global disease burden caused by schistosomiasis (King et al., 2005). Although recent research have adjusted the disease burden caused by schistosomiasis upwards (Hotez et al., 2014; Murray et al., 2012), the disease burden may still be considerably underestimated due to lack of a precise measuring basis for what has been called 'asymptomatic disease' (King, 2010, 2015).

2.2.3 Low coverage of chemotherapy

Preventive chemotherapy is the major intervention and coverage is the key issue of efficacy of control in most endemic countries. Among the 67 endemic countries in Africa and Asia, 50 need to MDA. Out of these countries, 44 are located in Africa as of 2012 (Fig. 2) (WHO, 2013). In 2012, only

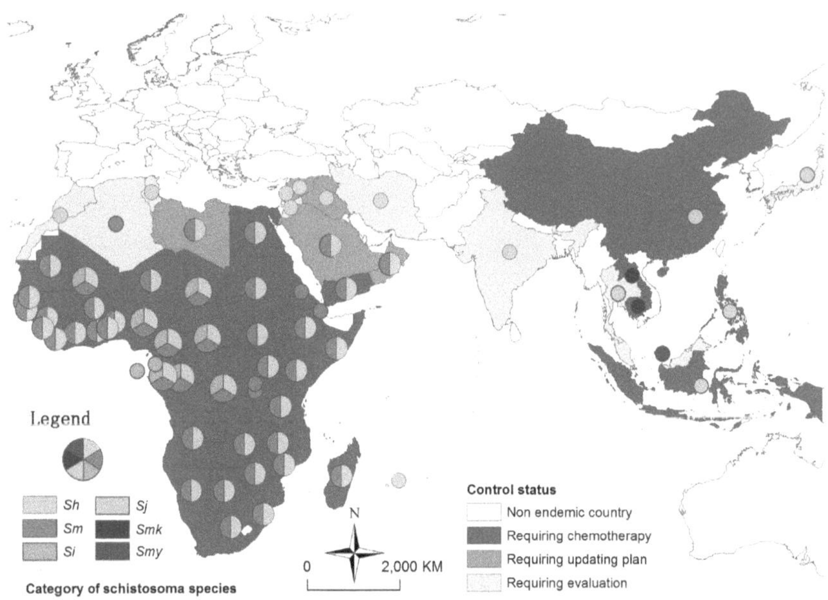

Figure 2 Geographical distribution of schistosomiasis and control status in Asia and Africa.

13.6%, 13.3% and 36.0% of people in need of preventive chemotherapy in the WHO regions of Africa, Eastern Mediterranean and Western Pacific, respectively, actually received treatment. Thus, a substantial number of patients were left at high risk (WHO, 2014). School-based MDA, the major approach in Africa, is regarded as a highly cost-effective approach, since at least 50% of those suffering from schistosomiasis there are school-aged children (Guyatt et al., 1994; Stothard et al., 2013b; Toure et al., 2008). However, as the proportion of school enrolment of children is low in most poor areas, and the high-risk population including fishermen, irrigation workers and preschool children account for a large part of all infected cases, there is a need to supplement with another drug delivery approach to increase coverage (Stothard et al., 2011, 2013a). Community-based approach is a good alternative that has been widely used in Asia (Chigusa et al., 2006; Inobaya et al., 2015). However, a recent report from the Philippines shows that the average coverage is only 48.3% in spite of various community-related control activities were introduced (Tallo et al., 2008). Ethnicity, incentives, ratio of population to available drugs, mode of distribution, infection status, etc. may have influenced the coverage (Dabo et al., 2013; Leslie et al., 2011; Massa et al., 2009; Mwinzi et al., 2012).

2.2.4 Inadequate coverage of safe water and sanitation

Chemotherapy cures infection, prevents morbidity and lowers prevalence but is unable to prevent reinfection. However, access to safe water and improved sanitation have interrupted transmission in many parts of previously endemic areas in The People's Republic of China through reducing the frequency of water contact with potentially contaminated water outside the home. This has reduced the contamination of schistosome eggs in the environment, which also improves control of other helminthiases transmitted by the faecal, urinary or oral route (Asaolu and Ofoezie, 2003; Huang and Manderson, 2005; Utzinger et al., 2003). The WHA 65.21 resolution underlines the importance of safe tap water, improved sanitation and public health education as means to control schistosomiasis. However, these approaches depend to a great extent on economic development (WHO, 2012b). By 2012, 89% of global population had gained access to improved drinking water, but more than 700 million people still lack access to drinking water of acceptable quality, 43% of them in SSA. Indeed, Southern Asia and SSA still have the lowest coverage of improved sanitation, the coverage in the latter being only 30% (WHO/UNICEF, 2014). Lack of investment, inadequate political will, inequity of access and difficulty in maintaining water supply are the main reasons. To improve these figures, sanitation services need to be upgraded in a large number of countries.

2.2.5 Lack of sectoral collaboration and stakeholders inclusion

Since schistosomiasis transmission involves natural, social and biological factors, sectoral cooperation is essential for progress in schistosomiasis control (King, 2009; Zhou et al., 2005). Although chemotherapy plays a crucial role by reducing prevalence and morbidity of schistosomiasis, while health education, supply of clean water and improved sanitation could interrupt the chain of infection (Rollinson et al., 2013). Poor knowledge with respect to behavioural change, treatment-seeking habits and sanitation have been observed (Musuva et al., 2014; Odhiambo et al., 2014; Worku et al., 2014). In addition, the construction of water conservancy projects without considering their impact on schistosomiasis has contributed to the spread of schistosomiasis in many parts of the world (Steinmann et al., 2006). Intersector cooperation and collaboration are essential to implement each intervention in an equitable and harmonized way, but most African and Asian countries lack mechanisms to deal with this situation, in particular if financial support is lacking coupled with insufficient enforcement of policies and absence of political will.

2.3 Opportunities

2.3.1 Interest in global health issues by the Chinese government

After its entry into World Trade Organization in 2001, The People's Republic of China has joined a large majority of other UN specialized agencies and multilateral health foundations. The number of Chinese experts participating in WHO's global normative work has increased significantly in the latest decade. Chinese funding for health-related aid has been augmented with an average of $4.8 billion per year during the period 2010–2012, 51.8% of which was received by African countries and 30.5% by Asian countries (Liu et al., 2014). Since 2000, The People's Republic of China has hosted a series of triennial meetings (forums) on China–Africa Cooperation (FOCACs), with each forum announcing and focussing on different topics related to health aid, eg, hospital construction, malaria control, high-education scholarships, health worker training, artemisinin drug donation and the Brightness Action campaign (FOCAC, 2012; King, 2006). Since 2005, in the field of parasitic diseases, The People's Republic of China had set up 30 antimalaria centres in African countries including a joint border malaria control project with Myanmar, Laos and Vietnam (Liu et al., 2014; Xu and Liu, 2012). At the fifth China–Africa Cooperation Forum in July 2012, The People's Republic of China made a promise to increase its investment continuously, extend cooperation to fields such as health care and disease control as well as carry out joint pilot schistosomiasis control and prevention projects through international cooperation with African countries (FOCAC, 2012).

2.3.2 New and sensitive tools

Regular monitoring and evaluation are necessary to ensure that programmes are efficiently implemented and receive maximal benefit. Surveillance is important when the goal move from morbidity control to elimination. This is particularly challenging given the diversity of tools and indicators. With the deep understanding of the schistosome genome and its host compatibility (Berriman et al., 2009; Hu et al., 2003; Zhou et al., 2009), sensitive and quality-assured diagnostic tools based on the monoclonal antibody technique and molecular methods, new drug candidates have been identified, some of them already widely used in control programmes (Cnops et al., 2013; Colley et al., 2013; Pontes et al., 2002; Tong et al., 2015). Some vaccine candidates have also been explored and shown high efficacy against schistosomiasis (Curti et al., 2013; Da'dara et al., 2008, Riveau et al., 2012). With the development of geographic information systems

(GIS), global positioning systems and remote sensing (RS) systems, mathematical and statistical modelling based on spatial, temporal, spatial–temporal analysis have been developed and used for predicating schistosomiasis risk (Chipeta et al., 2013; French et al., 2010; Hurlimann et al., 2011; Simoonga et al., 2009; Wu et al., 2008).

2.3.3 Increased international interest elimination of schistosomiasis

Although schistosomiasis remains a public health problem, morbidity and prevalence of schistosomiasis have decreased in many countries due to long-term interventions and some countries moving towards schistosomiasis elimination, which should be possible in countries where the prevalence is low and adequate resources coupled with strong political commitment are available (Hotez et al., 2012; Melo et al., 2014; Rollinson et al., 2013; Xu et al., 2015). With the significant reduced price of PZQ, increased advocacy and resources for NTD control, the Bill & Melinda Gates Foundation, the US and UK governments and Merck Serono donated a large amount of PZQ tablets to African countries in the recent decade (Fenwick and Savioli, 2011). Large-scale preventive chemotherapy was implemented across several countries and millions of children were given single standard PZQ doses. The agreement on the WHO's roadmap (2012) raised optimism that many NTDs can indeed be eliminated (WHO, 2012a) and led to the signing the London Declaration (http://unitingtocombatntds.org/resource/london-declaration), which represents an unprecedented commitment to control or eliminate 10 diseases by the end of this decade by global health leaders, including the chief executive officers of major pharmaceutical companies, Bill Gates of the Bill & Melinda Gates Foundation, WHO and senior government officials from both endemic and donor countries (NTDs, 2012; Webster et al., 2014).

2.3.4 Rapid social and economic development

One of the Millennium Declaration Goals (http://www.un.org/millenniumgoals/) is to eliminate absolute poverty, hunger and diseases by 2015 (General Assembly, 2000). These goals need to be supported by economic growth. Indeed, the economic situation of African and Asian countries has increased substantially in the past decade. African exports rose in real terms at an annual rate of 5.2%, higher than that of global average rate of 4.8% in 2011 (UNCTAD, 2013), and in Asia, the growth rate in many countries remains above 6% (Asian Development Bank, 2014). Correspondingly, the living conditions in Africa and Asia have improved during the past decade. The coverage of safe water increased to 64% in 2012 in SSA and over 89% in Asia. The total sanitation coverage increased in SSA at a slower pace, from 25% in 1990 to 30% in 2012, but covered 71% and 89% of population in Southeast Asia and Western Asia, respectively (WHO/UNICEF, 2014). Meanwhile, health systems were strengthened or reformed in several countries including promulgation of laws related to health, establishment of primary health-care infrastructures and health information systems for health services monitoring, improving medical services and capacity of disease diagnosis, resulting in easier access to health services (Benatar, 2004; Frenk and Horton, 2006; Green, 2013; Lieberman et al., 2005; Liljestrand and Sambath, 2012; Sekwat, 2003).

2.4 Threats

2.4.1 Fragile security situation

The political situation is a key determinant of consecutive social and economic development. Although the Middle East remains in unrest and conflict, warfare in SSA and most of Asian countries is declining both in frequency and intensity since the late 2000s (Straus, 2012). While schistosomiasis control is continuously conducted in regions with recovering economies and strong political commitment, the chaos caused by war and political change present in other countries has a great impact on the sustainability of these activities (Kahler, 2013; Straus, 2012). The local health system in countries sinking into turmoil is difficult uphold as warfare and conflict influence external funding and other investments. Careful considerations of local sociocultural, economic and political situations are needed to determine the application and/or acceptance of control measures.

2.4.2 Imperfect health systems

WHO and many other international agencies have encouraged countries to take concrete steps to move towards universal health coverage, which is an ideal target. However, various factors apart from warfare, such as ethics, politics and economy, influence society including the health system (Rodrigo and Smith, 2012; Savedoff et al., 2012). Although the funds donated by western developed countries has increased nearly three times from $1.5 billion in 1990 to 4.24 billion in 2011, the health system in Africa is still fragile and the health conditions have not improved significantly. African key problems include lack of primary health staff, health insurance and a functioning health information system (OECD, 2013). Indeed, many endemic countries do not have the public health infrastructure or necessary resources to implement proper schistosomiasis control. Loss of skilled health workers migrating from Africa exacerbates the problems of an effectively functioning health-care system (Connell et al., 2007). In Asia, most staff working on schistosomiasis control are on part-time basis, which is not sufficient to fulfil the national control requirements. With nearly 2.5 times the number of schistosomiasis cases in The People's Republic of China, the Philippines has only 200 part-time staff to do what is needed, which amounts to only 1% of the number of full-time staff in The People's Republic of China (Ross et al., 2013).

2.4.3 Lack of political commitment

Schistosomiasis as well as other NTDs is commonly endemic in rural and poor regions in low-income countries (Hotez and Kamath, 2009). In most African and Asian countries, the schistosomiasis control programmes mainly depend on external funds. The experience from Mali and the Philippines shows that the diminishing or termination of funding often result in staff reductions in control agencies as well as rebound of the disease (Clements et al., 2009; Inobaya et al., 2015). Even if chemotherapy does not prevent reinfection, sustainable and integrated interventions could be cost-effective, resulting in morbidity control or even elimination of schistosomiasis (Rollinson et al., 2013; Ross et al., 2013). For this to function, however, strong policy commitment and continuous donor funding is necessary. The global economic recession that started with the setback of 2008 may increase the instability of financial support. Furthermore, limited engagement and involvement of senior policymakers in endemic countries may result in less political commitment for schistosomiasis control leading to less available internal funds and lack of collaboration with other stakeholders.

2.4.4 Inequity of access

Due to current insufficient availability of PZQ, full coverage of effective drug delivery cannot be achieved. School-aged children are normally targeted for chemotherapy as prevalence and intensity of disease in this age group are normally higher than in adults. Children less than 5 years of age are often neglected by national control programmes as formal legislation and suitable paediatric PZQ dosages so not exist (Stothard et al., 2011). 'New' foci where schistosomiasis may have been endemic for a long time can become known as enlarged surveys and/or use of more sensitive diagnostic tools are implemented. Whether a village or a region is included in schistosomiasis control can be a matter of political and religious intracommunity priorities, which obviously leads to inequity. People living in rural areas are more often ignored with respect to treatment than urban dwellers (Aagaard-Hansen et al., 2009). Inequity can also be due to geographically uneven economic development, availability of donated funds, ethnicity or religion, rich or poor background. Inequalities also exist within countries or regions with regard to access to drinking water and sanitation services.

3. PRIORITIES IN CHINA – AFRICA/ASIA COLLABORATION

The Chinese national schistosomiasis control programme has been sustained without interruption for six decades. It has not only terminated the development of morbidity due to schistosomiasis, but has also produced a significant reduction of prevalence and is now geared at elimination of this infection (Li et al., 2013). Various approaches, products, techniques applied by experienced professionals ensured the success of the strategies that shifted according to the social situation and scientific development, with interventions adjusted and recombined accordingly. To translate the successful experience with schistosomiasis control/elimination to Africa and other parts of Asia, The People's Republic of China would promote an approach consisting of a set of priority fields as follows:

1. Transmission mapping;
2. Population dynamics;
3. Modelling based on available data sets;
4. Sensitive and specific diagnostics;
5. Response packages tailored to different transmission settings and levels; and
6. Validation.

3.1 Coordination

Lack of coordination among different sectors hinders the development of schistosomiasis control in Africa and other parts of Asia. Achievements gained in The People's Republic of China on coordinated schistosomiasis control are based on the close collaboration among different departments, including National Health and Family Planning Commission, State Forestry Administration, Ministry of Agriculture, Ministry of Water Resources, Ministry of Finance, Ministry of Land Resources, and the National Development and Reform Commission (Xu et al., 2015; Zhou et al., 2005). The State Council on schistosomiasis control is responsible for the coordination between different departments. The The People's Republic of China CDC, health bureaus and hospitals at all levels collaborate to manage and implement disease control activities. Regional collaboration has been strengthened via platforms such as RNAS+ and research programmes supported by the Canada's International Development Research Center (Zhou et al., 2015). The People's Republic of China could disseminate its experience on collaboration mechanisms and strengthen capacity building of management systems through training courses. International advocacy workshops and stakeholder meetings at the national or regional level are needed.

3.2 Risk mapping

Disease mapping has been given a high priority in The People's Republic of China as it can supply the needed, basic information for drafting control programmes and start-up activities (Guo et al., 2005; Yang et al., 2005). The addition of GIS and satellite-generated, remotely sensed environmental data and geostatistics to the arsenal in the last two decades has facilitated the understanding of the location of endemic and potentially endemic areas in a global warming scenario (Zhou et al., 2008). These new geospatial tools have been of critical importance for our understanding and prediction of the true distribution of schistosomiasis (Wu et al., 2008; Yang et al., 2006, 2013; Zhang et al., 2008). Such systematic, progressing input combined with data from surveys available in the *Atlas of Schistosomiasis Transmission in The People's Republic of China* that was recently updated (NIPD, 2013) present information on schistosomiasis in the form of thematic maps, diagrams and charts that are easy to understand. Annual risk mapping at the national, regional and county levels are regularly conducted to guide policy decisions. The People's Republic of China has now a cadre of skilled technicians with accumulated experience on disease mapping, communication, who can provide advanced training courses on disease mapping and be counted on to finalize the mapping in those countries which do not currently possess these tools.

3.3 Chemotherapy coverage

PZQ is the drug of choice for the treatment of all forms of schistosomiasis (Dömling and Khoury, 2010). It is an inexpensive, highly effective drug with low toxicity against all schistosome species and many other parasitic helminths. However, the quantity of existing donated PZQ is far short of the demand (Stothard et al., 2011). In addition, many cases could not receive treatment due to the absence of efficient drug delivery systems. Nanjing Pharmaceutical Factory (producing 50 tons of raw material annually corresponding to 100 million PZQ tablets at the strength of 200 mg/tablet) has improved the product by a film-coated form to increase the compliance rate of medication (Xu et al., 2009). This production can rapidly be upgraded to cover the needed amounts of drug. Community-based approach is the main delivery system in The People's Republic of China with the collaboration of the local hospital or rural doctors with the CDC or schistosomiasis stations. This way of distribution works well together with a reporting system, which is in operation nationwide to reflect the timing of chemotherapy guarantees the high coverage and efficacy (Zhou et al., 2012). The amounts of PZQ tablets needed, even at the international scale, can thus be supplied and thus increase the current coverage of chemotherapy in Africa and elsewhere. The Chinese government and nongovernmental organizations (NGOs) could use this new source of available PZQ to fill the gaps through drug donations. The People's Republic of China could also disseminate its experience through training programmes at the district level designed for persons administering pharmaceuticals and health-care personnel for improving the skills of drug delivery and supervision of local staff. Reporting systems for drug delivery could also be supported by Chinese experience.

3.4 Snail control

Control or eliminate snails will benefit to control or eliminate schistosomiasis. Different from the scarce snail control activities in Africa and other part of Asia, varieties of environmental modification were developed and implemented in The People's Republic of China, integrated with projects of other sectors such as land resources, agriculture, water conservancy, forestry through activities of reclaiming wetlands, environmental management (digging new ditches and filling up the old ones that would kill the amphibious snails), changing rice paddies into dry crops, etc. (Chen, 1999; Yuan et al., 2005). In addition, there are many various forms of molluscicides, the most common and effective being 50% niclosamide ethanolamine formulated as powder, granules, suspension concentrate, retarder, etc. were developed adopting to the local situation of the snail-infested areas (Xin and Dai, 2010; Yang et al., 2012a). Since the efficiency does not reach 100%, repeated application could be considered to increase the effect (Yang et al., 2012a, 2010). Before the advent of PZQ, mollusciciding was a cornerstones of schistosomiasis control in Africa, and some of its former role may have to be resurrected there as PZQ alone cannot stop transmission. The People's Republic of China has a strong industrial capacity in molluscicide production, and the main Chinese companies manufacturing niclosamide could produce 1000 tons per year. To effectively control snails in African and Asian countries, training courses and exchange of senior scientists could be conducted to share the experience and technology. If the molluscicides made in The People's Republic of China pass WHO prequalification certification, The People's Republic of China would be willing to supply quality-assured molluscicides to other endemic countries.

3.5 Diagnostic tools

Accurate diagnosis is essential to obtain data regarding the distribution, prevalence and infection intensity of schistosomiasis in endemic area, and diagnostic approaches should differ at different stages of schistosomiasis control (Bergquist et al., 2009; Zhou et al., 2011). Based on laboratory and field assessment, quality-assured immunodiagnostics approved by the State Food and Drug administration have been integrated into the national control programme, while basic principles using appropriate diagnostics to monitor disease trends and assess the effectiveness and impact of interventions have been established for guiding treatment strategies at different thresholds of schistosomiasis transmission and for certifying elimination (Xu et al., 2011; Zhou et al., 2011). Other sensitive and specific techniques based on the monoclonal antibody technique to detect circulating antigen, as well as molecular methods, eg, the polymerase chain reaction and the loop-mediated isothermal amplification (LAMP) were also developed, supplying tools populations studies, surveillance of snails and diagnosis of individual cases (Guo et al., 2012; Hung and Remais, 2008; Tong et al., 2015; van Dam et al., 2015). A network for schistosomiasis diagnosis was constructed with the establishment of provincial reference laboratories and sentinel monitoring laboratories at the county level (Qin et al., 2013). These laboratories are responsible for diagnosis, verification and providing scientific evidences for schistosomiasis surveillance and response in the elimination stage (Zhu et al., 2013). As some kits produced in The People's Republic of China have shown high sensitivity and specificity for diagnosis of other schistosomiasis (Zhu et al., 2005, 2006), these kits could be supplied at a competitive cost or freely delivered to African and Asia countries. Experience on developing diagnostic assays, decision-making of using appropriate diagnostic tools as well as management of diagnostic quality control could be transferred through training programmes or academic activities.

3.6 Surveillance and response

To achieve control and/or elimination of communicable diseases, surveillance and response to detect pockets of transmission and reemergence of disease are needed as the final, long-term activity in the control chain. Resource-constrained countries, which generally carry heavy NTD burdens, schistosomiasis not the least, face a challenge in strengthening their health system. Effective tools tailored to local settings are needed for surveillance and response that should take place by collating the components according to the priorities mentioned previously under 'Priorities'. Thus an effective and rapid response, including an early warning mechanism, is the prerequisite for the efficient management of infectious diseases (Zhou et al., 2013). The People's Republic of China relies on a variety of monitoring systems with different aims in longitudinal or cross-sectional format. The contents of surveillance have been developed from simple mapping of endemicity to factors, such as environmental monitoring, water conservancy, dam construction, irrigation projects, climate change, etc. (Dang et al., 2014; Zhao et al., 2005; Zhu et al., 2011). As the prevalence of schistosomiasis decrease significantly, transmission interruption becomes the next hurdle to overcome. Regular surveillance is now conducted in The People's Republic of China, and early warning systems (EWS) have been set up based on research and experience (Sun et al., 2011; Wu et al., 2005; Xu et al., 2014). This and the involvement of acute schistosomiasis monitoring in a real-time reporting system have provided a solid foundation for decision-making. Built in 2010, the schistosomiasis information management system provides valuable source data at the village level to support management. At the same time, new technologies such as RS systems, GIS and predictive modelling including sentinel mice (Yang et al., 2012) are applied for schistosomiasis monitoring and surveillance (Yang et al., 2006, 2012b; Zhang et al., 2005). To improve the capacity of African and Asian countries of monitoring and surveillance of schistosomiasis, basic and higher-level training could be provided through Chinese scientist visitors or by computer-based remote education. With the help from Chinese scientists, an EWS could be set up for tracking information about the density and infection status of intermediate snail host species.

4. CURRENT STATUS

The Ebola outbreak as well as the threat of and other infectious diseases have exposed the fragility of the public health system in some areas of the world. Chinese engagement in global health has been increased and more experts are involving in global health governance. As one of the main components of The People's Republic of China's health activities, medical teams composed of clinical doctors or nurses have been sent to Africa and Asia, while lower-level public health staff are usually not included. Hospitals and clinics targeting individual patients will benefit from this service (Liu et al., 2014). The public health system needs reform, training of health providers and general strengthening. According to the Beijing Declaration produced during the Ministerial Forum of China–Africa Health Development in 2013 (NHFPC, 2013), The People's Republic of China aims to extend its cooperation to health care and disease control. Schistosomiasis, malaria, and HIV were given priority for pilot studies in Africa and Asia through multilateral cooperation.

To promote the control and elimination of schistosomiasis, WHO and some European countries have expressed willingness to facilitate bridging perceived gaps in the endemic countries and it has been pronounced that The People's Republic of China could play a crucial role for the scientific exchange of experience and lessons on schistosomiasis control. Supported by the Department for International Development (DFID) in United Kingdom, two China–UK Global Health Support programmes have been initiated in the last 2 years. The first programme aims to distil Chinese experience and lessons on schistosomiasis and malaria, exploring the possibility to conduct control based on Chinese experiences in low- and middle-income endemic countries. The other programme aims to establish a centre of excellence in The People's Republic of China to provide health aid emphasized on NTDs through capacity building and information dissemination. A memorandum of understanding to conduct joint activities among WHO, The People's Republic of China and Tanzania governments for schistosomiasis control in Tanzania was signed in May, 2014. To explore the priority for schistosomiasis control and research as well as establishing cooperation mechanism between The People's Republic of China and Africa, a China–Africa institutional cooperation of schistosomiasis elimination meeting was held in Malawi, supported by WHO in April 2015. Based on the experience of RNAS+, regarded as an excellent model for schistosomiasis cooperation between The People's Republic of China and other Asian countries, the institution-based network on China–Africa cooperation of schistosomiasis (INCAS) is coordinated by the National Institute of Parasitic Diseases (NIPD) and WHO.

Global health is an important component of The People's Republic of China's foreign policy, and the selection of counterparts for schistosomiasis control will be based on requests from other countries for schistosomiasis control and decisions by The People's Republic of China's Health and Family Planning Commission, Ministry of Foreign Affairs, and Ministry of

Finance. To ensure a successful collaboration, countries would be selected according to the following principles:

1. Existing trade, economic, cultural and medical cooperation with the Chinese government via economic and technical agreements;
2. Rural public health is a high-priority item on the counterpart country's government agenda;
3. Impact of the opportunities in collaboration with Chinese institutions is identified;
4. The counterpart country's government has identified schistosomiasis control/elimination as a target with ongoing activities; and
5. Preventive chemotherapy is implemented nationwide.

Recently, pilot study for malaria control has been conducted in Tanzania in 2015 supported by DFID, which will accumulate experience for China–Africa, China–Asia collaboration in public health field in future. In addition, strengthening the capacity of Chinese scientists involved in international health collaboration on schistosomiasis control and coordination with WHO regional offices and other experienced organizations in developed countries would facilitate the coordination and implementation of cooperation activities.

5. CONCLUSIONS

Programmes tacking schistosomiasis are increased worldwide but great challenges exist to meet the set goals of WHO roadmap. As schistosomiasis mainly affects and infects the poorest and marginalized people in subtropical and tropical regions, collaborating with other health and development activities to reduce poverty and break the life cycle of schistosomes will contribute schistosomiasis control and elimination. To help control and eliminate schistosomiasis, The People's Republic of China will need to establish partnerships with Ministries of Health in African and other Asian countries, WHO regional offices, and existing NGOs at the international or national level, and collaborate closely to expand support for schistosomiasis programmes. Financial and technical support for training, designing national programme strategies and plans, intervention implementation, operational research, disease surveillance-response and production of health education materials should be provided. Coordination of INCAS, RNAS+ activities by NIPD and WHO would be helpful for strengthening the cooperation among institutions for basic and operational research and accelerate the process of schistosomiasis control in Africa and Asia. Governments, national or internationals foundations, as well as nonprofit organization are expected to take part in funding and supervising such kind of cooperation to maintain the sustainability of the cross-border monitoring of schistosomiasis risk.

ACKNOWLEDGEMENTS

This manuscript was granted by the (Grant no. GHSP-CS-OP1-01) National Special Science and Technology Project for Major Infectious Diseases of The People's Republic of China (Grant no. 2012ZX10004-220). We acknowledge partial financial support by the National Natural Science Foundation of The People's Republic of China (Grant no. 81301454).

REFERENCES

Aagaard-Hansen, J., Mwanga, J.R., Bruun, B., 2009. Social science perspectives on schistosomiasis control in Africa: past trends and future directions. Parasitology 136, 1747–1758.

Adewunmi, C.O., Furu, P., Christensen, N.O., Olorunmola, F., 1991. Endemicity, seasonality and focality of transmission of human schistosomiasis in 3 communities in southwestern Nigeria. Trop. Med. Parasitol. 42, 332–334.

Alebie, G., Erko, B., Aemero, M., Petros, B., 2014. Epidemiological study on *Schistosoma mansoni* infection in Sanja area, Amhara region, Ethiopia. Parasit. Vectors 7, 15.

Asaolu, S.O., Ofoezie, I.E., 2003. The role of health education and sanitation in the control of helminth infections. Acta Trop. 86, 283–294.

Attwood, S.W., 2001. Schistosomiasis in the Mekong region: epidemiology and phylogeography. Adv. Parasitol. 50, 87–152.

Attwood, S.W., Fatih, F.A., Campbell, I., Upatham, E.S., 2008a. The distribution of Mekong schistosomiasis, past and future: preliminary indications from an analysis of genetic variation in the intermediate host. Parasitol. Int. 57, 256–270.

Attwood, S.W., Fatih, F.A., Upatham, E.S., 2008b. DNA-sequence variation among *Schistosoma mekongi* populations and related taxa; phylogeography and the current distribution of Asian schistosomiasis. PLoS Negl. Trop. Dis. 2, e200.

Asian Development Bank, 2014. Growth Hesitates in Developing Asia [Online]. Available: http://www.adb.org/sites/default/files/publication/151010/ado-supplement-december-2014.pdf.

Barkia, H., Barkia, A., Nhammi, H., Belghyti, D., 2011. Schistosomiasis in Morocco: from discovery to after elimination. East Mediterr. Health J. 17, 250–256.

Bayne, C.J., 2009. Successful parasitism of vector snail *Biomphalaria glabrata* by the human blood fluke (trematode) *Schistosoma mansoni*: a 2009 assessment. Mol. Biochem. Parasitol. 165, 8–18.

Benatar, S.R., 2004. Health care reform and the crisis of HIV and AIDS in South Africa. N. Engl. J. Med. 351, 81–92.

Bergquist, R., 2013. Closing in on 'perhaps the most dreadful of the remaining plagues': an independent view of the multidisciplinary alliance to optimize schistosomiasis control in Africa. Acta Trop. 128, 179–181.

Bergquist, R., Johansen, M.V., Utzinger, J., 2009. Diagnostic dilemmas in helminthology: what tools to use and when? Trends Parasitol. 25, 151–156.

Berriman, M., Haas, B.J., Loverde, P.T., Wilson, R.A., Dillon, G.P., Cerqueira, G.C., et al., 2009. The genome of the blood fluke *Schistosoma mansoni*. Nature 460, 352–358.

Blanton, R.E., Barbosa, L.M., Reis, E.A., Carmo, T.M., Dos Santos, C.R., Costa, J.M., et al., 2015. The relative contribution of immigration or local increase for persistence of urban schistosomiasis in Salvador, Bahia, Brazil. PLoS Negl. Trop. Dis. 9, e0003521.

Blas, B.L., Rosales, M.I., Lipayon, I.L., Yasuraoka, K., Matsuda, H., Hayashi, M., 2004. The schistosomiasis problem in the Philippines: a review. Parasitol. Int. 53, 127–134.
Brooker, S., Kabatereine, N.B., Gyapong, J.O., Stothard, J.R., Utzinger, J., 2009. Rapid mapping of schistosomiasis and other neglected tropical diseases in the context of integrated control programmes in Africa. Parasitology 136, 1707–1718.
Chandiwana, S.K., Christensen, N.O., Frandsen, F., 1987. Seasonal patterns in the transmission of *Schistosoma haematobium, S. mattheei* and *S. mansoni* in the highveld region of Zimbabwe. Acta Trop. 44, 433–444.
Chen, M.G., 1999. Progress in schistosomiasis control in China. Chin. Med. J. Engl. 112, 930–933.
Chen, M.G., Feng, Z., 1999. Schistosomiasis control in China. Parasitol. Int. 48, 11–19.
Chen, M.G., Mott, K.E., 1988. Progress in assessment of morbidity due to *Schistosoma japonicum* infection. Trop. Dis. Bull. 85, R1–R45.
Chen, X.Y., Wang, L.Y., Jiming, C., Zhou, X.N., Zheng, J., Guo, J.G., et al., 2005. Schistosomiasis control in China: the impact of a 10-year World Bank Loan Project (1992–2001). Bull. World Health Organ 83, 43–48.
Chigusa, Y., Ohmae, H., Otake, H., Keang, H., Sinuon, M., Saem, C., et al., 2006. Effects of repeated praziquantel treatment on schistosomiasis mekongi morbidity as detected by ultrasonography. Parasitol. Int. 55, 261–265.
Chipeta, M.G., Ngwira, B., Kazembe, L.N., 2013. Analysis of schistosomiasis haematobium infection prevalence and intensity in Chikhwawa, Malawi: an application of a two part model. PLoS Negl. Trop. Dis. 7, e2131.
Chitsulo, L., Engels, D., Montresor, A., Savioli, L., 2000. The global status of schistosomiasis and its control. Acta Trop. 77, 41–51.
Clements, A.C., Bosqué-Oliva, E., Sacko, M., Landouré, A., Dembélé, R., Traoré, M., et al., 2009. A comparative study of the spatial distribution of schistosomiasis in Mali in 1984–1989 and 2004–2006. PLoS Negl. Trop. Dis. 3, e431.
Clements, A.C., Garba, A., Sacko, M., Toure, S., Dembele, R., Landoure, A., et al., 2008. Mapping the probability of schistosomiasis and associated uncertainty, West Africa. Emerg. Infect. Dis. 14, 1629–1632.
Clerinx, J., Van Gompel, A., 2011. Schistosomiasis in travellers and migrants. Travel Med. Infect. Dis. 9, 6–24.
Cnops, L., Soentjens, P., Clerinx, J., Van Esbroeck, M., 2013. A *Schistosoma haematobium*-specific real-time PCR for diagnosis of urogenital schistosomiasis in serum samples of international travelers and migrants. PLoS Negl. Trop. Dis. 7, e2413.
Colley, D.G., Binder, S., Campbell, C., King, C.H., Tchuem Tchuente, L.A., N'goran, E.K., et al., 2013. A five-country evaluation of a point-of-care circulating cathodic antigen urine assay for the prevalence of *Schistosoma mansoni*. Am. J. Trop. Med. Hyg. 88, 426–432.
Connell, J., Zurn, P., Stilwell, B., Awases, M., Braichet, J.M., 2007. Sub-Saharan Africa: beyond the health worker migration crisis? Soc. Sci. Med. 64, 1876–1891.
Croce, D., Porazzi, E., Foglia, E., Restelli, U., Sinuon, M., Socheat, D., et al., 2010. Cost-effectiveness of a successful schistosomiasis control programme in Cambodia (1995–2006). Acta Trop. 113, 279–284.
Curti, E., Kwityn, C., Zhan, B., Gillespie, P., Brelsford, J., Deumic, V., et al., 2013. Expression at a 20L scale and purification of the extracellular domain of the *Schistosoma mansoni* TSP-2 recombinant protein: a vaccine candidate for human intestinal schistosomiasis. Hum. Vaccin. Immunother. 9, 2342–2350.
Dömling, A., Khoury, K., 2010. Praziquantel and schistosomiasis. Chem. Med. Chem. 5, 1420–1434.
Da'dara, A.A., Li, Y.S., Xiong, T., Zhou, J., Williams, G.M., Mcmanus, D.P., et al., 2008. DNA-based vaccines protect against zoonotic schistosomiasis in water buffalo. Vaccine 26, 3617–3625.

Dabo, A., Bary, B., Kouriba, B., Sankare, O., Doumbo, O., 2013. Factors associated with coverage of praziquantel for schistosomiasis control in the community-direct intervention (CDI) approach in Mali (West Africa). Infect. Dis. Poverty 2, 11.

Dang, H., Xu, J., Li, S.Z., Cao, Z.G., Huang, Y.X., Wu, C.G., et al., 2014. Monitoring the transmission of *Schistosoma japonicum* in potential risk regions of China, 2008–2012. Int. J. Environ. Res. Public Health 11, 2278–2287.

Davis, A., Wegner, D.H., 1979. Multicentre trials of praziquantel in human schistosomiasis: design and techniques. Bull. World Health Organ 57, 767–771.

Day, J.H., Grant, A.D., Doherty, J.F., Chiodini, P.L., Wright, S.G., 1996. Schistosomiasis in travellers returning from sub-Saharan Africa. BMJ 313, 268–269.

Ebisawa, I., 1998. Epidemiology and eradication of schistosomiasis japonica in Japan. J. Travel Med. 5, 33–35.

Erfe, J.M., Belizario, V.Y., Chua, P.L., Naig, J.R., 2013. Validating the WHO dose pole in the Philippines for school-based mass drug administration of praziquantel for morbidity control of schistosomiasis. Trans. R. Soc. Trop. Med. Hyg. 107, 620–626.

Fenwick, A., Rollinson, D., Southgate, V., 2006. Implementation of human schistosomiasis control: challenges and prospects. Adv. Parasitol. 61, 567–622.

Fenwick, A., Savioli, L., 2011. Schistosomiasis elimination. Lancet Infect. Dis. 11, 346 author reply 346–347.

Fenwick, A., Webster, J.P., Bosque-Oliva, E., Blair, L., Fleming, F.M., Zhang, Y., et al., 2009. The Schistosomiasis Control Initiative (SCI): rationale, development and implementation from 2002–2008. Parasitology 136, 1719–1730.

Focac, 2012. The Fifth Ministerial Conference of the Forum on China-Africa Cooperation Beijing Action Plan, July 23th, 2012 [Online]. Available: http://www.focac.org/eng/zxxx/t954620.htm.

French, M.D., Churcher, T.S., Gambhir, M., Fenwick, A., Webster, J.P., Kabatereine, N.B., et al., 2010. Observed reductions in *Schistosoma mansoni* transmission from large-scale administration of praziquantel in Uganda: a mathematical modelling study. PLoS Negl. Trop. Dis. 4, e897.

Frenk, J., Horton, R., 2006. Evidence for health-system reform: a call to action. Lancet 368, 3–4.

General Assembly, 2000. United Nations Millennium Declaration [Online]. Available: http://www.un.org/millennium/declaration/ares552e.pdf.

Garba, A., Toure, S., Dembele, R., Bosque-Oliva, E., Fenwick, A., 2006. Implementation of national schistosomiasis control programmes in West Africa. Trends Parasitol. 22, 322–326.

Garjito, T.A., Sudomo, M., Abdullah, Dahlan, M., Nurwidayati, A., 2008. Schistosomiasis in Indonesia: past and present. Parasitol. Int. 57, 277–280.

Green, A., 2013. Kenya's new president promises health system reform. Lancet 381, 1348–1349.

Greer, G.J., Ow-Yang, C.K., Yong, H.S., 1988. *Schistosoma malayensis*: a *Schistosoma japonicum*-complex schistosome from Peninsular Malaysia. J. Parasitol. 74, 471–480.

Guo, J.G., Vounatsou, P., Cao, C.L., Utzinger, J., Zhu, H.Q., Anderegg, D., et al., 2005. A geographic information and remote sensing based model for prediction of *Oncomelania hupensis* habitats in the Poyang Lake area, China. Acta Trop. 96, 213–222.

Guo, J.J., Zheng, H.J., Xu, J., Zhu, X.Q., Wang, S.Y., Xia, C.M., 2012. Sensitive and specific target sequences selected from retrotransposons of *Schistosoma japonicum* for the diagnosis of schistosomiasis. PLoS Negl. Trop. Dis. 6, e1579.

Guyatt, H., Evans, D., Lengeler, C., Tanner, M., 1994. Controlling schistosomiasis: the cost-effectiveness of alternative delivery strategies. Health Policy Plan 9, 385–395.

Hisakane, N., Kirinoki, M., Chigusa, Y., Sinuon, M., Socheat, D., Matsuda, H., et al., 2008. The evaluation of control measures against *Schistosoma mekongi* in Cambodia by a mathematical model. Parasitol. Int. 57, 379–385.

Hotez, P.J., Alvarado, M., Basanez, M.G., Bolliger, I., Bourne, R., Boussinesq, M., et al., 2014. The global burden of disease study 2010: interpretation and implications for the neglected tropical diseases. PLoS Negl. Trop. Dis. 8, e2865.
Hotez, P.J., Kamath, A., 2009. Neglected tropical diseases in sub-Saharan Africa: review of their prevalence, distribution, and disease burden. PLoS Negl. Trop. Dis. 3, e412.
Hotez, P.J., Savioli, L., Fenwick, A., 2012. Neglected tropical diseases of the Middle East and North Africa: review of their prevalence, distribution, and opportunities for control. PLoS Negl. Trop. Dis. 6, e1475.
Hu, G.H., Hu, J., Song, K.Y., Lin, D.D., Zhang, J., Cao, C.L., et al., 2005. The role of health education and health promotion in the control of schistosomiasis: experiences from a 12-year intervention study in the Poyang Lake area. Acta Trop. 96, 232–241.
Hu, W., Yan, Q., Shen, D.K., Liu, F., Zhu, Z.D., Song, H.D., et al., 2003. Evolutionary and biomedical implications of a *Schistosoma japonicum* complementary DNA resource. Nat. Genet. 35, 139–147.
Huang, Y.X., Manderson, L., 2005. The social and economic context and determinants of schistosomiasis japonica. Acta Trop. 96, 223–231.
Hung, Y.W., Remais, J., 2008. Quantitative detection of *Schistosoma japonicum* cercariae in water by real-time PCR. PLoS Negl. Trop. Dis. 2, e337.
Hurlimann, E., Schur, N., Boutsika, K., Stensgaard, A.S., Laserna De Himpsl, M., Ziegelbauer, K., et al., 2011. Toward an open-access global database for mapping, control, and surveillance of neglected tropical diseases. PLoS Negl. Trop. Dis. 5, e1404.
Inobaya, M.T., Olveda, R.M., Tallo, V., Mcmanus, D.P., Williams, G.M., Harn, D.A., et al., 2015. Schistosomiasis mass drug administration in the Philippines: lessons learnt and the global implications. Microbes Infect. 17, 6–15.
Ishikawa, H., Ohmae, H., 2009. Modeling the dynamics and control of transmission of *Schistosoma japonicum* and *S. mekongi* in Southeast Asia. Korean J. Parasitol. 47, 1–5.
Kabatereine, N.B., Tukahebwa, E., Kazibwe, F., Namwangye, H., Zaramba, S., Brooker, S., et al., 2006. Progress towards countrywide control of schistosomiasis and soil-transmitted helminthiasis in Uganda. Trans. R. Soc. Trop. Med. Hyg. 100, 208–215.
Kahler, M., 2013. The Rise of Emerging Asia: Regional Peace and Global Security. Peterson Institute for International Economics Working Paper.
Kato-Hayashi, N., Yasuda, M., Yuasa, J., Isaka, S., Haruki, K., Ohmae, H., et al., 2013. Use of cell-free circulating schistosome DNA in serum, urine, semen, and saliva to monitor a case of refractory imported schistosomiasis hematobia. J. Clin. Microbiol. 51, 3435–3438.
King, C.H., 2009. Toward the elimination of schistosomiasis. N. Engl. J. Med. 360, 106–109.
King, C.H., 2010. Parasites and poverty: the case of schistosomiasis. Acta Trop. 113, 95–104.
King, C.H., 2015. Health metrics for helminth infections. Acta Trop. 141, 150–160.
King, C.H., Dickman, K., Tisch, D.J., 2005. Reassessment of the cost of chronic helmintic infection: a meta-analysis of disability-related outcomes in endemic schistosomiasis. Lancet 365, 1561–1569.
King, K., 2006. Aid Within the Wider China-Africa Partnership: A View from the Beijing Summit [Online]. Available: http://www.cctr.ust.hk/materials/conference/China-Africa/papers/King,Kenneth.pdf.
Kirinoki, M., Chigusa, Y., Ohmae, H., Sinuon, M., Socheat, D., Matsumoto, J., et al., 2011. Efficacy of sodium metaperiodate (SMP)-ELISA for the serodiagnosis of schistosomiasis mekongi. Southeast Asian J. Trop. Med. Public Health 42, 25–33.
Knopp, S., Mohammed, K.A., Ali, S.M., Khamis, I.S., Ame, S.M., Albonico, M., et al., 2012. Study and implementation of urogenital schistosomiasis elimination in Zanzibar (Unguja and Pemba islands) using an integrated multidisciplinary approach. BMC Public Health 12, 930.

Laymanivong, S., Hangvanthong, B., Keokhamphavanh, B., Phommasansak, M., Phinmaland, B., Sanpool, O., et al., 2014. Current status of human hookworm infections, ascariasis, trichuriasis, schistosomiasis mekongi and other trematodiases in Lao People's Democratic Republic. Am. J. Trop. Med. Hyg. 90, 667–669.

Lei, Z.L., Zhou, X.N., 2015. Eradication of schistosomiasis: a new target and a new task for the national schistosomiasis control program in the People's Republic of China. Chin. J. Schistosomiasis Control 27, 1–4.

Leonardo, L., Rivera, P., Saniel, O., Antonio Solon, J., Chigusa, Y., Villacorte, E., et al., 2015. New endemic foci of schistosomiasis infections in the Philippines. Acta Trop. 141, 354–360.

Leonardo, L., Rivera, P., Saniel, O., Villacorte, E., Lebanan, M.A., Crisostomo, B., et al., 2012. A national baseline prevalence survey of schistosomiasis in the Philippines using stratified two-step systematic cluster sampling design. J. Trop. Med. 2012, 936128.

Leonardo, L.R., Acosta, L.P., Olveda, R.M., Aligui, G.D., 2002. Difficulties and strategies in the control of schistosomiasis in the Philippines. Acta Trop. 82, 295–299.

Leonardo, L.R., Bergquist, R., 2002. Regional network on Asian schistosomiasis. Trends Parasitol. 18, 434–436.

Leonardo, L.R., Rivera, P., Saniel, O., Villacorte, E., Crisostomo, B., Hernandez, L., et al., 2008. Prevalence survey of schistosomiasis in Mindanao and the Visayas, the Philippines. Parasitol. Int. 57, 246–251.

Leslie, J., Garba, A., Oliva, E.B., Barkire, A., Tinni, A.A., Djibo, A., et al., 2011. Schistosomiasis and soil-transmitted helminth control in Niger: cost effectiveness of school based and community distributed mass drug administration [corrected]. PLoS Negl. Trop. Dis. 5, e1326.

Li, S.Z., Luz, A., Wang, X.H., Xu, L.L., Wang, Q., Qian, Y.J., et al., 2009. Schistosomiasis in China: acute infections during 2005–2008. Chin. Med. J. Engl. 122, 1009–1014.

Li, S.Z., Zheng, H., Gao, J., Zhang, L.J., Zhu, R., Xu, J., et al., 2013. Endemic status of schistosomiasis in People's Republic of China in 2012. Chin. J. Schistosomiasis Control 25, 557–563.

Lieberman, S.S., Capuno, J.J., Van Minh, H., 2005. Decentralizing health: lessons from Indonesia, the Philippines, and Vietnam. East Asia Decentralizes: Making Local Government Work 155–178.

Liese, B., Rosenberg, M., Schratz, A., 2010. Programmes, partnerships, and governance for elimination and control of neglected tropical diseases. Lancet 375, 67–76.

Liljestrand, J., Sambath, M.R., 2012. Socio-economic improvements and health system strengthening of maternity care are contributing to maternal mortality reduction in Cambodia. Reprod. Health Matters 20, 62–72.

Liu, F., Lu, J., Hu, W., Wang, S.Y., Cui, S.J., Chi, M., et al., 2006. New perspectives on host-parasite interplay by comparative transcriptomic and proteomic analyses of *Schistosoma japonicum*. PLoS Pathog. 2, e29.

Liu, P., Guo, Y., Qian, X., Tang, S., Li, Z., Chen, L., 2014. China's distinctive engagement in global health. Lancet 384, 793–804.

Massa, K., Olsen, A., Sheshe, A., Ntakamulenga, R., Ndawi, B., Magnussen, P., 2009. Can coverage of schistosomiasis and soil transmitted helminthiasis control programmes targeting school-aged children be improved? New approaches. Parasitology 136, 1781–1788.

Mazigo, H.D., Nuwaha, F., Kinung'hi, S.M., Morona, D., Pinot De Moira, A., Wilson, S., et al., 2012. Epidemiology and control of human schistosomiasis in Tanzania. Parasit. Vectors 5, 274.

Melo, E.V., Costa, W.D., Conceicao, M.J., Coura, J.R., 2014. A comparative cross-sectional study on the prevalence and morbidity of schistosomiasis in a community in northeastern Brazil (1979–2010). Mem. Inst. Oswaldo Cruz 0, 0.

Murray, C.J., Vos, T., Lozano, R., Naghavi, M., Flaxman, A.D., Michaud, C., et al., 2012. Disability-adjusted life years (DALYs) for 291 diseases and injuries in 21 regions, 1990–2010: a systematic analysis for the Global Burden of Disease Study 2010. Lancet 380, 2197–2223.

Musuva, R.M., Awiti, A., Omedo, M., Ogutu, M., Secor, W.E., Montgomery, S.P., et al., 2014. Community knowledge, attitudes and practices on schistosomiasis in western Kenya – The SCORE Project. Am. J. Trop. Med. Hyg. 90, 646–652.

Muth, S., Sayasone, S., Odermatt-Biays, S., Phompida, S., Duong, S., Odermatt, P., 2010. *Schistosoma mekongi* in Cambodia and Lao People's Democratic Republic. Adv. Parasitol. 72, 179–203.

Mwakitalu, M.E., Malecela, M.N., Mosha, F.W., Simonsen, P.E., 2014. Urban schistosomiasis and soil transmitted helminthiases in young school children in Dar es Salaam and Tanga, Tanzania, after a decade of anthelminthic intervention. Acta Trop. 133, 35–41.

Mwinzi, P.N.M., Montgomery, S.P., Owaga, C.O., Mwanje, M., Muok, E.M., Ayisi, J.G., et al., 2012. Integrated community-directed intervention for schistosomiasis and soil transmitted helminths in western Kenya – a pilot study. Parasit. Vectors 5, 182.

NHFPC, 2013. Beijing Declaration of the Ministerial Forum of China-Africa Health Development [Online]. Available: http://www.nhfpc.gov.cn/gjhzs/s3590/201308/da8ad62e487a481f987e631e1318c6fc.shtml (accessed 21.03.14.).

NIPD, 2013. Altas of schistosomiasis transmission in China. China map publishing house; Beijing.

Nordin, P., Poggensee, G., Mtweve, S., Krantz, I., 2014. From a weighing scale to a pole: a comparison of two different dosage strategies in mass treatment of Schistosomiasis haematobium. Glob. Health Action 7, 25351.

Obeng, B.B., Aryeetey, Y.A., De Dood, C.J., Amoah, A.S., Larbi, I.A., Deelder, A.M., et al., 2008. Application of a circulating-cathodic-antigen (CCA) strip test and real-time PCR, in comparison with microscopy, for the detection of *Schistosoma haematobium* in urine samples from Ghana. Ann. Trop. Med. Parasitol. 102, 625–633.

Odhiambo, G.O., Musuva, R.M., Atuncha, V.O., Mutete, E.T., Odiere, M.R., Onyango, R.O., et al., 2014. Low levels of awareness despite high prevalence of schistosomiasis among communities in Nyalenda informal settlement, Kisumu city, western Kenya. PLoS Negl. Trop. Dis. 8, e2784.

OECD, 2013. Aid to the Health [Online]. Available: http://www.oecd.org/dac/stats/health (accessed 06.01.15.).

Ohmae, H., Sinuon, M., Kirinoki, M., Matsumoto, J., Chigusa, Y., Socheat, D., et al., 2004. Schistosomiasis mekongi: from discovery to control. Parasitol. Int. 53, 135–142.

Omedo, M., Ogutu, M., Awiti, A., Musuva, R., Muchiri, G., Montgomery, S.P., et al., 2014. The effect of a health communication campaign on compliance with mass drug administration for schistosomiasis control in western Kenya – the SCORE project. Am. J. Trop. Med. Hyg. 91, 982–988.

Palha De Sousa, C.A., Brigham, T., Chasekwa, B., Mbuya, M.N., Tielsch, J.M., Humphrey, J.H., et al., 2014. Dosing of praziquantel by height in sub-Saharan African adults. Am. J. Trop. Med. Hyg. 90, 634–637.

Pontes, L.A., Dias-Neto, E., Rabello, A., 2002. Detection by polymerase chain reaction of *Schistosoma mansoni* DNA in human serum and feces. Am. J. Trop. Med. Hyg. 66, 157–162.

Prter, J., Webbe, G., Sturrock, R.F., 1993. Human Schistosomiasis. CAB International, Wallingford, UK.

Qin, Z.Q., Xu, J., Feng, T., Zhu, H.Q., Li, S.Z., Xiao, N., et al., 2013. Strategic thinking of the construction of national schistosomiasis laboratory network in China. Chin. J. Schistosomiasis Control 25, 329–332.

Riveau, G., Deplanque, D., Remoue, F., Schacht, A.M., Vodougnon, H., Capron, M., et al., 2012. Safety and immunogenicity of rSh28GST antigen in humans: phase 1 randomized

clinical study of a vaccine candidate against urinary schistosomiasis. PLoS Negl. Trop. Dis. 6, e1704.
Rodrigo, M.-S., Smith, P.C., 2012. Does progress towards universal health coverage improve population health? Lancet 380, 917–923.
Rollinson, D., Knopp, S., Levitz, S., Stothard, J.R., Tchuem Tchuente, L.A., Garba, A., et al., 2013. Time to set the agenda for schistosomiasis elimination. Acta Trop. 128, 423–440.
Ross, A.G., Olveda, R.M., Acosta, L., Harn, D.A., Chy, D., Li, Y., et al., 2013. Road to the elimination of schistosomiasis from Asia: the journey is far from over. Microbes Infect. 15, 858–865.
Rozendaal, J.A., 1997. Vector Control. Methods for Use by Individuals and Communities. WHO, Geneva.
Savedoff, W.D., Ferranti, D.D., Smith, A.L., Fan, V., 2012. Political and economic aspects of the transition to universal health coverage. Lancet 380, 924–932.
Savioli, L., Gabrielli, A.F., Montresor, A., Chitsulo, L., Engels, D., 2009. Schistosomiasis control in Africa: 8 years after World Health Assembly Resolution 54·19. Parasitology 136, 1677–1681.
Sekwat, A., 2003. Health financing reform in sub-Saharan Africa: major constraints, goals, and strategies. J. Health Care Finance 29, 67–78.
Simoonga, C., Utzinger, J., Brooker, S., Vounatsou, P., Appleton, C.C., Stensgaard, A.S., et al., 2009. Remote sensing, geographical information system and spatial analysis for schistosomiasis epidemiology and ecology in Africa. Parasitology 136, 1683–1693.
Steinmann, P., Keiser, J., Bos, R., Tanner, M., Utzinger, J., 2006. Schistosomiasis and water resources development: systematic review, meta-analysis, and estimates of people at risk. Lancet Infect. Dis. 6, 411–425.
Stothard, J.R., Chitsulo, L., Kristensen, T.K., Utzinger, J., 2009. Control of schistosomiasis in sub-Saharan Africa: progress made, new opportunities and remaining challenges. Parasitology 136, 1665–1675.
Stothard, J.R., Sousa-Figueiredo, J.C., Betson, M., Bustinduy, A., Reinhard-Rupp, J., 2013a. Schistosomiasis in African infants and preschool children: let them now be treated! Trends Parasitol. 29, 197–205.
Stothard, J.R., Sousa-Figueiredo, J.C., Betson, M., Green, H.K., Seto, E.Y., Garba, A., et al., 2011. Closing the praziquantel treatment gap: new steps in epidemiological monitoring and control of schistosomiasis in African infants and preschool-aged children. Parasitology 138, 1593–1606.
Stothard, J.R., Sousa-Figueiredo, J.C., Navaratnam, A.M.D., 2013b. Advocacy, policies and practicalities of preventive chemotherapy campaigns for African children with schistosomiasis. Expert Rev. Anti Infect. Ther. 11, 733–752.
Straus, S., 2012. Wars do end! Changing patterns of political violence in sub-Saharan Africa. Afr. Aff. 1–23.
Sturrock, R.F., Diaw, O.T., Talla, I., Niang, M., Piau, J.P., Capron, A., 2001. Seasonality in the transmission of schistosomiasis and in populations of its snail intermediate hosts in and around a sugar irrigation scheme at Richard Toll, Senegal. Parasitology 123 (Suppl.), S77–S89.
Sudomo, M., Pretty, M.D.S., 2007. Schistosomiasis control in Indonesia. Bul. Penelit. Kesehat. 35, 36–45.
Sun, L.P., Liang, Y.S., Wu, H.H., Tian, Z.X., Dai, J.R., Yang, K., et al., 2011. A Google Earth-based surveillance system for schistosomiasis japonica implemented in the lower reaches of the Yangtze River, China. Parasit. Vectors 4, 223.
Tallo, V.L., Carabin, H., Alday, P.P., Balolong Jr., E., Olveda, R.M., Mcgarvey, S.T., 2008. Is mass treatment the appropriate schistosomiasis elimination strategy? Bull. World Health Organ 86, 765–771.

Tong, Q., Chen, R., Zhang, Y., Yang, G., Kumagaid, T., Shimogawarad, R., et al., 2015. A new surveillance and response tool: risk map of infected *Oncomelania hupensis* detected by loop-mediated isothermal amplification (LAMP) from pooled samples. Acta Trop. 141, 170–177.

Toure, S., Zhang, Y., Bosque-Oliva, E., Ky, C., Ouedraogo, A., Koukounari, A., et al., 2008. Two-year impact of single praziquantel treatment on infection in the national control programme on schistosomiasis in Burkina Faso. Bull. World Health Organ 86, 780–787 (A).

Uniting to Combat Neglected Tropical Diseases, 2012. The London Declaration [Online]. Available: http://unitingTocombatntds.org/sites/default/files/resource_file/london_declaration_on_ntds.pdf.

UNCTAD, 2013. Economic Development in Africa Report 2013-Intra-African Trade: Unlocking Private Sector Dynamism (UNCTAD/ALDC/AFRICA/2013) [Online]. Available: http://unctad.org/en/pages/PublicationWebflyer.aspx?publicationid=604.

Urbani, C., Sinoun, M., Socheat, D., Pholsena, K., Strandgaard, H., Odermatt, P., et al., 2002. Epidemiology and control of mekongi schistosomiasis. Acta Trop. 82, 157–168.

Utzinger, J., Bergquist, R., Shu-Hua, X., Singer, B.H., Tanner, M., 2003. Sustainable schistosomiasis control – the way forward. Lancet 362, 1932–1934.

Utzinger, J., Raso, G., Brooker, S., De Savigny, D., Tanner, M., Ornbjerg, N., et al., 2009. Schistosomiasis and neglected tropical diseases: towards integrated and sustainable control and a word of caution. Parasitology 136, 1859–1874.

Van Dam, G.J., Xu, J., Bergquist, R., De Dood, C.J., Utzinger, J., Qin, Z.Q., et al., 2015. An ultra-sensitive assay targeting the circulating anodic antigen for the diagnosis of *Schistosoma japonicum* in a low-endemic area, People's Republic of China. Acta Trop. 141, 190–197.

Wang, L.D., Utzinger, J., Zhou, X.N., 2008. Schistosomiasis control: experiences and lessons from China. Lancet 372, 1793–1795.

Webster, J.P., Molyneux, D.H., Hotez, P.J., Fenwick, A., 2014. The contribution of mass drug administration to global health: past, present and future. Philos. Trans. R. Soc. Lond B Biol. Sci. 369, 20130434.

WHA, 2012. Elimination of Schistosomiasis. WHO, Geneva [Online]. Available: http://www.who.int/neglected_diseases/mediacentre/WHA_65.21_Eng.pdf (accessed 12.07.15.).

WHO, 2012a. Accelerating Work to Overcome the Global Impact of Neglected Tropical Diseases: A Roadmap for Implementation [Online]. Available: http://www.who.int/neglected_diseases/NTD_RoadMap_2012_Fullversion.pdf (accessed 15.08.15.).

WHO, 2012b. Key issues and challenges arising out or the Sixty-fifth World Health Assembly and the 130th and 131st sessions of the WHO Executive Board. Elimination of schistosomiasis (WHA 65.21). In: Sixty-fifth Session SEA/RC65/17. Yogyakarta, Indonesia.

WHO, 2013. Schistosomiasis: Progress Report 2001–2011 and Strategic Plan 2012–2020 [Online]. World Health Organization, Geneva.

WHO, 2014. Schistosomiasis: number of people receiving preventive chemotherapy in 2012. Wkly. Epidemiol. Rec. 89, 21–28.

WHO/UNICEF, 2014. Progress on Drinking Water and Sanitation [Online]. Available: Http://www.who.int/water_sanitation_health/publications/2014/jmp-report/en/2014.

Worku, L., Damte, D., Endris, M., Tesfa, H., Aemero, M., 2014. *Schistosoma mansoni* infection and associated determinant factors among school children in Sanja town, Northwest Ethiopia. J. Parasitol. Res. 2014, 792536.

Wu, X.H., Chen, M.G., Zheng, J., 2005. Surveillance of schistosomiasis in five provinces of China which have reached the national criteria for elimination of the disease. Acta Trop. 96, 276–281.

Wu, X.H., Zhang, S.Q., Xu, X.J., Huang, Y.X., Steinmann, P., Utzinger, J., et al., 2008. Effect of floods on the transmission of schistosomiasis in the Yangtze River valley, People's Republic of China. Parasitol. Int. 57, 271–276.
Xin, Y.T., Dai, J.R., 2010. Progress of research on molluscicide niclosamide. Chin. J. Schistosomiasis Control 22, 504–508.
Xu, J., Guo, J.G., Wu, X.H., Zeng, X.J., Yang, W.P., Yang, G.B., et al., 2009. Efficacy and adverse effects of film coated praziquantel for treatment of schistosomiasis japonica. Chin. J. Prev. Med. 43, 718–722.
Xu, J., Liu, H., 2012. The challenges of malaria elimination in Yunnan Province, People's Republic of China. Southeast Asian J. Trop. Med. Public Health 43, 819–824.
Xu, J., Peeling, R.W., Chen, J.X., Wu, X.H., Wu, Z.D., Wang, S.P., et al., 2011. Evaluation of nine immunoassays for the diagnosis of *Schistosoma japonicum* infection using archived sera. PLoS Negl. Trop. Dis. 5, e949.
Xu, J., Xu, J.F., Li, S.Z., Zhang, L.J., Wang, Q., Zhu, H.H., et al., 2015. Integrated control programmes for schistosomiasis and other helminth infections in P.R. China. Acta Trop. 141, 332–341.
Xu, J., Yang, K., Li, S.Z., Zhou, X.N., 2014. Surveillance system after transmission control of schistosomiasis in P.R. China. Chin. J. Schistosomiasis Control 26, 1–5.
Xu, J., Yu, Q., Tchuem-Tchuenté, L.A., Bergquist, R., Sacko, M., Utzinger, J., et al., 2016. Enhancing collaboration between China and African countries for schistosomiasis control. Lancet Infect. Dis. http://dx.doi.org/10.1016/S1473-3099(1015)00360-00366. Published Online: February 03, 2016.
Yang, G.J., Li, W., Sun, L.P., Wu, F., Yang, K., Huang, Y.X., et al., 2010. Molluscicidal efficacies of different formulations of niclosamide: result of meta-analysis of Chinese literature. Parasit. Vectors 3, 84.
Yang, G.J., Sun, L.P., Hong, Q.B., Zhu, H.R., Yang, K., Gao, Q., et al., 2012a. Optimizing molluscicide treatment strategies in different control stages of schistosomiasis in the People's Republic of China. Parasit. Vectors 5, 260.
Yang, G.J., Vounatsou, P., Tanner, M., Zhou, X.N., Utzinger, J., 2006. Remote sensing for predicting potential habitats of *Oncomelania hupensis* in Hongze, Baima and Gaoyou lakes in Jiangsu province, China. Geospat Health 1, 85–92.
Yang, G.J., Vounatsou, P., Zhou, X.N., Utzinger, J., Tanner, M., 2005. A review of geographic information system and remote sensing with applications to the epidemiology and control of schistosomiasis in China. Acta Trop. 96, 117–129.
Yang, K., Li, W., Sun, L.P., Huang, Y.X., Zhang, J.F., Wu, F., et al., 2013. Spatio-temporal analysis to identify determinants of *Oncomelania hupensis* infection with *Schistosoma japonicum* in Jiangsu province, China. Parasit. Vectors 6, 138.
Yang, K., Sun, L.P., Huang, Y.X., Yang, G.J., Wu, F., Hang, D.R., et al., 2012b. A real-time platform for monitoring schistosomiasis transmission supported by Google Earth and a web-based geographical information system. Geospat. Health 6, 195–203.
Yuan, Y., Xu, X.J., Dong, H.F., Jiang, M.S., Zhu, H.G., 2005. Transmission control of schistosomiasis japonica: implementation and evaluation of different snail control interventions. Acta Trop. 96, 191–197.
Zhang, Z., Carpenter, T.E., Chen, Y., Clark, A.B., Lynn, H.S., Peng, W., et al., 2008. Identifying high-risk regions for schistosomiasis in Guichi, China: a spatial analysis. Acta Trop. 107, 217–223.
Zhang, Z.Y., Xu, D.Z., Zhou, X.N., Zhou, Y., Liu, S.J., 2005. Remote sensing and spatial statistical analysis to predict the distribution of *Oncomelania hupensis* in the marshlands of China. Acta Trop. 96, 205–212.
Zhao, G.M., Zhao, Q., Jiang, Q.W., Chen, X.Y., Wang, L.Y., Yuan, H.C., 2005. Surveillance for schistosomiasis japonica in China from 2000 to 2003. Acta Trop. 96, 288–295.

Zhou, X.N., Bergquist, R., Tanner, M., 2013. Elimination of tropical disease through surveillance and response. Infect. Dis. Poverty 2, 1.
Zhou, X.N., Jiang, Q.W., Guo, J.G., Lin, D.D., Zhu, R., Yang, G.J., et al., 2012. Road map for transmission interruption of schistosomiasis in China. Chin. J. Schistosomiasis Control 24, 1–4.
Zhou, X.N., Olveda, R., Sripa, B., Yang, G.J., Leonardo, L., Bergquist, R., 2015. From gap analysis to solution and action: the RNAS(+) model. Acta Trop. 141, 146–149.
Zhou, X.N., Yang, G.J., Yang, K., Wang, X.H., Hong, Q.B., Sun, L.P., et al., 2008. Potential impact of climate change on schistosomiasis transmission in China. Am. J. Trop. Med. Hyg. 78, 188–194.
Zhou, X.N., Wang, L.Y., Chen, M.G., Wu, X.H., Jiang, Q.W., Chen, X.Y., et al., 2005. The public health significance and control of schistosomiasis in China – then and now. Acta Trop. 96, 97–105.
Zhou, X.N., Xu, J., Chen, H.G., Wang, T.P., Huang, X.B., Lin, D.D., et al., 2011. Tools to support policy decisions related to treatment strategies and surveillance of schistosomiasis japonica towards elimination. PLoS Negl. Trop. Dis. 5, e1408.
Zhou, Y., Zhen, H., Chen, Y., Zhang, L., Wang, K., Guo, J., et al., 2009. The *Schistosoma japonicum* genome reveals features of host-parasite interplay. Nature 460, 345–351.
Zhu, N., 2013. China to Strengthen Cooperation with Africa on Health. Xinhua Newspaper, Beijing [Online]. Available: http://news.xinhuanet.com/english/china/2013-08/16/c_132637291 (accessed 05.05.15.).
Zhu, R., Qin, Z.Q., Feng, T., Dang, H., Zhang, L.J., Xu, J., 2013. Assessment of effect and quality control for parasitological tests in national schistosomiasis surveillance sites. Chin. J. Schistosomiasis Control 25, 11–15.
Zhu, R., Zhao, G.M., Li, H.Z., Guo, J.G., 2011. Development and prospect of surveillance network of schistosomiasis in China. Chin. J. Schistosomiasis Control 23, 14–17.
Zhu, Y., Hassen, S., He, W., Cao, G., 2006. Preliminary study on detection of schistosomiasis mansoni with dipstick dye immunoassay (DDIA) kit. Chin. J. Schistosomiasis Control 18, 419–421.
Zhu, Y.C., Socheat, D., Bounlu, K., Liang, Y.S., Sinuon, M., Insisiengmay, S., et al., 2005. Application of dipstick dye immunoassay (DDIA) kit for the diagnosis of schistosomiasis mekongi. Acta Trop. 96, 137–141.

INDEX

'*Note*: Page numbers followed by "f" indicate figures and "t" indicate tables'.

A

B

Q

R

S

T

X

Y

Z

CONTENTS OF VOLUMES IN THIS SERIES

Volume 46

Volume 47

Volume 48

Volume 49

Volume 50

Volume 51

Volume 52

Volume 53

Volume 54

Volume 55

Volume 56

Volume 57

Volume 58

Volume 59

Volume 60

Volume 61

Volume 62

Volume 63

Volume 68

Volume 69

Volume 70

Volume 71

Volume 72

Volume 73

Volume 74

Volume 75

Volume 76

Volume 77

Volume 78

Volume 79

Volume 80

Volume 81

Volume 82

Volume 87

Volume 88

Volume 89

Volume 90

Volume 91

FSC
www.fsc.org
MIX
Papier | Fördert
gute Waldnutzung
FSC® C083411

Kolibri 360 GmbH
Ferdinand-Jühlke-Straße 7
99095 Erfurt, Deutschland
produktsicherheit@kolibri360.de